Current Controversies
in
Cardiovascular Disease

EDITED BY

ELLIOT RAPAPORT, M.D.

Professor of Medicine, University of California, San Francisco;
Chief of Cardiology, San Francisco General Hospital,
San Francisco, California

1980

W. B. SAUNDERS COMPANY
Philadelphia · London · Toronto

W. B. Saunders Company: West Washington Square
Philadelphia, PA   19105

1 St. Anne's Road
Eastbourne, East Sussex BN21 3UN, England

1 Goldthorne Avenue
Toronto, Ontario M8Z 5T9, Canada

Library of Congress Cataloging in Publication Data

Main entry under title:

Current controversies in cardiovascular disease.

1. Cardiovascular system – Diseases.   I. Rapaport, Elliot.
  [DNLM: 1. Cardiovascular diseases. WG100 C976]

RC667.C87   616.1   79–64600

ISBN 0–7216–7459–3

Current Controversies in Cardiovascular Disease   ISBN   0-7216-7459-3

Last digit is the print number: 9   8   7   6   5   4   3   2   1

CONTRIBUTORS

WALTER H. ABELMANN, M.D.
Professor of Medicine, Harvard Medical School; Beth Israel Hospital, Boston, Massachusetts

FORREST H. ADAMS, M.D.
Emeritus Professor of Pediatrics (Cardiology), University of California, Los Angeles, School of Medicine, Los Angeles, California

ROBERT J. ADOLPH, M.D.
Professor of Medicine, Division of Cardiology; Director, Cardiac Research Laboratory, University of Cincinnati College of Medicine, Cincinnati, Ohio

EZRA A. AMSTERDAM, M.D.
Professor of Medicine; Director, Coronary Care Unit, Department of Cardiovascular Medicine, University of California, Davis, School of Medicine, Davis, California

DANIEL S. BERMAN, M.D.
Director, Nuclear Cardiology, Department of Nuclear Medicine, Cedars-Sinai Medical Center; Assistant Clinical Professor of Radiology, University of California at Los Angeles, Los Angeles, California

WILLIAM J. BOMMER, M.D.
Assistant Professor of Medicine; Co-Director, Echocardiography and Non-Invasive Cardiology, Section of Cardiovascular Medicine, University of California, Davis, School of Medicine, Davis, California

EUGENE BRAUNWALD, M.D.
Hershey Professor of Theory and Practice of Physic (Medicine), Harvard Medical School; Physician-in-Chief, Peter Bent Brigham Hospital, Boston, Massachusetts

J. DAVID BRISTOW, M.D.
Professor of Medicine, University of California, San Francisco; Chief, Cardiology Section, Veterans Administration Hospital, San Francisco, California

GEORGE E. BURCH, M.D.
Emeritus Henderson Professor of Medicine, Tulane University

iii

School of Medicine; Consultant, Charity Hospital of New Orleans and the Veterans Administration Hospital, New Orleans, Louisiana

HOWARD B. BURCHELL, M.D.

Emeritus Professor of Medicine, University of Minnesota; Senior Cardiologic Consultant, Northwestern Hospital, Minneapolis, Minnesota

AGUSTIN CASTELLANOS, M.D.

Professor of Medicine; Director of Electrophysiology, University of Miami; Jackson Memorial Hospital, Miami, Florida

KANU CHATTERJEE, M.B., F.R.C.P.

Professor of Medicine; Associate Chief, Cardiovascular Division; Director, Coronary Care Unit, University of California, San Francisco, School of Medicine, San Francisco, California

MELVIN D. CHEITLIN, M.D.

Professor of Medicine, University of California, San Francisco, School of Medicine; Acting Chief of Medicine; Associate Chief, Cardiology Service, San Francisco General Hospital, San Francisco, California

LEONARD A. COBB, M.D.

Professor of Medicine, University of Washington; Director, Division of Cardiology, Harborview Medical Center, Seattle, Washington

JAY N. COHN, M.D.

Professor of Medicine; Head, Cardiovascular Division, University of Minnesota School of Medicine; Veterans Administration Medical Center, Minneapolis, Minnesota

CESAR CONDE, M.D., F.A.C.C.

Associate Clinical Professor of Cardiology, University of Miami; Jackson Memorial Hospital, Miami, Florida

C. RICHARD CONTI, M.D.

Professor of Medicine; Director of Cardiovascular Medicine, University of Florida College of Medicine, Gainesville, Florida

JAMES E. DALEN, M.D.

Professor and Chairman, Department of Medicine, University of Massachusetts Medical School; Physician-in-Chief, University Hospital, Worcester, Massachusetts

MICHAEL E. DEBAKEY, M.D.

President and Chancellor; Chairman, Cora and Webb Mading Department of Surgery; Director, National Heart and Blood Vessel Research and Demonstration Center, Baylor College of Medicine, Houston, Texas

ANTHONY N. DeMARIA, M.D.

Associate Professor of Medicine; Director, Cardiac Non-Invasive Laboratory, University of California, Davis, School of Medicine; UCD Medical Center, Davis, California

HARRIET P. DUSTAN, M.D.

Professor of Medicine, University of Alabama School of Medicine; Director, Cardiovascular Research and Training Center, University of Alabama Medical Center; Attending Physician, University of Alabama Hospitals and Clinics, Birmingham, Alabama

PAUL EBERT, M.D.

Professor and Chairman, Department of Surgery, University of California Medical Center, San Francisco, California

L. HENRY EDMUNDS, JR., M.D.

William Maul Measey Professor of Surgery; Chief, Cardiothoracic Surgery, University of Pennsylvania; Chief, Cardiothoracic Surgery, University of Pennsylvania Hospital; Chief, Cardiothoracic Surgery, Children's Hospital of Philadelphia, Philadelphia, Pennsylvania

FRANK A. FINNERTY, JR., M.D.

Clinical Professor of Medicine, George Washington University School of Medicine; Director, Hypertension Center of Washington, D.C., Washington, D.C.

NICHOLAS J. FORTUIN, M.D.

Associate Professor of Medicine, The Johns Hopkins University School of Medicine; Attending Physician, The Johns Hopkins Hospital, Baltimore, Maryland

NOBLE O. FOWLER, M.D.

Professor of Medicine; Director, Division of Cardiology, University of Cincinnati College of Medicine; Member, Directing Medical Staff, Cincinnati General Hospital; Consultant in Cardiology, Veterans Administration Hospital of Cincinnati, Cincinnati, Ohio

HARRY A. FOZZARD, M.D.

Otho S.A. Sprague Professor of Medical Sciences; Joint Director of Cardiology, University of Chicago School of Medicine; Attending Cardiologist, University of Chicago Hospitals and Clinics, Chicago, Illinois

MEYER FRIEDMAN, M.D.

Director Emeritus, Harold Brunn Institute, Mount Zion Hospital and Medical Center, San Francisco, California

EDWARD D. FROHLICH, M.D.

Vice President, Education and Research, Alton Ochsner Medical Foundation; Director, Division of Hypertensive Diseases, Ochsner Clinic, New Orleans, Louisiana

ALFRED P. HALLSTROM, Ph.D.

Research Assistant Professor, Department of Biostatistics, University of Washington, Seattle, Washington

E. WILLIAM HANCOCK, M.D.

Professor of Medicine (Cardiology), Stanford University School of Medicine; Attending Physician, Stanford University Hospital, Stanford, California

WARREN D. HANCOCK

Developer-Scientist, Hancock Laboratories, Inc., Anaheim, California

MICHAEL V. HERMAN, M.D.

Dr. Arthur M. and Hilda A. Master Professor of Medicine, Mt. Sinai School of Medicine; Chief, Division of Cardiology, Mt. Sinai Medical Center, New York, New York

W. DUDLEY JOHNSON, M.D.

Associate Clinical Professor of Medicine, Department of Thoracic and Cardiovascular Surgery, The Medical College of Wisconsin; Chief, Cardiovascular Surgery, Mount Sinai Medical Center, Milwaukee, Wisconsin

JAMES A. JOYE, M.D.

Assistant Professor of Medicine; Director, Nuclear Cardiology, Section of Cardiovascular Medicine, University of California, Davis, School of Medicine, Davis, California

JOSEPH A. KISSLO, M.D.

Associate Professor of Medicine; Director, Clinical Cardiology Laboratory, Duke University Medical Center, Durham, North Carolina

ROBERT A. KLONER, M.D., Ph.D.

Assistant Professor of Medicine, Harvard Medical School; Attending Cardiologist, Peter Bent Brigham Hospital, Boston, Massachusetts

CHARLES E. KOSSMANN, M.D.

Professor Emeritus of Medicine, University of Tennessee College of Medicine, Memphis, Tennessee

NICHOLAS T. KOUCHOUKOS, M.D.

Professor of Surgery, Division of Cardiovascular and Thoracic Surgery, Department of Surgery, University of Alabama, Birmingham, Alabama

JOHN H. LARAGH, M.D.

Master Professor of Medicine, Cornell University Medical College; Director, Cardiovascular Center; Chief, Division of Cardiology, New York Hospital–Cornell Medical Center, New York, New York

GARRETT LEE, M.D.

Assistant Professor of Medicine; Director, Cardiac Catheterization Laboratory, University of California, Davis, School of Medicine, Davis, California

A. JAMES LIEDTKE, M.D.

Professor of Medicine, Pennsylvania State University; Attending Cardiologist, Milton S. Hershey Medical Center, Pennsylvania State University, Hershey, Pennsylvania

DWIGHT C. McGOON, M.D.

Professor of Surgery, Mayo Medical School; Head, Section of Thoracic, Cardiovascular, and General Surgery, Mayo Clinic and Mayo Foundation, Rochester, Minnesota

HENRY D. McINTOSH, M.D.

Adjunct Professor of Medicine, Baylor College of Medicine, Houston, Texas; Clinical Professor of Medicine, University of Florida School of Medicine, Gainesville, Florida; Cardiology Section, Watson Clinic, Lakeland, Florida

JOHN C. MANLEY, M.D., F.A.C.C.

Associate Clinical Professor of Medicine, Medical College of Wisconsin; Director, Cardiac Rehabilitation and Exercise Stress Laboratory, St. Luke's Hospital, Milwaukee, Wisconsin

PETER R. MAROKO, M.D.

Director, Cardiovascular Research, Deborah Heart and Lung Center, Browns Mills, New Jersey

DEAN T. MASON, M.D.

Professor of Medicine; Professor of Physiology; Chief, Cardiovascular Medicine, University of California, Davis, School of Medicine, Davis, California

ALVARO MAYORGA-CORTES, M.D.

Clinical Assistant Professor of Medicine, University of Miami School of Medicine; Attending Cardiologist, University of Miami Medical Center, Miami, Florida

JAMES C. MELBY, M.D.

Professor of Medicine; Head, Section of Endocrinology and Metabolism, Boston University School of Medicine, Boston, Massachusetts

JOSEPH V. MESSER, M.D.

Professor of Medicine, Rush Medical College; Director, Section of Cardiology; Senior Attending Physician, Rush-Presbyterian-St. Luke's Medical Center, Chicago, Illinois

SHEILA C. MITCHELL, M.D.

Medical Planning Consultant, Princeton, New Jersey; Research Associate, The Biostatistics Center, George Washington University, Washington, D.C.; Lecturer in Pediatrics, The Johns Hopkins University, Baltimore, Maryland

HOWARD E. MORGAN, M.D.

Evan Pugh Professor and Chairman of Physiology, Pennsylvania State University; Hershey Medical Center, Hershey, Pennsylvania

JAMES J. MORRIS, JR., M.D.

Professor of Medicine, Division of Cardiology, Duke University School of Medicine; Duke University Medical Center, Durham, North Carolina

JAMES E. MULLER, M.D.

Assistant Professor of Medicine, Harvard Medical School; Jr. Associate in Medicine; Assistant Director, Samuel A. Levine Cardiac Unit, Peter Bent Brigham Hospital, Boston, Massachusetts

ROBERT J. MYERBURG, M.D.

Professor of Medicine and Physiology; Director, Division of Cardiology, University of Miami School of Medicine, Miami, Florida

ALBERT OBERMAN, M.D.

Professor, Department of Public Health; Associate Professor, School of Medicine, University of Alabama in Birmingham, Birmingham, Alabama

OGLESBY PAUL, M.D.

Professor of Medicine, Harvard Medical School; Physician, Peter Bent Brigham Hospital, Boston, Massachusetts

ROBERT G. PETERSDORF, M.D.

Professor and Chairman, Department of Medicine, University of Washington School of Medicine; Chairman, Department of Medicine, University Hospital, University of Washington, Seattle, Washington

ALFRED PICK, M.D.

Professor of Medicine Emeritus, Pritzker School of Medicine, University of Chicago; Senior Consultant, Cardiovascular Institute; Senior Attending Physician, Department of Medicine, Michael Reese Hospital and Medical Center, Chicago, Illinois

BERTRAM PITT, M.D.

Professor of Internal Medicine, University of Michigan School of Medicine; Director, Cardiology Division, University Hospital, Ann Arbor, Michigan

RICHARD L. POPP, M.D.

Associate Professor of Medicine; Director, Non-Invasive Laboratory, Cardiology Division, Stanford University Medical Center, Stanford, California

THOMAS A. PRESTON, M.D.

Associate Professor of Medicine, Division of Cardiology, University of Washington School of Medicine; Co-Director, Division of Cardiology, United States Public Health Service Hospital, Seattle, Washington

SHAHBUDIN H. RAHIMTOOLA, M.B., F.R.C.P.

Professor of Medicine, University of Oregon Health Sciences Center, Portland, Oregon

LEON RESNEKOV, M.D., F.R.C.P.

Professor of Medicine, University of Chicago; Joint Director, Section of Cardiology, University of Chicago Medical Center, Chicago, Illinois

BENSON B. ROE, M.D.

Professor of Surgery; Co-Chief of Cardiothoracic Surgery, University of California, San Francisco, School of Medicine, San Francisco, California

ABRAHAM M. RUDOLPH, M.D.

Professor of Pediatrics, Physiology, Obstetrics-Gynecology and Reproductive Sciences; Neider Professor of Pediatric Cardiology, University of California, San Francisco, School of Medicine, San Francisco, California

DAVID A. RYTAND, M.D.

Arthur L. Bloomfield Professor of Medicine, Emeritus, Stanford University School of Medicine, Stanford, California; Chief, Division of Cardiology, Santa Clara Valley Medical Center, San José, California

MELVIN SCHEINMAN, M.D.

Professor of Medicine, University of California, San Francisco; Chief, Electrocardiography and Clinical Cardiac Electrophysiology Section, Moffitt Hospital, San Francisco, California

ARTHUR SELZER, M.D.

Clinical Professor of Medicine, University of California, San Francisco; Clinical Professor of Medicine, Emeritus, Stanford University School of Medicine, Stanford, California; Chief of Cardiology, Presbyterian Hospital of Pacific Medical Center, San Francisco, California

PRAVIN M. SHAH, M.D.

Professor of Medicine, University of California at Los Angeles; Chief, Cardiology Section, Wadsworth Veterans Administration Medical Center, Los Angeles, California

W. McFATE SMITH, M.D., M.P.H.

Clinical Professor of Medicine and Epidemiology, University of California at San Francisco; Chief, Research Branch, Division of Hospitals and Clinics, United States Public Health Service; Attending Physician, Moffitt Hospital and San Francisco General Hospital, San Francisco, California

JEREMIAH STAMLER, M.D.

Professor and Chairman, Department of Community Health and Preventive Medicine; Dingman Professor of Cardiology, Northwestern University Medical School, Chicago, Illinois

D. E. STRANDNESS, JR., M.D.

Professor of Surgery, Department of Surgery, University of Washington School of Medicine; Attending Physician, University Hospital and Veterans Administration Hospital, Seattle, Washington

NANETTE K. WENGER, M.D.

Professor of Medicine (Cardiology), Emory University School of Medicine; Director, Cardiac Clinics, Grady Memorial Hospital, Atlanta, Georgia

STANFORD WESSLER, M.D.

Professor of Medicine, New York University School of Medicine; Attending Physician, NYU Medical Center, University Hospital, and Bellevue Hospital, New York, New York

MYRON W. WHEAT, JR., M.D.

Clinical Professor of Surgery, University of Louisville School of Medicine, Louisville, Kentucky; Cardiovascular Surgeon, Cardiac Surgical Associates; Staff Member, Bayfront Medical Center and All Children's Hospital, St. Petersburg, Florida

JAMES WILLERSON, M.D.

Professor of Medicine; Director, Cardiology Division, University of Texas Southwestern Medical School and Parkland Memorial Hospital, Dallas, Texas

PREFACE

The inspiration for this volume arose from Volumes I and II of Ingelfinger, et al.: *Controversy in Internal Medicine.* These touched on some of the problems facing the practicing cardiologist, but it was clear that many more controversies exist in the cardiovascular field than could be accommodated by efforts devoted to the broad field of internal medicine. Thus, a separate volume devoted exclusively to the cardiovascular field seemed warranted.

In recruiting the various proponents and opponents to the controversies discussed in this book, I have asked each author to present his own experience and viewpoint without attempting to exaggerate the case for the sake of argument. As a result, there are times when one can sense agreement toward what constitutes a rational approach to the question being posed. In other cases, the data indicate that we suffer from inadequate knowledge in the area, and one is left to adopt his or her own prudent course of action based on little factual background.

Following each chapter, I have chosen to present my personal response to the arguments that have been expressed rather than to ask for the opinion of still a third authority in that particular area. Even though absolute answers may not be forthcoming, it is hoped that the delineation of the "controversy" will help one sharpen his or her perception of the issues. Some of you will undoubtedly come to different conclusions than I, as you are influenced to a lesser or greater degree.

Finally, I wish to thank the authors who have contributed to this volume. Their assistance in helping to frame the questions being presented is acknowledged, and we have all gained from the clear exposition of their approach to these important and complex problems.

ELLIOT RAPAPORT, M.D.

CONTENTS

One

Are We Overproducing Cardiology Trainees Who Are Also Untrained to Handle Common Clinical Cardiologic Problems?

ARE THERE TOO MANY CARDIOLOGISTS AND ARE
THEY DOING THE WRONG THING?

Thomas A. Preston, M.D., and Robert G. Petersdorf, M.D.

WE ARE OVERPRODUCING CARDIOLOGY TRAINEES
WHO ARE ALSO UNTRAINED TO HANDLE COMMON
CLINICAL CARDIOLOGIC PROBLEMS: AN OPPOSING VIEWPOINT

Walter H. Abelmann, M.D.

COMMENT

Are There Too Many Cardiologists and Are They Doing the Wrong Thing?

THOMAS A. PRESTON, M.D.

Co-Director, Division of Cardiology, United States Public Health Service Hospital, Seattle, and Associate Professor of Medicine, Division of Cardiology, University of Washington, Seattle, Washington

ROBERT G. PETERSDORF, M.D.

Professor and Chairman, Department of Medicine, University of Washington School of Medicine, Seattle, Washington

At the present time, there is a surplus of cardiologists trained to perform cardiac catheterization and other technically oriented tests and a deficit of physicians well trained in the common clinical cardiologic problems. Furthermore, it is likely that cardiology training programs in their present form are likely to increase this imbalance. The reasons for the imbalance and the discrepancy between the apparent or imagined need and the actual need for care of patients by specialists are complex and deep-seated. Although "doctor shortage" and "health care crisis" have become familiar terms in recent years and have led to the popular opinion that they express reality, there is increasing evidence that nearly all types of medical and surgical specialists in this country exist in excess of what is required to provide for the health care needs of society. In this article, we will examine the need for and availability of one type of medical specialist, the cardiologist.

Number of Cardiologists

There is no precise inventory of the number of practicing cardiologists in the U.S. today. The last comprehensive study of the subject was reported

3

in 1974 and supplies data assembled prior to December, 1971.[1] This "Profile of the Cardiologist" listed 10,691 cardiologists in active practice, exclusive of trainees. Of this number, 5661 spent 50 per cent or more of their time in cardiology and were defined as "primary" cardiologists. In addition, there were 979 cardiologists in training, 8.4 per cent of the total cardiologist pool of 11,670. An estimated 617 cardiology trainees completed their training in 1971, 791 in 1973,[2] and approximately 1000 trainees completed their training in 1976.[3] Assuming that 95 per cent of these graduate's entered and have remained in the total pool of primary cardiologists, there has been infusion of about 4075 primary cardiologists during the period from 1972 to 1976. Unfortunately, there are no data on the number of secondary cardiologists (internist-cardiologists) added to the pool during the same time interval. Allowing an attrition rate of six per cent per year, an estimated 1600 primary cardiologists left active practice during the 1972–76 period, resulting in a total of approximately 8136 active primary cardiologists at the end of 1976; this represents a net increase of 44 per cent during this five-year period. This figure is remarkably close to the 7498 respondents to an A.M.A. questionnaire who listed themselves as cardiovascular specialists.[5] We emphasize that these figures are estimates, because precise data are not available. However, if these figures are reasonably accurate, and we believe they are, we are producing primary cardiologists at an annual rate of about 12 per cent of the existing supply.

We can only estimate the change in number of secondary cardiologists since 1971. Assuming a growth rate equivalent to that of all physicians in the country (about 18 per cent in five years from 1971 to 1976), there were at least 5935 secondary cardiologists in 1976.

In 1971, active cardiologists constituted 3.7 per cent of all physicians in active practice;[1] at the end of 1976, the figure was approximately 4.5 per cent. In 1971, there were approximately 2.7 primary cardiologists and about 2.4 secondary cardiologists per 100,000 population in the U.S.[1] In 1976, there were about 3.9 primary cardiologists and about 2.7 secondary cardiologists per 100,000 population, a total of about 6.6 cardiologists per 100,000. The number of cardiologists certified by the Subspecialty Board on Cardiovascular Disease was about 10 per cent of all primary and secondary cardiologists in 1971,[1] and an additional 1881 were certified during the 1972–76 period.[4] Assuming that all those with subspecialty certification are primary cardiologists, in 1976 approximately 25 per cent of all primary cardiologists had been certified by the Subspecialty Board. Although the above data are not precise, they do provide a reasonably accurate profile of the available manpower pool in cardiology.

Need for Cardiologists

What is the actual need for cardiologists in 1979? Although the precise need is less clearly defined than the present supply, there is considerable opinion that there are already too many cardiologists in active practice and that the number in training is excessive.[3, 6] Even cardiologists do not discern a need to increase their numbers; the Cardiologists' Training Survey indicated that 70 to 80 per cent of cardiologists believe that the number of cardiologists in practice today is about right. The American College of Cardiology "Profile of the Cardiologist" study (ACC study) did not make a firm numerical recommendation, but based projected needs for cardiologists on an arbitrary ratio of 6.0 cardiologists per 100,000 population.[7] This recommendation was derived from an analysis of estimates of present physician ratios per 100,000 population according to nine different geographical sections of the country. The ratio of 6.0 cardiologists per 100,000 population assumed that in 1972 only two of nine geographic sections had a sufficiently high ratio and that a "gap" existed in the remaining areas. In order to elevate all regions to the ratio of 6.0 per 100,000, it was estimated that an additional 4568 new cardiologists (primary and secondary) would be needed during the interval from 1972 to 1976.[7] Although some of us would have thought this number to be excessive, we have produced this number of new cardiologists and the national ratio now does, in fact, exceed 6.0 cardiologists per 100,000 population. However, it is very unlikely that these new cardiologists have settled only in those areas that had "gaps" in 1972. We have also attained an additional goal of the ACC study by graduating 900 new trainees per year. In the view of many, this goal was excessive. Be that as it may, in sheer numbers, we have met the goal of the ACC study.

However, as noted in the ACC study, and in most other studies dealing with needs for medical manpower, analysis of the number of physicians alone can be very misleading. In assessing the need for cardiologists, we find that there are different types of cardiologists and that many cardiologists should be designated "internist-cardiologists." These include most of the primary and secondary cardiologists in private practice who do not perform cardiac catheterizations. The ACC study estimated that in 1972 approximately 4500 physicians were cast in this role and that "more might be needed." This type of cardiologist is primarily a consultant who may or may not perform cardiac catheterizations. Apparently, there are insufficient data to assess further need for this type of physician. On the other hand, the ACC study concluded that present training programs are adequate to provide enough "cardiac specialists" (coronary angiographers), but complained that there are too few "academic cardiologists" (teachers and researchers). We doubt, however, that this dearth of academic cardiologists is due to inadequate training opportunities; it is much more likely that the financial lure to private practice keeps well-trained fledgling cardiologists from pursuing academic careers.

The need for cardiology manpower first must be defined by the *type* of cardiologist that should be trained, and not just by an arbitrary cardiologist-to-population ratio. If a large percentage of trainees becomes cardiac specialists and they devote much of their time to coronary angiography, increasing the cardiologist-to-population ratio would serve no useful purpose. Moreover, although present and future manpower needs are usually assessed by use of number of personnel, the lack of a precise definition of who really is a cardiologist confuses the subject. In the A.M.A. classification, specialists are largely self-designated, and certified cardiologists constitute only a minority of all active cardiologists, although their number is increasing rapidly. At present, however, it is difficult to be sure of the actual supply of cardiologists.

Estimating need is even more difficult, and two assumptions are made, neither one of which may be correct. These are that the number is accurate and that present standards will predict future needs. Moreover, the lack of correlation between the number of physicians and the quality of health care is well known. For example, the ratio of physicians to population has been virtually constant since 1900; yet it is clear that the quality of health care has improved. Moreover, analysis of physician-to-population ratios of different countries as well as the U.S. shows that health care statistics such as morbidity and mortality correlate poorly with the physician:population ratio. The statistic physician:population ratio is one of the more fallacious health care indexes to which we have been subjected.[3] The arbitrary goal of 6.0 cardiologists per 100,000 population was based on an increased need due to technical advances,[7, 8] an assumption that seems justified by past experience but that may reflect more the needs of technology than the needs of patients.

The entire issue of what the optimal number of physicians really is, is poorly defined and may depend more on our *perception* of needs rather than a proven relationship between the health of the population and the supply of medical services. For example, for white males there is a high correlation between the cardiologist-to-population ratio and the death rate from coronary artery disease, but we do not know whether such patients attract cardiologists, whether cardiologists overdiagnose the condition, whether the availability of cardiologists is causally related to the death rate, or whether, as seems likely, there are other factors accounting for this correlation. The most rational criterion for the optimal number of cardiologists should reflect the most effective outcome of the cardiac therapy rather than the need to sustain technology or to equalize ratios in different parts of the country. Unfortunately, the information upon which these decisions must be based is not at hand, and as is usual when true indications are not known, estimates are derived primarily from professional perception of need and past levels of activity. Until better data are available, we should acknowledge that it is impossible to state with certainty that the present supply is short, adequate, or overabundant.

FACTORS THAT INFLUENCE APPARENT NEED FOR CARDIOLOGISTS

GEOGRAPHIC MALDISTRIBUTION

It is apparent from most health manpower studies that any existing deficiencies in cardiology manpower are as much the result of inefficient utilization of specialists as of insufficient numbers. An example of this is geographic maldistribution. There is a wide disparity in the ratio of cardiologists to population in the nine sections of the United States, ranging from a ratio of 8.0 cardiologists per 100,000 population in the Middle Atlantic states to a ratio of 2.5 in the East South Central area.[7] The common assumption is that the optimum ratio is at or near the highest level in the country and that deficiencies exist in all other areas. This is not necessarily correct.

The reasons for this geographic maldistribution are imperfectly understood but include complex economic, social, demographic, educational, and cultural factors.[3] Most young physicians, especially specialists, choose not to settle in rural areas and prefer to remain close to the cities because of the opportunities for professional and social stimulation, imagined or real. This has resulted in the phenomenon, observed in almost every large and even medium-sized city, of newly trained cardiologists settling farther and farther from the center of the city in the suburbs in order to remain in a desirable urban setting, despite an obvious surfeit of cardiologists in the area. Not all cities, however, attract cardiologists equally; the ratio per 100,000 population is 17.0 in Miami, 11.0 in New York, 3.3 in Louisville, and 2.7 in Norfolk–Newport News. There may be even more striking differences within geographic areas.

Because of this marked geographic maldistribution, the solution to filling the "gaps" in the low-ratio regions would be to redistribute cardiologists, not simply to produce more. In the ACC study, the projected need for cardiologists was based upon increasing the number of cardiologists in low-ratio areas but not decreasing the number in high-ratio areas. Such an approach is conceptually unsound, and impractical as well. Simply to train more cardiologists is not the answer, because there is no evidence that newly graduated trainees will not follow the old distribution patterns. Indeed, most younger cardiologists are more likely to settle in the already high-ratio areas, thereby increasing the maldistribution, and there is additional evidence that present governmental planning policies will increase the gaps even more.

A number of arguments pertaining to the maldistribution of cardiologists are fallacies. The first fallacy is that training more cardiologists will correct the distribution of services. It would be impossible to distribute evenly a relatively scarce and expensive resource across a country as large as the United States, which has diverse social, economic, and regional differences. The problem of geographic maldistribution is probably not solvable within a social structure that permits free movement of physicians.

The second fallacy is that geographic maldistribution is inherently bad for the delivery of health care. Maldistribution is not a condition unique to medicine. It occurs in almost every other profession, in higher education, and in recreational activities. The concentration of politicians in the federal and state capitals produces a continuing maldistribution of that resource. Is maldistribution of cardiologists really a problem? Are cardiac specialists needed everywhere? Although the maldistribution among cardiologists is probably about the same for primary as secondary cardiac specialists, regional differences are probably greater for cardiac specialists, i.e., those doing cardiac catheterization. Just as other professions or businesses tend to concentrate in certain areas, there is no reason that specific medical services should not be highly concentrated in relatively few medical centers. For example, for years patients have traveled from all over the country to Cleveland or Houston for open heart surgery because of the advanced technical work done at these centers. Similarly, cardiac transplantation, bone marrow transplantation, high-powered cancer chemotherapy, and other specialty services are localized in a few centers of expertise, providing much needed efficiency. It is certainly highly desirable that primary care of common cardiologic problems be provided by competent physicians, distributed evenly on the basis proportional to population. Uniform distribution of specialists who handle less common cardiac conditions would, and does, necessarily entail inefficiencies inherent in duplicating technology and equipment.

There is little to be gained by manipulating personnel to attain uniform distribution along political, social, or demographic lines. It is much more important to assure access to needed medical care, and it is a fact that an Eskimo living north of the Arctic Circle in Alaska has easier access (through the Public Health Service) to a cardiac specialist than many inhabitants of inner sections of our large cities. Moreover, there is evidence that geographic distribution of specialist cardiac care tends to increase the indirect factors that produce overutilization of resources.[10]

UTILIZATION OF CARDIOLOGISTS

The second important factor in an analysis of the need for cardiologists is the utilization of available personnel. In addition to geographic maldistribution, there is also maldistribution by specialties. It is widely contended that in the United States, we are overproducing specialists of all types, particularly in comparison to the number of primary care physicians.[3, 11, 12] In support of this contention is the SOSSUS (Study of Surgical Specialties in the United States), which has shown clearly that there is an excess of general surgeons as well as of surgical subspecialists.[13] The cardiologist-to-population ratio correlates better with other medical specialists and surgeons than with any other known variable;[8] this suggests that if surgeons and other medical specialists exist in oversupply, so also do cardiologists. Moreover, within the subspecialty of cardiology, maldistribution exists because there appear to be too many "catheter-oriented" and procedure-oriented cardiac specialists and too few academic cardiologists.

There is also a maldistribution in the activities of cardiologists. The general feeling that there are too many cardiologists performing cardiac catheterization (particularly coronary angiography)[3, 6, 7] is supported by the recommendation that there be no more than 1000 to 2000 physicians of this type.[7] Although the exact number of physicians doing cardiac catheterization (radiologists also perform the procedure, particularly coronary angiography) is not known, the number almost certainly exceeds 3000. Almost all of the more than 4000 primary cardiologists trained since 1972 are well trained in cardiac catheterization, and we are producing an additional 1000 physicians per year who can perform this and related invasive procedures. Although not all of those trained in the technique subsequently use it, the total number trained in cardiac catheterization appears to be excessive. As the ACC study shows, young, recently trained cardiologists who increasingly are certified by the Subspecialty Board on Cardiovascular Disease are utilizing both invasive and non-invasive procedures to a progressively greater extent than older cardiologists; hence, they are developing a different cardiologic practice. This procedure-oriented practice of cardiology results in more and more time spent in performing increasingly complex procedures and in less utilization of time for direct patient care.

At the other end of the spectrum, there is also the question of whether the specialist is being utilized properly. In areas with many specialists, there is tendency for primary care physicians to refer more patients whose problems fall into the category of a specialty; when this happens the cardiologist frequently is inappropriately occupied with minor cardiac problems that do not require his special talents.[15] As an approximation,[8] we have learned from the ACC study that each cardiologist encountered an average of 12 patients a day for an average of 10 minutes each, and of these encounters, 40 per cent dealt with cardiovascular problems. An extrapolation of these data shows that the average cardiologist spent 48 minutes a day in direct encounters with patients having problems within the realm of his specialty. Of course, such an extrapolation based upon imprecise data cannot be taken as an exact measurement of physician activity, but it suggests that there is an under-utilization of the specific expertise of cardiologists, and probably of all other specialists. The corollary is that even if there were a need for more cardiologists, the need could be met by better utilization of existing personnel.

PATTERNS OF HEALTH CARE DELIVERY

One of the factors that influences utilization of specialists is the mode of health care delivery. There is evidence that fewer operations are performed on patients who receive health care in a group practice, regardless of method of payment,[16] and that solo surgeons seem to be either not working at full capacity or doing more surgery than is necessary.[17, 18] It is probable that cardiologists' use of procedures follows the same pattern, and that cardiologists in group practice are used primarily to practice their specialty, while cardiologists in solo practice are more likely to be under-utilized or are performing too many procedures. Therefore, group practice is probably a more efficient way to deliver specialty medical care, a point that might well be noted by health policy planners.

The differences in utilization are even more striking when examined in the milieu of prepaid health plans. Although this introduces economic factors, which will be discussed subsequently, analysis of prepaid health care systems illustrates a striking difference in utilization compared to other health care delivery systems. The Group Health Cooperative of Puget Sound, a prepaid health care system, now has four cardiologists (two internist-cardiologists and two cardiac specialists) for a subscriber population of 220,000. This is a ratio of 1.8 cardiologists per 100,000 population, or less than one third of the recommended ratio of 6.0. The Health Insurance Plan of New York and the Southern California Kaiser Permanente plans have similarly low cardiologist-to-population ratios. There is no reason to believe that the subscribers of these prepaid health plans receive inferior care or have poorer health statistics than patients not enrolled in such plans. Although the use of prepaid health care plans to judge the need for cardiologists may not be entirely appropriate because the populations served may have different characteristics, this type of analysis has considerably more credibility than specialty needs defined by training program directors, specialty boards, or past and present national cardiologist-to-population ratios. Part of the lower ratio for the prepaid health plans is probably attributable to a lower utilization of open heart surgery, specifically coronary artery surgery.[10]

Probably the most fundamental factor in the utilization of specialists is how professionals relate to each other and to their patients.[6] In a system such as ours, in which roles are vaguely defined at best, there is a tremendous overlap in the activities of primary care physicians, secondary cardiologists, and primary cardiologists. Under-utilization of specialty skills for the necessary care of common cardiac problems and over-utilization of specialists and their resources for less indicated but more complex technical services requires a large pool of cardiologists. In contrast, in the British National Health Service there is a very clear demarcation of the roles of primary and specialist physicians, allowing a much greater utilization of specialty skills. By controlling the number of trainees and the number of consultant (specialty) positions, the ratio of specialists to population has been kept an order of magnitude lower than in the United States. Although opinions vary about whether the National Health Service offers sufficient access to cardiac surgery, in the absence of valid indications for coronary artery surgery in particular, this is largely a social and economic question, and there is little to indicate that patient needs for valid cardiac problems are less well met in the United Kingdom than in the United States. Because the U.K. seems to have a sufficient number of cardiologists, there are relatively few registrar (resident) positions in cardiology, and the cardiology trainee in the National Health Service runs a considerable risk of not obtaining a speciality position, especially in the location of his choice. A comparison of the British system with our own makes it clear that in the U.K. the relationship between the specialist and the primary care physician, and to his patients, is the most important determinant of the number of specialists. Before we can make an intelligent assessment of the number of cardiologists needed in the United States, it is imperative that we define these interprofessional working relationships more clearly.

ECONOMIC FACTORS

There is no doubt that economic factors play an important role in creating a "need" for cardiologists, or for that matter any other type of specialist. The experience of the prepaid health care systems demonstrates that there is a marked reduction in the number of specialists when there is an economic disincentive to use them and their services. Whether the prepaid plans use too few cardiologists or the fee-for-service system uses too many cannot be determined from this difference, but assuming that there are no other obvious major differences between prepaid and fee-for-service medicine, it is reasonable to conclude that the economic variable produces the disparity in the number of cardiologists. Moreover, in the fee-for-service system, the usual rules of supply and demand do not exist. In the marketplace sense, the physician is both purchaser and seller, because he decides on the need for a service and then provides it. The patient's most important decision in such a transaction is the solicitation of the physician contact; once that contact has been made, the usual patient-doctor relationship deems it proper that the patient acquiesce in most, if not all, of the physician's decisions. Indeed, it is implicit in the understanding between patient and physician that the patient is incapable of making a wise decision (despite informed consent) and that the physician is superbly qualified to do so. This unusual relationship, in the business sense, enables the physician to control the specific purchases of his time and services, provided he has sufficient patient contact and the patients do not bolt the system.

The physician is, therefore, in a unique position to obtain a maximum economic return for his time. Given a choice of services that he can supply and great latitude in the indications for service provided to any given patient, it is easy and natural within the fee-for-service system to choose that service which brings the greatest remuneration, as long as that service provides proper and acceptable medical care for the patient. In virtually all segments of medicine, income per unit time is greatest for performance of procedures. For a long time, most procedures were operations, performed by surgeons or general practitioners. But procedures, or the use of procedures to obtain maximum income, has its place in virtually every medical specialty as well. The medical fee structure, supported by every form of insurance, favors procedures to the extent that most physicians can realize several times the fee for a simple procedure than for a complete history and physical examination, for time spent in talking to patients and their families, or for a life-saving maneuver that does not involve the use of a knife, tube, or needle. Endoscopy, bronchoscopy, needle biopsies, dialysis, x-rays, scans, and even skin testing provide devices for amplification of income; witness the flourishing activity in these procedures. For the cardiologist, known as the surgeon of the internists, procedures include electrocardiograms, echocardiograms, other non-invasive measurements, and cardiac catheterization. Although a physician can earn a comfortable living just reading electrocardiograms or echocardiograms, it is cardiac catheterization and, particularly, coronary angiography that have become the bread-and-butter procedures of the cardiologist. As with all procedures, the economic incentive is a temptation to stretch the indications for coronary angiography or an echocardiogram. Cardiologists, like all others, tend to do what they know how to do best and, given a suitable setting and technical expertise, perform more and more procedures, almost surely to excess. As was asked in a recent symposium on training of cardiologists, "Does not the mastery of the skill put pressure on the physician to maintain the skill and use it for a means of earning a living?"[19] If this is so, is it not possible that the goal of maintaining competence in a skill or to use it to earn a living will tend to obfuscate the medical indications for using this skill? Does it make the need for maintaining the technical skill and incidentally generating income a stronger rationale than the need for the procedure by the patients?

Do the financial rewards of procedurism increase the "need" for procedure-oriented cardiologists? The answer is almost certainly yes, and any assessment of need for future personnel based upon present levels of activity must take this factor into account. What would the effect on future need for cardiologists be if the fee for coronary angiography was reduced to 100 dollars (as in Canada) instead of 400 dollars, as is presently the case in the U.S.?

In evaluating the legitimacy of the present number of cardiologists as a guide to future needs, we must consider the well-known fact that doctors, especially specialists, create their own demand for services.[3, 6, 8-10, 20] There is widespread evidence that the number of non-emergent operations is proportional to the number of surgeons who can perform them,[9, 16, 21] that is, the surgical rate is not altogether a function of patient need or medical indications but is determined to a large extent by the number of surgeons offering the service. Similarly, the rate at which coronary angiography is performed is probably also, to a significant extent, a function of the number of angiographers. Moreover, there is nothing to suggest that as the number of cardiologists exceeds demand for their services, the cost of these procedures will drop. From the surgical analogy, if an excess of physicians develops, some or many work shorter hours, but the fees for procedures do not come down. The support level of third-party payments ensures against decreasing prices. It is a well-known dictum that even in areas that appear to be saturated by cardiologists (or other subspecialists), there is always "room for one more," further increasing the demand for their services. Cardiologists' incomes also influence the distribution of cardiologists in private practice. At a time when highly trained teams of cardiologists and cardiac surgeons are under-utilized in a number of large metropolitan centers, we are seeing the phenomenon of new cardiac surgical centers being created in smaller communities, when adherence to sound principles of regionalization would deem them unnecessary. While this dispersion of cardiac facilities may solve the problem of geographic maldistribution, in economic terms it is disadvantageous for society as a whole. Indeed, these peripheral centers provide considerable financial incentives to those who set them up — physicians and hospitals. The resulting proliferation of many smaller centers, each aspiring to become a big-time operation, creates a demand for patients, who in turn demand and receive services far in excess of what would occur under a system of well-ordered regionalization in which there would be fewer medical centers with better facilities and better trained personnel.

PROFESSIONAL, POLITICAL, AND SOCIAL FACTORS

Regardless of societal need, as is true with all specialists in medicine, the number of new cardiologists is, in fact, determined by the number of trainees who enter the approximately 350 cardiology training programs presently extant in this country. The size of these training programs bears no relationship to either local or national needs for cardiologists, but reflects the need of the institutions maintaining the training programs, particularly as those needs are perceived by the program directors. For example, despite an excess of surgeons and surgical subspecialists in active practice, in a study of specialists in the Pacific Northwest, every residency program director of a surgical specialty indicated a need for more individuals to be trained in his specialty.[22] Not only are the number and types of trainees determined by the hospital division or department, but once these training positions have been determined, and trainees have been recruited, and the program is operating smoothly, any attempt to alter the number or characteristics of the trainees, except to increase their number, results in tremendous pressure against such change. Trainees are integrated, productive members of the medical staff, and any suggestion that reduces the size of the medical staff is seen as a threat to the professional integrity — in the ecologic, not moral, sense — of the department or division in question. There is always the desire, appropriate or not, of sections to grow in size and economic importance. The easiest way to enlarge a section is to increase the number of trainees, which in turn creates a need for more permanent staff members to handle the increased activity.

Cardiologists as a group and program directors in particular want to create trainees in the image of the trainers. The non-invasive clinical cardiologist sees a great need for more of the same; the angiographer specialist argues that trainees must spend more time in the cath lab; the researcher decries the abundance of clinicians and the dearth of well-trained investigators; and the electrophysiologist's primary concern is over the lack of electrophysiology in the training program. However, allocation of the trainee's time to a given activity is almost invariably governed by institutional needs. Those activities that are most essential to the hospital, e.g., cardiac catheterization, are assigned top priority. Trainees in specialty programs are a source of relatively low-cost labor who provide a very specialized and often expensive service. Cardiology trainees are essential in teaching hospitals to perform catheterizations and other time-consuming procedures, which otherwise would divert faculty from other activities, notably research. Even in private practice settings, it is financially advantageous to develop a training program for the purpose of providing low-cost assistance for procedures and after-hours coverage in the hospital. Trainees, the "graduate assistants" of clinical services, are also highly desirable as cheap and proficient (and often very bright) research assistants for the faculty.

U.S. Public Health Service training grants have been a strong stimulus in promoting an increase in the number of clinically trained cardiologists. Although the purpose of these grants may have been to create academic or research cardiologists, there is ample evidence that one of their major effects was to greatly increase the number of clinical cardiologists, particularly cardiac specialists (angiographers). By encouraging clinical research programs that involve invasive analysis of cardiac anatomy and pathophys-

iology, the various federal grants and contracts have produced a generation of technically oriented cardiologists who now want to increase their
number. This is not to argue that much of the clinical research performed
under the aegis of these grants is not very important. There is also no evidence that the recent decrease in the National Institutes of Health training grants has reduced the number of clinical fellowships. Faced with loss
of grant support, cardiology training program directors have shown a remarkable ingenuity in obtaining support from other sources. While the
recent renaissance of cardiology training programs contains safeguards that
are aimed at having the trainee remain in academic cardiology, it seems
unlikely to us that these safeguards will be effective. It is axiomatic that the
factors that regulate the number of trainees today determine the number of
cardiologists tomorrow. Experience has shown clearly that the ability to formulate the type of cardiologist produced by a training program by attaching
strings such as pay-back time to it will exert only a limited effect.

The ever-expanding number of medical school graduates places further
pressure on training programs to increase the number of trainees. Unless
there is a reduction in the overall ratio of specialists to primary care physicians, cardiology training programs will have to expand to accept the increased number of medical residents seeking specialty training. Moreover,
the curricula of medical schools and medical residency programs favor specialization. In many departments of medicine, for example, there is a great
emphasis on subspecialty medicine, and few departments have strong programs in general medicine. Likewise, few members of the faculty are
strong general internists, making it difficult for house officers to find appropriate role models for a career outside of a medical specialty.

The increased demand of medical residents for subspecialty training
may be aided and abetted by the certification process. The very existence
of certification makes it a major goal for many medical residents because
certification appears to confer upon the bearer a higher position in the hierarchy of the profession. In addition, there exists what the former President
of the National Board of Medicine Examiners has termed the "catalyst"
function of certification.[15] Once a specialty develops and gains recognition,
certification becomes a permit to practice the specialty. Recognition of specialty status for one group implies lack of knowledge and expertise for all
others who wish to practice that particular specialty. The nonspecialists
then begin to doubt their competence in that specialty and accelerate their
referrals of both simple and complex problems within that specialty to the
certified specialist. This, in turn, begets more feelings of incompetence because of decreased exposure to clinical problems in the speciality, and soon
the primary care physician refers most cases within the specialty to the
specialist. Then even very simple cases are referred, leading to a suspicion
on the part of the specialist that the primary care physician is indeed in-
competent in the field. The primary physician's fear is reinforced by his
experiences in medical school and residency training, where he is surrounded by specialists. This fear has kept many students from choosing a nonspe-
cialist career, which they perceive will lead to early atrophy of knowledge
and skills and will result in incompetence. For all its positive features,
therefore, certification tends to be self-serving because it endows incompe-

tence upon the uncertified. "Jack of all trades, master of none" is not a desirable position in modern medicine.

The drive for specialization within internal medicine, which has been most rampant in cardiology, may be motivated in part by the fear that future government control may favor the specialist. The expectation is that under a more controlled system of medicine, such as exists in the United Kingdom, specialists will be a notch higher than generalists in the professional hierarchy and pay scale. Specialization is seen as a form of insurance against a loss of professional mobility in the future, when a more tightly controlled system that is likely to keep a physician in his original track will be in force. There is among some trainees an urgency to reap the financial rewards of private practice now, before being "forced" into a controlled system. To many trainees, the best means of attaining that goal is through specialization.

Professional societies, also, tend to overestimate the need for their own members' services, thereby increasing the supply of specialists. An example of this was provided by the American Board of Dermatology. This group argued that because approximately 10 to 20 per cent of the diseases seen by primary care physicians have dermatologic implications, a similar proportion of physicians trained must be dermatologists; therefore, there was obviously a major lack of dermatologists.[23] If this sort of reasoning were applied to cardiology, calculations show that we would need five times the present number of cardiologists in order to see each patient with cardiovascular disease just once a year.[8] Similar ill-conceived chauvinism leads to the all-too-common practice that every medium- or large-sized hospital must have complete diagnostic and surgical facilities, including, of course, suites for cardiac catheterization and cardiac surgery. There is great pressure from local hospital boards and civic organizations to procure all forms of modern facilities and treatment modalities, which, in turn, require the appropriate number of specialists. The drive of more and more communities to have facilities for coronary angiography and surgery, and the burgeoning number of cardiac surgeons able to do the surgery, are strong factors in reinforcing the apparent need for more cardiologists today.

RELATIONSHIP BETWEEN INTERVENTION AND HEALTH STATUS

Of all the factors that determine the apparent need for cardiologists, the one least discussed, least studied, and least understood deals with the relationship between the interventions or services provided by cardiologists and the health status of their patients. Increasingly, the role of cardiologists has become procedure-oriented, which in itself creates a need for cardiologists to perform the procedures. In order to justify the large number of cardiologists required to perform the procedures presently available and those that will appear in the future and will probably be more complex, time-consuming, and costly, we must seriously address the question of whether these procedures are in the best interest of patients. For instance, as was asked in a study of medical practice in Vermont, does performing six times as many electrocardiograms in one area compared to another result in greater improvement of health for the population of the first area?[9] Are there not less expensive methods that will not compromise the health status of patients? In modern medicine, all of us find it difficult to avoid use of the newest technical, diagnostic, and theapeutic procedures, but what data can be mustered to support the contention that these devices actually improve patient health? Without cardiac catheterization, echocardiography, and isotope imaging, the modern cardiologist would feel relegated to the Dark Ages, but what evidence is there that the increased information provided by these interventions actually improves or prolongs life, particularly on the scale with which they are applied? No one can deny that modern cardiac surgery, with its remarkable achievements and benefits, depends on accurate diagnostic assessment that most often requires technical interventions. In the case of congenital heart disease and most valvular abnormalities, the need for intervention is generally indisputable. However, the great number of cardiologists now practicing are applying these interventions in ever-increasing quantity and for reasons that in many cases lie outside valid indications. The problem of excess interventions arises because so little is known about the relationship between interventions and health status; hence, indications for procedures can be broadened to cover many possibilities or contingencies. We should not project a greater need for cardiologists to provide more services when we do not know that the services are in the public interest, despite our own beliefs of benefit. We must know much more about the effects of cardiac catheterization and cardiac surgery before we can assert that more manpower is needed to perform more of these procedures.

In the last decade, the procedure contributing most to the apparent need for cardiologists has been the coronary artery bypass operation. Approximately 75,000 of these operations are performed every year in the United States, requiring approximately 225,000 coronary angiograms to evaluate and screen patients for the surgery. The prevalence of coronary artery disease is about 4,000,000, or about two per cent of the population of the United States, all of whom are potential candidates for this operation.[24] Many surgeons and cardiologists openly advocate and use the operation prophylactically, a practice which, if applied universally, would increase their activity fiftyfold. This increased frequency of coronary artery surgery has been supported by cardiologists despite any scientific validation of its efficacy in prolonging life or preventing myocardial infarction and despite the evidence provided by five controlled studies demonstating that the operation does not attain these objectives.[19, 25] This intervention is more responsible for the projected need for cardiologists in this country than any other single factor, and yet the best data fail to show major benefit in health status as a result of the intervention. In 1971, about 35 per cent of all cardiologists' contacts with patients were for problems relating to coronary artery disease.[14] The number of coronary artery operations per year has almost quadrupled since then, and although we do not have data detailing time spent in various activities, it is probable that primary cardiologists as a group spend more than one fourth of their time in contact with patients performing cardiac catheterizations, primarily coronary angiography. The total time spent in all activities related to coronary artery surgery is even greater. Until we acquire scientific data showing a positive correlation between coronary artery surgery and health status, the true indication for cardiologists' time to be spent in this endeavor will remain unknown, and a further increase in cardiologists who will contribute to the increased use of this unproven therapy, however optimistic we may be about it, is not justified. If well-controlled scientific studies do demonstrate the benefit of present or future forms of coronary artery surgery, we should then make an assessment of whether widespread application of such therapy is in the public interest, considering total cost and all other factors.

Similar arguments should be applied to the burgeoning use of echocardiography and isotope angiography. Are there real benefits to patients from these procedures, or are the gains primarily professional? Although we do not have answers to these questions, surely we are remiss not to consider them in assessing the future need for cardiology manpower.

NEGATIVE ASPECTS OF SPECIALIZATION

Although specialization is probably indispensible for the rapid technological advances to which we have become accustomed, disadvantages do accrue from overspecialization. The overabundance of specialists makes it difficult for patients to obtain primary care. Indeed, one of the most important reasons for the crescendo of complaints about the present health delivery system is overspecialization in all fields of medicine, which makes it more difficult to gain access to ambulatory care, emergency care, and even to the medical system itself.[26] The preponderance of specialists in some areas also increases the difficulty in gaining access to the proper specialist, because without easy access to a primary care physician, the patient often encounters difficulty in determining which specialist is appropriate. Also, without referral from a primary care physician, it is frequently difficult to get an appointment with a specialist. The only solution to the problem of having too few primary care physicians is to lessen the ratio of specialists to generalists.[11, 12] This will not occur if cardiologists and other specialists continue to increase their number in proportion to the total physician pool.

Excessive specialization also leads to fragmented care.[27] All too frequently, patients end up visiting regularly four or five specialists for multiple system disorders or complaints, when one competent primary care physician, perhaps with an occasional consultation, could do the total job better. Each specialist refers the patient to another specialist for a problem outside his domain; the net result is excessive doctoring and "medicine by committee." Moreover, this type of practice breeds specialists, further exacerbating the imbalance between primary care and specialty physicians.

Lack of Contact with Common Cardiologic Problems

Because today's cardiology trainees spend so much time learning the skills of the new technology and are oriented away from direct patient care, there is considerable opinion that they are inadequately trained in the common cardiac problems, such as management of arrhythmias, hypertension, and congestive heart failure. The one extant analysis of American cardiology training programs tends to support the hypothesis that too much training time is spent in learning laboratory procedures, and proportionately too little time is spent in mastering the more common skills needed for direct patient care.[2] In averaging the data defining the activities of two-year training programs, in 1971 more trainee time was spent in laboratory diagnostic techniques (35 per cent) than in cardiac patient care (32 per cent). Cardiac catheterization and angiography accounted for 18 per cent of all training time, as opposed to 15 per cent for research or 10 per cent for laboratory and classroom instruction in basic sciences and clinical disease. Undoubtedly, the time spent in the catheterization laboratory and other laboratory procedures is proportionately even greater today than it was in 1971.

The percentage of trainee time spent in patient management in a coronary care unit and in treatment of arrhythmias is limited compared to time spent learning technical procedures. Trainees spent 2.5 times as many hours in the catheterization laboratory than in electrocardiography.[2]

The influence of Board certification in determining trainee activities is difficult to judge, but the most important effect of certification is probably the requirement that two years of cardiology training is necessary. It is very likely that a clinical cardiologist can be well trained, exclusive of technical procedures, with just one year of specialty training following proper training in internal medicine[28] and that the compulsory second year for attainment of certification adds time that is devoted almost entirely to technical procedures. As has been pointed out above, once having acquired these technical skills, it seems wasteful for the trainee not to use them. Therefore, the certification requirement of two years of training has the net effect of producing more cardiac specialists than the internist-cardiologists who are likely to be the most needed. Incidentally, the ACC study showed that fewer than half of all trainees had fulfilled the full requirements for Internal Medicine Board certification before beginning training in cardiology,[2] a finding not in keeping with the recommendations of the study. The structure of and requirements for specialty and subspecialty Board certification strongly favor enrollment of the internal medicine resident in a subspecialty program, including cardiology.

Emphasis on subspecialty training programs in teaching hospitals detracts from the subspecialty training of residents in primary care programs, either in family practice or internal medicine. The commitment to teaching by the cardiology faculty is too frequently restricted to cardiology trainees, and very few cardiology program directors have much interest in directing portions of their programs specifically at noncardiology residents. The overall effect is that usually the noncardiology trainees receive insufficient training in cardiology to function well as internist-cardiologists. At present, neither cardiology trainees nor medicine residents are receiving the type of instruction that will make them effective internist-cardiologists.

Conclusions and Recommendations

In 1979 there is no need for more cardiologists, and it is probable that there are too many cardiologists in practice today. The projections that contend that an increased need for cardiologists exists are arbitrary and based on the existing number of cardiologists and on present professional and demographic practices. A more global view of the health care system mandates the training of more primary care physicians and fewer specialists. In terms of the specialty of cardiology, there is a need for more internist-cardiologists and fewer cardiac specialists. The old issues of physician-to-population ratios and geographic maldistribution are largely fallacious in determining true need. The proper issue is not how many cardiologists, but what kind and for what purpose. There are certainly enough well-trained cardiologists today to handle all problems requiring a subspecialist, if only there were better utilization of personnel. The present economic, professional, and certification incentives combine to favor the training of an excess number of cardiologists, particularly because it is perceived by many that their services appear to have made a positive impact on total health care status. It is imperative to assess the real effect of modern technological intervention before we muster more cardiologists to do more of the same thing.

The only solution to the problem of too few primary care physicians and too many specialists is to reduce the number of specialist trainees, including cardiologists. Contrary to the continued trend of increasing the number of trainees or of keeping programs at their present level, both the *number* and *size* of programs should be reduced. In order to stem the tide of increasingly applying new technology, we must train fewer cardiac specialists; that is, fewer cardiologists should be trained in cardiac catheterization and coronary angiography. To attain this end, teaching hospitals may have to hire additional faculty to take the place of the inexpensive labor provided by trainees.[3] Not unimportant to this argument is that containment of technological application (without restriction of technical advances) and overspecialization are two important ways to contain health care costs.

In order to better prepare the primary care physicians who should provide most of the care for the common cardiac problems, cardiology training programs should include a higher percentage of one-year trainees, and there should be more willingness to provide cardiology training to general medicine residents. It is especially important to check the insidious trend toward three-year cardiology programs, except for a few clearly committed academic cardiologists.

Although it would be heartening to think that cardiologists would themselves regulate the number and type of trainees so as to bring into balance the supply of cardiologists and the true need of patients, unless there are major changes in some of the powerful incentives to specialization, this is unlikely to happen. If self-regulation does not work, as appears to be the case, the only recourse is external regulation, which, while less satisfactory, seems in the present atmosphere more likely.

References

1. Adams FH, and Mendenhall RC (eds): Profile of the cardiologist: Training and manpower requirements for the specialist in adult cardiovascular disease. Am J Cardiol. 34:389–456, 1974.

2. Fowler NO, Hultgren HN, and McIntosh HD: Training programs in cardiovascular disease. Am J Cardiol 34:429–438, 1974.
3. Petersdorf RG: Health manpower: Numbers, distribution, quality. Ann Intern Med 82:694–701, 1975.
4. Source: American Board of Internal Medicine.
5. Source: American Medical Association, Center for Health Services Research and Development, Chicago, 1977.
6. Ginzberg E: Manpower for cardiology: No easy answers. Am J Cardiol 37:955–958, 1976.
7. Pritchard WH, and Abelmann WH: Future manpower needs in cardiology. Am J Cardiol 34:444–448, 1974.
8. Abelmann WH: Cardiologic manpower resources and their distribution: A challenge for the future. Am J Cardiol 36:550–554, 1975.
9. Wennberg J, and Gittlesohn A: Small area variations in health care delivery. Science 182:1102–1108, 1973.
10. Preston TA: *Coronary Artery Surgery: A Critical Review.* New York, Raven Press, 1977, Chapter 9.
11. Cooper T: The government's concerns regarding postgraduate training and health care delivery. Am J Cardiol 36:555–557, 1975.
12. Relman A: The responsible role of a chairman of the department of medicine in postgraduate training. Am J Cardiol 36:563–564, 1975.
13. The American College of Surgeons and the American Surgical Association: *Surgery in the United States.* Baltimore, Lewis Advertising Co., 1975.
14. Swan HJ, and Gifford RW: Current profile of the professional activities of the American cardiologist. Am J Cardiol 34:417–428, 1974.
15. Chase RA: Proliferation of certification in medical specialties: Productive or counterproductive. N Engl J Med 294:497–499, 1976.
16. Bunker JP: Surgical manpower: A comparison of operations and surgeons in the United States and in England and Wales. N Engl J Med 282:135–144, 1970.
17. Roemer MI, and DuBois DM: Medical costs in relation to the organization of ambulatory care. N Engl J Med 280:988–993, 1969.
18. Fuchs VR: *Who Shall Live? Health, Economics, and Social Choice.* New York, Basic Books, Inc, 1974, p 72.
19. McIntosh HD: Responsible leadership in the training of the cardiologists of tomorrow. Am J Cardiol 36:547–549, 1975.
20. McGregor M: Cardiology in a system of socialized medicine: Canadian experience. Am J Cardiol 36:560–562, 1975.
21. Vayda E: A comparison of surgical rates in Canada and in England and Wales. N Engl J Med 289:1224–1229, 1973.
22. Clawson DK, Bennett RL, and Steen MK: Planning residency programs based on physician projections. A paper presented to the American Medical Association Symposium on Distribution of Health Manpower, San Francisco, June 17, 1972.
23. Senior B, and Smith BA: The number of physicians as a constraint on delivery of health care. JAMA 222:178–183, 1972.
24. Preston TA: *Coronary Artery Surgery: A Critical Review.* New York, Raven Press, 1977, p 4.
25. Preston TA: *Coronary Artery Surgery: A Critical Review.* New York, Raven Press, 1977, Chapter 8.
26. Fuchs VR: *Who Shall Live? Health, Economics, and Social Choice.* New York, Basic Books, Inc, 1974, p 68.
27. Petersdorf RG: Internal medicine 1976: Consequences of subspecialization and technology. Ann Intern Med 84:92–94, 1976.
28. Marcus F: Discussion: Responsible leadership in the training of the cardiologists of tomorrow. Am J Cardiol 36:572, 1975.

We Are Overproducing Cardiology Trainees Who Are Also Untrained to Handle Common Clinical Cardiologic Problems: An Opposing Viewpoint

WALTER H. ABELMANN, M.D.

Department of Medicine and Thorndike Laboratory, Beth Israel Hospital, and Professor of Medicine, Harvard Medical School, Boston, Massachusetts

The responsibilities of a cardiovascular specialist toward his patient, the patient's family, and the patient's primary health care professionals comprise the detection and diagnosis of any cardiovascular disease that may be present, as well as prevention of cardiovascular disease or disability. Furthermore, the cardiovascular specialist is responsible for assessing the life situation of the patient and for making recommendations to use the available resources for rehabilitation of the patient toward optimal self-care and physical and mental activity. To the extent that a cardiovascular specialist may find himself responsible for the primary care of his patients — in some instances for brief periods in the course of cardiovascular disease and in others for longer periods, if not the entire course, he may become responsible not only for formulating the primary care plan, but also for implementing it. Furthermore, patients with cardiovascular disorders are also liable to have or develop other medical problems, so that the cardiovascular specialist must be sufficiently conversant with general medicine in order to recognize and plan management of such additional

21

disorders or infirmities. The authors of the preceding article of this controversy state that "we are overproducing cardiology trainees who are also untrained to handle common clinical cardiologic problems." This statement may be interpreted in two ways. The first takes the statement as a whole as indicating that too many cardiologists are being trained who are not able to handle common cardiologic problems. Whereas, according to this interpretation, the statement does not address itself to the question of whether we are overproducing cardiologists in general, a second interpretation would hold that we are also training an excessive number of cardiologists. Let us address the first interpretation.

If freestanding cardiovascular training, and especially training addressing itself predominantly to invasive and non-invasive procedures, were available and led to certification in the specialty of cardiovascular diseases, then one could and should doubt seriously whether cardiology trainees would have the training and experience in cardiovascular and general medicine that would equip them to "handle common clinical cardiologic problems" and take on the responsibilities for consultative and occasional primary care as defined above. However, cardiovascular training and certification in cardiovascular disease in the United States is not freestanding, but is conditional upon prior training and qualification for certification in internal medicine. Furthermore, most training programs form an integral part of an academic department of medicine.

Thus, a physician entering upon training in cardiology, after having been carefully selected as an appropriate candidate for the M.D. degree, almost always has taken four semesters of clinical courses of active participation in patient care as a prerequisite for the M.D. degree and has completed an internship and at least one, and often two, years of residency in medicine.

On general medical services in the United States, approximately one third of the in-patient population has been hospitalized because of cardiovascular problems, and approximately another third has clinically significant cardiovascular disease in addition to the medical problems that led to hospitalization. It is evident that it would be exceedingly difficult for a cardiovascular trainee to evade in-depth exposure to cardiovascular disease and responsibility for management of cardiovascular patients.

Thus, the cardiology trainee whose training has conformed to the guidelines for training in cardiovascular disease proposed by the Subspecialty Board on Cardiovascular Disease should be well prepared to handle common clinical cardiologic problems. However, we may not ignore three pathways by which physicians have entered cardiology in the past and must ask ourselves whether they remain operative. *First,* as of 1972–1973, 27 per cent of the 329 identified cardiology training programs offered only one year of training in cardiology. Their trainees, thus, do not fulfill the standards referred to. It is unknown to what extent and at what rate these programs will comply with the current guidelines. *Second,* physicians trained abroad have in the past entered cardiology training in the United States in large numbers, often to remain in this country. Many of these individuals have specialized in invasive and non-invasive subspecialty areas and have not been fully trained or experienced in internal medicine and general cardiology, and thus the title statement of this chapter may well apply. However, the current visa and immigration laws have made it exceedingly difficult for foreign physicians to enter the United States for postgraduate training and to remain here subsequently. *Third,* physicians in general medicine or internal medicine may enter cardiology after a number of years in practice, either by independent study and experience or, occasionally, by way of a part-time or full-time training fellowship. These physicians, however, are likely to have had in-depth experience in the delivery of health care to cardiovascular patients.

Ultimately, the question as to the ability of a given cardiovascular subspecialist (e.g., electrocardiographer, echocardiographer, catheterizer) to function as a complete cardiologist would have to be answered by the evaluation of his performance and its outcome. However, such evaluation is difficult and lacks established methodology. Furthermore, an accessible data base to permit comprehensive evaluation of performance in relation to training does not exist. We do, however, have data with respect to the prevalence of and morbidity from heart disease. These suggest strongly that mortality from heart disease has decreased significantly from 1968 to 1975, a decrease that is generally attributed to advances in the prevention and treatment of acute myocardial infarction, hypertension, and congestive heart failure.

Let me now address the question, "Are we overproducing cardiologists?" This question can only be answered if we know the number of cardiologists presently active, the number of cardiologists being trained, and the number needed. The first two are known fairly accurately for 1972–73, but the latter is at best an estimate. A nationwide study of cardiology manpower in 1973 revealed that there were 5.1 active cardiologists per 100,000 population in the United States. However, cardiologists were very unevenly distributed, with ratios ranging from 8.0 per 100,000 population in the Middle Atlantic region to 2.5 in the East South Central region. Furthermore, cardiologists tended to be concentrated in some cities but scarce in others, with ratios ranging from 17.0 and 11.0 per 100,000 populatin in Miami and in New York, respectively, to 3.3 and 2.7 in Milwaukee and Norfolk–Newport News, respectively. There is no evidence that this striking maldistribution of cardiologists has changed significantly in the intervening years. Inasmuch as it is highly unlikely that cardiologists will redistribute themselves to correct this maldistribution, and even if it is admitted that there is an excess of cardiologists in certain parts of the country, a need for increasing the number of cardiologists to be trained is evident. In addition, consideration must be given to the needs for improving standards of care — including prevention and rehabilitation, to the needs created by the development of new diagnostic and surgical techniques, and to the effects of restriction on foreign medical graduates. The cardiology manpower report, taking cognizance not only of the need for geographical gap-filling, but also projecting the overall need for increasing the number of cardiologists, recommended that the then annual output of 800 graduates of cardiovascular training programs be increased to 900 per year.

The above arguments lead to the logical conclusion that we are not overproducing cardiology trainees and that current and future cardiology trainees are not untrained to handle common clinical cardiologic problems. Are we then to relax and conclude that all is for the best in the best of all possible worlds? Emphatically, such is not the case. Admittedly, we have trained individuals in cardiology who have not completed what is currently considered full training in internal medicine, and we have permitted the growth of cardiovascular technologists who limit their practice to sub-subspecialities such as electrocardiographic interpretation, cardiac catheterization and angiocardiography, or echocardiography. These developments have been facilitated by the endorsement of the marketplace and the associated financial rewards. Furthermore, it is quite possible that many of these professionals not only have responded to needs for their services, but also have actually created increased and not always justified demands for their services. We must be fully cognizant of these developments and see to it that the present guidelines for graduate education in cardiology are accepted and implemented in all cardiovascular training programs.

Many current cardiovascular training programs are deficient in one or more respects. Pharmacology, pathology, pulmonary disease, vascular disease, research, behavioral sciences, and ambulatory cardiology are areas of training and experience often insufficiently emphasized. The structure of the curriculum in many training programs is determined more by the institution's manpower requirement than by consideration of optimal distribution of time and emphasis among the many disciplines and skills that must be covered. More consideration must also be given to achieving the kind of flexibility in programs that would permit curricula designed to fit the individual trainee's career goals. Levels of competence reached, rather than arbitrary length of service, should determine the time assigned to a given rotation. Such considerations logically lead to the need to develop mechanisms for ongoing evaluation of trainees' knowledge and performance during the training period.

Selected References

Abelmann WH, and Adams FH: Cardiology manpower. Ninth Bethesda Conference of the American College of Cardiology. Am J Cardiol 37:941–983, 1976.

Adams FH, and Mendenhall RC (eds): Profile of the cardiologist: Training and manpower requirements for the specialist in adult cardiovascular disease. Am J Cardiol 34:389–456, 1974.

McIntosh HD (ed.): Symposium: Responsible leadership in the training of the cardiologists of tomorrow. Am J Cardiol. 36:547–549, 1975.

Subspecialty Board on Cardiovascular Disease of the American Board of Internal Medicine: Guidelines for training in cardiovascular disease. Am J Cardiol 39:617–620, 1977.

Comment

As an academic cardiologist, it is perhaps inappropriate for me to comment on this controversy since I share a natural bias with my colleagues that favors the opposing position. Despite this bias, I am impressed with the arguments marshalled by Drs. Preston and Petersdorf. They have focused on many issues facing the cardiologic community, and it would be well for all of us to examine these carefully and thoughtfully.

Both sides of this controversy have recognized that there is a need for an increase in academic cardiologists. In my judgment, this reflects a discouragement among many young graduates as to the future of academic cardiology in light of the general cutback that is apparent in both training and research support by the federal government and by the affiliates of the American Heart Association as well. This, however, involves but a small block of cardiologists; it is not the central problem addressed by Drs. Abelmann, Preston, and Petersdorf. I think there is also agreement that a need exists to insure that the primary care physician, who is not a cardiologist or internist-cardiologist, needs some exposure to cardiovascular training; this is a responsibility that academic cardiology training programs must meet. It is part of the problem that internal medicine residency programs face in insuring that the family practice resident obtains adequate exposure to the discipline of internal medicine.

Preston and Petersdorf make a compelling argument that the practice of cardiology has become increasingly procedure-oriented and suggest that evidence is lacking that this improves health care. This is provocative food for thought, and I share with them an uneasiness that we have become excessive in our desire to perform laboratory cardiologic investigations of all types in lieu of a few critical determinations. Such zealousness does require a greater manpower pool, and there are some data to support the contention that the creation of the specialist encourages unnecessary procedures.

Nevertheless, despite the above, I do feel that there are too few cardiologists who currently are trained to meet many of the cardiologic health care needs of our population. In particular, there appears to be a need for cardiologists, both primary and secondary, who can manage the common problems of cardiology, most of which revolve around the field of coronary artery disease as well as the management of hypertension, heart failure, and arrhythmias. Myocardial infarction, angina pectoris, and the other manifestations of coronary heart diseases are not limited to urban centers. Small community hospitals in rural areas often have coronary care units and reasonable diagnostic facilities. I believe internist-cardiologists, or even primary cardiologists, if the population base is large enough, should care for these patients, utilizing the latest skills, including appropriate knowledge of electrocardiography, myocardial imaging, echocardiography, and the bedside use of the Swan-Ganz catheter. These techniques are fundamental today to the care of many patients and must be taught in our cardiology training programs. I share, however, Dr. Preston and Dr. Petersdorf's feeling that the number of coronary arteriographers and those knowledgeable in cardiac catheterization is adequate and that each community does not need physicians versed in these areas. It is quite reasonable to regionalize such diagnostic centers together with regionalization of the cardiac surgeons for whom such procedures are a supportive service.

The problems stated in this controversy defy simplistic answers. It seems to me, however, that continual re-examination of our cardiologic health care needs and the relevance of our training programs to these needs is a fundamental responsibility of our academic cardiology centers. We must continually be on our guard that our training programs do not simply create replicas of ourselves.

ELLIOT RAPAPORT, M.D.

Two

Does Exercise Prevent Coronary Artery Disease?

The Role of Exercise in Preventing Coronary Heart Disease

ALBERT OBERMAN, M.D., M.P.H.

Director, Division of Preventive Medicine, The University
of Alabama in Birmingham, Birmingham, Alabama

With few exceptions, population studies of risk factors repeatedly show an inverse association between physical activity and coronary heart disease (CHD). Other evidence indicates that periodic exercise enhances physical capabilities, general well-being, and physiologic adaptations favorable to longevity. Such results led to the widespread assumption that an increasingly sedentary existence increases the vulnerability to CHD. In response, millions of Americans walk, jog, swim, or otherwise exercise, primarily to improve their health.

Others report that available evidence is not at the same level of confidence or magnitude as that concerning major risk factors. Comparisons between conductors and bus drivers, mailmen and postal clerks, and others provided the initial documentation of less CHD among more active workers within specific occupations.[1] However, different kinds of persons seek sedentary tasks in preference to manual labor for many reasons, including those related to health. Job selection, transfer, and retirement are not random processes. The problem of selection bias reaches the extreme in studies of men who were athletes in their youth. It is reasonable to assume that longitudinal studies of former athletes will detect the extent of protection against CHD provided by sustained physical activity. Unfortunately, unique genetic endowments, health attitudes, and other traits distinguishing athletes from non-athletes confound the relationship with CHD. One possible conclusion may be that those who are sick and at high risk of CHD select themselves out of the active group, leading to an artificial correlation between sedentary activities and CHD.

On the other hand, a number of factors severely limit the ability to demonstrate strong associations between physical activity and CHD. Job titles may be grossly misleading as indices of actual duties. Protection from CHD most likely requires vigorous physical effort; yet, energy expenditure has become uniformly low among most workers. Occupational class is a

29

poor surrogate for assessment of vigorous physical activity. Even so, few investigators attempt to evaluate leisure activities to appropriately classify individuals as active or inactive. Substitution variables (caloric intake, obesity, vital capacity, handgrip strength, and so on) have been used as indices of physical activity. The relationship of these variables to physical activity is complex, not necessarily direct, and insures a low-order association with CHD. Little can be expected from rudimentary studies of physical activity based on occupational class or superficial estimates of energy expenditure. An analogous situation would be to attempt to demonstrate an association between cholesterol and CHD by measuring food intake. Such analyses have met with little success despite the well-established relationship between cholesterol and CHD.

The physical activity hypothesis can best be evaluated in a clinical trial; but prospects remain dim for a randomized controlled study to test the role of physical activity in preventing CHD. Implementation requires recruitment of large numbers of men, extensive exercise testing, exercise facilities, assurance of safety, adherence by participants to various training routines, avoidance of crossover from control to training groups or vice versa, and long-term surveillance of the total population. In the absence of definitive data and with the likelihood of such a trial remote, the physician must judge the relative merits of an exercise program for the individual patient.

It is the purpose of this report to demonstrate " . . . that it is not necessary to become either a bus conductor or an athlete in order to improve cardiovascular health, and possibly achieve some protection against coronary heart diseases, merely to heed the wisdom of the ages on the body's need for adequate exercise."[2]

Incidence Studies

As noted in Table 1, not all long-term studies of men initially healthy at entry show a relationship between CHD incidence and occupational class. Although several of the countries participating in the Seven Countries Coronary Disease Study had more favorable CHD rates for the physically active, the overall results for the initial five years of follow-up did not corroborate this relationship. The high rates of CHD in the vigorously active Finns are most frequently cited as contradictory to the physical activity hypothesis. However, these people are at high risk for multiple factors, and the protective effect of activity may not always suffice in this situation. It should be pointed out that Finnish lumberjacks had fewer electrocardiographic abnormalities, even Q waves, than persons in other occupations in the same locale. These findings — unaccounted for by other factors — support, not refute, the importance of physical activity. Employees of the People's Gas Company showed no differential for CHD by occupational class, but of 1329 men followed for 12 years, only 169 were engaged in moderate work and *none* in heavy work. Follow-up after eight years in the Western

Table 1. *Recent Incidence Studies of Factors Related to Coronary Heart Disease (CHD)*

STUDY (PRINCIPAL INVESTIGATOR)	REPORT	COMPARISON GROUPS	RELATIONSHIP BETWEEN PHYSICAL INACTIVITY AND CHD
Western Electric Co. (Paul)	Am J Cardiol 23:303, 1969	Within and between shop workers and office workers	None
Seven Countries (Keys)	Circulation 41:Suppl 1, 1970	Active and sedentary occupations	None overall, but relationship noted in some countries
Evans County (Cassel)	Arch Intern Med 128:920, 1971	Farmers and non-farmers	Positive
Framingham (Kannel)	Cardiol Digest 6:28, 1971	Overall sedentary, moderate, and heavy activity levels	Positive
People's Gas Co. (Stamler)	The Pathogenesis of Atherosclerosis. Baltimore, Williams and Wilkins, 1972, pp. 77–80	Blue-collar and white-collar workers	None
British Civil Servants (Morris)	Lancet 1:333, 1973	Vigorous and non-vigorous leisure activity	Positive
Israeli Kibbutzim (Brunner)	J Chronic Dis 27:217, 1974	Active and inactive workers	Positive
Gotesburg (Tibblin)	Am J Cardiol 35:514, 1975	Sedentary, moderate, and heavy work and leisure activity	None, but apparent trend with leisure time
Longshoremen (Paffenbarger)	N Engl J Med 292:545, 1975	High, medium, and low caloric output at work	Positive
Western Collaborative (Rosenman)	JAMA 233:872, 1975	Regular and non-regular exercise habits	Positive in group aged 50–59 at entry
Harvard Alumni (Paffenbarger)	CVD Epidemiology Newsletter 22:46, 1977	Low and high energy expenditure	Positive
Whitehall Civil Servants (Rose)	Lancet 1:105, 1977	Inactive, moderately active, and active leisure time	Positive in men without ischemic heart disease at entry

Electric Company of Chicago revealed no difference in CHD rates, even though caloric expenditure was shown to differ among small samples of shop workers. In Gotesburg, a trend was noticed between CHD and reduced effort during leisure time, apart from occupational activity. The Western Collaborative group found after 8.9 years of follow-up that men aged 50 to 59 reporting regular exercise habits had less CHD than those with occasional or no avocational activities. With lack of sufficient variability in physical activity, limited depth of study, and dependence on inadequate methodology, these past evaluations of exercise and development of CHD were imprecise and statistically weak.

Among numerous studies unequivocally reporting less CHD for physically active individuals, several deserve detailed consideration. In the classic Framingham Study, 5127 men and women were followed over 16 years to identify precursors of CHD. At the fourth biennial exam, a weighted index of hours spent at physical activity during leisure time and work was calculated for each participant. This index represents the sum of the hours of activity per usual 24-hour day weighted by a factor of 1.0 (basal) to 5.0 (heavy). After 10 years of follow-up, the most sedentary men had an incidence of CHD almost twice that of those most active (Fig. 1).

In the Evans County Study, a gradient was found for CHD, with the highest rates in the most sedentary occupations. A marked difference appeared in the incidence of CHD among white farmers; the most sedentary

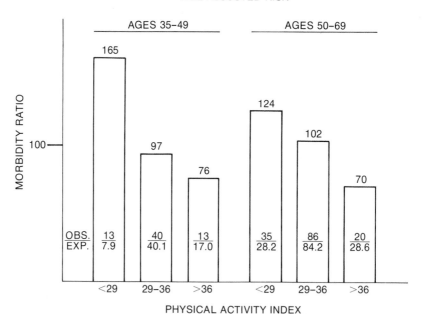

Figure 1.   Risk of coronary heart disease (10 years) according to age and physical activity status for men 35 to 69 at Exam 4: Framingham Study. In each age group, the most sedentary men had approximately twice the coronary disease incidence of the most active. (Data adapted from Kannel WB, Gordon T, Sorlie P, and McNamara PM: Physical activity and coronary vulnerability: The Framingham Study. Cardiol Digest 6:28, 1971.)

farm owners had an incidence of CHD three times the rate of the active sharecroppers. Despite greater saturated fat intake and more hypertension, blacks had less CHD than the less active whites in every group except sharecroppers. Genetic factors are unlikely to account for both the differences between blacks and whites and those between white sharecroppers and farmers. The possibility that men with coronary disease might leave the more physically demanding occupations cannot explain the difference, because the incidence study was based on classification according to occupation seven years before. While it is possible that such differences may be due to characteristics other than physical activity, no such factor has yet been identified to account for these differences. The investigators concluded that sustained physical activity above a certain threshold was protective against CHD.

The Kibbutzim or communal settlements in Israel provided a unique setting in which to study the role of exercise. All inhabitants shared a uniform lifestyle, even eating in a common dining room. The more active, requiring more calories, probably consumed relatively less meat and rich food because of restrictions on these items but not on other foodstuffs. Yet, there were no significant differences in cholesterol values between the groups. Therefore, the setting provided a valuable experimental situation. The sedentary group who spent at least 80 per cent of their work day sitting had two to four times the 15-year incidence of CHD than the more active men in all age brackets. These data, from a population with a single standard of living and free from various types of bias found in other studies, provide strong evidence of the value of physical work, other factors being equal.

Recent studies focus on more appropriate measures of physical activity in order to determine whether or not it is truly a risk factor for CHD. Realizing the commonality of energy expenditure on the job, Morris and coworkers recorded the leisure-time activities of 16,882 male civil servants in the United Kingdom between 1968 and 1970. Investigators relied on the supposition that some of these middle-aged sedentary workers exercised vigorously outside of work and that their habits were sufficiently stable to sample a short period of time, a Friday and Saturday. No activities were categorized during working hours, as the men were almost entirely sedentary during the work day. The investigators identified those men likely to expend peaks of energy output of 7.5 kilocalories or more per minute, equivalent to an oxygen consumption of 1.5 liters per minute (Table 2). Such activities constitute "heavy work" exceeding usual levels of industrial work. Preliminary analyses showed each episode of heavy work must continue for at least 30 minutes, or a total of one hour or more, during the sample period to protect against CHD. Work loads below this threshold did not discriminate for CHD. Only 11 per cent of the men who sustained a coronary event reported this level of peak activity, while 26 per cent of the matched controls did so, a relative risk of approximately one-third. The relative risk was similar for fatal and nonfatal coronary events. If the findings were due to relative inactivity of the men because they were subclinically ill, the advantage would be apparent only for coronary events early in this

Table 2. *Relative Risk of Coronary Heart Disease (CHD) in Civil Servants, 1968–1972, for Various Forms of Vigorous Exercise. The Protective Effect of Exercise is Apparent, Most Notably in the "Vigorous Getting About/or Climbing 500+ Stairs" Group*[1]

FORMS OF VIGOROUS EXERCISE	MEN HAVING A FIRST ATTACK OF CHD N = 214	MATCHED CONTROLS N = 428	RATIO OF OBSERVED TO EXPECTED FREQUENCY
Active recreations	5	15	0.67
Keep fit	3	15	0.40
Heavy physical work	17	73	0.47
Vigorous getting about/or Climbing up 500+ stairs	1	26	0.08
Men doing vigorous exercise°	23	111	0.41
Men not doing vigorous exercise	191	317	1.21

°Three cases and 16 controls did two forms of vigorous exercise; one control did three.

[1]Source: Morris JN, et al.: Vigorous exercise in leisure time and the incidence of coronary heart disease. Lancet *1*:333, 1973.

study. Such was not the case. Furthermore, results are unaltered when men with chest pain at the initial evaluation are excluded from further analyses. Habitual, vigorous exercise protected these middle-aged civil servants against fatal myocardial infarction and other initial clinical manifestations of CHD. There is no other likely explanation. Results are also available from a five-year mortality follow-up for men aged 40 to 64 in the Whitehall study of civil servants. In a sample of those men without evidence of ischemic disease at the outset and reporting little leisure activity in response to a simple question, there was 1.6 times the CHD mortality as those reporting such activity. In this study, the trend was reversed in those men showing manifestations of ischemia at entry into the study.

The most comprehensive evaluation of occupational physical activity to date has been accomplished in a series of San Francisco longshoremen by Paffenbarger and colleagues. This is one of the few studies in which not only heavy physical demands are made on some of the workers, but accurate detailed records of job assignments were kept over a long period of time. Work energy requirements were determined from actual measurement of oxygen consumption on the job. Assignments of these longshoremen were checked annually to account for job transfers and changes in work energy ouput. With extended follow-up for 22 years, the age-adjusted coronary death rates were 26.9, 46.3, and 49.0 per 10,000 work years for those in the high, medium, and low caloric output jobs, respectively (Fig. 2). The least active group differed by approximately 600 and 1000 kilocalories in work-day expenditure from the more active groups. High- and low-energy-output workers were comparable in terms of risk at the outset of the study in 1951. These results connote a protective threshold effect, and the investigators concluded that these repeated periods of high energy

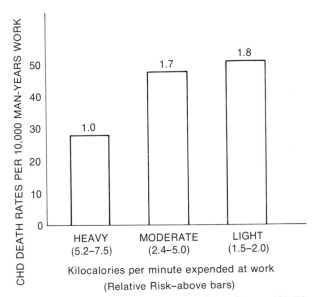

Figure 2. Age-adjusted death rates from coronary heart disease (CHD) among San Francisco longshoremen, 1951–1973, by caloric expenditure at work. This mortality pattern suggests a threshold effort of physical activity above which risk of CHD decreases significantly. (Data adapted from Paffenbarger RS Jr and Hale WE: Work activity and coronary heart mortality. N Engl J Med 292:545, 1975.)

expenditure protected against coronary mortality. Selection of ill workers for transfer to light jobs may produce a gradient with CHD, but it is unlikely to produce the threshold effect noted. The relationship was greatest for sudden unexpected death, a situation unlikely to be preceded by a job transfer because of symptoms. Deaths were charged against a job held six months earlier to avoid bias from transfers. Even excluding those men with job transfers does not alter the relationship, implying that any change of occupation for health reasons could not be of major importance in these analyses. Cohort analyses of these data for fatal heart attack support earlier findings and indicate low energy output, heavy smoking, and high blood pressure in combination increase the risk of fatal heart attack by as much as twentyfold. The association between energy expenditure and CHD held for all ages throughout the 22 years of the study, and the strength of the association, was greater than that for other personal characteristics studied. It is concluded that the strong inverse association between work and energy level of fatal heart attack demonstrated a genuine protective influence.

In a parallel study, Paffenbarger and coworkers surveyed the habitual energy output, mainly outside of work, for over 36,000 Harvard alumni to determine the risk of heart attack after six to ten years of follow-up. Multivariate estimates of heart attack risks were adjusted for age, systolic blood pressure, cigarette smoking, history of hypertension, obesity, and parental history of heart attack. Alumni were classified by hours per week of sports activities, stairs climbed, and blocks walked, expressed as kilocalories per week. When the group is divided on the basis of 2000 or more kilocalories per week in energy expenditure, the relative risk for the more sedentary group was significantly greater, 1.5 times for nonfatal CHD and 1.9 times for fatal CHD.

Possible Mechanisms for Prevention

Long-term exercise may prevent CHD through multiple postulated mechanisms. The possibilities can be grouped into (1) factors that retard atherosclerosis and (2) factors that protect against clinical manifestations of CHD.

FACTORS THAT RETARD ATHEROSCLEROSIS

Physical activity may either directly influence various factors predisposing to CHD or serve as an adjunct to the management of others.[3] Although a number of reports indicate a decrease in cholesterol with increased physical activity, most studies fail to demonstrate a significant lowering independent of dietary changes and weight reduction. However, the distribution of total cholesterol among plasma lipoproteins may shift with strenuous exercise. The ratio of cholesterol in high-density compared to low-density lipoprotein is greater after increased physical activity. This finding may prove to be an important consideration because of the well-documented *inverse* correlation between high-density lipoproteins and CHD and may also explain in part the discrepancies in the literature regarding the effect of exercise on cholesterol. With rare exception, triglycerides and plasma-free fatty acid levels fall in response to continuous physical activity, though physical activity must be continued or the triglycerides will revert to baseline values. There is preferential utilization of lipids for fuel in trained individuals. Glucose metabolism is altered as well. Longstanding data indicate exercise improves glucose tolerance. Also, training can induce a marked decrease in insulin values independent of changes in blood glucose values.

Although obesity is not a major risk factor, weight reduction can lead to reduced cholesterol and blood pressure and improved glucose tolerance, resulting in a lowered risk for CHD. For many individuals, obesity results from inactivity rather than excessive food intake. Contrary to widespread impressions, moderate levels of physical activity may suppress rather than enhance appetite. Long-term exercise and consequent caloric expenditures can be a valuable adjunct to a weight control program. Even in those showing no weight change, there is favorable alteration in body composition as fat tends to diminish and lean body mass to increase with chronic exercise.

Reports vary concerning the efficacy of habitual activity in lowering systolic and diastolic blood pressure. Accumulated data indicate that elevated systolic and diastolic blood pressure may be reduced, but these data require further corroboration. It is difficult to interpret the blood pressure studies because of many confounding variables and lack of controlled, blinded observations. Nevertheless, a reduction in heart rate and blood pressure at submaximal work loads remains one of the most tangible effects of a training program. It is not unreasonable to infer that trained persons demonstrate a similar lessened blood pressure response to stress during daily activities. Higher heart rates, inevitably lowered with long-term training, have been considered a risk factor for CHD, though the mechanism and, consequently, the value of intervention are unclear.

Published data on cessation of cigarette smoking in conjunction with a training program suggest potentiation, but are not conclusive. It is certainly conceivable that simultaneous modification of several health-related factors provides reinforcement and may be more powerful than the more traditional approach of attempting one behavioral change at a time.

Probably the least understood but most important and universal benefits of a regular exercise program are the associated behavioral changes. Innumerable reports confirm that persons in physical activity programs develop a sense of well-being, increased tolerance to anxiety and various psychologic stresses, and an improved self-image. These acquired characteristics may lessen the propensity toward CHD or strengthen other health habits, such as cessation of smoking, modification of diet, and general health behavior.

FACTORS THAT PROTECT AGAINST CLINICAL MANIFESTATION OF CHD

Habitual stimulation by exercise work loads leads to adaptive improvement in the functional capacity of multiple organ systems. Those adaptations induced by physical activity generally at levels requiring 65 per cent or more of maximal oxygen uptake constitute the physical training effect. The response is governed by age, sex, previous fitness, health status, and genetic traits, among other variables. Optimal physiologic function can only be achieved by periodic overload of the musculoskeletal, the nervous, and the cardiovascular systems. Such training enables an individual to respond to imposed work loads without taxing the circulation and possibly compromising myocardial oxygen needs. In trained individuals, the need for myocardial oxygen, estimated by heart rate–systolic blood pressure products, decreases at submaximal work loads.

The potential for vigorous exercise depends on the upper limits of the oxygen transport system, determined primarily by the cardiovascular system. Major cardiovascular adaptations include increased stroke volume and greater arteriovenous oxygen differences. Other changes include increased heart size and possibly increased total hemoglobin, blood volume, and oxygen delivery through a decrease in oxyhemoglobin affinity. Studies in rats subjected to moderate training programs demonstrate that physical training enhances myocardial contractility and cardiac work capacity. Increased contractile responses and faster relaxation phases in conditioned rats suggest modification of excitation-contraction coupling and relaxation.[4] Superior performance of skeletal muscles after training results from enlargement of existing muscle fibers, enhanced blood flow per unit mass of muscle, higher muscle myoglobin, and local adaptive changes in the capacity for aerobic metabolism.

Another potentially valuable benefit of vigorous exertion is the increase in myocardial vascularity. Improved myocardial perfusion results from the increment in the size and extent of the coronary vasculature, as well as increased capillary density in the myocardium after controlled exercise, especially in younger animals. Isolated pathologic studies support the experimental findings of increased coronary artery size with physical activity but require further substantiation. Conditioning also confers partial resistance to myocardial hypoxia, apparently due to improved efficiency and energy utilization. Probably the most cited animal work is that demonstrating retrograde or collateral flow potentiated by exercise after surgical constriction of the coronary arteries. In some studies, without prior narrowing of the circumflex artery, acute ligation did not significantly alter the maximum rate of retrograde flow of exercised dogs, but total retrograde flow appeared to increase. Even with cessation of exercise, the capillary-to-fiber ratio and cross-sectional areas of collateral arteries may remain increased in hearts of previously conditioned rats.[4] Human studies of collateral circulation and physical activity have proved disappointing. Arteriographic techniques may not be sensitive enough to reflect these changes, but new methods of determining myocardial perfusion should resolve this problem.

Indirect evidence for improved cardiovascular function include reversion of aberrant ballistocardiographic wave forms and electrocardiographic ST segments toward "normal" after regular exercise. The frequency of ectopic ventricular activity, supposedly a harbinger of sudden death, has been shown to be reduced in individuals who participate in a regular exercise program. This finding may be of therapeutic importance to those individuals without overt cardiovascular disease for whom physicians are reluctant to use long-term anti-arrhythmic agents to control ectopic ventricular beats. It is unlikely that these clinical findings can be explained by avoidance of activity for health reasons related to ischemic disease.

Other mechanisms by which physical activity may reduce the occurrence of CHD include alterations in platelet adhesiveness, fibrinolysis, thyroid hormone metabolism, and a lessened adrenergic response to stress, with decreased catecholamine production in trained individuals.[3]

Possible Adverse Effects

As with any therapeutic intervention, there are likely to be associated sequelae, not necessarily beneficial. The risk of musculoskeletal disability and precipitation of myocardial infarction or sudden death as a direct result of physical exertion cannot be accurately estimated from available data. Proper advice on beginning a training program, especially for the middle-aged man who has not exercised, can circumvent many of the minor side effects. The serious danger of unfit persons undertaking prolonged strenuous exercise in adverse environments cannot be overemphasized. Age, general risk of CHD, extent of coronary atherosclerosis, and method of physical exertion undoubtedly determine the likelihood of such an occurrence. However, data from exercise testing and supervised exercise programs even of relatively high intensity indicate a low order of risks for serious cardiovascular morbidity and mortality.

Physical training can induce physiologic changes generally thought associated with disease states. At one time it was believed that the resulting "athlete's heart" was deleterious. However, cardiac hypertrophy is a natural consequence of long-term training, and hemodynamic studies of persons with such hypertrophy reveal no compromise of cardiovascular function. Athletic training has been associated with various electrocardiographic alterations — prolonged PR interval, early repolarization, high voltage, and conduction and rhythm disturbances. There is no indication that any of these changes alter one's health unfavorably, though in different context some of these may be risk indicators for CHD in the population.

Comments

Data from a variety of sources give reasonably consistent support for an association between the lack of vigorous physical activity and the subsequent development of CHD. There is some question whether the protection comes from physical activity or from coincidentally associated differences between active and sedentary persons. Recent incidence studies of CHD among longshoremen, Harvard alumni, British civil servants, workers at the Israeli Kibbutzim, and participants in the Evans County and Framingham Studies suggest it is the physical activity that is responsible.

Application of better methods for estimating energy expenditure for long periods of time and in multiple environments undoubtedly will strengthen such data. Objective assessment of energy expenditure at work and at leisure is within the realm of possibility. Evaluation of cardiovascular fitness using the physiologic response to exercise and estimates of functional adaptation to physical activity can provide additional data. Use of such measurements in populations with a broad range of physical activity will take us further toward understanding the association between habitual physical activity and the reduced risk of coronary disease. As with any risk factor, the association implies, but does not guarantee, that intervention or assumption of physical activity can reduce the risk of CHD. Obviously, certain kinds of persons are more likely to be energetic during their leisure time. This is not to say that large numbers of inactive individuals cannot be convinced to exercise. They can. Witness the current popularity of exercise.

But, will such individuals benefit? It appears that there is an approximately twofold relative risk for inactive men compared to their more vigorous peers with regard to the occurrence of CHD. Although there are multiple possibilities, the mechanism whereby physical activity protects against CHD is uncertain. Despite the inconsistent findings between habitual activity and major risk factors for CHD, exercise undoubtedly modifies some risk factors to more optimal levels. Chronic exercise lowers triglycerides, raises the alpha-to-beta cholesterol ratio in lipoproteins, and can be used to advantage in weight control programs. Either directly or indirectly through weight changes, physical activity may lower total cholesterol levels and blood pressure. Most individuals at high risk for CHD are so because of several risk factors rather than a single extremely abnormal risk factor. Such persons would benefit most from a physical activity program. Yet, these particular benefits of exercise probably do not represent the main effect of vigorous exercise on the incidence of CHD. Those large-scale studies that have shown a reduced risk for the physically active inevitably have demonstrated that exercise operates independently of the major risk factors.

Multiple studies now document a threshold effect for physical activity. The relationship between energy expenditure and CHD appears to be curvilinear. Implicit in this concept is that the intensity of exercise must be enough to stress the cardiorespiratory system. Physiologic adaptations to exercise are more likely to occur from bouts of high energy outputs. This presence of a threshold and lack of a linear gradient suggest the protective mechanism results from a direct effect on the cardiovascular system. Heightened myocardial performance, alterations in myocardial perfusion, reduced myocardial oxygen, or some combination of these and other possible mechanisms might be responsible for the favorable CHD rates. Men in middle age share these benefits of exercise, although experimental data indicate adaptations to exercise may be facilitated at younger ages. In addition to age, training effects are a function of intensity, duration, and frequency of exercise, as well as the prior level of fitness. Training effects require heart rate levels at 70 per cent to 85 per cent of the maximum attainable. It is desirable to achieve such levels in not less than 30 minutes of exercise at least three times per week. If the current data are accurate, activities at the level of six to seven METS (digging, a fast walk, hand lawn mowing, and so on), representing a target heart rate of approximately 130 to 150 beats per minute for the middle-aged man, would suffice. Though useful for weight loss, modification of risk factors, and musculoskeletal fitness, less strenuous levels of exercise probably do not confer significant levels of protection against CHD in the general population.

It is altogether too easy to conclude that more evidence is needed, but the physician must advise his patients now. There is probably much to be gained and little to be lost from a rational exercise program. Excellent guidelines are available to physicians for advising patients on exercise.[5]

Conclusion

Generally, population studies utilizing adequate measures of energy expenditure demonstrate that physical activity protects against CHD. The possibility of a primary CHD prevention trial of exercise is remote. There are those who insist on such a trial before recommending exercise. If the same standards were applied to other therapeutic modalities, many with greater toxic effects, much of our so-called "therapeutic armamentarium" would have to be discarded.

A consensus is growing that mild, prolonged exercise does not suffice for the healthy individual. Prevention demands more strenuous exertion with peaks of energy output to stress the cardiorespiratory system. This effort beyond a threshold supports a mechanism of protection through a direct effect on the cardiovascular system. Noncompetitive, graduated energy expenditure at levels sufficient for training effects can be accomplished at little risk to the general population, with appropriate safeguards. Patients should be advised as to the appropriate exercise for preventing heart attacks. The sum of evidence from experimental, clinical, and population studies decisively indicates that vigorous physical activity protects against CHD. Sufficient rationale and documentation now exist for action.

I gratefully acknowledge the helpful comments of Drs. John O. Holloszy and Charles Gilbert and Mr. Steven D. Spivey.

References

1. Froelicher VF, and Oberman A: Analysis of epidemiologic studies of physical inactivity as risk factors for coronary artery disease. Prog Cardiovasc Dis 15:41, 1972.
2. Morris JN: Physical inactivity and coronary heart disease. Acta Cardiol (Suppl) 20:95, 1974.
3. Fox SM, Naughton JP, and Gorman PA: Physical activity and cardiovascular health. Mod Concepts Cardiovasc Dis 41:17, 1972.
4. Scheuer J, and Tipton CM: Cardiovascular adaptations to physical training. Ann Rev Physiol 39:221, 1977.
5. The Committee on Exercise: Exercise Testing and Training of Apparently Healthy Individuals: A Handbook for Physicians. New York, American Heart Association, 1972.

Exercise and the Prevention of Coronary Artery Disease: The Evidence Is Inconclusive

OGLESBY PAUL, M.D.

Professor of Medicine, Harvard Medical School, Boston, Massachusetts; Physician, Peter Bent Brigham Hospital, Boston, Massachusetts

Anyone who preaches against exercise is clearly speaking against a cherished, albeit relatively recent, faith of the American public. What could be more healthful than the encouragement of walking, golf, tennis, swimming, and so on to provide clear heads, good hearts, strong muscles, and trim waistlines. It is not my purpose to decry exercise. I also agree on the pleasurable nature of physical activity, on its value in providing a desirable mental change of pace, on its contribution to weight control, and on its usefulness to our musculoskeletal system. I advise most of my patients with heart disease to exercise regularly, as I consider that this promotes a sense of well-being and self-confidence, and when angina is present, it may be useful in the control of this symptom.

The purpose of this brief essay is quite different, namely, to view some of the evidence relating to the purported benefits of physical activity in relation to *coronary artery disease* (not the normal heart) and to point out that the evidence is not all convincing. We as physicians must not look only for researches supporting current popular beliefs; we must also at least be informed as to the limitations of the data behind such beliefs, since such limitations periodically lead to new emphases in health practices. After all, it was not very long ago that physicians, school health officials, and nutritionists were vigorously promoting a diet containing eggs, whole milk, and butter — not egg substitutes, skimmed milk, and margarines. It was only a few years ago that leading cardiologists advised many weeks and months of rest and very limited exercise after any type of acute coronary event. I recall very clearly that I was interrogated for my Massachusetts State medical licensure after World War II by one of the greatest American internists, who was horrified that I would not advise a minimum of six weeks of strict bed rest after myocardial infarction.

One may inquire first as to the mechanisms by which exercise may prevent or minimize coronary atherosclerosis and its complications. Surely, one mechanism might be the stimulation of coronary collateral development. However, our information in this area is far from satisfactory. In a recent comprehensive, authoritative review of coronary collateral development, Gregg[1] wrote: "Very little is known about the vascular changes, their time course, and the mechanisms responsible for the early and delayed development of the protective coronary circulation." He also observed: "Unfortunately, there is no experimental evidence that physical exertion improves the collateral circulation of the normal heart" and indicated that the work of Eckstein[2] on dogs 20 years ago was "the only experimental evidence that exercise as a postcoronary insufficiency procedure enhances the coronary collateral procedure." Animal investigations by Burt and Jackson[3] and by Stevenson et al.[4] did not provide support for the concept that continued exercise stimulated coronary collateral growth or increased coronary artery size. Dehn and Mullins[5] also recently stated:

Very little evidence exists of a significant change in the coronary vasculature (development of collaterals or an expanded cross-sectional area) as a result of exercise, except in selected patients. Improvement — if any — in coronary blood flow at a given work load appears to be more likely related to the increased perfusion time associated with reduced submaximal heart rates rather than any change in coronary anatomy.

This comment would appear to be consistent with the report of Helfant, Vokonas, and Gorlin,[6] which failed to find evidence in 119 patients studied by coronary arteriography of an association between the magnitude of coronary collateral development and a simple questionnaire regarding level of physical exercise.

Is there then a persuasive argument that if the collateral circulation is not definitely better developed by physical exercise, that in any case coronary atherosclerosis as such is favorably modified? Unfortunately, here, too, one must agree with a further statement of Dehn and Mullins[5] that "insufficient data are available to pass judgment" on the relation between physical exercise and the primary prevention of atherosclerotic heart disease. This question was reviewed by the Report by the National Heart and Lung Institute Task Force on Arteriosclerosis,[7] which assessed postmortem studies and concluded on the basis of the then available studies that "they agree on one fundamental point, that there is no major difference in the degree of coronary arteriosclerosis in sedentary as compared to physically active individuals." Rose[8] has also reviewed the evidence and has stated that "physical activity probably does not affect atherosclerosis," and Paul,[9] in a similar survey, reached the same conclusion.

It might be argued that somehow risk factors associated with premature coronary artery degeneration are favorably modified by physical activity. This has not in general received much support in the past, and Kannel[10] has commented that "physical activity has not been shown to be a major determinant of the chief contributors to accelerated atherogenesis." There would appear to be no question that individuals who are engaged in physical fitness programs tend to be health-conscious and thus tend to smoke less or not at all as compared with persons not engaged in such undertakings. They may also be less obese. As regards cigarette smoking as such, it has not been shown that it becomes an innocuous habit if counterbalanced by regular physical exertion, although Paffenbarger[11] has concluded that its deleterious influence is blunted by the physically active employment of working as a longshoreman as contrasted with sedentary employment. However, he noted that cigarette smoking far outranked sedentary work as a risk factor. It has not been consistently observed that regular exercise as such effectively lowers the blood pressure in hypertensive persons or prevents the development of hypertension, although if it contributes to weight loss such might be the case. Taylor,[12] in a broad international survey, did not find that blood pressure and physical activity levels were significantly correlated. Hickey et al.[13] and also Leren et al.[14] reported that heavy leisure physical activity appeared to be associated with lower blood pressures than were encountered among those with lesser leisure physical activity, but the former also reported less overweight subjects in his active group. Furthermore, in the study of Leren et al.,[14] men with the greatest physical activity at work actually had higher blood pressures than those in more sedentary occupations. The same study also found higher serum cholesterol levels among those in physically active employment than in those in less active work, although the reverse was true if leisure physical activity only was considered. Indeed, the whole matter of lipid levels and exercise is characterized by highly conflicting reports. Salzman et al.[15] studied a group of Cleveland businessmen, made comparisons with data from Finland, and concluded that "diet, rather than the level of habitual physical activity, predominantly determines the serum cholesterol level." Hickey et al.[13] described lower serum cholesterol levels among men with heavy leisure physical activity but not with heavy work physical activity. Rose[8] could not ascertain any relation of serum cholesterol values to duration of walking to work. Mann[16] found very minimal (three per cent) improvement in serum cholesterol, and the blood pressure changes strongly suggested only a regression toward the mean in men participating in a supervised exercise program. Indeed, this whole area of purported favorable influence of degree of physical activity on risk factors (cigarette smoking, elevated blood lipids, and elevated blood pressure) is far from a simple negative correlation.

The epidemiological reports of population groups and the prevalence of heart attacks, sudden death, and total coronary mortality in relation to physical exercise at work and/or leisure are numerous. The tendency is to believe that they overwhelmingly support the role of physical activity in minimizing coronary attack rates. Such is not the case, although there are indeed excellent studies[17, 18] reaching that conclusion. There are reports that fail to demonstrate any protective effect. Elmfeldt et al.[19] described 299 men who had survived their first myocardial infarction and compared them to a control group; physical activity at work was not different in the two groups, although the infarct cases reported less leisure physical activity. Paul[9] did not encounter significant differences in rates for angina pectoris, myocardial infarction, or coronary deaths in relation to physical effort on the job among 1718 industrial workers followed for eight years. Rosenman et al.,[20] in a prospective study of over 3000 men followed for eight and one-half years, stated that the development of clinical coronary heart disease was not significantly related to the history of physical activity at work or to exercise habits. The Report by the National Heart and Lung Institute Task Force on Arteriosclerosis[21] listed 12 epidemiological studies confirming the presence of physical inactivity as a risk factor for coronary artery disease and 11 studies failing to confirm this. Haskell,[22] in a critique of this problem, commented:

> A closer look at the physical activity classifications in several studies reveals that the greatest difference in coronary heart disease frequency or severity between groups with different activity levels occurs between groups classified as sedentary and those classified as only slightly more active; . . . It is surprising how little physical activity at a low intensity a sedentary individual would have to perform in order to be placed in the more favorable intermediate group, in some cases no more than about 100 calories per day.

However, Morris et al.[17] found no advantage of lighter exercise and no apparent protective effect related to overall activity; rather, vigorous leisure-time exercise was needed to demonstrate a beneficial influence on coronary rates.

It is beyond the scope of this review to enumerate all the pros and cons on the exercise issue. There is little doubt that much may be said in favor of regular physical activity as being of value in total physical fitness and in relation to cardiovascular health in particular. There is also little doubt that there are those with severe coronary heart disease for whom any strenuous exercise is not merely unwise, but dangerous. It is unfortunate that, as yet, the dimensions of the value of physical activity in preventing or postponing coronary events is unclear. Does activity on the job play a role? Or must it be only leisure-time exercise? Should it be mild or moderate, or must it be vigorous to be effective? Is it possible to dissociate adequately the possibility that the person who indulges in regular moderate or vigorous exercise does so because he has indeed good coronary arteries to start with, whereas the person who already has some coronary atherosclerosis with a marginal coronary flow under unusual stress finds exercise difficult and unpleasant and consciously or unconsciously avoids it? Can we clearly identify the tendency of those who like to exercise in leisure time to pay more attention to good health habits, such as avoidance of overweight and cigarette smoking? Has anyone examined the benefits of non-physically active or mildly active recreation, such as regularly playing a piano or violin, playing chess, and so on?

These are some of the questions that it will be desirable to answer with time. It is to be hoped that eventually, an exercise prescription may be confidently written, justified by a greatly expanded and solid base of scientific knowledge.

Summary

There is much to recommend regular physical activity as one component in a healthful way of life. In relation specifically to the prevention of coronary heart disease, there is need for a better understanding of mechanisms, magnitude of protection, and form of exercise required for a beneficial effect. As yet, the evidence for promotion of coronary collateral development, for a lessening of coronary atherosclerosis, or for a modification of other risk factors as a result of physical exercise is far from impressive. Further research is needed, although many excellent studies have been reported.

References

1. Gregg DE: The natural history of coronary collateral development. Circ Res 35:335–344, 1974.
2. Eckstein RW: Effect of exercise and coronary artery narrowing on coronary collateral circulation. Circ Res 5:230–235, 1957.
3. Burt JJ, and Jackson R: The effects of physical exercise on the coronary collateral circulation of dogs. J Sports Med Phys Fitness 5:203–206, 1965.
4. Stevenson JAF, Feleki V, Rechnitzer P, and Beaton JR: Effect of exercise on coronary tree size in the rat. Circ Res 15:265–269, 1964.
5. Dehn MM, and Mullins CB: Physiological effects and importance of exercise in patients with coronary artery disease. Cardiovasc Med 2:365–387, 1977.
6. Helfant RH, Vokonas PS, and Gorlin R: Functional importance of the human coronary collateral circulation. N Engl J Med 284:1277–1281, 1971.
7. Arteriosclerosis. A Report by the National Heart and Lung Institute Task Force on Arteriosclerosis. DHEW Publication No. (NIH) 72-219, Volume II, 1971 (June), p 111.
8. Rose G: Physical activity and coronary heart disease. Proc R Soc Med 62:1183–1187, 1969.
9. Paul O: Physical activity and coronary heart disease. Am J Cardiol 23:303–306, 1969.
10. Kannel WB: Physical exercise and lethal atherosclerotic disease (editorial). N Engl J Med 282:1153–1154, 1970.
11. Paffenbarger RS, Laughlin ME, Gima AS, and Black RA: Work activity of longshoremen as related to death from coronary heart disease and stroke. N Engl J Med 282:1109–1114, 1970.
12. Taylor HL, Blackburn H, Brozek J, Parlin RW, and Puchner T: Railroad employees in the United States. Acta Med Scand (Suppl) 460:55–115, 1967.
13. Hickey N, Mulcahy R, Bourke GJ, Graham I, and Wilson-Davis K: Study of coronary risk factors related to physical activity in 15,171 men. Br Med J 3:507–509, 1975.
14. Leren O, Askevold E-M, Ross OP, Frølili A, et al: The Oslo Study. Cardiovascular disease in middle-aged and young Oslo men. Acta Med Scand (Suppl) 588:1–38, 1975.
15. Salzman SH, Hellerstein HK, Feil GH, and Marik S: Serum cholesterol and capacity for physical work of middle aged sedentary males. Lancet 1:1348–1351, 1967.
16. Mann GV, Garrett HL, Farhi A, Murray H, et al: Exercise to prevent coronary heart disease. Am J Med 46:12–27, 1969.
17. Morris JN, Chave SPW, Adam C, Sirey C, et al: Vigorous exercise in leisure-time and the incidence of coronary heart disease. Lancet 1:333–339, 1973.
18. Paffenbarger RS Jr, and Hale WE: Work activity and coronary heart mortality. N Engl J Med 292:545–550, 1975.
19. Elmfeldt D, Wilhelmsson C, Verdin A, Tibblin G, and Wilhelmsen L: Characteristics of representative male survivors of myocardial infarction compared with representative population samples. Acta Med Scand 199:387–398, 1976.
20. Rosenman RH, Brand RJ, Jenkins CD, Friedman M, Straus R, and Wurm M: Coronary heart disease in the Western Collaborative Group Study. JAMA 233:875–877, 1975.
21. Arteriosclerosis. A Report by the National Heart and Lung Institute Task Force on Arteriosclerosis. DHEW Publication No. (NIH) 72-219, Volume II, 1971 (June), p 111.
22. Haskell WL: Physical activity and the prevention of coronary heart disease: What type exercise might be effective. J SC Med Assoc 65:41–45, 1969.

Comment

This controversy has implications for all of us. To what extent can one decrease the likelihood of developing coronary heart disease through a consistent exercise program? As a result of the attention focused on the benefits of bicycle riding by Dr. Paul D. White many years ago, the American public has become increasingly engaged in pursuing various forms of exercise such as jogging, bicycling, marathon running, and so on. The rationale claimed for these programs by exercise enthusiasts is that they decrease the likelihood that one will subsequently suffer from coronary heart disease.

Dr. Paul presents evidence from both pathological and epidemiological studies that fail to confirm the thesis that exercise protects against the subsequent development of coronary heart disease. Dr. Oberman presents the results of studies that suggest otherwise. Thus, the data are controversial and conflicting, and as a result, the protective value of exercise today remains undefined. Furthermore, it is unlikely that any definitive answers will be forthcoming in the near future, since the type of prospective study that is required would be so expensive and difficult to perform that it is unlikely to be done.

Despite the statements above, several points emerge. First, there is no evidence that exercise among the general public without coronary heart disease is seriously detrimental to health. Although certain musculoskeletal problems have surfaced due to jogging programs, these have not been of life-threatening or serious consequence. Second, it is also clear that those who engage in repetitive exercise enjoy psychological benefits as well as improved physical conditioning. Thus, it appears to be prudent advice to recommend exercise to the general public as part of a better, healthful way of life. All of us should be engaging in those kinds of exercise that we enjoy. I do not believe it is appropriate to suggest to someone that he should jog daily when, in fact, such effort is looked upon by him with dread and foreboding. On the other hand, a person should be encouraged to do the kinds of activities and sports that give him pleasure, help him relax and forget the mental stresses of daily life, and improve his physical conditioning. If physical activity such as jogging or marathon running are greatly enjoyed by an individual, all the better. But it would not appear justified at this point in time for us to coerce the public into such a program based upon the assertion that participation in such a program will reduce the likelihood of subsequent coronary heart disease.

ELLIOT RAPAPORT, M.D.

47

Three

Should Low-Cholesterol, Low–Saturated-Fat Diets Be Routinely Started in Childhood to Prevent Future Coronary Heart Disease?

THE CASE FOR ROUTINE PRIMARY PREVENTION OF ATHEROSCLEROTIC DISEASES IN CHILDREN
Forrest H. Adams, M.D.

LOW-CHOLESTEROL, LOW–SATURATED-FAT DIETS SHOULD *Not* BE ROUTINELY STARTED IN CHILDHOOD TO PREVENT FUTURE CORONARY HEART DISEASE
Sheila Mitchell, M.D.

COMMENT

The Case for Routine Primary Prevention of Atherosclerotic Diseases in Children

FORREST H. ADAMS, M.D.

Professor of Pediatrics (Cardiology), Emeritus, UCLA School of Medicine, Los Angeles, California

I believe prophylaxis against adult coronary artery disease, atherosclerosis, stroke, and hypertension should be started routinely in childhood because it is a *reasonable objective* based upon considerable strong evidence. In such a prophylactic program, emphasis should be placed upon

1. Eating healthy, nutritious foods (the prudent diet).
2. Maintenance of proper weight for height.
3. Refraining from smoking cigarettes.
4. Maintenance of systolic blood pressure below 110 mmHg.
5. Development of good, regular leisure-time activities.

Since the etiology of adult coronary heart disease is likely multifactorial, prevention also needs to be multifaceted. Such a concept is not peculiar to this condition, but exists as well for many other diseases, such as rheumatic fever, tuberculosis, and congenital heart disease. At this time, our information and knowledge do not permit us to assign a specific weight to *the role of diet* in the etiology of adult cardiovascular disease; however, research indicates that it is an important contributor along with the other factors mentioned.

In almost all areas of clinical medicine, physicians possess incomplete knowledge regarding the etiology and/or proper treatment of disease. Furthermore, for any particular issue, one can always find striking differences of opinion among so-called experts in the field. These statements are true for most forms of cancer, for hypertension, for collagen diseases, for certain endocrine diseases, and for many congenital defects, including congenital heart disease.

Thus, physicians have only partial knowledge and partial solutions to most medical problems. This, however, does not prevent doctors from prac-

51

ticing medicine with the expectation of giving relief of pain and suffering, of ameliorating signs and symptoms, and of preventing diseases from occurring when the etiology is known. The etiology and therefore the prevention of coronary heart disease definitely belong in the category of incomplete knowledge. Some facts are known, however, that do not require further substantiation.

Known Points About Coronary Heart Disease

PREVALENCE OF ATHEROSCLEROSIS IN THE UNITED STATES

All agree about the magnitude of the problems created by atherosclerosis in the United States. Atherosclerosis and two closely related problems, stroke and hypertension, have been the major causes of disability and death for several decades.[1] It would appear also that atherosclerosis is not as common a cause of disability and/or death in certain countries and regions of the world, such as Japan, France, Sweden, Italy, Switzerland, the Netherlands, Norway, Yugoslavia, and Greece.[1]

CORONARY RISK FACTORS

The concept of coronary risk factors has been derived from a number of population studies, including those from Framingham[2] and Tecumseh.[3] These factors, singly or in combination, have been found to be predictive of the development of coronary heart disease. Although the presence of a particular factor does not imply that it is a causal agent, its presence does alter the probability of coronary disease.

From the populations studied,[2, 3] three major risk factors were found: hypercholesterolemia, smoking, and hypertension. Other risk factors identified were obesity, diabetes mellitus, some psychological factors, a family history of coronary heart disease, and physical inactivity. In combination, these factors were cumulative, adding to the risk of coronary heart disease. Furthermore, there was no evidence of a critical level of serum cholesterol, which separates high-risk individuals from low-risk individuals. Populations in countries with a high intake of saturated fat and high serum cholesterol levels had more severe atherosclerotic lesions than did populations in countries with low saturated-fat intake and low serum cholesterol levels.[1]

PREMATURE ATHEROSCLEROSIS IN FAMILIAL HYPERLIPIDEMIA

It has been known for a number of years that some families have a premature form of atherosclerosis and coronary heart disease, with associated high levels of cholesterol and other lipids in the blood. The adults are known to die at relatively young ages, and in rare instances, their offspring have died of heart disease during adolescence. Sophisticated genetic and biochemical studies have been performed only recently on such families.

Goldstein et al.[4] have described five distinct lipid disorders in families of patients with coronary heart disease. Three of these — familial hypercholesterolemia, familial hypertriglyceridemia, and familial combined hyperlipidemia — appeared to represent dominant expression of three different autosomal genes, occurring in about 20 per cent of survivors below 60 years of age. Two other disorders — polygenic hypercholesterolemia and sporadic hypertriglyceridemia — affected about six per cent of survivors.

The homozygous form of familial hypercholesterolemia is characterized by profound elevations of serum cholesterol beginning in infancy, the appearance of tendon and tuberous xanthoma in infancy or childhood, and rapidly progressive atherosclerotic coronary heart disease with death by the third decade. In the heterozygous state, the hypercholesterolemia can also be identified in infancy,[5] but the other clinical manifestations usually do not appear until the third to the fifth decades.

Familial combined hyperlipidemia was the most common form of hyperlipidemia found in the families of subjects with myocardial infarction.[4] Affected family members have elevated levels of both cholesterol and triglycerides; however, it usually does not cause difficulty until the fourth or fifth decade, when coronary artery disease is the most common associated disorder.

CORONARY ARTERY DISEASE IN U.S. SOLDIERS

Although the symptoms of atherosclerosis seldom occur in children, there are indications that the origins of adult atherosclerosis have their beginnings during childhood. The evidence is suggested from the autopsy studies performed on young soldiers killed in the Korean and Viet Nam wars.[6-8] Even though the average age of the casualties studied in Korea was only 22 years, gross coronary atherosclerosis was seen in 77 per cent of these young men who had no known clinical evidence of coronary disease (Table 1).

PRODUCTION OF ATHEROSCLEROSIS IN ANIMAL MODELS

Many animal studies have been reported in the past suggesting the relationship of cholesterol intake in the diet to serum cholesterol and to the

Table 1. *Autopsy Findings in U.S. Soldiers Killed in Korean War**

Number examined	300
Average age	22
Age range	18–48
Gross arteriosclerosis in	77%

*Modified from Enos WF, Holmes RH, and Beyer J: Coronary disease among United States soldiers killed in action in Korea. JAMA 152:1090, 1953.

development of atherosclerosis. A recent study in monkeys[9] seems to me to be the most convincing. In a well-controlled study, monkeys fed increased amounts of cholesterol and saturated fat in their diet for six months developed hypercholesterolemia and mild atherosclerosis of the major coronary arteries; the small coronary branches were not involved. In contrast, the coarcted, hypertensive monkeys fed the same atherogenic diet for the same length of time developed severe coronary atherosclerosis that involved not only the major coronary arteries, but the small ones as well. Isolated hypertension alone did not produce atherosclerosis in the monkeys.

Thus, in animal models, the role of a high-cholesterol, high-fat diet seems to be well established. Alteration of the diet toward a low cholesterol and low fat intake seemed to result in a reduction of the atherosclerotic process.[9]

DIETARY REDUCTION OF SERUM CHOLESTEROL

If one assumes that in some individuals an increased amount of cholesterol and saturated fat consumed in the diet can affect the serum cholesterol in an adverse way, the question still remains: Is it possible to reverse the process, particularly in healthy, nonhospitalized children? A recent study[10] of 144 adolescent males, ages 12 to 18, indicates that the introduction of a modified diet (low in cholesterol and saturated fat) will promptly result

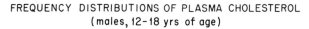

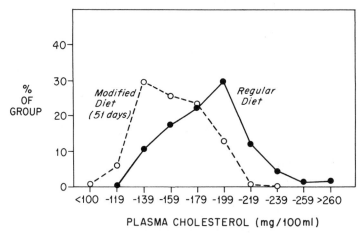

modified from Store et al 1973

Figure 1. Distribution of cholesterol values in 144 adolescent healthy males on a regular diet and then after 51 days on a modified, low-cholesterol, low–saturated-fat diet.[10] Note an overall 15 per cent decrease in plasma cholesterol.

in an overall 15 per cent decrease in the serum cholesterol, as shown in Figure 1. These authors recommended:[10]

1. The use of low-fat milk with extra skim-milk solids.
2. Replacement of butter with highly polyunsaturated margarine.
3. Use of polyunsaturated oils and shortenings in baked goods and for frying.
4. Use of low-cholesterol or cholesterol-free egg products, particularly in baking.
5. Fewer eggs and more cereals.
6. Use of a low-fat ice cream.
7. Frequent use of fish, veal, poultry, and carefully trimmed beef.

Unknown Points About Coronary Heart Disease

PATHOGENESIS OF ATHEROSCLEROSIS

As stated earlier in this essay, the exact pathogenesis of atherosclerosis, like that of many other disease conditions afflicting man, is not fully understood at this time. The role of the various risk factors is only surmised from the various epidemiological and animal studies. Current research efforts attempt to define the cellular or enzymatic defects in familial hyperlipidemia; the role of fatty streaks in the development of the fibrous plaque; basic steps in the metabolism of fat and its precursors; factors that produce blood vessel wall injury (particularly stress and abnormal clotting mechanisms); the role of smooth muscle cells in the intima of vessels; and so on.

OPTIMAL LEVELS OF BLOOD LIPIDS

As stated earlier, no evidence exists at present to indicate that there is a critical level of serum cholesterol that separates high-risk from low-risk individuals. The risk appears to increase as a continuum from low to high levels of serum cholesterol, particularly that portion carried by low-density lipoproteins (LDL). On the other hand, an increase in the high-density lipoprotein fraction (HDL) may offer some protective effect against the development of atherosclerosis.

It is my opinion that the lower the serum cholesterol can be maintained, the lower is the risk for atherosclerosis. Levels of total cholesterol below 180 mg/dl are sought and preferred. There is no evidence at present that levels above 200 mg/dl are normal. Cross-sectional population studies in the United States of children and young adults aimed at determining the serum cholesterol values are worthless for getting some notion of normal values, since atherosclerosis is such a common problem in our country. Only studies from populations and regions of the world where atherosclerosis is uncommon will give us some notion of optimal levels of blood lipids. Unfortunately, there are too few such studies.

DOES LOWERING OF BLOOD LIPIDS AFFECT OR PREVENT ATHEROSCLEROSIS?

Unfortunately, in man, we do not know the answer to the question, "Does lowering of blood lipids (especially cholesterol) reverse or prevent the development of atherosclerosis?" Animal studies would suggest that the answer is yes, but can we extrapolate the animal studies to man? In many other areas of research in medicine we extrapolate, but the purists say we cannot. This is why we currently have a national study of adult man under way to answer the question. It will take many years to answer only that part of the question dealing with reversing the atherosclerosis that already exists. It would take a number of decades to determine if lowering the blood lipids *prevents* atherosclerosis from developing.

The Practical Dilemma

One group of scientists contends that since we do not have enough information in the field of atherosclerosis, we should not proceed at this time with a general national policy for children aimed at preventing future coronary heart disease. A second group of scientists contends that we already have a great deal of information that should allow us to make some overall recommendations to the general public, especially with regard to children. Are there any risks in making such recommendations for children? I think not. We know that the strict dietary recommendations for lowering the serum cholesterol in patients with familial hypercholesterolemia are well tolerated by them in terms of normal growth and development. No deficiency states have yet been observed in patients on such a strict diet.

The Subcommittee on Atherosclerosis of the American Heart Association has confused the issue on the pediatric aspects of prevention of adult atherosclerosis.[11] They correctly identified the magnitude of the problem for adults, but incorrectly made recommendations for identifying and treating *only children with Type II hyperlipoproteinemia,* an infrequent cause of adult coronary artery disease. It now appears likely that Type II hyperlipoproteinemia (or familial hypercholesterolemia) is due to a cellular defect and that the serum cholesterol is not significantly altered by dietary manipulation, as shown by our studies (Fig. 2) as well as others.

Thus, for the time being, if pediatricians are to make a contribution toward "preventing future coronary heart disease," they should identify and treat the risk factors that exist in their patients. Better still, they should embark upon a prophylactic program of preventing all the risk factors from occurring in their patients as outlined in the beginning of this essay.

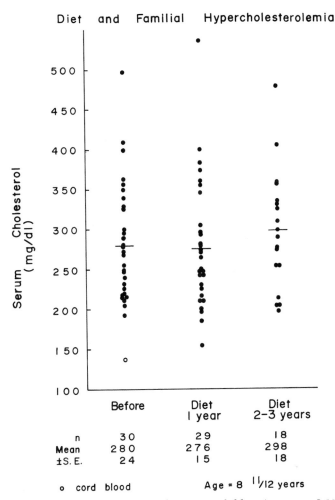

Figure 2. Distribution of cholesterol values in 30 children (mean age 8 11/12 years) with definite familial hypercholesterolemia (Type II) before starting strict diet. Note no significant change in mean values after one year, and after two to three years on diet.

References

1. Stamler J, Beard RR, Connor WE, et al: Primary prevention of the atherosclerotic diseases. Circulation 42:A55, 1970.
2. Truett J, Cornfield J, and Kannel W: A multivariate analysis of the risk of coronary heart disease in Framingham. J Chronic Dis 20:511, 1967.
3. Deutscher S, Ostrander LD, and Epstein FH: Familial factors in premature coronary disease. Am J Epidemiol 91:233, 1970.
4. Goldstein JL, Schrott HG, Hazzard WR, Bierman EL, and Motolsky AG: Hyperlipidemia in coronary heart disease: genetic analysis of lipid levels in 176 families and delineation of a new inherited disorder, combined hyperlipidemia. J Clin Invest 52:1544, 1973.
5. Glueck CJ, Heckman F, Schoenfeld M, Steiner P, and Pearce W: Neonatal familial type II hyperlipoproteinemia: cord blood cholesterol in 1800 births. Metabolism 20:597, 1971.

6. Enos WF, Holmes RH, and Beyer J: Coronary disease among United States soldiers killed in action in Korea. JAMA 152:1090, 1953.
7. Enos WF, Beyer JC, and Holmes RH: Pathogenesis of coronary disease in American soldiers killed in Korea. JAMA 158:912, 1955.
8. McNamara JJ, Molot MA, Stemple JF, and Cutting RT: Coronary artery disease in combat casualties in Viet Nam. JAMA 216:1185, 1971.
9. Hollander W, Madoff I, Paddock J, and Kikpatrick B: Aggravation of atherosclerosis by hypertension in a subhuman primate model with coarctation of the aorta. Circ Res 38(Suppl II):II-63, 1976.
10. Ford CH, McGandy RB, and Stare FJ: An institutional approach to the dietary regulation of blood cholesterol in adolescent males. Prev Med 1:426, 1972.
11. Mitchell S, Blount SG, Blumenthal S, Jesse MJ, and Weidman WH: The pediatrician and atherosclerosis. Pediatrics 49:165, 1972.

Low-Cholesterol, Low–Saturated-Fat Diets Should *Not* Be Routinely Started in Childhood to Prevent Future Coronary Heart Disease

SHEILA MITCHELL, M.D.

Medical Planning Consultant, Princeton, New Jersey

The children in this country are *not* the most unhealthy population in the world.[1]

The argument that the prevention of arteriosclerosis must be accomplished in childhood rests upon two reputed facts: one, that arteriosclerosis begins in childhood; and two, that arteriosclerosis is often first manifested in an irreversible *clinical* event, such as a massive stroke or sudden cardiac death. No one argues with the clinical findings. All the epidemiologic and clinical evidence, as well as the vital statistics, support this "fact." And since there may be no warning of impending disaster, all hope must lie with prevention. And if the first "fact," that of onset in childhood, were an equally well-established fact, then prevention for all children would be highly desirable; but it has not been so established. It has been, in the main, deduced by clinicians from studies of pathology, studies that have been of varying reliability.

The autopsy studies of American personnel who died during the Korean conflict, but not as a direct result of acts of war,[2] appear to be the most quoted and the least read of any pathology reports in recent times relevant to cardiovascular disease. As quoted, these studies attest that most young, i.e., 20- to 30-year-old, American males have severe arteriosclerosis, particularly of their coronary arteries. As read, the studies are extremely difficult to interpret and, at best, suggest that possibly five per cent of this study population had serious, unrecognized coronary arteriosclerosis. Similar study design and presentation problems plague other investigations of coronary disease in young, asymptomatic males.[3, 4]

Well-designed, comparative, geographic pathology studies conducted by Strong and McGill[5] show that all children, wherever they reside, display fatty streaks in their aortas during the first and second decades of life. These data also suggest, although inevitably they are point-prevalence data, that *some,* but far from all, of these fatty streaks progress to become arteriosclerotic lesions. Furthermore, the data obtained in this extensive global study, while confirming the geographic clinical findings of an increased incidence of coronary heart disease in adult Americans, in no way support the conclusion that all Americans show precursors of arteriosclerosis in childhood.[6]

But since the clinical findings of sudden cardiac death and irreversible stroke are irrefutable and irremediable, there has been a diligent search for etiologic agents of arteriosclerosis. In this quest, the following *correlates* of arteriosclerosis have been found: elevated serum cholesterol; elevated blood pressure; excessive cigarette smoking;[7] an aggressive, hostile, time-hounded personality;[8] and living in an affluent society.[9] Some of these factors, such as elevated serum cholesterol and elevated blood pressure,[10–12] have been found to cluster in families, suggesting the possibility of a genetic influence. Some of the data suggest that many of these correlates may be associated with particular life-styles.[13, 14]

Possibly because generations of parents — and most investigators are of parental age — have labored to inculcate particular eating habits, social habits, and life-styles in their offspring, it has become an accepted folk belief that "as the twig is bent, so the tree will grow." For some this may be true. For some, a desired effect may be produced at certain ages. But careful investigation fails to substantiate the generality of this idea.[15] These same studies suggest that the opinions held by a six-year-old with regard, for example, to smoking may relate in no way to the opinions and actions of that same youngster at 16.

The belief still persists, however, that lifelong habits may be established in childhood and, once established, may be difficult to change. This, coupled with the belief that coronary heart disease may begin insidiously during these same years of growth and development, has convinced many that adult risk factors should be attacked during childhood and that all children should be protected from risk factors.

We are concerned here only with cholesterol and saturated fats as risk factors and with the effects of proposed dietary changes to alter these in *all* children. However, we do have a real concern that for lipid levels, as for other correlates of premature* coronary heart disease, eliminating the risk factors may not eliminate the risk.

---

*Premature is customarily taken to mean clinical coronary heart disease before age 65.

In considering the possibility of altering the diet of every child, it must be remembered that, important as it is, coronary heart disease is not the only health problem that children in our ƙociety face. Nor is it the only social problem with which our society must deal. If mass action, effective mass action, were to be taken to change the diet of all Americans, then we might find that adding guilt to the lunch pail was not, overall, a plus. Making every meal a hassle is apt to do at least as much harm as good.

Apart from any potential psychological problems, there are economic ones attendant upon universal dietary change, and these are not trivial in nature. While medicine has traditionally ignored economics, the economic implications of altering the American diet "en masse" cannot be ignored. Switching every child from full to skim milk, limiting each person to one or two eggs per week, persuading all to eschew well-marbled beef and to forego spare ribs and chicken skin could seriously upset certain segments of the domestic economy and might well make the diet of some families worse. In this connection, it is well to remember that 339,000 people are earning their living in the meat products industry alone, and this figure does not include the farmers and cattlemen. For these wage earners and their families, jobs today far outweigh potential illness tomorrow.[16]

Apart from jobs for the "producer," there are serious considerations for the "consumer." At the present time, the cost of milk is calculated on the butterfat content. If skim milk were to be made virtually mandatory, then the cost of milk would perforce be calculated on the protein content. This in turn would raise the cost of skim milk, so that the poor, who now find one of their best sources of protein in skim milk, would be worse off than before.*

Some of the dietary changes that have evolved over the past two or three generations have been changes for the better. Rickets, scurvy, malnutrition predisposing to chronic infection, iron-deficiency anemia, and goiter are uncommon among today's children. These children are bigger and presumably stronger than their forefathers. It would require a brave, and possibly foolish, man to risk jettisoning all these real benefits for the possibility of improving the outlook for those now destined to suffer premature coronary disease.

Clearly, a balance must be struck between the economics of industry — i.e., the wages of many family supporters and the economics of consumers, as indicated above — and the environment, both internal and external, which will be optimum for those who are particularly susceptible to arteriosclerosis. In attempting to strike this balance, one must first determine who is highly susceptible to arteriosclerosis. This in turn necessitates defining who is not susceptible; who is normal and who is abnormal. Somewhat to

---

*While some may try, it is not possible to apply these arguments to the tobacco industry. Smoking has never been shown to promote or improve good health. Its elimination from the economy would release land for the production of health-producing foodstuffs: rich, tillable, well-watered land close to areas of dense population; land that is becoming increasingly scarce. Costs incurred in retraining and retooling the tobacco production industry might well be offset by savings in medical costs of those afflicted with clearly established smoking-related diseases — lung cancer, emphysema, and chronic obstructive respiratory disease, not to mention the social costs of providing smoking and nonsmoking areas in all public facilities.

the surprise of many physicians, this task is far from easy.[17] Fortunately, a number of recent studies have shed some light upon this problem, at least as far as serum cholesterol, serum triglycerides, and concomitant dietary cholesterol, saturated fats, and carbohydrates are concerned.

Point-prevalence studies, and intensive studies of families where one member has already succumbed to a premature arteriosclerotic event, suggest that 230 to 250 mg per cent is probably the *upper* limit of normal serum cholesterol for youngsters of both sexes, both black and white, throughout the first half of the teen years.[10, 18, 19] If we knew for certain that each of these youngsters would maintain his own level of serum cholesterol throughout adult life, then we could be reasonably certain who would be at slight risk and who at high risk of coronary artery disease. But we do not know this. Some youngsters must move out of their adolescent cholesterol "track" into the higher levels, since an extensive sampling of the adult population shows that the upper limit of "normal," i.e., the ninety-fifth percentile, rises with age, being approximately 280 mg per cent at 50 years of age.[11]

Clearly, we need more data, especially longitudinal data, since measurements in addition to random serum cholesterol or serum triglyceride determinations are needed to ascertain who is at high risk of premature coronary heart disease and who is not. Fortunately, one of the measurements that is needed is easily and cheaply obtained. This is the family history. Any youngster who has a first-degree relative with a history or clinically documented evidence of premature coronary heart disease should be considered as being at increased risk of arteriosclerotic heart disease, regardless of his or her current lipid levels. Obviously, any youngster who is found to have a serum cholesterol level repeatedly in excess of the "normal" level should also be considered at high risk. Repeated measurements are essential, since it has been demonstrated that an individual's serum cholesterol can vary by as much as 30 mg per cent from day to day.[18]

All the members of the family of a youngster classified in either of these two ways as being at increased risk of premature coronary heart disease should have a thorough investigation, including blood lipid determinations. Depending upon the levels found, practical advice with regard to diet should be given, with or without the cholesterol-lowering assistance of an appropriate drug. A workable drug regimen has been carefully described by Lloyd.[20]

The long-term effects of drug therapy are, at this time, completely unknown; but the effects of premature coronary heart disease are well known. Consequently, it seems prudent for the individual child at high risk to take an unknown risk in order to forestall a known risk. However, the physician should fool neither himself nor his patient as to the basis of his therapeutic recommendations. There are no data at present that prove that altering ingested cholesterol or saturated fats or lowering the serum cholesterol artificially will, in fact, reduce the chance of a premature heart attack. However, it is also well to remember that much of medicine, and much that was therapeutically efficacious, has been conducted on the basis of equal or less evidence.

This then raises the point as to what is the best method of ascertaining, in the general population, and particularly among those not receiving regular medical care, who is at high risk. It has been suggested that the family history is an excellent way of making such a determination, but to obtain a family history one must see at least one family member in a health or treatment setting. Accordingly, many have recommended mass screening. Recent experience, however, has suggested that this is not only expensive, but ineffective. For mass screening to be effective, there must be readily available, good medical follow-up that will provide appropriate therapy for those truly at risk and discharge as healthy those who are not. Unfortunately, once a label has been applied to a patient, it is difficult to remove it. Then, too, if adequate medical facilities are available for follow-up, it is more cost-effective to educate the population as to the availability of these than it is to go out and screen all the population for a specific laboratory sign. While the sign may be detected with more or less accuracy, other evidence of other disorders will be missed that could be readily picked up while taking a good clinical history and performing a general physical examination. Patients, after all, are people with medical problems. It is these problems we are trying to treat or forestall. The alteration of laboratory signs is a means, not an end.

All the evidence to date, then, suggests that the best preventive medicine for premature coronary heart disease is to identify through good family histories and judicious laboratory investigation those who show the correlates of increased risk of coronary heart disease and then, specifically and individually, to treat these patients and these families to reduce their risk. This regimen has all the earmarks of the best possible therapy for the patient and the fewest side effects for society at large. It also bears the least loss of credibility to the medical profession should other, equally compelling correlates of premature coronary heart disease be found in the future.

Accordingly, then, to prevent coronary heart disease we need two things in addition to more knowledge about arteriosclerosis and its development: good medical facilities to which the people will readily come and widespread knowledge as to where they are and how best they can be utilized. It is within these facilities, at the present time, that high-risk patients can best be identified. It is here that ongoing care can be provided that may reduce these risks while insuring that other health problems are not neglected. In contrast, changing every child's diet, routinely providing low-cholesterol, low–saturated-fat diets for all children, has many of the earmarks of King Herod's approach to preserving his throne. It may miss the high-risk child, damage those at low risk, and adversely affect our society. Our children, who may indeed be among the healthiest in the world, should not be denied this potential through well-intentioned but premature, and possibly erroneous, advice.

References

1. Mission Budgeting and Priorities. A Hearing before a Subcommittee of the Committee on Appropriations, United States Senate, 94th Congress, Second Session, Special Hear-

ing, Department of Health, Education and Welfare as represented by Dr. Theodore Cooper, Assistant Secretary for Health, Office of the Secretary. GPO publication 75-5480, 1976, p 33.

2. Enos WF, Holmes RH, and Beyer J: Coronary disease among U.S. soldiers killed in action in Korea. JAMA 152:1090, 1953.

3. McNamara JJ, Molot MA, Stremple JF, et al: Coronary artery disease in combat casualties in Vietnam. JAMA 216:1185–1187, 1971.

4. Rigal RD, Lovell FW, and Townsend FM: Pathologic findings in the cardiovascular systems of military flying personnel. Am J Cardiol 6:19, 1960.

5. Strong JP, and McGill HC Jr: The pediatric aspects of atherosclerosis. J Atheroscler Res 9: 251–265, 1969.

6. McMillan GC: Development of arteriosclerosis. Am J Cardiol 31:542–546, 1973.

7. Truett J, Cornfield J, and Kannel W: A multivariate analysis of risk of coronary heart disease in Framingham. J Chronic Dis 20:511–524, 1967.

8. Jenkins CD: Psychologic and social precursors of coronary disease. N Engl J Med 284:244–255, 307–317, 1971.

9. Krueger DE, and Morijama IM: Mortality of the foreign born. Am J Public Health 57:496–503, 1967.

10. Blumenthal S, Jesse MJ, Hennekens CH, Klein BE, Ferrer PL, and Gourley JE: Risk factors for coronary artery disease in children of affected families. J Pediatr 87:1187–1192, 1975.

11. Johnson BC, Epstein FH, and Kjelsberg MO: Distributions and familial studies of blood pressure and serum cholesterol levels in a total community — Tecumseh, Michigan. J Chronic Dis 18:147–160, 1965.

12. Kwiterovich PO: Pediatric Aspects of Hyperlipoproteinemia. In Rifkind B, and Levy RI (eds): Hyperlipidemia: Diagnosis and Treatment. New York, Grune and Stratton, 1977, Chapter 12.

13. Schull WJ, Harburg E, Erfurt JC, et al: A family set method for estimating heredity and stress. II. Preliminary results of the genetic methodology in a pilot survey of Negro blood pressure, Detroit, 1966–67. J Chronic Dis 23:83–92, 1970.

14. Keys A: Coronary Heart Disease in Seven Countries. American Heart Association Monograph No 29, 1970.

15. Leventhal H: Changing attitudes and habits to reduce risk factors in chronic disease. Am J Cardiol 31:571–580, 1973.

16. Caudill HM: Night Comes to the Cumberlands. Boston, Little, Brown and Co, 1962.

17. Murphy EA: The normal. Am J Epidemiol 98:403–411, 1971.

18. Lauer RM, Connor WE, Leaverton PE, Reiter MA, and Clarke WR: Coronary heart disease risk factors in school children: The Muscatine Study. J Pediatr 86:697–706, 1975.

19. Frerichs RR, Srinivasan SR, Webber LS, and Berenson GS: Serum cholesterol and triglyceride levels in 3446 children from a biracial community: The Bogalusa Heart Study. Circulation 54:302, 1976.

20. Lloyd JK: Hyperlipidemia in children. Br Heart 37:105–114, 1975.

21. Ahrens EH, and Connor WE: An evaluation of the evidence relating national dietary patterns to disease. Am J Clin Nutr. In press, 1979.

Comment

This controversy highlights a disagreement that exists among pediatricians regarding recommendations on the lipid content in the diet of the young child and adolescent. There is no fundamental disagreement in the facts presented by Drs. Mitchell and Adams. The basic issue is the philosophical one as to whether we are entitled to make a rather sweeping public-health recommendation to the American people on the diet of young persons based upon incomplete, but nevertheless suggestive, data.

I find myself leaning more toward the side of Dr. Adams on this issue. It is difficult for me to accept that end-stage coronary disease manifested by calcified atheromatous plaques will regress with dietary or any other management designed to lower serum cholesterol. At best, at this stage, I believe one may retard the rate of development of new or further progression of existing atherosclerotic plaques. If lowering of cholesterol and saturated fats in the diet is to prevent atherosclerosis, it should be initiated at a time when atherosclerosis is still in its formative stage, that is, early in the natural history of the disease.

I have no difficulty in recommending a prudent diet, low in cholesterol and saturated fats, to the general population of children and adolescents. As long as our dietary recommendations are kept reasonable, reduction of cholesterol and saturated fats in the diet should not impose undue hardships on the population as a whole. One can hardly call the American Heart Association's current recommendation of less than 35 per cent of total calories in the diet as fat, with no more than one-third from saturated fat and no more than 300 mg of cholesterol a day, a stringent, nutritionally deficient, or unpalatable diet to thrust upon the pediatric or the adult population. Many population groups in the world normally consume far fewer total calories as saturated fat and cholesterol without evidence of harm being done to the young-aged population.

It is likely that we will not see in the near future the kind of long-term prospective study that is necessary to answer definitely whether reduction in the fat and cholesterol consumption of the pediatric age group will reduce the prevalence of future coronary heart disease. Nevertheless, in light of animal studies and the large body of clinical and epidemiological data that have been amassed, I think it is a reasonable recommendation for the overall population.

ELLIOT RAPAPORT, M.D.

65

Four

Is Type A Behavior a Serious Risk Factor for the Future Development of Coronary Heart Disease?

TYPE A BEHAVIOR AND ISCHEMIC HEART DISEASE

Meyer Friedman, M.D.

TYPE A BEHAVIOR PATTERN: AN ESTABLISHED MAJOR RISK FACTOR FOR CORONARY HEART DISEASE? THE KEY LIFE-STYLE TRAIT RESPONSIBLE FOR THE CORONARY EPIDEMIC?

Jeremiah Stamler, M.D.

COMMENT

Type A Behavior and Ischemic Heart Disease

MEYER FRIEDMAN, M.D.

Director Emeritus, Harold Brunn Institute, Mount Zion Hospital
and Medical Center, San Francisco, California

In the past 18 years since Rosenman and I[1] first observed the close association of a specific behavior pattern (Type A) with clinical ischemic heart disease (IHD), we have amassed clinical, epidemiological, and experimental data that strongly suggest that this behavior pattern plays a major role in hastening the onset of clinical IHD.

Although diverse descriptions of Type A behavior have been given by psychologists and psychiatrists, I believe that it is most comprehensively and correctly described as an emotion-action complex that is exhibited (or is possessed but sometimes concealed) by individuals who are engaged in a chronic and incessant struggle to achieve more and more in less and less time, thus giving rise to a sense of time urgency or hurry sickness,[2] and who usually exhibit a free-floating but well-rationalized hostility. The Type B behavior pattern is totally lacking in these signs or symptoms so suggestive of struggle.

We have published data[3] indicating that elevation in serum cholesterol is often invoked by Type A behavior; this has been confirmed by other investigators.[4-6] We have also demonstrated experimentally that not only can the serum cholesterol of the rabbit and the rat be elevated by alterations in the functions of the central nervous system, but the course of experimental atherosclerosis can be worsened. We have demonstrated that Type A subjects, long before they develop overt clinical IHD, may have increased clotting propensities, *postprandial sludging*, increased production of norepinephrine, an increased plasma level of corticotropin, a hyperinsulinemic response to a glucose challenge, and an apparent functional deficiency in growth hormone.

Epidemiological studies of 3154 initially well men[7-9] have demonstrated that subjects exhibiting Type A behavior are far more prone to develop overt clinical IHD than Type B subjects. These findings have been either directly or indirectly confirmed by more than a score of investigators, as Jenkins has stated in his review of the psychological and social risk factors for coronary disease.[10]

69

Despite the widespread confirmation of most of our studies relating Type A behavior to the prevalence and incidence of IHD, there still remain investigators who are reluctant to accept such a posited relationship; they seem reluctant even to address themselves to any studies that might confirm or negate such an association. Dr. R. F. Klein was probably correct when, in reviewing our recent book on Type A behavior,[2] he wrote, "when the history of the pandemic of ischemic heart disease is written . . . one fact will stand clear. The gap between medicine and psychiatry has hindered recognition and research of the behavioral and psychosomatic aspects of the disease."[11] He concluded that at this future date, our work on Type A behavior and its relationship to IHD will seem "like a voice crying in the wilderness." I hope that it will not be too long before our voice emerges from this wilderness, since possibly hundreds of thousands of coronary patients may also be crying for effective treatment!

From the beginning of this century, at least a few distinguished physicians had strongly suspected that excessive drive or aggression played an important part in the pathogenesis of coronary atherosclerosis. Osler, in 1897[12] and again in 1910,[13] insisted that he could diagnose the presence of IHD in a new patient by the speed and drive with which the latter entered his consultation room. Later the Menningers[14] and Dunbar[15] strongly suspected a psychogenic element at play in the few coronary patients they studied. Kemple[16] described some of the typical identifying Type A personality traits in several coronary patients he had studied.

The first reason that the opinions of these few distinguished physicians failed to draw attention to the personality of coronary patients was the fact that the leading Boston cardiologists (Drs. Paul White and Samuel Levine) and English cardiologists (Drs. James Mackenzie and Thomas Lewis) concentrated so heavily on the physical signs and studying the polygraphic and electrocardiographic abnormalities associated with various cardiac disorders that they failed to perceive not only the emotional nuances, but also the specific psychomotor manifestations exhibited by most coronary patients.

Distinguished as these pioneer cardiologists undoubtedly were in their general diagnostic acumen, they nevertheless probably harbored a rather large blind spot when considering relationships between the personality and any form of heart disease. I note this because the possible emotional precursors of IHD were not the only emotional aberrations connected with heart diseases that escaped the recognition of these cardiologists.

For example, although both Lewis and Levine were chosen by their respective governments in World War I to study the cause of what Lewis called the "Effort Syndrome,"[17] Levine, "Neurocirculatory Asthenia,"[18] and White, "The Soldier's Irritable Heart,"[19] neither cardiologist suspected that the disorder resulted from a personality disturbance.* If they had studied the faces as carefully as they had studied the hearts, arteries, and veins of

---

*When the central nervous system etiology of this disorder was first considered, I suggested that the name be changed to "functional cardiovascular disease." Paul Wood also concluded that this syndrome was due to a personality disorder. He considered observation of the facial expression helpful for diagnosis. In his textbook, *Diseases of the Heart Circulation*,[20] he reproduced an oil portrait of a patient suffering from functional cardiovascular disease. It is in the museum of the Postgraduate Medical School in London.

their soldier patients, they might have detected, as we had, the woe and agony displayed there.

If White, working later with Gertler, had studied the faces of the 100 young coronary patients he had under investigation as carefully as he had measured the bulk and contour of their musculature, he might have detected the telltale signs of struggle or hostility so often present, particularly in young coronary patients. If he had then correlated this clinical finding with the peculiar medical history given to him by these 100 patients, he might have concluded that it was a disturbed personality, rather than mesomorphy, that distinguished his coronary patients from his normal control subjects.*

A second reason for the delayed recognition of the possible involvement of Type A behavior in the causation of IHD was the gradual and essentially unnoticed increase in the intensity of environmental factors (e.g., urbanization and densification of the American population; the increased employment of persons in service industries; the increasing speed of transportation and communication; and the increasing intrusion, as Toynbee so acutely observed,[21] of acceleration in almost all phases of human activity) that has occurred over the past seven decades and that we believe has hastened the occurrence of Type A behavior in greater numbers of Americans. For example, while we found that somewhat over half of the Bay Area population in 1960 exhibited some degree of Type A behavior, I observed 17 years later, in a personally studied large sample of persons from the same urban area, that well over 75 per cent of these individuals now exhibit Type A behavior.**

A third reason many cardiologists have not seriously suspected Type A behavior as a major accelerant of coronary atherosclerosis is the fact that almost all cardiologists themselves suffer from Type A behavior. Blankenhorn et al.,[22] in a study of cardiologists attending a convention, found that these cardiologists exhibited Type A behavior in such an extreme degree that they suggested that cardiologists avoid direct contact with their patients and employ paramedical aides for that purpose. But whether or not this advice should be followed is debatable, for if a process seizes both the doctor and his patient, the former cannot easily detect and label this process a pathological entity. This, of course, becomes even more difficult if both persons are not only proud of possessing this disorder, but are also inclined to attribute to it some of the successes both may have attained in their respective careers.

A fourth and very important reason for the delay in a broad investigation of the role of Type A behavior in the pathogenesis of IHD has been the trend of turning to epidemiologists for help in finding clues to the causal agents of IHD. Unfortunately, however, few of these investigators pre-

---

*In 1974, Dr. George Griffith wrote to me (personal communication) that Paul White had recently told him that he had begun to believe that Type A behavior probably did play some part in hastening the onset of clinical IHD.

**I do not believe, however, that this large difference is solely due to an increase in the prevalence of Type A behavior. In 1960–1961, lacking knowledge of many of the psychomotor manifestations presently used to diagnose this behavior pattern, we probably did not detect its presence in a large proportion of this earlier population.

viously had been trained in either the laboratory or clinical techniques of cardiovascular research. Rather, they were knowledgeable in or they were able to use other individuals who were skilled in statistical techniques. Such training and experience, of course, led these researchers to investigate only those possibly pathogenic items that could be measured.

Thus, scores of studies now have been done on the measurable factors associated with clinical IHD. Some of these measurable factors are important, such as the serum cholesterol, glucose and triglyceride, blood pressure, family history of IHD, or number of cigarettes smoked. But other measurable factors, such as the number of cups of coffee drunk, number of hours slept, amount of salt ingested, or number of hours of physical exercise, are either trivial, irrelevant, or secondary to other primary agents.

But because Type A behavior does not easily lend itself to quantitative manipulations of primary computerized transactions and, perhaps even more importantly, since its detection involves a clinical investigative stance rather than acumen in computative processes, its role in accelerating the course of IHD was totally neglected in most major epidemiological studies.

In this omission and concentration on the tabulation of some of the measurable factors above, the leaders of these studies may have mistakenly labeled some agents as primary risk factors, when actually they may be secondary to a risk factor they failed to investigate — that is, Type A behavior. It is too late to salvage the damage done to these epidemiological studies by their omission of the study of the personality of their cohorts. This flaw cannot be rectified by a post hoc dispatch of questionnaires to their surviving cohorts, since the detection of Type A behavior cannot be accurately assessed by pencil and paper; it must be done by clinical scrutiny.

A fifth reason for not accepting a relationship between Type A behavior and the pathogenesis of IHD has been the tendency of many psychologists investigating this relationship to attempt to discern and isolate the emotional aberrations that make up the Type A behavior pattern and to discover which are more and which are less pathogenetically important. Thus, they have singled out such entities as the following for investigation (usually by paper and pencil tests):

1. obsessive-compulsive disturbances;
2. speed and impatience;
3. excessive job involvement;
4. hard driving;
5. excessive ambition;
6. anxiety;
7. hysteria;
8. status incongruity;
9. cultural mobility;
10. sleep disturbances;
11. work dissatisfaction;
12. "emotional drain."

It seems almost quixotic for one group of investigators (i.e., the psychiatrists and psychologists) to concern themselves so seriously with studies to determine which emotional components of the total Type A behavior pattern might bear the greatest relevance in the pathogenesis of coronary atherosclerosis, while another group (i.e., contemporary epidemiologists) very seriously doubts if any part of this behavior pattern plays a part in accelerating or aggravating the course of coronary atherogenesis. I think it best to continue to view Type A behavior in a global manner as a form of continuous struggle. And when this struggle is viewed more widely as having major relevance in the pathogenesis of IHD (as I am certain it will),* it then will be more appropriate to analyze the intrinsic and extrinsic factors responsible for this continuous struggle.

A sixth and final reason for the reluctance of some cardiologists to accept Type A behavior as a major pathogen in IHD is the fact that although it has a close predictive association with IHD, association does not prove causation. Thus, Type A behavior, like hypertension and hypercholesterolemia, still requires specific demonstration that its presence or absence directly influences the course of coronary atherosclerosis. We are now beginning such a study. We shall attempt to alter, modify, or if possible, even eliminate Type A behavior in a large fraction of postinfarction patients. If Type A behavior bears not only an associative, but also a causal, relationship to clinical IHD, then those postinfarction patients who succeed in altering the intensity of their behavior patterns will demonstrate unequivocally that Type A behavior plays a very significant role in the onset of premature IHD.

Modification of Type A Behavior

Should we not attempt to alter or modify the Type A behavior pattern until its causal role in clinical IHD is established beyond all possible criticism? I see no greater reason to delay such attempts than to postpone attempts to lower elevated serum cholesterol or blood pressure levels in afflicted subjects. In fact, in Type A behavior subjects who have already suffered myocardial infarction, there may be far more justification for attempting behavior modification than attempting to alter these other risk factors. Reduction of serum cholesterol has been found to be useless in preventing recurrence of myocardial infarction, and reduction of the blood pressure of hypertensive patients has been found to be similarly useless in forestalling the initial advent of myocardial infarction.

Irrespective of the data accumulated in the future, it still may take a long time to convince all our colleagues of the pathogenic importance of the Type A behavior pattern. In this connection, it should not be forgotten that distinguished physicist Max Planck once declared that new concepts

---

*On December 4, 1978, a review panel assembled by the National Heart, Lung, and Blood Institute concluded that the available body of scientific data suggested an association between IHD and Type A behavior pattern. The panel also concluded that the risk presented by this pattern was of the same order of magnitude as the relative risk associated with other risk factors, such as hypercholesterolemia or smoking.

rarely get accepted by rational persuasion of the opponents. He believed that sometimes one simply has to wait until the opponents die out.

I have found it extremely difficult to alter Type A behavior in any person who has not succumbed to the clinical onset (i.e., angina pectoris or infarction) of IHD. I suspect that it is usually the conviction of even my highest-risk patients (i.e., hypercholesterolemic, heavily smoking, hypertensive, Type A subjects) that somehow it will be other high-risk patients, not they, who will succumb to clinical IHD.

I believe, therefore, that behavior modification might most profitably be confined to Type A behavior persons who have already suffered from and survived a myocardial infarction. Approximately 75 per cent of these persons are susceptible to behavior modification.

This type of behavior can be altered in probably the majority of postinfarction patients. Such modification, I believe, will be almost routinely attempted by thousands of cardiologists before another decade has passed. And it will be accomplished not just by cardiologists alone, but by cardiologists working with psychiatrists, clinical psychologists, or suitably trained paramedical personnel who will aid them in modifying Type A behavior.

References

1. Friedman M, and Rosenman RH: Association of specific overt behavior pattern with blood and cardiovascular findings. JAMA 169:1286, 1959.
2. Friedman M, and Rosenman RH: Type A Behavior and Your Heart. New York, Alfred A Knopf, Inc, 1974.
3. Friedman M, Rosenman RH, and Carroll V: Changes in the serum cholesterol and blood-clotting time in men subjected to cyclic variation of occupational stress. Circulation 17:852, 1958.
4. Dreyfuss F, and Czaczkes JW: Blood cholesterol and uric acid of healthy medical students under stress of an examination. Arch Intern Med 103:708, 1959.
5. Grundy SM, and Griffin AC: Effects of periodic mental stress on serum cholesterol levels. Circulation 19:496, 1959.
6. Wertlake PT, Wilcox AA, Haley MI, and Peterson JE: Relationship of mental and emotional stress to serum cholesterol levels. Proc Soc Exp Biol Med 97:163, 1958.
7. Rosenman RH, Friedman M, Straus R, Wurm M, Jenkins D, Messinger HB, Kositchek R, Hahn W, and Werthessen NT: Coronary heart disease in the Western collaborative group study: A follow-up experience of two years. JAMA 195:86, 1966.
8. Rosenman RH, Brand RJ, Jenkins CD, Friedman M, Straus R, and Wurm M: Coronary heart disease in the Western collaborative group study: Final follow-up experience of 8½ years. JAMA 233:872, 1975.
9. Brand RJ, Rosenman RH, Sholtz RI, and Friedman M: Multivariate prediction of coronary heart disease in the Western collaborative group study compared to the findings of the Framingham study. Circulation 53:348, 1976.
10. Jenkins CD: Recent evidence supporting psychologic and social risk factors for coronary disease. N Engl J Med 294:987 and 1033, 1976.
11. Klein RF: Type A behavior and your heart. Circulation 50:411, 1974.
12. Osler W: Lectures on Angina Pectoris and Allied States. New York, D Appleton and Co, Inc, 1897.
13. Osler W: The Lumleian Lectures on Angina Pectoris. Lancet 1:839, 1910.
14. Menninger KA, and Menninger WC: Psychoanalytic observations in cardiac disorders. Am Heart J 11:10, 1936.
15. Dunbar HF: Psychosomatic Diagnosis. New York, Paul B Hoeber, 1943.

16. Kemple C: Rorschack method and psychosomatic diagnosis. Personality traits of patients with rheumatic disease, hypertensive cardiovascular disease, coronary occlusion, and fracture. Psychosom Med 7:85, 1945.
17. Lewis T: *The Soldier's Heart and the Effort Syndrome*. New York, Paul B Hoeber, 1919.
18. Oppenheimer BS, Levine SA, Morrison RA, Rothschild MA, St Lawrence W, and Wilson FN: Report on neurocirculatory asthenia and its management. Med Surg 42:409, 1918.
19. White PD: The soldier's irritable heart. JAMA 118:270, 1942.
20. Wood P: *Diseases of the Heart and Circulation*, 2nd ed. Philadelphia, JB Lippincott Co, 1956.
21. Toynbee A: *A Study of History*, vol 12. London, Oxford University Press, 1961, p 603.
22. Blankenhorn DH, Jenkins CD, Insull W Jr, and Weiss B: Type A physicians and coronary risk education. Ann Intern Med 81:700, 1974.

Type A Behavior Pattern: An Established Major Risk Factor for Coronary Heart Disease? The Key Life-Style Trait Responsible for the Coronary Epidemic?

JEREMIAH STAMLER, M.D.

Professor and Chairman, Department of Community
Health and Preventive Medicine, and Dingman Professor
of Cardiology, Northwestern University Medical School,
Chicago, Illinois

This paper explores two key questions concerning Type A behavior: First, do the available data meet the criteria for designating Type A behavior as one of the established major risk factors for coronary heart disease (CHD)? Second, do the data warrant the inference that Type A behavior is *the* key life-style characteristic accounting for the epidemic of CHD in the U.S.A. and other "Western" industrialized countries in the twentieth century?

76

Does Type A Behavior Meet the Criteria for an Established Major CHD Risk Factor?

The literature on Type A behavior is now extensive, and recent reviews are available, including the valuable *Proceedings of the Forum on Coronary-Prone Behavior* held in mid-1977 under the sponsorship of the National Heart, Lung, and Blood Institute.[1-3] These show clearly that the decisive data on the relationship of Type A behavior to CHD are epidemiologic in nature, more precisely from observational — i.e., nonexperimental (noninterventional) — epidemiologic research. No large-scale, randomized, controlled trials have been reported testing whether sustained modification of Type A behavior is possible in large numbers of Type A people and whether it results in the primary and/or secondary prevention of CHD. Therefore, judgment as to whether Type A behavior is an established major risk factor for CHD, i.e., whether it is a component in the multifactorial *causation* of this disease, must be based first and foremost on the observational epidemiologic data.

Established criteria are available to assess whether epidemiologic associations are etiologically significant.[4, 5] They are succinctly summarized by the Advisory Committee to the Surgeon General in the landmark *Report to the Surgeon General on Smoking and Health.*[6] In up-dated form they are:

1. *Strength* of the association;

2. *Graded nature* of the association, i.e., the more marked the suspected trait (e.g., Type A behavior), the greater the risk of disease (e.g., CHD);

3. *Temporal sequence,* i.e., does the presumed etiologic factor precede the disease?

4. *Consistency* of the findings in multiple studies;

5. *Independence* of each of the associations, one from the other;

6. *Predictive capacity,* i.e., ability based on the findings in one or more sets of populations to predict events in other different populations.

7. *Coherence* of the findings in two senses, i.e., consistency of the epidemiologic findings with those from other research methods (animal experimentation, clinical and pathologic investigation), and coherence in the sense that reasonable pathogenetic mechanisms are known, indicating pathways whereby the etiologic agents act to produce the disease.

By definition, a risk factor is a habit or trait associated with *future* risk of developing a disease, that is, persons with the characteristic (in the present case, the Type A behavior pattern), currently free of evidence of the disease under study (here CHD), are more likely to develop the disease subsequently. (For persons who already have the disease, the risk factor may also relate to proneness to future recurrent episodes and/or death from the disease.) Therefore, in the application of the foregoing criteria, *prospective* epidemiologic data are crucial. To date, prospective findings on Type A behavior and CHD risk have been reported from two investigations, the Western Collaborative Group Study (WCGS) and the Framingham Study.[1-3, 7-12] The latter study presented prospective data in March, 1978, to the annual scientific meeting of the Council on Epidemiology of the American Heart Association, but has not yet published a definitive report.[12]

As noted in the *Proceedings of the Forum on Coronary-Prone Behavior*, the WCGS data are "the cornerstone of the evidence regarding the association between the incidence of coronary heart disease and A-B behavior...."[13] They are the results of 8.5 years of follow-up of 3154 men aged 39 to 59 at entry, who were originally free of clinical evidence of definite CHD and characterized extensively at baseline in regard to many habits and traits, including Type A-B behavior, by a structured interview.[1-3, 7-9] In univariate and multivariate analyses, the WCGS data reaffirmed that the established major risk factors—hypercholesterolemia, hypertension, and cigarette smoking[4, 5, 14-19]—were independently and significantly related to CHD incidence. Type A behavior pattern was related to CHD incidence as well (Table 1).[7] For men aged 39 to 49 at entry, the incidence rates for Type A and Type B men were 10.5 and 5.0 per 1000 per year, respectively, i.e., a univariate risk ratio of 2.1, and an absolute excess risk (attributable risk) of 5.5 per 1000 per year for Type A men. For those originally aged 50 to 59, the rates were 18.7 and 8.9, respectively; the risk ratio was again 2.1; and the absolute excess risk for Type A men was 9.8 per 1000 per year.[7] For "hard" CHD, for example, nonfatal or fatal myocardial infarction (MI), the findings were similar.

In addition to bivariate cross-classification findings (Table 1), multiple logistic regression analysis data — based on the same 8.5-year follow-up experience — have also been published by the WCGS investigators (Tables 2 and 3).[8, 9] They permit a point-by-point evaluation as to whether the findings fulfill criteria 1, 2, 3, and 5 noted earlier. From all the WCGS data sets, the relationship of Type A behavior to CHD risk is a *strong* one. In the bivariate cross-classification analyses (Table 1), the risk ratios are in the range 1.7 to 2.8 for the group aged 39 to 49 at entry (ignoring the findings for men smoking one to 15 cigarettes per day at entry), and 1.4 to 8.2 for men aged 50 to 59. (Given the small numbers for some of the strata, many of these ratios have large confidence intervals.) The overall risk ratio of 2.1 is somewhat smaller than the risk ratio for hypercholesterolemic men — 2.4 for men with entry values ≥260 mg/dl compared to those with <260 mg/dl, and 3.6 for these men compared to those with <220 mg/dl. It is somewhat larger than that for hypertensive men (1.9) and of about the same order of magnitude as that for cigarette smokers compared to those who never smoked (2.2).

The standardized coefficients from the multiple logistic analyses (Tables 2 and 3) and the standardized risk ratios (Table 3) lead to similar conclusions.[8, 9] With the eight variables considered simultaneously in Table 2, four variables are significantly and independently related to CHD risk for both age groups — behavior pattern, serum cholesterol, systolic pressure, and cigarette use. The size of a standardized coefficient is a measure of the relative strength of the independent relationship of a given variable to CHD risk, compared to other variables. For men aged 39 to 49 at entry, the coefficient for behavior pattern is smaller than that for serum cholesterol, about the same as that for cigarette smoking, and larger than that for systolic pressure. For the group aged 50 to 59 at baseline, the coefficients

Table 1. *Univariate and Bivariate Cross-Classification Data Type A-B, Major Risk Factors and 8.5-Year CHD Incidence by Age at Entry, Western Collaborative Group Study†*

BASELINE FINDINGS	AGE 39–49							AGE 50–59						
	Type A			Type B				Type A			Type B			
	At Risk	CHD	Rate	At Risk	CHD	Rate	Risk Ratio	At Risk	CHD	Rate	At Risk	CHD	Rate	Risk Ratio
Serum Cholesterol														
<220 mg/dl	486	24	5.8	670	11	2.1	2.76	211	20	11.2	148	6	4.8	2.33
220–259	352	32	10.7	376	20	6.3	1.70	179	36	23.7	142	10	8.3	2.86
≥260	226	39	20.3	195	19	11.5	1.77	130	27	24.4	90	13	17.0	1.44
Risk Ratio			3.50△ / 2.57△△			5.48 / 3.11				2.18 / 1.44			3.54 / 2.62	
Diastolic Pressure														
<95 mm Hg	970	81	9.8	1100	45	4.8	2.04	448	64	16.8	344	25	8.5	1.98
≥95	97	14	17.0	82	5	7.2	2.36	74	19	30.2	39	4	12.1	2.50
Risk Ratio			1.73			1.50				1.80			1.42	
Smoking														
Never Smoked	221	11	5.9	315	8	3.0	1.97	90	10	13.1	89	5	6.6	1.98
Pipe or Cigar	191	11	6.8	216	6	3.3	2.06	81	17	24.7	78	2	3.0	8.23
Former Cigarette	110	11	11.8	129	5	4.6	2.57	91	10	12.9	41	2	5.7	2.26
Current Cigarette	545	62	13.4	522	31	7.0	1.91	260	46	20.8	175	20	13.4	1.55
1–15/day	95	3	3.7	119	8	7.9	0.47	65	8	14.5	43	1	2.7	5.37
≥16	450	59	15.4	403	23	6.7°	2.30	195	38	22.9	132	19	16.9	1.36
Risk Ratio			2.27° / 2.61°°			2.33 / 2.23				1.59 / 1.75			2.03 / 2.56	
All	1067	95	10.5	1182	50	5.0	2.10	522	83	18.7	383	29	8.9	2.10

All rates are average annual rates per 1000 per year. °In the original table, incorrectly given as 11.4.

° $\dfrac{\text{Current Cigarette}}{\text{Never Smoked}}$

°° $\dfrac{\geq 16}{\text{Never Smoked}}$

△ $\dfrac{\geq 260}{<220}$

△△ $\dfrac{\geq 260}{<260}$

†From Rosenman RH, Brand RJ, Jenkins D, Friedman M, Straus R, and Wurm M: Coronary heart disease in the Western Collaborative Group Study: Final follow-up experience of 8½ years. JAMA 233:872–877, 1975.

Table 2. *Coefficients and Standardized Coefficients from Multiple Logistic Analysis, by Age at Entry, 8.5-Year CHD Incidence Data, Western Collaborative Group Study†*

VARIABLE	MEN AGE 39–49			MEN AGE 50–59		
	Coefficient	Std. Deviation of Variable	Standardized Coefficient	Coefficient	Std. Deviation of Variable	Standardized Coefficient
Serum Cholesterol	0.0120[***]	43.123	0.5175	0.0086[***]	41.429	0.3563
Systolic Pressure	0.0150[*]	14.155	0.2123	0.0202[***]	16.544	0.3342
Cigarette Smoking	0.2429[***]	1.244	0.3022	0.2990[***]	1.222	0.3654
Behavior Pattern	0.6396[***]	0.497	0.3179	0.7430[**]	0.491	0.3648
Age	0.0902[**]	3.079	0.2777	0.0615	2.721	0.1673
Relative Weight	0.0103	— — —[△]	0.107[°]	0.0185	— — —[△]	0.191[°]
Hematocrit	0.0326	— — —[△]	0.085[°]	0.0147	— — —[△]	0.042[°]
ECG	−0.4242	— — —[△]	−0.104[°]	0.1007	— — —[△]	0.030[°]

[*]$p < 0.05$ [**]$p < 0.01$ [***]$p < 0.001$
[△]Not available in published papers.
[°]From a WCGS handout available to the author.
Standardized coefficient is the coefficient multiplied by the standard deviation of the variable.

†From Rosenman RH, Brand RJ, Sholtz RI, and Friedman M: Multivariate prediction of coronary heart disease during 8.5-year follow-up in the Western Collaborative Group Study. Am J Cardiol 37:903–910, 1976; and Brand RJ, Rosenman RH, Sholtz RI, and Friedman M: Multivariate prediction of coronary heart disease in the Western Collaborative Group Study compared to the findings of the Framingham Study. Circulation 53:348–355, 1976.

for these four factors are of a very similar size. The findings are similar from the analysis with a set of 11 variables (Table 3). Thus, the WCGS data indicate that the relationship between Type A behavior pattern and CHD is *strong* and is *independent* of the three established major risk factors. The criterion of *temporal sequence* is also met, since the WCGS made the assessment of behavior pattern at baseline for its 3154 men free of overt evidence of definite CHD at that point, and CHD incidence was recorded for a subsequent 8.5 years.

The criterion of a *graded relationship* — i.e., the greater the degree of the possible risk factor at entry, the greater the subsequent incidence of CHD — cannot be assessed from these data, since all the cited analyses involved dichotomizing the cohort into Type A or Type B men based on the structured interview technique used at entry, i.e., no findings are given for gradations of behavior pattern. However, the initial A-B classification was made at four levels, A_1, A_2, B_3, and B_4, and it has been reported that men classified as A_1 and A_2 had comparable risk, as did men classified B_3 and B_4 (at about half the level of A_1 and A_2 men).[3, 20] Thus, "no convincing dose-response relationship was observed. . . ."[21]

Furthermore, in regard to this criterion of graded relationship, in 1965 — four to five years after the baseline examinations of the WCGS — 2750 CHD-free men completed a 61-item multiple choice questionnaire as-

Table 3. *Coefficients, Standardized Coefficients, and Standardized Relative Risk from Multiple Logistic Analysis, by Age at Entry, 8.5-Year CHD Incidence Data, Western Collaborative Group Study†*

VARIABLE	MEN AGE 39–49				MEN AGE 50–59			
	Coefficient	Std. Dev. of Variable	Stdized. Coeff.	Stdized. Rel. Risk△	Coefficient	Std. Dev. of Variable	Stdized. Coeff.	Stdized. Rel. Risk
Serum Cholesterol	0.010***	43.123	0.4312	1.57	0.008***	41.429	0.3314	1.40
Systolic Pressure	0.017**	14.155	0.2406	1.27	0.020****	16.544	0.3309	1.40
Cigarette Smoking	0.223***	1.244	0.2774	1.32	0.285***	1.222	0.3483	1.42
Behavior Pattern	0.628***	0.497	0.3121	1.37	0.774***	0.491	0.3800	1.46
Age	0.079**	3.079	0.2401	1.28	0.053	2.721	0.1442	1.16
Corneal Arcus	0.458*	0.434	0.1988	1.22	– – –△△	– – –	– – –	– – –
Parental CHD	0.356	0.386	0.1374	1.15	– – –△△	– – –	– – –	– – –
Schooling	–0.146	0.930	–0.1358	0.87	–0.214	0.907	–0.1941	0.82
Lipoprotein Ratio	0.112	1.046	0.1172	1.12	– – –△△	– – –	– – –	– – –
Body Mass Index	– – –△△	– – –	– – –	– – –	0.071	2.515	0.1786	1.20
Exercise Habits	– – –△△	– – –	– – –	– – –	–0.348	0.450	–0.1566	0.86

* p < 0.05   ** p < 0.01   *** p ≤ 0.001

△The approximate relative risk (odds ratio) for a change in the risk factor by an amount equal to its standard deviation.

△△Not among variables in the analysis for this age group.

Standardized coefficient is the coefficient multiplied by the standard deviation of the variable.

†From Rosenman RH, Brand RJ, Sholtz RI, and Friedman M: Multivariate prediction of coronary heart disease during 8.5-year follow-up in the Western Collaborative Group Study. Am J Cardiol 37:903–910, 1976; and Brand RJ, Rosenman RH, Sholtz RI, and Friedman M: Multivariate prediction of coronary heart disease in the Western Collaborative Group Study compared to the findings of the Framingham Study. Circulation 53:348–355, 1976.

sessing behavior pattern, the Jenkins Activity Survey (JAS).[22] Responses to this questionnaire were scored according to four scales, including a Type A scale that best discriminated men judged to be Type A from those judged to be Type B by the clinical, structured interview. This cohort was then followed for an additional four years, and JAS scores were found to relate significantly to CHD risk in a prospective case-control analysis (120 CHD cases, 524 control men). With division of the men into three groups — JAS score <-5.0 (Type B), -5.0 to $+5.0$, or $>+5.0$ (Type A), annual CHD incidence rates were 8.0, 10.7, and 14.3 per 1000, respectively. Linear regression analysis showed a significant relationship indicating that risk was graded, i.e., the greater the JAS score, the greater the risk. No multivariate analyses were reported; hence it is not clear whether JAS score is related to CHD risk in a graded fashion independent of the established major risk factors. At this juncture, therefore, it seems reasonable to conclude, as did the Forum on Coronary-Prone Behavior,[21] that further studies are essential to clarify whether the criterion of graded relationship is or is not met.

A key criterion is assessing whether an association reflects a causative relationship is *consistency* of findings in multiple studies, particularly prospective investigations. Here data are still sparse. Until the recent report from the Framingham Study,[12] there were no findings from longitudinal studies other than the WCGS. In 1965–67, an extensive life-history questionnaire was administered to 1674 CHD-free persons in Framingham. From the many questions, a set was selected by a panel of experts and validated in three separate studies as yielding a scale of Type A behavior. Based on an eight-year follow-up for men aged 55 to 64 in 1965–67, Type A men were over two times as likely to develop CHD as Type B men, with relative risks of 3.4, 2.1, and 2.1 for uncomplicated angina (AP), MI, and all CHD, respectively. For Type A women aged 45 to 64, relative risks for AP and CHD were 3.8 and 2.1, respectively. In multivariate analyses, these associations remained significant when controlled for the established major risk factors. For men, the association of Type A behavior with CHD incidence was significant for white-collar but not blue-collar workers. For women, the associations were noted for both housewives and employed women, being slightly stronger for the former.

This set of findings from Framingham represents an important advance in regard to the criterion of consistency for this variable. To my knowledge, at least three other prospective investigations will eventually be reporting data on behavior pattern and CHD: the Chicago Heart Association Detection Project in Industry study (CHA), the U.S. Multiple Risk Factor Intervention Trial (MRFIT), and the Brussels Controlled Multifactorial Prevention Trial.[23-26] Their results will be important in regard to this key criterion.

In the interim, additional data relevant to the consistency criterion have been reported by several cross-sectional (i.e., nonlongitudinal) studies, most in the U.S.A. and a few in Europe, generally using the JAS Type A scale.[2, 3, 11, 23] (See particularly references 2, 3, and 11 for citations of the literature.) Scores were reported to be consistently related to CHD; one review cites 24 of 25 papers as supporting a positive association.[2] As noted in the Summary Statement of the *Proceedings of the Forum on Coronary-*

Prone Behavior on the Association of the Coronary-Prone Behavior Pattern and Coronary Heart Disease:

However, since response bias and sample selection can, in many ways, influence the results and interpretations in case-control studies, these replications take on added meaning. They assume greater significance in that they speak to the following issues: (1) random phenomena rarely replicate; (2) a variety of population groups were studied, and not simply narrowly defined and selected cases vs. controls; and (3) epidemiological studies have often found that replicated associations based on prevalence data are prospectively related as well.[27]

Nevertheless, the possibility exists that in populations in industrialized countries, many persons who have developed clinical CHD perceive themselves as having been hard-driving, excessively competitive, striving, aggressive, beset by time urgency, engaged in chronic and excessive struggle, and so on prior to their MI and relate this to their disease — that is, the popularly held view that "stress" contributes to risk of heart attack may have led some persons who were not really Type A individuals before developing clinical CHD to describe themselves afterwards as having Type A behavioral traits, thus repeatedly introducing bias into studies that are not prospective. Given this possibility, it seems reasonable to conclude, despite the consistent results of the two prospective and several cross-sectional epidemiologic studies, that the crucial criterion of consistency is *not* at this juncture met in a fully satisfactory way. In arriving at this judgment, I hasten to add what should be obvious but may not be: This is not and cannot be a criticism of the pioneers in the Type A-B concept and research, Drs. M. Friedman and R. Rosenman. Clearly, responsibility for testing the reproducibility of their findings, particularly the critically important results from the large-scale prospective WCGS, was not and could not be primarily theirs. If the undertaking of studies to assess replicability of the Type A-B data has been a slow process, and I believe it has been, the rest of the cardiovascular epidemiologic community — and the granting agencies — must be self-critical.

As to the criterion of *predictive capacity,* in one sense, this has been met to a degree by the results of the two prospective studies, WCGS and Framingham — that is, the prior hypothesis was clearly formulated that characterizing men with CHD as to Type A behavior would prospectively predict risk of CHD independent of the major established risk factors, and that is what was, in fact, found. However, there is another aspect of this criterion, as set down under criterion 6 above: When the quantitative findings on risk factors from one population are applied independently to another population to predict CHD risk, how good is the agreement between the observed and the predicted? Specifically, in regard to the issue at hand, will inclusion of information about behavior pattern — for example, from the WCGS or Framingham multivariate analyses — give better multivariate prediction (e.g., for the CHA, MRFIT, or Brussels cohorts) than the established major risk factors alone? To my knowledge, no data on this matter are as yet available. They should be forthcoming in the years ahead.

With regard to the seventh criterion, *coherence:* First, in the sense of consistency of the epidemiologic findings with those from other research methods (clinical and pathologic investigation and animal experimentation), the WCGS research group reported in 1968 on autopsy findings of 51 of 82 decedents in the first six years of their study: 35 of them were assessed at entry to be Type A and 16 Type B, seven of the former and none of the latter with a positive history of CHD at baseline.[28] Of the 35 Type A decedents, 22 died of CHD; of the 16 Type B, two died of CHD. Eleven of the Type A men showed evidence of old MI; none of the Type B men did. Eight of the Type A men showed evidence of new MI; one of the Type B men did. Severity of coronary atherosclerosis was greater in Type A than Type B decedents overall and for the 13 Type A men compared to the 13 Type B men dying of noncardiac causes. Correspondingly, results of four studies are reported as consistently indicating that score on the JAS Type A scale is related to severity of coronary atherosclerosis as assessed angiographically.[29-33] However, a fifth such study yielded no evidence of an association.[34]

As to animal experimental work, Type A behavior is an all-too-human trait, so that its direct reproduction in other species in the laboratory is a difficult challenge. Nonetheless, it has been stated that ". . . behavior patterns seen in certain individuals under natural circumstances can be elicited in laboratory situations and can be elicited in experimental animals."[35] A review and assessment of the literature basic to this conclusion is beyond the scope of this paper and is not critical for its conclusions concerning the issue under discussion, since it is my estimate that in regard to a human personality-behavior pattern like Type A-B, its induction in nonhuman species is not an absolute prerequisite for its establishment as an independent, etiologically significant risk factor.

As to the criterion of coherence in its other sense, reasonable pathogenetic mechanisms linking the trait with the underlying disease, such pathways — neuroendocrine in nature — have been proposed, and several reports have presented data comparing Type A and Type B men. They encompass such findings as increased serum level of corticotropin in Type A compared to Type B men; subnormal corticoid secretion in response to exogenous ACTH; reduced serum level of growth hormone both prior to and after arginine challenge when Type A men are studied in their typical working milieu; hyperinsulinemic response to a glucose challenge (without an abnormal glucose tolerance in most instances); increased norepinephrine secretion and high serum level of this hormone when Type A men are studied in their usual working milieu or engaged in a competitive contest; accelerated blood clotting; higher platelet counts in whole blood; less of a decrease in platelet aggregation in response to noradrenalin after exercise; a shorter platelet aggregation time in response to ADP; higher serum triglycerides prior to and for many hours after a fat meal; and increased erythrocyte sludging with postprandial hypertriglyceridemia.[36, 37] Most of the data of this kind on neuroendocrine-metabolic-hematologic responses of Type A compared to Type B men have been reported by Friedman and colleagues; hence independent replication of the findings is needed. It has also been stated that hypercholesterolemia is more common in Type A than Type B men.[38, 39] In fact, in the WCGS cohort there was modest support for this conclusion only for the men aged 39 to 49 at entry: Prevalence rates were 211 and 165 per 1000 for Type A and B men, respectively, with a cutpoint ≥260 mg/dl, and 542 and 483 per 1000, respectively, with a cutpoint ≥220 mg/dl (Table 1).[7] However, for those aged 50 to 59 at baseline, Type A and Type B men had very similar rates of hypercholesterolemia with these two cutpoints: 249 and 235 per 1000, respectively, and 592 and 606 per 1000, respectively. For the subcohort of 3611 generally healthy white men and women aged 25 to 64 with JAS scores in the Chicago Heart Association Detection Project in Industry, no association between score and serum cholesterol was found for men or women aged 25 to 44 or 45 to 64.[23] Similarly, no such association was found in the Framingham population.[10]

As noted in the *Proceedings of the Forum on Coronary-Prone Behavior,* "... There are very few published studies documenting a difference between Type A and Type B subjects in psycho-physiological response to environmental stimulation."[38] Thus, in regard to this matter of pathogenetic pathways and mechanisms, much remains to be clarified, and much work is needed. Nonetheless, for years it has been, in my judgment, a reasonable hypothesis that, given the impact of "rich" diet and cigarette smoking (plus the sedentary habit as well) as established aspects of mid–twentieth-century life style for tens of millions in the "Western" industrialized countries, and given the related high prevalence rates of hypercholesterolemia and hypertension, Type A behavior and other psycho-social incongruities also made widely prevalent by modern society add insult to injury in regard to CHD risk.

In summary on this first question, the data available to date, particularly the prospective epidemiologic findings from the Western Collaborative Group Study and the Framingham Study, indicate that the criteria of strength of the relationship, temporal sequence, independence, and coherence are more or less reasonably met in regard to assessing the etiologic significance of the Type A–CHD association. More data, particularly data from *prospective* epidemiologic studies, are needed to determine the graded nature of the association, its consistency in a range of populations, and the enhanced capacity to predict CHD risk when Type A behavior is considered along with the established major risk factors. If this evaluation is sound, it is reasonable at this point, according to what is presently known, to designate Type A behavior pattern as a *possible or probable independent CHD risk factor, but not yet an unequivocally established major risk factor.*

Is Type A Behavior the Key Life-Style Trait Responsible for the Coronary Epidemic in the "Western" Industrialized Countries?

Given the foregoing assessment, it is arguable that there is no need to deal with this second question; it is rendered moot. Nonetheless, it needs to be discussed, since the original developers of the concept of the Type A coronary-prone behavior pattern have time and again, in writings addressed to both the scientific community and the general public, more or less explicitly propounded the thesis that Type A behavior is *the* key factor responsible for the mid–twentieth-century epidemic of premature CHD in the "Western" industrialized countries.[40-42] A recent example is the opening presentation by Dr. R.H. Rosenman at the Forum on Coronary-Prone Behavior.[43] A detailed referenced critique of this statement would convert this article into a lengthy review; however, a brief examination of the main propositions set down by Dr. Rosenman may be useful. He begins with the statement, "In the early 1950's, there was a widespread belief that coronary atherosclerosis was simplistically caused by intimal deposition of cholesterol from the blood and derived from dietary sources."[43] If this statement is meant as an evaluation of "belief" among researchers in the field, then I must respectfully disagree. In the early 1950's, for example, I co-authored a monograph with Dr. Louis N. Katz that reviewed the extant literature on atherosclerosis.[44] In contains major sections on the interplay in atherogenesis between nutritional and other factors, including the secretions of the anterior pituitary, adrenal cortex, and adrenal medulla. It cites, for example, the work of Anitschkow made available in English in 1933, including (among many) experiments in rabbits involving repeated injection of adrenalin, with and without concomitant feeding of cholesterol-fat.[45] The relevant point here is that not only in the 1950's, but also in the 1930's and before, serious investigators of this problem clearly recognized the possibility and the likelihood that multiple factors were involved. A few quotations from Anitschkow are revealing:

> In human patients we have probably to deal with a primary disturbance of the cholesterin metabolism, which may lead to atherosclerosis even if the hypercholesterolemia is less pronounced, provided only that it is of long duration and associated with other injurious factors, of which more later on. The etiology and nature of this metabolic disturbance underlying human atherosclerosis has not yet been cleared up. But on the basis of the experimental results we are certainly justified *in stating that atherosclerosis belongs to the "metabolic diseases," and that cholesterin is the "materia peccans."*[45]

Again, two paragraphs later:

> On the basis of all these experimental results, it may therefore be regarded as definitely established that cholesterin, or rather a disturbance of cholesterin metabolism, is of decisive significance as far as the genesis of atherosclerosis is concerned. But, to say it again, it would be wrong if, on the basis of these experimental results, we were to regard this factor as *of exclusive etiologic significance*. On the contrary, all pertinent observations recorded in these experiments point to the probability that *several factors* contribute to the genesis of atherosclerosis — factors both of a general and of a local nature.[45]

Anitschkow then goes on to discuss some of these other factors — mechanical conditions in the arterial system, especially blood pressure variations and hypertension; general metabolic factors; hormonal influences; local factors; and dietary factors other than cholesterol-fat. He cites his own experiments showing that in cholesterol-fed animals hypertension intensified atherogenesis. He then goes on to make this seminal comment:

Although these experiments have shown that increased blood pressure, or variations of the same, play an important role in the etiology of atherosclerosis, no one has yet been able to produce typical atherosclerotic changes merely by increasing the blood pressure *without cholesterin feeding* (see above). On the other hand, *cholesterin feeding is in itself* alone sufficient to produce very pronounced atherosclerotic changes in experimental rabbits. We are therefore justified in regarding this etiologic factor (the increased cholesterol content of the organism) as the *exciting cause* of the disease. The increased blood pressure rather plays the part of a *predisposing cause* inasmuch as it furthers the entrance of the lipids into the arterial wall and their deposition in the intima.[45]

This is indeed a modern formulation! (The contemporary terminology would be *primary* or *essential* cause and *secondary* or *adjuvant* cause.)

Other major reviews document the non-simplistic approaches to the atherosclerosis problem extant at mid-century, such as that by Hueper in 1944–45, for example, which included, by the way, a section on "psychic strain."[46]

The argument that in the early 1950's a simplistic view was widespread about the etiology of atherosclerosis is ill-founded. Asserting it serves no scientific purpose and brings no scientific credit to the founders of the Type A-B concept. Their original contribution is clear without it, especially if it is ultimately confirmed in full. They have no need to put forth such a distortion and should drop it.

In the second paragraph of his presentation, Dr. Rosenman makes three broad assertions. Two are crucial to the issue of whether Type A behavior is *the* key life-style trait causing the coronary epidemic and, hence, must be briefly discussed here.

During the next several years, we found that the blood level of cholesterol is not regulated by the input of cholesterol from either endogenous sources or from the diet, but primarily by its rate of egress from the plasma.[43]

On its face, this statement is at best ambiguous and misleading. In regard to *groups*, it is patently incorrect. The mean level of serum cholesterol of populations is unquestionably regulated — and critically regulated — by the mean level of cholesterol in the habitual diet, as well as by the level of saturated and polyunsaturated fatty acids, the calorie balance, and probably by other nutritional factors (e.g., pectins). This is crystal clear from both international and intranational comparisons of populations (e.g., within the U.S.A., vegetarians vs. omnivores); from the results of metabolic ward studies (e.g., by the research groups headed by Connor, Hegsted, Keys, and Mattson); and from the findings of intervention studies in institutionalized and free-living groups (e.g., the Finnish and Minnesota mental hospital studies, the Los Angeles Veterans Administration domiciliary facility study, the Chicago Coronary Prevention Evaluation Program, the Oslo diet studies, the National Diet-Heart Study, and the Multiple Risk Factor Intervention Trial.[4, 5, 14, 16, 17, 47] It is further confirmed by experimental research in animals, including investigations in nonhuman primates. As to *individuals*, it is clear that habitual dietary lipid intake is one among a set of factors regulating serum cholesterol level. It is not the sole factor, as is evident from metabolic ward experience, in which with diets of identical composition fed under isocaloric conditions to healthy men of similar age, intra-individual differences in serum cholesterol are sizable (e.g., standard deviations of the group mean of about 30 to 35 mg/dl). But when diet change is effected, e.g., from a diet of U.S. lipid composition to one of Italian or Japanese composition, virtually all people experience a decrease in serum cholesterol, indicating the role of dietary lipid in regulation. Under these varying circumstances, individuals tend to retain their position in the distribution around the group mean. These intra-individual differences reflect endogenous metabolic regulatory mechanisms, interacting with the exogenous (dietary) factor. Undoubtedly, these endogenous mechanisms, not yet well delineated with regard to their specific pathways, are under polygenic influence. Whether behavior pattern also plays a long-term role in the stable differences among people is not clear, although the weight of the evidence currently available indicates a negative answer to this question (see the discussion above on Type A-B behavior and serum cholesterol level). (Evidence is available indicating that short-term intense Type A behavior may induce acute rises in serum cholesterol.) In any case, *both for individuals and groups, dietary lipid composition, including level of cholesterol intake, is an important component of the regulation of serum cholesterol level.*

The other sweeping statement in the second paragraph of Dr. Rosenman's paper at the Forum on Coronary-Prone Behavior that is highly questionable is the following:

> Finally, we realized that international population comparisons had many faults of methodology, with many exceptions to the relationship between dietary fat, blood cholesterol level, and prevalence of CHD set forth by Keys and others.[43]

Since no specifics whatsoever are given, it is difficult to come to grips with this evaluation. What "faults of methodology," in what studies? In general, four types of international comparisons have been reported in the literature. First, there are the analyses of data on foods and nutrients available for consumption for sets of countries and their relationship to CHD mortality rates, using data available from the UN Food and Agriculture Organization (FAO) and from the World Health Organization (WHO). Data from at least 10 such studies are now available, and a number appeared in the 1950's, all consistently showing significant positive associations between dietary lipid composition and CHD mortality.[4, 5, 16, 48]

Second, there are the studies involving international comparisons of findings at autopsy, again several in number, with the International Atherosclerosis Project being the most extensive.[4, 5, 14, 16, 17, 47-49] Here again the data have been consistently positive in showing a relationship between dietary lipid composition and the disease, assessed in autopsy studies as severity of coronary atherosclerosis. Several reports were already in the literature on this matter in the 1950's.[5, 48] The International Atherosclerosis Project (IAP) quantified the degree of atherosclerosis of the aorta and coronary arteries in over 31,000 persons from ages 10 to 69 years who died during 1960–65 in 15 communities throughout the world, two of them (New Orleans and Oslo) in higher-income, industrialized nations, the remainder in lower-income, developing countries of Africa, Asia, and Latin America.[49] Marked geographic differences in the occurrence of severe coronary atherosclerosis were recorded. The IAP assessed not only the relationship between dietary fat and severity of atherosclerosis, but also average serum cholesterol levels of the populations under study and severity of atherosclerosis, and showed a significant positive relationship among these.

The third type of international comparison has involved studies of samples of living populations. Again, significant data were available in the 1950's.[5, 48] Again, extensive further information has been accrued in the last 20 years.[4, 5, 14, 16, 17, 47] One of the most important investigations of this kind is the Seven Countries Study under the leadership of Ancel Keys.[50, 51] This prospective international study of 18 population samples in seven countries (Finland, Greece, Italy, Japan, the Netherlands, the United States, and Yugoslavia) dealt with observations of approximately 12,000 men, originally ages 40 to 59 years. Marked population differences in the prevalence and incidence of CHD were recorded; in particular, much higher rates for the northern European and U.S. samples than for the southern European and Japanese. In extensive analyses, significant relationships were demonstrated among baseline mean dietary saturated fat, median serum cholesterol level, and five-year CHD incidence rates.[51] Ten-year data, which have recently become available, confirm these findings.[52] (Dietary cholesterol was not measured in this study.) Blood pressure and smoking levels of the populations were also shown to be predictively related to CHD incidence in multivariate analyses.[51]

The fourth type of international study has involved assessment of the effects of migration. Again, data were available in the 1950's, e.g., on Italians in Naples and Boston, on Israelis of various geographic origins, and on people of Japanese ancestry in Japan and the United States.[5, 48] Probably the most comprehensive investigation of this type is the Ni-Hon-San study, involving sizable populations of middle-aged men of Japanese ethnicity in Japan, Hawaii, and the San Francisco Bay area.[53–59] The Japanese in Japan were found to differ markedly from the Japanese-Americans in Hawaii and San Francisco in dietary habits, with conspicuously lower levels of total fat and saturated fat intake for the former, and a lower mean level of cholesterol and sugar intake as well. The Japanese men were also significantly less obese than the Japanese-Americans. Correspondingly, serum cholesterol levels were markedly different, i.e., means of 181, 218, and 228 mg/dl, respectively, for the three samples, and a prevalence rate of gross hypercholesterolemia ($\geq$260 mg/dl) of only 32/1000 for the Japanese men, compared to 124 and 163/1000, respectively, for the two Japanese-American samples. Mean fasting serum triglycerides varied correspondingly, as did CHD prevalence and mortality rates. The age-adjusted CHD incidence rate of the Japanese men in Japan was less than half that of the Hawaiian Japanese-American men and less than one-third that of the Californian Japanese-Americans. Multivariate logistic analyses revealed serum cholesterol to be significantly related to CHD incidence as an independent risk factor (along with blood pressure) for the two populations reported to date, i.e., the Japanese men in Japan and the Hawaiian Japanese-Americans.

Again, this is not to infer that high dietary cholesterol–saturated fat is the sole factor influencing CHD incidence and mortality, or even the sole dietary factor. Nor is it to infer that the influence of diet on serum cholesterol of populations is the sole mechanism whereby habitual nutritional patterns influence CHD (e.g., calorie imbalance, high salt intake, and heavy alcohol consumption are almost certainly important, too; low complex carbohydrate intake may also be; and high animal-protein intake needs further evaluation). Nor is it to infer that "rich" diet is the sole significant life-style factor or high serum cholesterol the sole significant personal trait. Clearly, both cigarette smoking and high blood pressure have repeatedly been shown to be massively implicated *when the essential nutritional-metabolic prerequisites are operative in the population*. And the data from the Ni-Hon-San study also indicate that sociocultural and psychosocial factors also play a role under this critical circumstance.[60]

The main point, given Dr. Rosenman's sweeping deprecation of the international epidemiologic research, is that a wide range of methodologic approaches, used in scores of international studies of the four cited types, all demonstrate positive significant relationships among dietary lipid composition, serum cholesterol level, and CHD incidence-mortality rates of populations. The findings of these investigations constitute one of the several sets of data demonstrating that "rich" diet is a primary causative factor among the constellation of modern life-styles producing the coronary epidemic in the "Western" industrialized countries.

As to the matter of "exceptions," if by this Dr. Rosenman means that not every population falls exactly on the line best fitting the significant relationship for a group of populations, that is an expected finding. The reasons for this are elementary. First of all, there is the matter of characterizing a population only once, at a given point in time, in regard to such complex, dynamic, independent variables as dietary pattern and serum cholesterol level. Clearly, this is by no means an exhaustive assessment of these two key variables and their operation in populations over a lifetime. It is also evident that different populations have had different experiences over these decades of the twentieth century in regard to these variables — for example, marked differences in the effects of World War II and the post-War years;[4, 5, 16, 47, 48] hence, it is all the more remarkable that positive significant correlations are recorded over and over again by a variety of research methodologies. Furthermore, it is generally agreed that the disease is multifactorial in etiology; hence no one-to-one relationship can be expected between any one etiologic factor and CHD rates. In terms of life-styles, both habitual dietary habits and patterns of use of cigarettes are definitely involved, and sedentary life-styles and behavior patterns are probably playing a role as well. Inevitably, therefore, a one-to-one relationship between any single one of these traits and CHD incidence rates could be expected only if all of them were perfectly intercorrelated. While evidence is available indicating some intercorrelation among them, reflecting the fact that each trait is in turn correlated to a degree with national levels of affluence (as reflected by per capita national income), these associations are far from one-to-one. For example, in a recent analysis of 20 economically more developed countries, using data for 1954–65, saturated fatty acids available per person for consumption and tobacco use per person correlated significantly at the level of 0.656; dietary cholesterol with tobacco at 0.725.[5] Similar significant correlations, but also a good deal less than 1.000, are also demonstrable for groups of countries between other income-related variables, e.g., between dietary variables and indices probably reflecting level of habitual physical activity (for example, motor cars per 100 persons). Thus, several factors all related to socioeconomic development are significantly intercorrelated, but by no means at the 1.000 level. Therefore, evaluation of any single factor and its relationship to CHD is bound not to show a perfect association, i.e., the countries will not fall exactly on the curve (linear or curvilinear) representing the significant relationship between the two. Some countries may even be quite exceptional in departing from the curve of a univariate relationship, even if the data are entirely valid — as they may well not be, even at any one point in time, let alone as reflections of decades of experience. Therefore, the real issue is not of a one-to-one or perfect relationship between any one of these factors and CHD incidence, but whether or not there is a significant, independent association. Massive amounts of data demonstrate that the answer in that regard is clearly yes.

As to certain exotic, isolated populations at times cited as meaningful exceptions (e.g., the Masai in East Africa and the Eskimos), a thorough discussion of this matter, which is beyond the scope of this paper, has been presented previously.[16] In brief, it is not at all clear that any such truly exceptional populations have indeed been identified. If they *were* actually identified, their exceptional status is scientifically explicable without any need to regard it as a refutation of sound etiologic inferences based on masses of data throughout the world, further supported by evidence from metabolic ward and other clinical investigations and by animal experimental findings, all showing a strong independent relationship among habitual dietary lipid composition, serum cholesterol level, and CHD risk.

Clearly, any attempt to dismiss the extensive findings on this matter amassed by international epidemiologic research on grounds of either "faults of methodology" and/or "exceptions" is unwarranted.

Dr. Rosenman begins the third paragraph of his presentation with the statement,

> It was apparent that although coronary atherosclerosis had always occurred in man, the clinical incidence of CHD was rather rare until the second or third decade of the 20th century.[43]

Again, it is difficult to come to grips briefly with such a sweeping generalization. What literally is meant by "always"? Nothing is really known about the occurrence of atherosclerosis in man over the hundreds of thousands of years of human evolution prior to the ancient Egyptians. Studies of mummies indicate that aortic atherosclerosis (severity and clinical significance? concomitant coronary lesions?) was present in upper-class Egyptians.[48] There are also reports in the literature of the ancient world suggesting that sudden death of the type occurring in persons with CHD may have transpired.[5] Beyond that, nothing can be said about prehistoric or ancient man, or medieval man for that matter, with regard to CHD. The earliest materials of any scope are from the most recent centuries, and they permit no quantitative statement about trends of incidence of CHD in populations over these centuries and no quantitative statement about trends of age-sex-specific prevalence of the crucial underlying pathologic process, *severe* coronary atherosclerosis. The only real time lines available are for the CHD mortality rates for a handful of industrialized countries, and these go back only to about 1940, not to the second and third decades of this century.[61] Further inferences as to time trends earlier in this century are derived from evaluating mortality data for the broad category of all cardiovascular diseases. Given this necessary qualification of the foregoing sweeping generalization, it can be stated that evidence *is* available indicating increased mortality rates for premature CHD in the industrialized countries (including the United States) in this century.[48, 61] It is this phenomenon that Dr. Rosenman then focuses on in inferring that the emergence of Type A behavior — "modern 'stress' factors" — is of key importance in the causation of the CHD epidemic.

In general, Dr. Rosenman's line of reasoning is sound on this difficult problem of the relationship between time trends of life-style and time trends of CHD incidence, a problem that is difficult essentially because of the paucity of data on time trends for the multiple factors of concern.[48] He properly notes that any true increase in incidence of this mass disease in the population must be a by-product of changes in living habits. "In the middle 1950's we searched for factors that had really changed in the twentieth century environment and that might causally relate to the modern epidemic."[43] He then argues, "We were aware that the lowest rates of CHD were observed in farming communities in the U.S.A. and in Great Britain, despite their habitual exposure to high saturated fat intakes."[43] The implication is clear: marked differences between urban and rural populations in CHD, despite similar or like diets of presumably atherogenic composition, demonstrating that diet is not a key factor; as the nation has evolved from predominantly rural to predominantly urban, the proportion of the population manifesting Type A behavior has increased substantially, and this is the main factor — or does Dr. Rosenman mean to imply the sole factor? — accounting for the coronary epidemic. No mention is made of data on prevalence rates of Type A behavior in rural and urban Americans now, or 20 or 50 or 100 years ago. Do any such exist? But even if the reasonable impression were accepted that the prevalence rate of Type A behavior is lower (markedly lower?) in rural than urban American populations, the facts about CHD in rural vs. urban Americans do not lend much weight to this line of reasoning. In actuality, available data indicate that rural-urban CHD differences are small. Thus, for the years 1959–61, the age-adjusted CHD mortality rate for white males residing in metropolitan counties with a central city was 16 per cent higher than for white males residing in non-metropolitan counties. The findings were similar with regard to age-specific rates, e.g., for white males aged 45 to 54 and 55 to 64 and for the other three major sex-color strata of the U.S. population.[61] This is hardly impressive support for the argument.

In the next sentences of the same paragraph, Dr. Rosenman departs from a discussion of populations and time trends for populations to deal with individuals. He reports the following observations:

... Most coronary patients had dietary habits that were the same as or were similar to individuals with good longevity who never exhibited clinical disease.
 ... There was indeed little relationship in most individuals between dietary fat intake and their blood cholesterol level.

In a number of such individuals, we also observed wide fluctuations of serum cholesterol, occasionally over short periods of time, that clearly could not be ascribed to changes in diet.[43]

From these three observations about contemporary patients, Dr. Rosenman drew the following inference: "This led us to believe that the diet was not the *sine qua non* of the epidemic."[43]

Here the problem is one of fallacious reasoning. The fact that at any given age people eating similarly may or may not have CHD, may or may not have hypercholesterolemia, in no way refutes the conclusion that a certain habitual pattern of diet is a *sine qua non* for the epidemic occurrence of CHD. For almost every disease, there are no one-to-one relationships between etiologic agents and disease occurrence. For example, it is now fully appreciated that millions of people are exposed to the polio virus, with only a small percentage, in the pre-immunization era, developing paralytic polio. Similarly, millions of children are infected repeatedly by group A beta-hemolytic streptococcal infection, but only a few get rheumatic fever; and only a proportion of the victims of rheumatic fever get rheumatic heart disease. In neither case is this lack of a one-to-one relationship a valid basis for concluding that the agent is not etiologically related to the disease. All that such findings prove — and the same applies to the relationship among dietary lipid, serum cholesterol, and CHD — is that in most diseases the relationship between cause and effect is not simple and one-to-one, i.e., different individuals react in different ways, over a broad spectrum, to the causative agent. Such findings do not permit dismissal of the role of the causative agent; rather, they only indicate that simple unifactorial concepts of causation are invalid. Clearly, as discussed above, diet does indeed influence serum cholesterol, both for populations overall and, necessarily, for individuals within populations, but it is not the only factor influencing serum cholesterol (as further indicated by studies on acute fluctuations of serum cholesterol with acute changes in behavior). As to the failure in some studies to find a correlation of dietary lipid composition and serum cholesterol in *individuals*, this is chiefly a result of methodologic limitations of the published reports, as has recently been set down in detail elsewhere.[4, 5, 62]

As to the main thrust of the argument on this issue, the implication that diet changes in the twentieth century cannot account for the emergence of epidemic premature CHD, I have the following comment on that complex issue: Only limited statistical data are available for populations. For example, for the United States, long-term time trend data are extant from the United States Department of Agriculture only for the period 1909 to the present, and only on foods available for consumption per capita per year for the whole population, without data by age, sex, race, ethnicity, income, region, and so on. But these data do in fact show important changes in the twentieth century, changes that added up to a marked increase in the percentage of calories from total fat and saturated fat and in dietary cholesterol from the period 1909–13 to the mid-century years (Table 4 and Fig. 1).[63, 64] Total fat rose from about 32 to 42 per cent of calories (+23.8%), saturated fat increased by a similar percentage, and dietary cholesterol by about 13 per cent.

The sources of these increases are generally evident from Table 4, but a few words of explanation may be helpful. First, there is the marked increase in

Table 4. *The Changing United States Diet, 1909–1976**

FOOD ITEM, PER PERSON PER YEAR	YEAR								
	1909–13	1925–29	1935–39	1947–49	1957–59	1965	1970	1975	1976
Meat	141	129	120	141	144	148	165	158	165
Poultry	18	17	16	22	34	41	49	49	53
Fish	13	14	13	13	13	14	15	15	15
Meat, Poultry, Fish	172	159	149	176	192	203	228	222	233
Eggs	37	40	36	47	45	40	40	35	35
Dairy Products, Excluding Butter△	177	191	202	236	239	235	226	216	222
Butter	18	18	17	11	8	6	5	5	4
All Fats and Oils△△	41	48	49	46	49	51	56	57	59
Citrus, Fresh	17	31	47	52	33	28	28	28	29
Citrus, Processed	0	#	2	14	25	23	35	46	47
Other Fruits, Melons, Fresh	151	139	127	112	87	77	77	74	78
Other Fruits, Melons Processed	8	18	23	30	37	38	39	34	34
All Fruits, Melons△△△	176	188	199	208	182	166	178	181	188
Vegetables									
Dark Green, Yellow, Fresh	14	24	27	27	19	17	17	18	18
Dark Green, Yellow, Processed	#	1	2	4	6	6	7	7	7
Other, Including Tomatoes, Fresh	172	166	171	157	130	124	124	125	127

Other, Including Tomatoes, Processed	17	25	31	43	54	60	64	66	62
Total	203	217	231	232	209	206	212	217	213
Potatoes									
White, fresh	182	142	128	111	88	68	59	58	54
White, Processed	#	#	#	#	6	12	19	22	22
Sweet, Fresh	23	20	19	12	7	5	4	4	4
Sweet, Processed	#	#	#	#	1	1	1	2	2
Total	205	162	147	123	101	86	83	84	80
Dry Beans, Peas, Nuts, Soy Products	16	17	19	17	17	16	16	18	18
Flour and Cereal Products	291	237	204	171	148	144	141	139	140
Sugar and Other Sweeteners	89	119	110	110	106	112	120	114	119
Miscellaneous	10	13	16	19	15	15	14	12	12

All quantities are in pounds except for dairy products, which are in quarts; 1976 data are preliminary.
△Milk equivalent based on calcium content.
△△Includes butter.
#0.05 lb.

*From Page L, and Friend B: The changing United States diet. BioScience 28:192–197, 1978; and Select Committee on Nutrition and Human Needs, United States Senate: *Dietary Goals for the United States.* Washington, DC, US Government Printing Office, February, 1977.

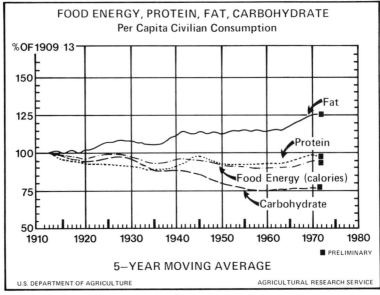

Figure 1

meat and poultry consumption, especially in the years after the Great Depression and World War II, paced by mounting beef use, up from 55 lbs/person/year available for consumption in 1940 to 117 in 1974 (+112.7%).[4, 5, 47] Here the transformation of beef production must also be kept in mind, i.e., the development in recent decades of the feedlot, resulting in marbled, high-fat

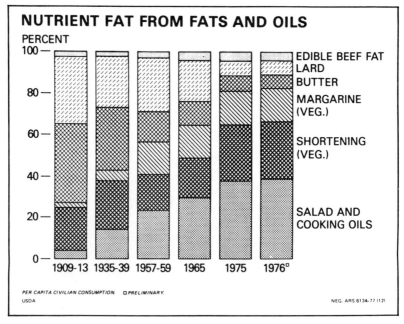

Figure 2

beef, a major determinant of both saturated fat and cholesterol intake. Next, there is the egg trend, significantly correlated with total cholesterol intake, given the high cholesterol content of egg yolk, with egg intake up by 21 per cent from 1909–13 to 1947–49, then gradually going down again. There is the dairy product trend, with dairy product intake up 33 per cent from 1909–13 to 1947–49. While butter and lard use tended to go steadily and markedly downward in the 1940's, through the 1960's, the use of vegetable margarine and shortening, developed after the invention of the catalytic hydrogenation process earlier in the century, more than made up the difference (Fig. 2).[63] Until very recently, these were exclusively "hard" margarines and shortenings, i.e., high in saturates, not in unsaturates (mono or poly).

These are the major components producing the sizable increases in total fat, saturated fat, and cholesterol intake in the American diet from 1909–13 to the 1950's, the period referred to by Dr. Rosenman. Clearly, the diet had become more atherogenic in terms of its lipid composition. Clearly, too, it was even in 1909–13 far from optimal in that regard (e.g., with about 13 per cent of calories from saturates, about 500 mg/person/day of dietary cholesterol on the average) compared, for example, to southern European or Far Eastern diets (Table 5).[5] But it *is* a fact that the American diet became significantly worse after 1909–13 in lipid composition, and in other respects as well, possibly of significance in terms of the CHD epidemic and its genesis — e.g., the decrease in percentage of calories from carbohydrates (replacement of carbohydrate by fat) (Fig. 1) and the marked change in the *type* of carbohydrates, i.e., the absolute and relative increase in simple sugars and decline in complex carbohydrates from potatoes and grains, a continuation in the twentieth century of a long-term trend beginning in the nineteenth century (Table 4 and Fig. 3).[4, 5, 48, 63–65] For Americans, bread has ceased to be the staff of life. Today, 95 per cent of the domestic grain supply goes not directly for human consumption here, but to animals (the feedlot phenomenon), to come to us as marbled animal products.[47, 66]

Much more could be said about the transformation in diet in the U.S. and other industrialized countries from the late nineteenth century on as a result of the mechanical and chemical revolutions of this era, and many other data sets and references could be cited, and have been elsewhere.[5, 16, 47, 48] Suffice it to note that for the masses of the populations of the industrialized nations, i.e., their poorer economic classes, regular availability of sizable amounts of animal products — "living off the fat of the land" — is a historically new and unprecedented phenomenon (as yet unknown to the great majority of mankind in Africa, Asia, and Latin America). *Only among populations experiencing this change is there epidemic premature CHD.* Correspondingly, only such a change, i.e., a shift to a diet high in cholesterol and satured fat, can produce severe atherosclerosis in experimental animals, including nonhuman primates.[4, 5, 14, 16, 44, 47, 48] Hypertension, cigarette chemicals, and psychological stresses by themselves do not. Hence, it is sound to designate "rich" diet as an essential and primary cause of the epidemic, its *sine qua non.* Dr. Rosenman has fallaciously dismissed this conclusion on totally inadequate grounds.

Lest there be misunderstanding, I hasten to add that "rich" diet is a *necessary but not sufficient* cause for the CHD epidemic. Thus, many persons

Table 5a. *Sources of Calories, Foods Available for Consumption per Person per Day, U.S.A., Italy, Japan, 1954–65* [*]

VARIABLE	CALORIES AND PER CENT OF TOTAL CALORIES/PERSON/DAY					
	U.S.A.		Italy		Japan	
Total Calories	3127	100.0[△]	2697	100.0	2226	100.0
Butter	69	2.2	34	1.3	0	0.0
Dairy Products (including butter)	478	15.3	214	7.9	39	1.8
Eggs	78	2.5	36	1.3	24	1.0
Meats, Poultry	573	18.3	134	5.0	19	0.9
Dairy, Eggs, Meats, Poultry	1129	36.1	384	14.2	82	3.7
Fish, Shellfish	23	0.7	23	0.8	81	3.6
Fruits, Non-starchy Vegetables	190	6.1	193	7.2	130	5.8
Grains, Starchy Vegetables	790	25.3	1484	55.0	1652	74.2
Fruits, Non-starchy Vegetables, Grains, Starchy Vegetables	980	31.3	1677	62.2	1782	80.1
Oils, Nuts	168	5.4	320	11.9	97	4.4
Sugar, Syrup	505	16.1	222	8.2	160	7.2

[△]Per cent of total calories.

[*]From Stamler J: Population studies. *In* Levy RI, Rifkind BM, Dennis BH, and Ernst ND (eds): *Nutrition, Lipids and Coronary Heart Disease — A Global View.* New York, Raven Press, 1979, pp 25–88.

Table 5b. *Nutrients Available for Consumption per Person per Day, U.S.A., Italy, Japan, 1954–65* [*]

VARIABLE	NUTRIENTS PER PERSON PER DAY					
	U.S.A.		Italy		Japan	
Total Calories	3127	100.0[△]	2697	100.0	2226	100.0
Total Protein, gm.	94	12.0	79	11.7	68	12.2
Animal Protein, gm.	68	8.7	27	4.0	16	2.9
Total Carbohydrate, gm.	372	47.6	423	62.7	425	76.4
Total Fat, gm.	135	38.9	77	25.7	25	10.1
Saturated Fatty Acids, gm.	49	14.1	21	7.0	5	2.0
Monounsaturated Fatty Acids, gm.	54	15.5	33	11.0	6	2.4
Polyunsaturated Fatty Acids, gm.	16	4.6	13	4.3	7	2.8
Cholesterol, mg.	586	– –	246	– –	129	– –
Calcium, mg.	998	– –	573	– –	377	– –
Iron, mg.	17	– –	18	– –	19	– –
Niacin, mg.	21	– –	20	– –	20	– –
Riboflavin, mg.	2.7	– –	2.0	– –	0.8	– –
Thiamine, mg.	1.9	– –	2.2	– –	2.1	– –
Ascorbic Acid, mg.	125	– –	127	– –	100	– –

[△]Per cent of total calories.

[*]From Stamler J: Population studies. *In* Levy RI, Rifkind BM, Dennis BH, and Ernst ND (eds): *Nutrition, Lipids and Coronary Heart Disease — A Global View.* New York, Raven Press, 1979, pp 25–88.

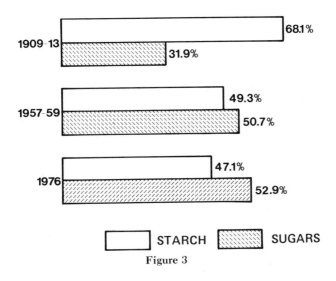

CARBOHYDRATE FROM STARCH AND SUGARS

1909-13 68.1% 31.9%

1957-59 49.3% 50.7%

1976 47.1% 52.9%

STARCH   SUGARS

Figure 3

escape its potential consequences, and many others are victimized only when other factors (e.g., cigarette use) are concurrently at work. Similarly, these changes in the diet in the U.S. in the twentieth century are *by themselves* probably insufficient in degree to account for the sharp increase in male death rates from CHD, for example, in the 1940's.[4, 5, 47, 61, 67]

This brings us to the next points in Dr. Rosenman's argument implying that Type A behavior is the key factor behind the modern CHD epidemic:

> But again it became clear to us that physical activity level was not the *sine qua non* of the present epidemic. Smoking has increased and clearly is related to the increased CHD incidence, but again we could not find it to be a major culprit. Finally, we were unable to find evidence of any significant increase in prevalence either of hypertension or hypercholesteremia that might explain what happened.[43]

Let us explore these arguments briefly. While a considerable body of evidence exists implicating sedentary life style as a coronary risk factor, it is indeed true that there are inconsistencies in the data, both from intra-U.S. and international studies. Therefore, in my judgment, this common aspect of contemporary life-style in the "Western" industrialized countries must be regarded as a possible or probable, but not a definitely established, major risk factor. But if the focus is on trends in the twentieth century, as Dr. Rosenman's is, then the change in the level of habitual physical activity that the populations of the industrialized countries have undergone, due both to replacement of human by nonhuman energy at work and emergence of the automobile-TV sedentary culture at leisure, must be recognized as an unprecedented modern phenomenon, unique in man's course on earth. Its possible or probable role as a contributory cause of the CHD epidemic cannot be readily dismissed, even though it is not its *sine qua non*.

As to the twentieth-century habit of cigarette smoking, in the U.S. it has been a mass phenomenon only since World War I (Fig. 4),[68] and in several other industrialized countries only since World War II.[47] On what grounds does Dr. Rosenman declare the upward spiral of cigarette use *not* to be "a major culprit"? He gives no reasons. As the data in Tables 1 to 3 clearly show, the Western Collaborative Group Study found cigarette use to be a powerful independent risk factor for CHD, as has study after study of populations in "Western" industrialized countries where the nutritional-hygienic prerequisites exist for large-scale occurrence of premature severe coronary atherosclerosis. Why then does Dr. Rosenman reject the generally held conclusion that cigarette smoking is a key contributory cause of the coronary epidemic, an established major risk factor? Is it not likely that the sharp rise in CHD mortality rates in the 1940's reflects the emergence into middle age of the generation of men who took up smoking around World War I?

As to inability " . . . to find evidence of any significant increase in prevalence either of hypertension or hypercholesterolemia that might explain what happened,"[43] I am unaware of any data on trends of hypertension and hypercholesterolemia over the decades prior to the 1950's in the U.S. population or any other population. Can Dr. Rosenman cite data one way or another on this intriguing question? Or is not the fact of the matter that inability to find any significant increase in prevalence merely reflected lack of any data, so that Dr. Rosenman's formulation, implying no increase, is a bit misleading? Once again, it is necessary to state: The insoluble problem of the difficulty of getting good data sets to evaluate long-term trends must not be ignored.

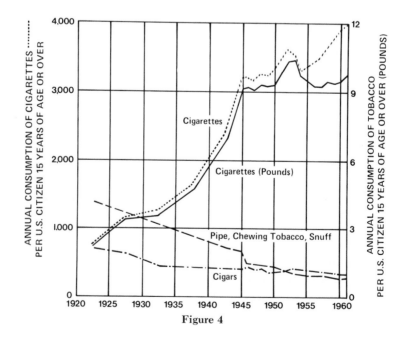

Figure 4

There is very recent evidence from several population studies of a downturn in the 1970's in mean serum cholesterol levels of U.S. adults, paralleling decreases (however modest) in intake of dietary cholesterol and saturated fat and increases in intake of polyunsaturated fats.[5] From these data, it may be inferred by extrapolation backward (but it cannot be proved) that mean serum cholesterol levels of the population rose from 1909–13 levels to those recorded in the 1950's, just as it may be inferred (but cannot be proved) that the major decline in mortality rates from premature CHD over the 1968–76 period may be a result, at least in part, of the noted changes in diet and serum cholesterol, the recent decreases in cigarette use, and the improved control of hypertension.[4, 5, 47, 67, 69] Beyond that, little can be said. Dr. Rosenman is wrong in his implication concerning these major risk factors.

After his discussion of the trend data, Dr. Rosenman then presents this sweeping statement:

> During the 1950's, it also became clear to us that many population groups were being studied who exhibited a high fat diet, a lack of adequate physical activity, and a significant prevalence of hypertension and smoking, but still exhibited low serum cholesterol and a relative absence of CHD.[43]

Again, there is no elaboration. By the vague term "high fat diet" does Dr. Rosenman mean a habitual eating pattern high in cholesterol and saturated fat (rather than high in vegetable oil, e.g., olive oil, as in Greece)? If so, and this is a key point, then I respectfully request a list of "the many population groups" eating such a diet who have "low serum cholesterol," are inactive, and who have "a significant prevalence of hypertension and smoking" (cigarette smoking?)—and "a relative absence of CHD" (definition?). I am hard-put to name even *one* such population.

Among the several issues Dr. Rosenman addresses in this key summary paper, he fails to note one of relevance. As already stated, he correctly infers that the modern CHD epidemic in the industrialized countries is almost certainly caused by multiple factors that are new in the twentieth-century environment. He also infers that the Type A behavior pattern is one of these, i.e., a pattern emerging as widely prevalent in modern urban industrialized populations. From this he further infers, logically, that if Type A behavior is *a* key or *the* key factor responsible for the modern CHD epidemic (he never says outright what his concept is, *a* or *the* key factor?), CHD rates should be much lower in rural than urban populations. And he states this is indeed the case in the U.S., an assertion noted above to be at variance with available data.

But there is a further inference, not at all discussed by Dr. Rosenman, concerning social classes. Is it not reasonable to expect Type A behavior to be more prevalent among "upper"-class, white-collar entrepreneurs, executives, managers, professionals, and so on compared to "lower"-class, blue-collar, skilled, semi-skilled, and unskilled laborers? In fact, available data bear out this expectation, as shown, for example, in the highly significant independent correlations ($p < 0.001$) between socioeconomic status score (SES) and Type A behavior score (JAS) in all four age-sex groups of the Chicago Heart Association Detection Project in Industry cohort.[23] If Type A behavior is of key importance in the genesis of epidemic CHD, then the higher SES strata of the U.S.

population should have significantly higher CHD rates, unless other countervailing factors (diet, smoking, exercise?) are at work. The available data do not indicate higher rates for the higher SES strata. If anything, they indicate slightly lower rates, as shown, for example in the DuPont, Peoples Gas Co., and Western Electric Co. studies.[16] Certainly this apparent paradox must be considered further in assessing the role of Type A behavior in the etiology of CHD.

With this in mind, it is relevant to cite the concluding statement in the paragraph from which the last citation was made: "Consequently, we wondered if modern 'stress' factors could be playing some pathogenetic role."[43] This is an intriguing formulation, of considerable importance, reaching directly to the issue under discussion here. Everything Dr. Rosenman set down up to that point implies that other aspects of life style and other traits — "rich" diet, cigarette smoking, sedentary habit, hypertension, and hypercholesterolemia — are *not* key factors in the modern epidemic, i.e., they are at most playing a secondary role (they are not the "*sine qua non*," not "major culprits"). But this last formulation has a different implication, possibly — that is, if the concept is of "modern 'stress' factors playing *some* pathogenetic role" in concert with and complementary to "rich" diet as a primary and necessary cause, cigarette smoking as a major secondary cause, sedentary habit as a possible additional secondary cause, then there is no issue. Will Dr. Rosenman please identify his real position on this cardinal matter?

The issue, please note, is not "just" a matter of theory, no mere esoteric, ivory-tower debate among researchers on Olympus. At stake are very practical matters of public policy for preventing and controlling the CHD epidemic, i.e., the soundness of recommendations made repeatedly by expert groups over the last two decades, in the United States and other countries, urging the people to improve their eating, drinking, and exercise habits, to be non-smokers, and to be aware of and act on hypertensive status.[4, 5, 14, 16, 17, 19, 47, 48] It is this crucial public-health and medical-care issue that makes it essential to rebut scientifically erroneous presentations implying that Type A behavior is *the* key factor in the modern coronary epidemic and that "rich" diet, hypercholesterolemia, hypertension, cigarette smoking, and sedentary habit are of secondary or minor importance.

Again, the comment is appropriate that the founders of the Type A concept have a firm foundation of scientific contribution to stand on. They should not undermine it by false implications.

Summary

1. The available data are sufficient to characterize the Type A behavior pattern as a possible or probable risk factor for epidemic CHD, but they are not yet sufficient to meet all the criteria necessary to designate it as a fully established major risk factor along with "rich" diet, hypercholesterolemia, hypertension, and cigarette smoking.

2. Any implication that Type A behavior is *the* key factor in the genesis of the modern CHD epidemic is unfounded in data and fallacious in reasoning.

References

1. Rosenman R: The role of behavior patterns and neurogenic factors in the pathogenesis of coronary heart disease. *In* Eliot RS (ed): *Stress and the Heart.* Mt. Kisco, NY, Futura Publishing Co, 1974, pp 123–141.

2. Jenkins CD: Psychologic and social risk factors for coronary disease. N Engl J Med 294:987–994 and 1033–1038, 1976.

3. Dembrowski TM (ed), Feinleib M, Haynes SG, Shields JL, and Weiss SM (assoc eds): Proceedings of the Forum on Coronary-Prone Behavior. Department of Health, Education, and Welfare, Public Health Service, National Institutes of Health, DHEW Publication No (NIH) 78–1451, Bethesda, Md, 1978.

4. Stamler J: Lifestyles, risk factors, proof and public policy. George Lyman Duff Memorial Lecture. Circulation 58:3–19, 1978.

5. Stamler J: Population studies. *In* Levy RI, Rifkind BM, Dennis BH, and Ernst ND (eds): *Nutrition, Lipids and Coronary Heart Disease — A Global View.* New York, Raven Press, 1979, pp 25–88.

6. Smoking and Health: Report of the Advisory Committee to the Surgeon General of the Public Health Service, U.S. Department of Health, Education, and Welfare. Public Health Service Publication No 1103, Superintendent of Documents, US Government Printing Office, Washington, DC, 1964.

7. Rosenman RH, Brand RJ, Jenkins D, Friedman M, Straus R, and Wurm M: Coronary heart disease in the Western Collaborative Group Study: Final follow-up experience of 8½ years. JAMA 233:872–877, 1975.

8. Rosenman RH, Brand RJ, Sholtz RI, and Friedman M: Multivariate prediction of coronary heart disease during 8.5-year follow-up in the Western Collaborative Group Study. Am J Cardiol 37:903–910, 1976.

9. Brand RJ, Rosenman RH, Sholtz RI, and Friedman M: Multivariate prediction of coronary heart disease in the Western Collaborative Group Study compared to the findings of the Framingham Study. Circulation 53:348–355, 1976.

10. Haynes SG, Levine S, Scotch N, Feinleib M, and Kannel WB: The relationship of psychosocial factors to coronary heart disease in the Framingham study. I. Methods and risk factors. Am J Epidemiol 107:362–383, 1978.

11. Haynes SG, Feinleib M, Levine S, Scotch N, and Kannel WB: The relationship of psychosocial factors to coronary heart disease in the Framingham study. II. Prevalence of coronary heart disease. Am J Epidemiol 107:384–402, 1978.

12. Haynes SG, Feinleib M, and Kannel WB: Psychosocial factors and CHD incidence in Framingham: Results from an eight-year follow-up study. Abstracts of the 18th Annual Conference on Cardiovascular Epidemiology, March 13–16, 1978, Orlando, Fla. Dallas, Texas, American Heart Association, Abstract #53, 1978.

13. Dembrowski TM (ed), Feinleib M, Haynes SG, Shields JL, and Weiss SM (assoc eds): Proceedings of the Forum on Coronary-Prone Behavior. Department of Health, Education, and Welfare, Public Health Service, National Institutes of Health, DHEW Publication No (NIH) 78–1451, Bethesda, Md, 1978, p. 20.

14. Inter-Society Commission for Heart Disease Resources, Atherosclerosis Study Group, and Epidemiology Study Group: Primary prevention of the atherosclerotic diseases. Circulation 42:A55–A95, 1970.

15. Blackburn H, Chapman JM, Dawber TR, Doyle JT, Epstein FH, Kannel WB, Keys A, Moore FE, Paul O, Stamler J, and Taylor HL: Revised data for 1970 ICHD Report (Letter to the editor). Am Heart J 94:539–540, 1977.

16. Stamler J: *Lectures on Preventive Cardiology.* New York, Grune and Stratton, Inc, 1967.

17. Stamler J, Berkson DM, and Lindberg HA: Risk factors: Their role in the etiology and pathogenesis of the atherosclerotic diseases. *In* Wissler RW, and Geer JC (eds): *Pathogenesis of Atherosclerosis.* Baltimore, Williams and Wilkins Co., 1972, pp 41–119.

18. McGee D, and Gordon T: The Framingham Study — An Epidemiological Investigation of Cardiovascular Disease. Section 31. The results of the Framingham study applied to four other US-based epidemiologic studies of cardiovascular disease. US Department of Health, Education and Welfare, DHEW Publication No (NIH) 76–1083, Washington, DC, April, 1976.

19. Pooling Project Research Group: Relationship of blood pressure, serum cholesterol, smoking habit, relative weight and ECG abnormalities to incidence of major coronary events: Final report of the Pooling Project. J. Chronic Dis 31:201–306, 1978.

20. Rosenman RH, Friedman M, Straus R, Jenkins CD, Zyzanski SJ, and Wurm M: Coronary heart

disease in the Western Collaborative Group Study — A follow-up experience of 4½ years. J Chronic Dis 23:173–190, 1970.

21. Dembrowski TM (ed), Feinleib M, Haynes SG, Shields JL, and Weiss SM (assoc eds): Proceedings of the Forum on Coronary-Prone Behavior. Department of Health, Education, and Welfare, Public Health Service, National Institutes of Health, DHEW Publication No (NIH) 78–1451, Bethesda, Md, 1978, p 22.

22. Jenkins CD, Rosenman RH, and Zyzanski SJ: Prediction of clinical coronary heart disease by a test for coronary-prone behavior pattern. N Engl J Med 290:1271–1275, 1974.

23. Shekelle RB, Schoenberger JA, and Stamler J: Correlates of the JAS Type A behavior pattern score. J Chronic Dis 29:381–394, 1976.

24. Multiple Risk Factor Intervention Trial Research Group: The MRFIT behavior pattern study. I. Study, design, procedures, and reproducibility of behavior pattern judgements. J Chronic Dis 32:293–305, 1979.

25. Kornitzer M, DeBacker G, Dramaix M, and Thilly C: Modification of cardiovascular risk in a controlled multifactorial prevention trial. Circulation 56 (Suppl III):III-114, 1977.

26. Kittel F, Kornitzer M, Zyzanski SJ, Jenkins CD, Rustin RM, and Degre C: Two methods of assessing the Type A coronary-prone behavior pattern in Belgium. J Chronic Dis 31:147–155, 1978.

27. Dembrowski TM (ed), Feinleib M, Haynes SG, Shields JL, and Weiss SM (assoc eds): Proceedings of the Forum on Coronary-Prone Behavior. Department of Health, Education, and Welfare, Public Health Service, National Institutes of Health, DHEW Publication No (NIH) 78–1451, Bethesda, Md, 1978, p 23.

28. Friedman M, Rosenman RH, Straus R, Wurm M, and Kositchek R: The relationship of behavior pattern A to the state of coronary vasculature — a study of fifty-one autopsy subjects. Am J Med 44:525–537, 1968.

29. Zyzanski SJ, Jenkins CD, Ryan TJ, Flessas A, and Everist M: Psychological correlates of coronary angiographic findings. Arch Intern Med 136:1234–1237, 1976.

30. Perosio AM, et al: Evolution of chronic coronary heart disease (Sp). La Prensa Med Argentina 64(2):27–32, 1977.

31. Frank KA, Heller SS, Kornfeld DS, Sporn AA, and Weiss MB: Type A behavior pattern and coronary angiographic findings. JAMA, 240:761–763, 1978.

32. Blumenthal JA, Williams RB Jr, Kong Y, Schanberg SM, and Thompson LW: Type A behavior pattern and coronary atherosclerosis. Circulation 58:634–639, 1978.

33. Jenkins D: Personal communication.

34. Dimsdale JE, Hackett TP, Block PC, Hutter AM Jr, and Catanzano DM: Influence of behavior pattern on coronary artery disease. J Psychosom Res, in press.

35. Dembrowski TM (ed), Feinleib M, Haynes SG, Shields JL, and Weiss SM (assoc eds): Proceedings of the Forum on Coronary-Prone Behavior. Department of Health, Education, and Welfare, Public Health Service, National Institutes of Health, DHEW Publication No (NIH) 78–1451, Bethesda, Md, 1978, p. 157.

36. Dembrowski TM (ed), Feinleib M, Haynes SG, Shields JL, and Weiss SM (assoc eds): Proceedings of the Forum on Coronary-Prone Behavior. Department of Health, Education, and Welfare, Public Health Service, National Institutes of Health, DHEW Publication No (NIH) 78–1451, Bethesda, Md, 1978, p. 158.

37. Simpson MT, Olewine DA, Jenkins CD, Ramsey FH, Zyzanski SJ, Thomas G, and Hames CG: Exercise-induced catecholamines and platelet aggregation in the coronary-prone behavior pattern. Psychosom Med 36:476–487, 1974.

38. Dembrowski TM (ed), Feinleib M, Haynes SG, Shields JL, and Weiss SM (assoc eds): Proceedings of the Forum on Coronary-Prone Behavior. Department of Health, Education, and Welfare, Public Health Service, National Institutes of Health, DHEW Publication No (NIH) 78–1451, Bethesda, Md, 1978, p 159.

39. Friedman M, Byers SO, Rosenman RH, and Elevitch FR: Coronary-prone individuals (type A behavior pattern) — some biochemical characteristics. JAMA 212:1030–1037, 1970.

40. Friedman M, and Rosenman RH: *Type A Behavior and Your Heart*. New York, Alfred A Knopf, Inc, 1974.

41. Rosenman RH: Type A behavior — pro and con. American Heart Association 2nd Science Writers Forum, Marco Island, Fla, January, 1975. New York, American Heart Association, 1975.

42. Rosenman RH, Stamler J, and Ross RS: Is there anything to heart disease and 'Type A' personality? Medical Opinion 4(4):56–63, 1975.

43. Rosenman RH: History and definition of the Type A coronary-prone behavior pattern. *In* Dembrowski TM (ed), Feinleib M, Haynes SG, Shields JL, and Weiss SM (assoc eds): Proceedings of the Forum on Coronary-Prone Behavior. Department of Health, Educa-

tion, and Welfare, Public Health Service, National Institutes of Health, DHEW Publication No (NIH) 78–1451, Bethesda, Md, 1978, pp 13–17.

44. Katz LN, and Stamler J: *Experimental Atherosclerosis.* Springfield, Ill, Charles C Thomas, Publisher, 1953.

45. Anitschkow N: Experimental arteriosclerosis in animals. *In* Cowdry EV (ed): *Arteriosclerosis.* New York, Macmillan, Inc, 1933, pp 271–322.

46. Hueper WC: Arteriosclerosis. Arch Pathol 38:162, 245, and 350, 1944 and 39:51, 117, and 187, 1945.

47. Stamler J: Introduction to risk factors in coronary artery disease. *In* McIntosh HD (ed): *Baylor College of Medicine Cardiology Series,* Vol 1, Part 3. Northfield, Ill, Medical Communications, Inc, 1978.

48. Katz LN, Stamler J, and Pick R: *Nutrition and Atherosclerosis.* Philadelphia, Lea and Febiger, 1958.

49. McGill HC Jr (ed): *Geographic Pathology of Atherosclerosis.* Baltimore, Williams and Wilkins Co, 1968.

50. Keys A, Aravanis C, Blackburn H, vanBuchem FSP, Buzina R, Djordjevic BS, Dontas AS, Fidanza F, Karvonen MJ, Kimura N, Lekos D, Monti M, Puddu V, and Taylor HL: Epidemiological studies related to coronary heart disease: Characteristics of men aged 40–59 in seven countries. Acta Med Scand, Suppl 460, 1966.

51. Keys A (ed): Coronary heart disease in seven countries. Circulation 41:Suppl 1, 1970.

52. Keys A: Mortality and coronary heart disease in the Mediterranean area. *In* Proceedings of the II International Congress on the Biological Value of Olive Oil. Torremolinos, Spain, 1976, pp 231–286.

53. Tillotson JL, Kato H, Nichaman MZ, Miller DC, Gay ML, Johnson KG, and Rhoads GG: Epidemiology of coronary heart disease and stroke in Japanese men living in Japan, Hawaii, and California: Methodology for comparison for diet. Am J Clin Nutr 26:177–184, 1973.

54. Kato H, Tillotson J, Nichaman MZ, Rhoads GG, and Hamilton HB: Epidemiologic studies of coronary heart disease and stroke in Japanese men living in Japan, Hawaii, and California: Serum lipids and diet. Am J Epidemiol 97:372–385, 1973.

55. Kagan A, Harris BR, Winkelstein W Jr, Johnson KG, Kato H, Syme SL, Rhoads GG, Gay ML, Nichaman MZ, Hamilton HB, and Tillotson J: Epidemiologic studies of coronary heart disease and stroke in Japanese men living in Japan, Hawaii, and California: Demographic, physical, dietary and biochemical characteristics. J Chronic Dis 27:345–364, 1974.

56. Marmot MG, Syme SL, Kagan A, Kato H, Cohen JB, and Belsky J: Epidemiologic studies of coronary heart disease and stroke in Japanese men living in Japan, Hawaii, and California: Prevalence of coronary and hypertensive heart disease and associated risk factors. Am J Epidemiol 102:514–525, 1975.

57. Worth RM, Kato H, Rhoads GG, Kagan A, and Syme SL: Epidemiologic studies of coronary heart disease and stroke in Japanese men living in Japan, Hawaii, and California: Mortality. Am J Epidemiol 102:481–490, 1975.

58. Robertson TL, Kato H, Rhoads GG, Kagan A, Marmot M, Syme SL, Gordon T, Worth RM, Belsky JL, Dock DS, Miyanishi M, and Kawamoto S: Epidemiologic studies of coronary heart disease and stroke in Japanese men living in Japan, Hawaii, and California: Incidence of myocardial infarction and death from coronary heart disease. Am J Cardiol 39:239–243, 1977.

59. Robertson TL, Kato H, Gordon T, Kagan A, Rhoads GG, Land CE, Worth RM, Belsky JL, Dock DS, Myanishi M, and Kawamoto S: Epidemiologic studies of coronary heart disease and stroke in Japanese men living in Japan, Hawaii, and California: Coronary heart disease risk factors in Japan and Hawaii. Am J Cardiol 39:244–249, 1977.

60. Marmot MG, and Syme SL: Acculturation and coronary heart disease in Japanese-Americans. Am J Epidemiol 104:225–247, 1976.

61. Moriyama IM, Krueger DE, and Stamler J: *Cardiovascular Diseases in the United States.* Cambridge, Mass, Harvard University Press, 1971.

62. Liu K, Stamler J, Dyer A, McKeever J, and McKeever P: Statistical methods to assess and minimize the role of intra-individual variability in obscuring the relationship between dietary lipids and serum cholesterol. J Chronic Dis 31:399–418, 1978.

63. Page L, and Friend B: The changing United States diet. BioScience 28:192–197, 1978.

64. Select Committee on Nutrition and Human Needs, United States Senate: *Dietary Goals for the United States.* Washington, DC, US Government Printing Office, February, 1977.

65. Lopez A, Krehl WA, Hodges RE, and Good EI: Relationship between food consumption and mortality from atherosclerotic heart disease in Europe. Am J Clin Nutr 19:361–369, 1966.

66. Pimentel D, Terhune EC, Dyson-Hudson R, Rochereau S, Samis R, Smith EA, Denman D, Reifschneider D, and Shepard M: Land degradation: Effects on food and energy resources. Science 194:149–155, 1976.

67. Cooper R, Stamler J, Dyer A, and Garside D: The decline in mortality from coronary heart disease, 1968–1975. J Chronic Dis 31:709–720, 1978.

68. Hammond EC: The effects of smoking. Sci Am 207:39–51, July 1962.

69. Byington R, Dyer AR, Garside D, Liu K, Moss D, Stamler J, and Tsong Y: Recent trends of major coronary risk factors and CHD mortality in the United States and other industrialized countries. In Havlik RJ, and Feinleib M (eds): Proceedings of the Conference on the Decline in Coronary Heart Disease Mortality. Department of Health, Education and Welfare, Public Health Service, National Institutes of Health, NIH Publication No 79-1610, May, 1979, pp 340–379.

Comment

Cardiologists have been slow to accept Type A behavior as a risk factor in the development of coronary heart disease. Some of the reasons for this are given in Dr. Friedman's presentation. However, in defense of the cardiologist, it should be pointed out that it is hard to accept a concept that is difficult to measure quantitatively. For many years, Drs. Friedman and Rosenman were the only investigators who classified Type A behavior in this manner, and thus we were dependent on their reports as to its significance. As other groups have started to look at behavior in a similar manner, additional supporting evidence has accumulated suggesting that Type A behavior is a risk factor for coronary disease. Dr. Stamler has already mentioned the corroborative findings of the Framingham Study. Other studies, including coronary arteriographic ones demonstrating the high incidence of Type A personality in patients with three-vessel coronary disease, are beginning to appear. It seems reasonable to assume at this stage of our knowledge that Type A behavior is an independent risk factor for coronary heart disease, although all of the required criteria enumerated by Dr. Stamler have not been fully met.

Much more controversial is the importance of Type A behavior in relationship to other known risk factors. Dr. Stamler takes issue in great detail with the arguments proposed by Dr. Rosenman in earlier publications which tend to deny the importance of other risk factors in comparison to that of behavior. It is unfortunate that this whole issue in the past has been surrounded by such emotional content, since it has tended to polarize positions in an area already plagued by difficulties in accumulating data. Clearly, many more data are needed in this field.

Of paramount interest will be the results of Friedman and Rosenman's efforts to modify Type A behavior and, thus, affect coronary heart disease by risk-factor intervention. Statistics in the United States over the past decade have shown a reduction of approximately 25 per cent in mortality from coronary heart disease. Although some of this probably reflects improvements in the medical and surgical management of clinical coronary heart disease, part undoubtedly reflects the results of traditional risk-factor intervention over many years designed to lower serum cholesterol by dietary and/or drug means, detect and treat hypertension, and eliminate cigarette smoking. Thus, traditional risk-factor intervention through public and professional education has been successful in contributing to a lowering of coronary heart disease mortality, although its effect on the prevalence of coronary artery disease is, unfortunately, unknown. During this time, societal behavioral changes presumably have not occurred in a direction that would have been expected to decrease coronary heart disease. If the work of Friedman and Rosenman is borne out

107

with further study, and if behavior can be successfully modified as well, we can hopefully look forward to further exploitation of the inroads that have led to the recent, encouraging decline in coronary heart disease mortality. If not, Type A behavior will be relegated to those unmodifiable categories such as age and family history.

ELLIOT RAPAPORT, M.D.

Five

Should Coronary Arteriography Be Performed in the Asymptomatic Patient With a Positive Stress Test?

CORONARY ARTERIOGRAPHY SHOULD BE PERFORMED IN THE ASYMPTOMATIC PATIENT WITH A POSITIVE STRESS TEST

Michael V. Herman, M.D.

CORONARY ARTERIOGRAPHY SHOULD BE PERFORMED IN THE ASYMPTOMATIC PATIENT WITH A POSITIVE STRESS TEST: AN OPPOSING VIEWPOINT

J. David Bristow, M.D.

COMMENT

Coronary Arteriography Should Be Performed in the Asymptomatic Patient With a Positive Stress Test

MICHAEL V. HERMAN, M.D.

Dr. Arthur M. and Hilda A. Master Professor of Medicine and Chief, Division of Cardiology, Department of Medicine, The Mount Sinai School of Medicine of the City University of New York.

In the assessment of individuals with potential coronary artery disease, two testing modalities have come into widespread use: exercise stress testing and coronary arteriography. Often these procedures are performed in tandem, and the functional and pathoanatomic data are integrated in a complementary fashion. In the patient with incapacitating angina and other definitive signs of underlying coronary disease, few would question the wisdom and value of these procedures. Controversy certainly exists, however, as to whether these procedures should be utilized for an asymptomatic person. Furthermore, questions have been raised as to whether a person without symptoms, who for one reason or another undergoes stress testing with a positive result, should have follow-up coronary arteriography. I favor the position that coronary arteriography should be performed in such a patient when a positive stress test has been identified.

Background

Exercise electrocardiographic stress testing is commonly accepted in the evaluation of chest pain syndromes.[1-4] Three methods for applying exercise stress are employed, the two-step or double Master's test, bicycle er-

111

gometry, and the treadmill. The latter two methods are the most useful for the multistaged tests that are currently employed. The end point for termination of the study is the development of a positive test, symptoms, or a target heart rate that is submaximal or maximal as predicted by age and body size. Strict criteria for a positive test are based on ST-segment depression that is horizontal or downsloping and at least 1.0 mm or more. The interpretation of a positive response also must take into account the blood pressure response, the achieved heart rate, and the duration and exercise load to produce the ST-segment change or the development of arrhythmias.

In the asymptomatic individual, indications for the performance of a stress test include job screening where public safety may be involved, the evaluation of individuals for exercise training programs, and the study of other cardiac findings (e.g., abnormal electrocardiogram). Mass screening of the general population with stress testing has been suggested, but has gained little acceptance. The accuracy and value of stress testing depends on a number of variables and the population being studied.[1-5] In men with typical angina pectoris, the predictive value approaches 85 to 90 per cent for the detection of underlying coronary artery disease. In young asymptomatic individuals, the predictive value may be as low as 25 per cent, with a large number of false positives to be explained. However, in this group, the conversion of a previous negative test to positive is very predictive.

Thus, the identification of a positive stress test has important *implications*. It may variably reflect myocardial ischemia due to significant coronary atherosclerosis. It may indicate myocardial ischemia due to some other cardiac condition, such as myocardial hypertrophy. It may be a "false positive" test and have a benign long-term outlook. The prognostic implications of a positive stress electrocardiogram are well documented.[3, 6, 7] Life insurance studies demonstrated that subjects with ST-segment depression of 2 mm or more on two-step testing had 16 times the mortality of those with a negative response.[6] A similar correlation was found in treadmill testing in a large series of asymptomatic subjects.[7] In addition, a markedly positive test (2 mm or greater ST-segment depression) has been associated with extensive angiographic disease with a high frequency of the left main stem or three-vessel coronary disease.[1, 8] Thus, a positive stress test needs definitive resolution in most cases, and this is best done with coronary arteriography and cardiac catheterization at the present time.

Currently, coronary arteriography is a procedure that can be performed with a high diagnostic yield at a very low mortality and morbidity.[9] The two general approaches to selective coronary arteriography, the retrograde brachial approach and the percutaneous femoral technique, are equally effective and safe in experienced hands. These studies provide a precise definition of the coronary anatomy and can clearly identify, localize, and assess obstruction lesions due to coronary atherosclerosis. Coronary arteriography is coupled with left ventriculography and hemodynamic studies to complete the total cardiac anatomic and functional evaluation. Coronary arteriography has provided a great deal of new knowledge about the natural history, pathophysiology, and therapy of coronary heart disease. The surgical treatment of coronary disease with revascularization follows directly from our ability to visualize coronary obstructive disease. The coronary arteriographic and ventriculographic findings provide important prognostic data about patients. It has been conclusively shown that prognosis is directly related to the number of coronary arteries with significant atherosclerotic involvement and to left ventricular function in patients referred for arteriography.[10-13] A patient with a significant single right coronary artery obstruction and normal ventricular function has an outlook similar to the general population of his age. On the other hand, only 10 per cent of patients with three-vessel disease and severe limitation of ventricular function will be expected to be alive five years after study.

Finally, coronary arteriography has demonstrated that not all chest pain is due to coronary atherosclerosis.[14] The syndrome of angina-like chest pain with normal coronary arteries has been identified and characterized as having a good long-term outlook. Other cardiac syndromes such as mitral valve prolapse and hypertrophic disease may mimic actual coronary artery disease and can be differentiated with catheterization and coronary arteriography, along with other ancillary cardiac tests such as the echocardiogram.

One aspect of the asymptomatic positive stress test deserves special comment — the concept of painless ischemia. It is now becoming quite clear that not all episodes of myocardial ischemia are associated with clinical angina pectoris.[15] We have found in patients with proven coronary disease that over 90 per cent of episodes of ST-segment alterations detected by Holter monitoring are asymptomatic.[16] It seems very probable that the threshold for anginal pain may vary from patient to patient — and not be exceeded in certain patients who would thus be included in the category of asymptomatic. When one also considers the fact that those "asymptomatic" individuals with underlying coronary artery disease and myocardial ischemia are candidates for sudden death[17] and the fact that about 10 per cent of myocardial infarctions are painless,[18] our traditional concept that the "asymptomatic" state connotes a benign outlook may have to be closely reexamined.

Conclusion

When one recommends coronary arteriography for the asymptomatic individual with a positive stress test, certain prerequisites should be followed:

1. The electrocardiographic interpretation of a positive stress test must follow strict criteria, i.e., 1.0 mm or greater ST-segment horizontal or downsloping depression, particularly at an early stage of the test (low work load).

2. The patient should not have any complicating diseases such as metastatic cancer, severe lung disease, and so on.

3. Equipment for cardiac catheterization or coronary angiography must be of the highest technical quality.

4. A skilled, competent team, including a well-trained angiographer, must be available for the studies. The interpretive skills of the team are crucial.

Therefore, a coronary arteriographic study is definitively indicated in the asymptomatic individual with a positive stress test:

1. It will establish firmly the presence or absence of coronary atherosclerosis.

2. If no cardiac disease is found, the patient can be reassured about his benign outlook.

3. If coronary disease is present, prognosis for that patient can be estimated from the number of vessels involved and the left ventricular functional status.

4. In the presence of extensive coronary disease (left main coronary involvement, three-vessel disease), one should consider surgical revascularization.

5. A recommendation for activity (exercise) can be based on the angiographic or catheterization findings.

References

1. Cohn PF, Vokonas PS, Most AS, Herman MV, and Gorlin R: Diagnostic accuracy of two-step postexercise ECG. Results in 305 subjects studied by coronary arteriography. JAMA 220:501, 1972.
2. Bruce RA, and McDonough JR: Stress testing in screening of cardiovascular disease. Bull NY Acad Med 45:1288, 1969.
3. Ellestad MH, and Wan MKC: Predictive implications of stress testing. Follow-up of 2700 subjects after maximal treadmill stress testing. Circulation 51:363, 1975.
4. Froelicher VF, Thompson AJ, Longo MR Jr, Triebwasser JH, and Lancaster MC: Value of exercise testing for screening asymptomatic men for latent coronary artery disease. Prog Cardiovasc Dis 18:265, 1976.
5. Erikssen J, Enge I, Forfang K, and Storstein, O: False positive diagnostic tests and coronary arteriographic findings in 105 presumably healthy males. Circulation 54:371, 1976.
6. Robb GP, and Marks HH: Post-exercise electrocardiogram in arteriosclerotic disease: Its value in diagnosis and prognosis. JAMA 200:918, 1967.
7. Doyle JT, and Kirch SH: The prognosis of an abnormal electrocardiographic stress test. Circulation 41:545, 1970.
8. Cohen MV, and Gorlin R: Main left coronary artery disease. Clinical experience from 1964–1974. Circulation 52:275, 1975.
9. Conti CR: Coronary arteriography. Circulation 55:227, 1977.
10. Bruschke AVG, Proudfit WL, and Sones FM Jr: Progress study of 590 consecutive nonsurgical causes of coronary disease followed 5–9 years. I. Arteriographic correlations. Circulation 47:1147, 1973.
11. Bruschke AVG, Proudfit WL, and Sones FM Jr: Progress study of 590 consecutive nonsurgical cases of coronary disease followed 5–9 years. II. Ventriculographic and other correlations. Circulation 47:1154, 1973.
12. Webster JS, Moberg C, and Rincon G: Natural history of severe proximal coronary artery disease as documented by coronary cineangiography. Am J Cardiol 33:195, 1974.
13. Burggraf GW, and Parker JO: Prognosis in coronary artery disease. Angiographic, hemodynamic and clinical factors. Circulation 51:146, 1975.
14. Herman MV, Cohn PF, and Gorlin R: Angina-like chest pain without identifiable cause. Ann Intern Med 79:445, 1973.
15. Gettes LS: Painless myocardial ischemia. Chest 66:612, 1974.
16. Kunkes SH, Kupersmith J, Pichard AD, Malanyaon E, Teichholz LE, and Herman MV: Silent ST segment changes and their relationship to coronary artery disease. (In preparation).
17. Liberthson RR, Nagel EL, Hirshman JC, Nussenfeld SR, Blackbourne BD, and Davis JH: Pathophysiologic observations in prehospital ventricular fibrillation and sudden death. Circulation 49:790, 1974.
18. Margolis JR, Kannel WB, and Feinleib M: Clinical features of unrecognized myocardial infarction — Silent and symptomatic. Eighteen year follow-up: The Framingham Study. Am J Cardiol 32:1, 1973.

Coronary Arteriography Should Be Performed in the Asymptomatic Patient With a Positive Stress Test: An Opposing Viewpoint

J. DAVID BRISTOW, M.D.

Chief, Cardiology, Veterans Administration Hospital, San Francisco, and Professor of Medicine, Department of Medicine and the Cardiovascular Research Institute, University of California, San Francisco

Should coronary arteriography be performed in the asymptomatic patient with a positive exercise test? Because of several unresolved problems, the present answer must be "no," especially if one asks that arteriography be generally, or always, done in this circumstance. From the discussion to follow, the reader should not infer that I am unenthusiastic about exercise testing. Its uses for evaluation of physical competence and therapy, to add an objective dimension to the history, and for diagnostic purposes are essential in contemporary cardiology. However, there are issues that seriously weaken the assertion that a positive test, *of itself*, is an indication for arteriography.

The questions include these: What goals are served by testing apparently healthy people? What is the quality of the usual exercise tracing? What diagnostic criteria should be chosen, i.e., what levels of confidence do we wish for case finding or exclusion of disease? How sensitive and specific are current criteria for interpretation of the test in an asymptomatic population? How many well people will be given a label of illness long before symptoms develop?

115

A very important role for study of an asymptomatic person would be to detect disease that was a potential threat and then to prevent death, suffering, or disability by effective treatment. The questions then follow: Can we prevent myocardial infarction, progression of coronary disease, congestive heart failure, arrhythmias, and sudden death by means that require knowledge of coronary arterial anatomy? Will coronary artery bypass surgery achieve these ends, or if one subscribes to risk-factor modification, can such measures be better advised or followed when the coronary patho-anatomy is known? Put another way, do risk-factor interventions require information from an arteriogram in order to be followed? If one is convinced that arteriographic information is essential for these goals, and that they can be achieved, how many normal people and those whose course *cannot* be changed must be studied to find those whose lives *could* be helped? Is the benefit sufficient to justify the discomfort, risk, and cost of proving that the normal patient with a positive stress test is really free of coronary disease after all?

The reasons I chose for the negative conclusion will be summarized as some of these questions are explored.

Quality of Records and Observer Variation

With usual electrocardiographic equipment, there is substantial variation in the interpretation of exercise tests by physicians. Diagnostic criteria can only be accurately evaluated and employed when the quality of the record is consistently high. As it now stands, muscle artifact and baseline movement can make some electrocardiograms during exercise impossible to read and make interpretation of others variable. Fortunately, much diagnostic information is found after exercise has been stopped. Although post-exercise records are very useful, tracings during exertion are also essential, yet are often difficult to interpret. Hope for the future is shown by the type of computer-processed records in Figures 1 and 2. Until such improve-

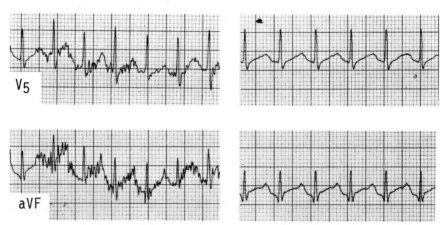

Figure 1. *Left:* Tracing during exercise, displaying muscle artifact and baseline drift. *Right:* Computer-processed display of the same record, allowing confident ST-segment evaluation. Such aids lend promise for better stress test interpretation.

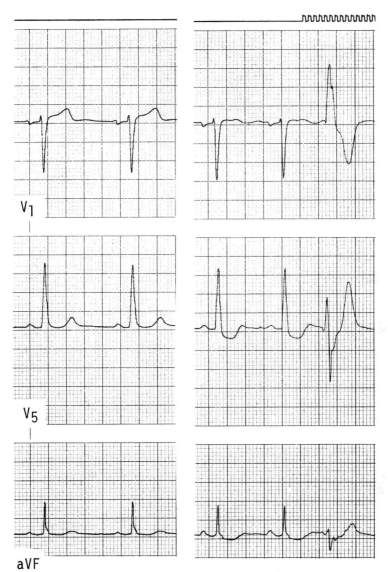

Figure 2. Records at rest and during mild exercise. Computer processing allows accurate assessment of ST segments, for example, in V_5. When a rhythm change occurs, a transient shift to real time is signaled at the top of the record and a premature beat recorded.

ments are widely used, up to 20 per cent of exercise records could be subject to interpretive error.[1] Indications for coronary angiography cannot be based solely on data of variable quality.

Choice of Leads and Test Protocols

A variety of leads have been used. Most employ a modified left precordial lead, although some investigators have used all 12 ECG leads during exercise, or orthogonal leads. Concern for inclusion of information from the frontal plane has led to inclusion of a modified aVF as a reflection of inferior wall forces. The variation in the pattern of ST-segment displacement that can be found in different leads during exercise in the same patient is shown in Figure 3.

Before one could recommend that all positive tests should be followed by coronary arteriography, agreement on standardized lead configurations is important, and they should be leads with diagnostic yield and reliability clearly understood.

There are similar concerns about uniformity of testing conditions. Continuous tests with steady or periodically increasing work loads using steps, treadmill, or bicycle ergometer are in use. Intermittent stages with a rest between lead levels are also employed. Termination of the test at 75 per cent of the maximum predicted heart rate or less, as opposed to stopping the test at the predicted maximum heart rate, introduces another variable from one exercise laboratory to another.

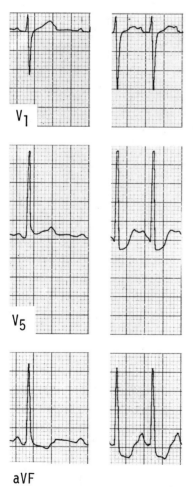

Figure 3. Demonstration of the problem of abnormality present at rest and different responses to exercise in different leads. Slow upsloping ST segments are present in V_5 during exercise (right-hand panel) and further downsloping in aVF. Interpretation may depend on which lead is chosen for analysis.

Reproducible exercise test criteria with a specific protocol are essential. It is not logical to take any criterion in any lead in any sort of test as an indication for arteriography in a patient who feels completely well.

Sensitivity, Specificity, and Test Criteria

A recent exchange of editorials has highlighted the problems of diagnostic accuracy.[2-4] *Sensitivity* expresses the ability of the test to find the patient with coronary disease. The percentage of sensitivity equals the proportion of patients who have coronary disease who manifest a positive test. If a test is 85 per cent sensitive, 85 persons out of 100 with the disease will have a positive test, and 15 would have a false negative result.

Specificity describes the problem of false positive tests. It is the proportion of people without coronary disease who have a negative test. If a test is 90 per cent specific, 90 out of 100 people without disease will have a negative test (and a false positive test would be found in 10 without disease).

The values found in the literature vary greatly. A positive test has been interpreted from ST-segment depression of 0.5, 1.0, 1.5, and 2.0 mm. The ST segment has been described at these levels as being horizontal, upsloping, or downsloping and has been evaluated at varying intervals from the J point (junction of the QRS complex and the ST segment). Furthermore, criteria have been proposed for tracings with abnormal ST segments or T waves at rest. Thus, up to nine categories of abnormal exercise ST-segment responses have been proposed.[5] It is entirely possible that sensitivity and specificity are different for each of these circumstances, but the values are not all known.

Published reports of sensitivity and specificity vary from about 35 per cent to 90 per cent, depending on diagnostic criteria used and the population studied. It is well established that the incidence of false positives increases (poorer specificity) as test criteria are made more liberal to improve sensitivity (better case finding). We do not appear able to avoid this trade-off at present.

Many of the earlier, classic studies of the predictive accuracy of exercise testing described an increased frequency of acute coronary events or death in the years following a positive test. However, what is not known is the status of the coronary arteries at the time of the original test. More direct relationships between exercise test results and coronary pathoanatomy are now beginning to be appreciated, and better information is on the way.

A recent step forward has been to provide arteriographic information for comparison with different test criteria.[6] When 1-mm depressed, flat, or downsloping ST segments were used to express positivity, sensitivity was 64 per cent and specificity was 93 per cent. Specificity increased to 99 per cent and sensitivity fell to 45 per cent when downsloping ST segments were required. The study provides an important guideline for varying degrees and configurations of ST-segment displacement and allows choices to be made at different levels of confidence (specificity and sensitivity). In addition, there is the possibility of estimating severity of coronary disease, using graded interpretation of the test.[6] As such approaches are extended, our diagnostic capability will continue to improve. Unanswered by this progress, however, is whether an asymptomatic patient with disease is helped by the information.

As recently discussed, the number of positive arteriograms in an asymptomatic population with a positive exercise test is likely to be small in contrast to the "yield" in a population with symptoms.[2] Well below 50 per cent of positive tests in an asymptomatic population could be true positives, whereas a high proportion of positive tests will be found in those with symptoms, a group with higher prevalence of coronary disease.

Thus, there is valid concern for those with a positive test and no coronary disease. They may represent a substantial or even the major proportion of an asymptomatic group with positive tests, especially if criteria for screening are extended. By the assertion advanced, normal patients who have a positive test must have an arteriogram to prove that they are not sick, when they felt well in the first place. The other problem, presented by the positive arteriogram in the asymptomatic patient, will be taken up subsequently.

With a literature replete with varying exercise methods, varying end points for the procedure, varying leads recorded, greatly varying diagnostic criteria, varying observer interpretation of the records, and varying populations studied with different prevalence of coronary disease, the day is not here to require an arteriogram for every exercise test that has been judged positive (Fig. 4).

Use of Arteriographic Information in an Asymptomatic Patient

Progress is being made in sorting out the problems summarized earlier. It is reasonable to expect broader use of standard test protocols, leads, and information about sensitivity and specificity of various test criteria, and in specific patient populations. Questions then must be faced about our ability to prevent progression of atherosclerosis and acute coronary events. What do we do with the information from abnormal arteriograms in an asymptomatic population?

RISK-FACTOR MODIFICATION

Although controversy continues about the therapeutic role of risk-factor intervention, there seems little argument that control of elevated blood pressure, abstinence from cigarettes, having an appropriate body weight, and perhaps achieving optimal blood lipid levels are desirable goals in our

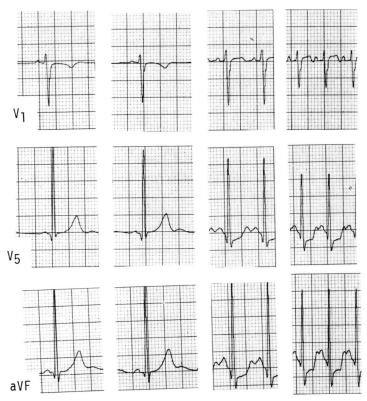

Figure 4. Computer-processed records at rest and at three levels of exercise, the last during stage V of the Bruce treadmill test, in a healthy 48-year-old man. The patient participates in regular, very heavy exertion. The physician must have effective therapy to justify putting the patient through a coronary arteriogram or to recommend changes in life-style for this single observation.

national attack on coronary disease. Does one need to know that the asymptomatic patient has anatomically demonstrable coronary disease in order to achieve appropriate risk-factor modification? Do patients who know that they have asymptomatic coronary lesions adhere to a risk-factor program better? Information is sketchy, but I conclude that knowing the coronary anatomy should not alter the recommendations one would make about prudent life patterns and risk-factor intervention, if one subscribes to the basic hypothesis concerning these risks and coronary disease.

KNOWING THE TRUTH

There is hardly justification for not being completely truthful with a patient about the presence of disease. But that is a different matter than searching out latent problems whose future is uncertain. I doubt that a life is better and happier if a person knows that he or she has asymptomatic coronary lesions. How rapidly does one need to get one's affairs in order because of a statistical probability for sudden death based on arteriographic, epidemiologic studies? How does an apparently well patient handle the information that he or she fits into a group with a 15 per cent chance of dying this year? The approach depends on one's philosophy in dealing with patients. I do not believe the physician has made a contribution to health and happiness by ferreting out latent disease in someone who feels well, unless he has something very good to offer. I think some patients have not been helped if we cannot prevent sudden death, arrhythmias, myocardial infarction or congestive failure. This raises the next topic for consideration, whether coronary surgery could achieve these goals.

CORONARY ARTERY SURGERY

This operation is frequently dramatic in its relief of symptoms and is often indicated for this goal. However, one of the important questions remaining to be answered about coronary surgery is its ability to prevent future myocardial infarction and death. At present, the question can be looked at in two populations, those with and without main left coronary arterial involvement.

Patients with disease of the main left coronary artery have a clear improvement of prognosis by coronary bypass grafting. The question then is whether one can do exercise testing in an asymptomatic patient, identify latent coronary disease, perform arteriography, find patients with main left coronary artery disease, and help them by surgery. The reasoning is logical until one looks at the details. The improvement in prognosis in main left coronary artery disease has been demonstrated in those with important or severe symptoms, very often unstable angina with pain at rest, not in latent disease. Asymptomatic, severe main left coronary artery disease no doubt occurs, but must be rare. Thus, broad-scale exercise testing to identify this small sub-population is not warranted, in my opinion.

It remains to be seen if coronary disease without main left coronary artery involvement can have its prognosis improved by coronary surgery. Opinions are easy to find, but carefully constructed studies are few. Those available have thus far failed to show differences in life expectancy with and without surgery in patients with symptoms. Virtually no information is available about the outlook with and without surgery in asymptomatic patients with arteriographically demonstrated coronary arterial pathology. The prospect for prevention of myocardial infarction or sudden death is of enormous importance, but it must be tested rigorously before embarking on a campaign of widespread testing of healthy people.

At this time, I do not believe the sequence of screening by exercise electrocardiography and coronary arteriography, leading to surgery for asymptomatic coronary arterial lesions, is justified. The view has been published recently that a positive test in an asymptomatic person should be used much as a risk factor in management.[7]

Conclusions

The rationale behind exercise testing of asymptomatic patients requires little defense. We *should* be looking for potential health problems we can treat to prevent disability and death. The problem is that our therapy is insufficient for this particular disorder. Furthermore, the detection of coronary disease by exercise testing has had variable results, and thus our confidence level is uncertain at present.

Arteriography will be negative in many asymptomatic patients who have positive exercise tests, and its performance would put our skyrocketing national health care costs even higher. Even if help for the patient were dependent upon knowing coronary artery anatomy, many normal patients would have to be examined. This trade-off requires concern about philosophical issues, i.e., pain and expense to many normal people in order to help find those who could be helped.

If coronary arteriograms are normal, the healthy patient can be reassured with confidence. However, the view could be taken that the patient could have been spared the anxiety of the test, as well as the discomfort, risk, and expense, if the stress test had not been performed in the first place. One worries that exercise testing sometimes provides more reassurance for the physician than the patient.

If criteria for a positive test interpretation are restrictive enough to provide high test specificity, then a case can be made for arteriography in those with a positive result, because of the high prospect of finding severe disease, such as main left coronary artery involvement. In an asymptomatic population, however, the number of such people remains unknown. My opinion is that it is low. We clearly need more information from the research realm.

Finally, the role of the most direct attack on the coronary arterial problem, coronary surgery, is unexplored in the asymptomatic patient. If the unanswered questions here are to be resolved, prospective research studies, not anecdotal approaches by individuals, will be necessary.

Although future data could give us much greater confidence or broader indications for study and management of patients, our knowledge as of this writing does not allow me to recommend that all patients with a positive exercise test have coronary arteriography.

References

1. Abbott JA, Tedeschi MA, and Cheitlin MD: Graded treadmill stress testing. West Med 126:173–178, 1977.
2. Redwood DR, Borer JS, and Epstein SE: Whither the ST segment during exercise. Circulation 54:703–706, 1976.
3. Sheffield LT, Reeves TJ, Blackburn H, Ellestad MH, Froelicher VF, Roitman D, and Kansal S: The exercise test in perspective. Circulation 55:681–682, 1977.
4. McHenry PL: The actual prevalence of false positive ST segment response to exercise in clinically normal subjects remains undefined. Circulation 55:683–685, 1977.

5. Ellestad MH: *Stress Testing. Principles and Practice.* Philadelphia, FA Davis Co, 1975, p 100.
6. Goldschlager N, Selzer A, and Cohn K: Treadmill stress tests as indicators of presence and severity of coronary artery disease. Ann Intern Med 85:277–286, 1976.
7. Bristow JD, Burchell HB, Campbell RW, Ebert PA, Hall RJ, Leonard JJ, and Reeves TJ: Report on the indications for coronary arteriography. Council on Clinical Cardiology, American Heart Association. Circulation 55:969A–974A, 1977.

Comment

The controversy discussed in this chapter has an unstated preamble, namely, that asymptomatic patients are subjected to exercise stress testing. This happens on occasions, particularly in the case of older individuals contemplating beginning a jogging program. Additionally, business executives undergoing routine examinations are occasionally subjected to exercise stress testing by their physicians. Nevertheless, I question the wisdom of stress testing asymptomatic patients in the first place. When one is dealing with an overall group in which the incidence of ischemic heart disease is relatively low and uses a test in which specificity is not 100 per cent, a significant number of false positives will contribute to the total group of patients who have a positive response. Thus, this controversy can be divided into two aspects: (1) Is the yield of patients in whom organic coronary artery disease will be verified sufficiently high as to warrant blanket coronary arteriographic examination among those in whom a positive exercise stress test is present? (2) Is the information revealed by a positive arteriogram likely to alter that patient's life-style or management or contribute information of such importance as to justify exposing him to a procedure with some cost, morbidity, and even mortality, albeit remote?

My own view of these two questions is that routine exercise stress testing of a given population group as a test to uncover coronary heart disease is unwarranted. The sensitivity and specificity are not great enough to prevent more false positive than true positive tests from occurring. Thus, not only may patients with coronary heart disease fail to be uncovered, but the majority of patients with a positive test may not even have coronary heart disease. It seems to me that the asymptomatic patient should not be subjected to exercise stress testing unless he is in a particularly sensitive occupation, such as an airline pilot, in which public safety may warrant unusual measures.

Coming back to the thesis of this controversy, I do not believe that routine coronary arteriography should be performed on patients with positive stress tests of 1-mm horizontal ST segment depression or lower as defined by Dr. Herman. However, I do believe that coronary arteriography should be done on occasion. There are, in my judgment, two major situations in which this applies. When a patient has a 2-mm or greater ST-segment depression, the likelihood of left main coronary artery disease becomes a significant possibility even though this lesion, in an asymptomatic patient, would be rather unusual. Nonetheless, if ST-segment depression of this magnitude is uncovered, particularly if it is associated with hypotension during exercise or comes early in the course of stress testing, immediate coronary arteriography is warranted. There appears to be sufficient evidence in the literature to suggest that this lesion should be treated surgically today, even if the patient is asymptomatic.

If a positive stress test is demonstrated in an asymptomatic patient in which ST-segment depression is only 1 mm or 1.5 mm, I feel that it would be desirable, under those circumstances, to repeat the test with a thallium perfusion scan performed during exercise and several hours later after redistribution. This should help to establish those cases that are true positives without having to resort to coronary arteriography solely for diagnostic confirmation.

There is one other circumstance for which I would recommend coronary arteriography be done on the asymptomatic patient, namely, in an extremely young patient (someone in his 20's or 30's) who demonstrates an abnormal stress test. Under these circumstances, the possibility of unusual anatomy, such as a congenital coronary artery lesion, warrants coronary arteriography, since surgery may be indicated, even though it would not be indicated were the patient to have the usual type of atherosclerotic coronary disease.

In summary, I believe that coronary arteriography is a valuable procedure that may influence management in a certain subset of patients who demonstrate a positive stress test even though they may be asymptomatic; however, I do not feel that it should be performed routinely.

ELLIOT RAPAPORT, M.D.

Six

Should Patients With Coronary Heart Disease Avoid Strenuous Physical Exertion?

PATIENTS WITH CORONARY ARTERY DISEASE SHOULD
AVOID STRENUOUS PHYSICAL EXERTION

Howard B. Burchell, M.D.

PATIENTS WITH CORONARY HEART DISEASE SHOULD
AVOID STRENUOUS PHYSICAL
EXERTION — ANTAGONIST POSITION

Nanette K. Wenger, M.D.

COMMENT

Patients With Coronary Artery Disease Should Avoid Strenuous Physical Exertion

HOWARD B. BURCHELL, M.D.

Professor of Medicine, Emeritus, University of Minnesota;
Senior Cardiologic Consultant, Northwestern Hospital,
Minneapolis, Minnesota

This essay pertains to patients *with* coronary disease and the theoretical or experimental benefit of their participation in *strenuous* exercise, not to the advantages of continued physical fitness nor the importance of some continued physical activity, as planned by physician and patient, in the patient with coronary disease.

The subject of exercise often incites controversial opinions in the profession regarding recommendations of physical activity for patients with coronary artery disease. The essential premises on which arguments have been launched in the past have not always been clear; whether lack of exercise is a risk factor for development of coronary disease, whether coronary "events" can be prevented by an exercise program, and whether progression of existing coronary disease might be affected favorably are *not* the crucial questions at issue. Simply stated, the questions are: For the coronary patient, is some exercise good? Is more better? How much more is needed? And is "strenuous" the ideal level?

I will define "patients" as everyone with coronary artery disease, without stratification into groups according to exercise tolerance. The word "strenuous" should also be defined. Obviously, an external work load that is strenuous for one person may be easy for another. The discriminating physician also will require some notion of the dynamic and isometric components of the exertion, of the level of exercise as a percentage of known or estimated maximum aerobic capacity, and of the symptoms allowable before the label "strenuous" is considered applicable. Additionally, there is the problem of equating sustained exercise, or "endurance," with one's concept and definition of strenuous exercise. I submit my definition: The

129

word *strenuous* implies physical exertion approaching the level of maximum O_2 uptake (VO_2 maximum) (about 80 per cent associated with *symptoms* probably at unpleasantness level). After listening to talks given by proponents of active exercise programs (or reading their papers), I have noted emphasis on the proper selection of patients and of a stratification of groups with respect to allowable levels of exercise. My conclusion is that there has not been a universal push for strenuous exercise in *all* patients with coronary disease, regardless of age and physical infirmity.

I have long been opposed to a basic regimen of rest as a panacea for people with heart disease. However, it seems prudent to individualize the amount of exercise in which any particular patient should participate. Hellerstein[1] emphasizes that the exercise prescription "requires the same care as the prescription of a potent drug." Physicians' attitudes vary toward exercise in patients with coronary disease, colored by the approach they have to their specialty, their training and experience, and their own habits. As each of us in the profession prescribes for patients with known coronary disease, an examination of our motives underlying our recommendations is in order; in what capacity are we acting? (What "hat" are we wearing?) I am not pointing my finger at anyone to place him or her in a rigid category; I ask only each of us think of the role he or she believes himself or herself to be playing in the patients' care.

1. *Epidemiologist.* Approaching the patient from this background, one might stand accused of being devoid of interest in the individual, of having an overall scientific delight only in the observation and accurate recording of events in controlled, randomized groups. With the collection of proper data, one would hope that events could be predicted in certain groups or, in reverse, that from the nature of the events, one could retrospectively categorize the individual predestined to have difficulty.

2. *Preventive Cardiologist.* Under this banner, one might have an epidemiologist's viewpoint, a clinician's cares, or an administrator's responsibilities in an exercise program, convinced of the value of his or her program. In repetition of the objectives of this essay, it is "secondary prevention" efforts, not "primary prevention" efforts, that are under study. Wenger has stated, "One crucial question is whether the institution of exercise after myocardial infarction can alter the natural course of the illness—and further research is required for this determination." Enthused by the benefits accomplished through one's worthy crusade, one could be relatively immune to grief from the occasional death resulting from a cherished program, believing that benefit would still have accrued to a larger number. There should be no disputing the statement that awareness of increasing physical fitness during convalescence from a myocardial infarction increases confidence and reduces anxiety.

3. *Clinical Physiologist.* To belong in this category, one could be the scientist who was interested in physiological maximums and the hemodynamic responses to exercise of subjects with all levels of impaired function, with or without medication. In one's experiments the ultimate fate of an individual might appear to be secondary to the research project, *per se.*

4. *A Specialist with Subtle Objectives.* As a member of this group, a

cardiovascular surgeon, to demonstrate the value of an operative procedure, might have encouraged maximum efforts from his patient. One might belong in this category if one had convictions (a condition that Bronowski has labeled a sense of "monstrous certainty") about a program. One might feel infallible regarding the value of special medications or the modification of a patient's life-style. Among us, there could be good physicians who had a vested interest in the subject's continued exercise; for example, a physician to a professional football player, a celebrity, a military commander, or a political leader, where it would seem more important for a subject to appear exceptionally physically fit at a specific time than to have to worry about possible long-range harm in the program.

   5. *A Private Physician.* Functioning as a primary practitioner, one often looks on the patient as a specific responsibility and may believe (sometimes deludedly) that one can recognize subtle differences in the patient's status and responses to life's challenges. Such a background encourages the conviction that one could plan a program tailored to the patient's particular needs and comforts which could, but would be unlikely to, include *vigorous* exercise. In instances where vigorous exertion is part of the program prescribed for patients with angina or a prior myocardial infarction, this doctor might first wish to have coronary arteriographic studies. In the development of a needed program (a ritual) by the private physician, the publicized accomplishments of patients in strenuous exertion programs may be utilized to encourage his patient's participation in a progressive rehabilitation program. There is no gainsaying the rapturous delight of some patients completing an hour of brisk jogging or a strenuous run, but this does not guarantee the same effect, nor is it possible, for all. An occasional claim to a transcendental experience is reminiscent of the euphoria of some subjects with hypoxia at high altitudes. It is pertinent to note that the primary physician will have the task of caring for the "dropouts" from programs, some of whom will be disconsolate from their failure through recurrent angina.

Individualism in Exercise Responses

   In any discussion of the advantages and disadvantages of exercise, personality differences, behavior patterns when young, and the severity of symptoms accompanying the exercise must be considered. A relatively small percentage of elderly patients will be capable of high work loads. Some will experience undesirable concomitant physiological stresses associated with strenuous effort, which are hazards not reflected in heart rate or level of oxygen uptake. For example, when lifting heavy objects, the patient may perform a Valsalva maneuver, and there may be severe hypertension in the post-straining period. With the continued strain of lifting, a hypertensive reflex (the isometric reflex) will also occur. In addition, a considerable emotional overlay may ensue, with frustration and anger, as in, for example, pushing an automobile stuck in the snow, shoveling heavy snow, or pulling a slain deer through the woods. One must be careful in indicting the hypertensive isometric response; to do so, there should be evidence that at least 30 per cent of maximum effort had been continuously maintained for 15 seconds or more. Likewise, when applying the physiological phenomena studied in lower animals to humans (such as the diving reflex), one must have restraints, though not discarding the possibilities of their application. Another aspect of severe exertion, which may be readily forgotten, pertains to hazards from a precipitously induced Herculean effort, i.e., an immediate jump from rest to a high level of exercise without any "warm-up" period. Tests during such activity have revealed electrocardiographic changes indicative of myocardial ischemia in healthy, physically fit men.[2] The advantages of the physiological changes accompanying development of physical fitness have been extensively investigated. That a person can do more at the same oxygen cost to his heart and feel generally better is well established. However, it is not as clear exactly how much exercise is required for the cardiac patient to maintain a reasonable level of physical fitness.

In contrast to the extensive data available on the advantages of exercise, the disadvantages, i.e., the harm that might result, are quantitatively undocumented. Much of what has been written is anecdotal. Information is scanty concerning the fate of patients within the population with coronary disease who have failed in the exercise rehabilitation programs. Evidence that ST-segment changes early after myocardial infarction presaged a poor prognosis is increasing,[3] but there are no data to prove that the trial of the exercise program worsened the patients' outlook as a group.

A disturbing finding in well-organized exercise rehabilitation programs is the drop-out rate. While it may be implied that the drop-outs occur because of psychological reasons or because of inadequate community facilities, one must wonder whether there is a self-selective process that has occurred, and whether some drop-outs could be related to a cardiac disability, with possible harm from the exercise not excluded. In the study of Wilhelmsen et al.,[4] of Goteborg, 75 per cent of those in the exercise program had discontinued the program within four years, and the meaning of the higher death rate for the drop-outs is not clear. As a corollary, for those who remained in the exercise group, it cannot be claimed that exercise was unequivocably the cause of the decreased mortality rate. Wilhelmsen et al. concluded that "the value of the training program seems more to be related to the quality of life than to longevity." In a report of the Cardiopulmonary Research Institute (CAPRI) program reported by Bruce et al.[5] comparing active participants and drop-outs, there was approximately a 60 per cent drop-out rate within nine months. There was a 4.7 per cent mortality rate in the drop-outs (number of deaths per person-years) compared with 2.7 per cent in the continuing participants. It is noteworthy that there were 11 instances of exertional arrest during class training, with all resuscitations successful. Bruce et al. state that "without this benefit of medical supervision there would have been little difference in mortality experience." In another report on the effect of long-range strenuous sports training for cardiac rehabilitation by Gottheimer,[6] the exercising group had about a third of the mortality rate of a non-exercising group. He stated that there were no deaths during the supervised exercise, but he did mention the death of a "beginner" participating in an athletic event. In another study in Finland by Palatsi,[7] post–myocardial infarction patients following an exercise program had a lower death rate than controls from a sequential group of patients. While the trend was impressive, the rates for recidivous infarctions and coronary deaths were not statistically significant. The drop-out rate at a year was approximately 30 per cent. In the prospective study by Rose et al.,[8] the subjects already demonstrating evidence of myocardial ischemia did not show evidence of different survival rates according to their activity. The authors caution against any conclusion from the data; and the proponents of exercise programs may wonder about the level of the exercise.

We are well acquainted with newspaper stories and case reports concerning individuals who have died from strenuous exercise during the hunting season or during heavy snowstorms. Blumgart[9, 10] noted the malevolent effect of exertion in some individuals and often illustrated his talks with lantern slides made from newspaper headlines following each snowstorm. It is a common observation that some patients have ventricular arrhythmias, hypertension, or hypotension during exercise tests or during the immediate recovery period. I have seen two instances of sudden onset of mitral regurgitation caused by chordal separation from the papillary muscle during exertion. It has long been known that following exercise, some individuals develop fourth heart sounds, reversed splitting of second sounds, and gross abnormal movement of the ventricular wall, revealed by apex-displacement recordings, all of which document that undesirable cardiac effects can result from exercise in patients with ischemic heart disease. A physiological subject that has recently become a popular topic for investigation is the effect of increased heart rate and shortened diastolic periods. A predictable steal of blood from the subendocardial area must occur when even moderate proximal coronary obstructive lesions are present. From a physiological viewpoint, tachycardia, systolic hypertension, increased intraventricular diastolic pressure, ventricular dilatation, and an increased catecholamine milieu have ill effects when there is coronary obstruction, particularly when hypertrophy coexists. A number of workers have stated to me conversationally that gross ST-segment shifts do not portend serious trouble in the absence of arrhythmia or pain. Patients demonstrating such shifts may have a benign course, but they are still at high risk for untoward cardiac events.

In general, the goal of the private physician is to have his patient happy and content while exercising. In any dialogue concerning strenuous exertion, I submit that in some instances the imposed drills are not associated with enjoyment, and more important, enjoyment does not always develop as one is forced to participate in an exercise program. With some types of physical activity, such as hiking and leisurely climbing, one can enjoy the accompanying beauty of the environment and/or conversation. Individualization of activity merits the attention of the physician; tennis, swimming, bicycling, hiking, or skating may fit the patient's wishes and needs. Effler[11] has recommended that coronary patients have a dog: "Regular walking exercise will be good for the animal at either end of the leash."

However, one should recall the exasperation that may be caused by the young dog that may escape from its leash.

Physical activity has long been noted to be a release from tension and anxiety, sometimes alleviating bulimic states and insomnia. Many physicians are wary of being identified as true believers in the hypothesis that mental stress is a factor in the aggravation of coronary disease, and some eschew it completely. The well-known phenomenon that tension or stress may be dissipated while exercising has recently been reviewed by Eliot et al.[12] In the recent updated Report of the Committee on Stress, Strain and Heart Disease[13] of the American Heart Association, psychological factors are downgraded more than my own convictions allow. It is pertinent to point out that jogging, by the dictionary, is not *strenuous* exercise. In the popular *Consumer's Guide to Medical Care* by Vickery and Fries,[14] the statement is made that "walking, jogging, swimming, and bicycling are easy and pleasant ways to put regular physical activity into your life." These recommendations are repetitive of hygienic codes and home care in kitchen medicine books through the ages but are directed toward goals of health maintenance, not treatment of the cardiac patient.

Jogging and Running

My observations have led me to believe that jogging should be encouraged for patients who enjoy it. Also, a large group of marathoners or cross-country skiers of a wide age range is an encouraging sight, for I believe in physical fitness as a national objective, and there is no reason why a cardiac patient might not be among them if he or she has been trained and finds it enjoyable. In the contributions of Kavanaugh and Shephard[15] in rehabilitation, demonstrating that patients who had recovered from a myocardial infarction could attain an aerobic capacity equal to or in excess of their sedentary counterparts, it must be noted the average age of these patients was about 45 and that very few had angina. We do not know the coronary-arteriographic findings.

Medicolegal Aspects of Exercise

There are medical-legal implications inherent in *prescribing* exercise for an individual patient, as opposed to *recommending* it for a general or specific population. The physician must be aware that the attitude of the courts with respect to accepting causative relations of exertion to a coronary event is likely to differ from his concepts, and it is immaterial that the action of the courts may be regarded as astoundingly wrong. I have noted that many of the reports of work-related incidents for which individuals have claimed harm and have been awarded damages have seemed characterized more by anger, frustration, or sudden effort during the episode when the heart damage was alleged to have occurred than by the level of activity. In relation to work compensation cases, the differentiation of "unusual" from "usual" in the events during work is often the point of argument, not the level of the work per se. I hope that the attitude of the courts will change, but the past decisions should inculcate sobering thoughts when one *prescribes* high levels of activity.

In rehabilitation programs, I have not thought it necessary for the patient to sign a consent form, but it may be noted that Bruce[16] has written, "Informed consent of the patient, and possibly of his spouse, is reasonable." I think that this consent should be inherent in the design of the regimen when the patient elects to follow it. Sagall,[17, 18] writing on malpractice aspects of medically prescribed exercise, is specific in recommending that the physician explain in detail to the patient the nature and risk of exercise "so that the consent to such procedures can be classified as valid and informed." One can only deplore such a need if it is the way of the future.

While it is important that members of the patient's family know that a properly metered activity may be more beneficial than harmful to the patient and that to die during exercise while happy may be preferred by the patient to dying discontented at rest (e.g., restricted to a veranda), is it fair for the individual to take undue risks by which he may unduly worry others or to endanger the lives of others who might be called for rescue operations? For example, is it reasonable for a patient with symptomatic coronary disease to participate in arduous mountain climbing or in highly competitive sports in which, perhaps, he or she pursues the images of past prowess or denies the appearance of significant symptoms? "Take it easy" is not necessarily bad advice; obviously, if it creates anxiety and inactivity, it is overtly bad, and if it creates relaxation and enjoyment in exercise, it is not. The attitude of the physician communicates more than the words. "Jogging" by original concept was "taking-it-easy" running, with one dictionary definition (Webster's, 3rd ed.) being "to go at a slow, easy, monotonous pace."

Physical Fitness, Strenuous Exertion, and Aging

As people age, they generally "slow down," and often their physical efforts are limited by a benign shortness of breath, awkwardness, joint aches, fatigue, or weakness of the legs. These symptoms frequently limit endurance and their level of peak performance. Obviously, these symptoms would not prevent them from participating in sudden exertion for which they are unprepared. It is noteworthy that in the report on the death of young soldiers from coronary disease by French and Dock,[19] there was a high percentage of sudden deaths during exercise. Many of these young soldiers were obese, thus *not* physically fit. It would be expected that they had autonomic imbalance, and it would be reflected in transient, inappropriate QT durations.

Interest in physical fitness appears to occur in cycles. For instance, at the turn of the century, following movements in Europe, physical education became emphasized in the schools in the United States. Interest in physical fitness was very high, as shown, for example, in the writings of R. Tait McKenzie.[20] This interest did not last, possibly in part because it was a rebellion against regimentation, or because of the sour attitude of some groups concerning a master race concept, or because some intellectuals were decrying it as "immature."

To recapitulate, I am an avid crusader for young adult sports programs, with continued activity into middle age and for many of the elderly, and a supporter of the recommendation of exercise for patients with coronary disease at mild to moderate levels. In a long-range program, there appears to be *no* mandate for strenuous exercise to ensure the maintenance of an enjoyable, long life. From the point of view of the private practitioner, one death in a thousand resulting from any *prescribed* strenuous program is one too many if the benefit to a large group has not been established.

There is no evidence that marathon running is the best therapy for individuals afflicted with coronary disease, despite the fact that many individuals have been successful at it. The number of letters to the editor[21] engendered by the report of one marathoner who died of what was said to be acute myocardial infarction (without coronary disease)[22] was large and revealed various types of bias and opinion.

The data supporting the view that strenuous exertion is harmful to groups of patients with coronary disease are difficult to assess, but harm to individuals can definitely be accepted because of the concurrence of events. The dreaded events related to coronary disease are ventricular tachyarrhythmias and heart failure, both of which have, on occasion, been precipitated by strenuous exercise. While the toll of coronary-related deaths is lamentably high in the young and middle-aged, the majority of patients who are cared for by the primary physician are over 60 years of age, and to initiate unaccustomed strenuous exertion for *all* members of this latter population lacks logic or experimental support. Despite the plethora of recent data on exercise and heart disease, the practitioner sees considerable support to the conclusions of one of the earliest students of the disease, Parry,[23] who stated nearly two centuries ago,

> But though organic diseases of the heart may be produced by violent exertions, it has been thought that they are counteracted by moderate bodily exercise ... it appears to me that the principle is well-founded and that nothing guards more certainly against irregular action of the heart than uniform and gentle bodily exertion.

I can leave the following thought with the reader: Is strenuous exercise for the patient with coronary disease usually "too much, too late"? In the past five years, we have progressed but little from an analysis of the problem made by a colleague in the *Controversies in Internal Medicine,* 1974 issue; Henry Blackburn[24] stated, "Widespread, large-scale treatment of sedentary middle-aged coronary patients with intensive exercise is not beyond the skills and facilities of the medical care system, while its risks are quite obvious and its preventive health is undemonstrated." Evidence favoring advantages of some exercise in patients accumulates, however, and more quantitative information regarding risks has become available; for instance, the 30-center survey made by Haskell,[25] in which there were 50 cardiac arrests among 13,570 participants.

Epilogue

As an epilogue, I venture to mention two literary references to exertion that highlight aspects of exercise. One is the account of the death of Doctor Zhivago, in which Boris Pasternak underscores the theory of tension as a causative factor in coronary disease and describes a final event: the struggle (isometric) to open the trolley window, the panic with failure to do so, followed by strenuous effort to get off the crowded trolley, and having reached the street, "collapsing on the stone paving and not getting up again." The second reference, in a light vein, is the short story of O. Henry, "Let Me Feel Your Pulse," an account of a man with an agitated anxiety depressive state, who regained his health by tramping over the hills with a physician, looking for a fictitious curative herb the doctor had conjured up as the objective of their walks. Both stories illustrate different types of exercise and should add awareness of the possible harm or benefit from the situation in which the effort is occurring.

Addendum

Since the manuscript was initially written, a number of reports on symposia and monographs on exercise have appeared. Some of these are listed below and are a source of further data concerning the many effects of exercise in patients with coronary disease.

1. Amsterdam EA, Wilmore SH, and DeMaria AN (eds): *Exercise in Cardiovascular Health and Disease.* New York, Yorke Medical Books, 1977.
2. Milvy P (ed): The marathon; physiological, epidemiological and psychologic studies. Ann N Y Acad Sci *301*, 1977.
3. Froelicher VF: Does exercise conditioning delay progression of myocardial ischemia in coronary atherosclerotic heart disease? Cardiovasc Clin 8:11–31, 1977.
4. James WE, and Amsterdam ED (eds): *Coronary Heart Disease. Exercise Testing and Cardiac Rehabilitation.* New York/London, Stratton Intercontinental Medical Book Corp, 1977.
5. Wenger NK (ed): Exercise and the heart. Cardiovasc Clin 9, 1978.
6. Kala R, et al: Physical activity and sudden cardiac death. Adv Cardiol 25:27–34, 1978.

References

1. Hellerstein HK: Exercise therapy in convalescence from acute myocardial infarction. Schweiz Med Wochenschr *103*:66, 1973.
2. Barnard RJ, MacAlpin R, Kattus AA, and Buckberg GD: Ischemic response to sudden strenuous exertion in healthy men. Circulation 48:936, 1973.
3. DeBusk RF, Domanico L, Luft S, and Harrison DC: Return to work following myocardial infarction: a medical and economic critique of the work evaluation unit. J Chronic Dis 30:325, 1977.
4. Wilhelmsen L, Sanne H, Elmfeldt D, et al: A controlled trial of physical exercise on risk factors, non-fatal infarction and death. Prev Med 4:491, 1975.

5. Bruce EH, Fredrick K, Bruce RA, and Fischer LD: Comparison of active participants and drop-outs in CAPRI rehabilitation program. Am J Cardiol 37:53, 1976.
6. Gottheimer V: Long-range strenuous sports training for cardiac reconditioning and rehabilitation. Am J Cardiol 22:426, 1968.
7. Palatsi I: Feasibility of physical training after myocardial infarction and its effect on return to work, morbidity and mortality. Acta Med Scand (Suppl 599), 1976.
8. Rose G, Hamilton PJS, Keen H, et al: Myocardial ischemia, risk factors and death from coronary disease. Lancet 1:105–109, 1977.
9. Blumgart HL: The relation of effort to attacks of myocardial infarction. JAMA 128:775, 1945.
10. Blumgart HL: Coronary disease: clinical pathological correlations and physiology. Bull NY Acad Med 27:693, 1951.
11. Effler DB: Personal communication.
12. Eliot RS: Aerobic exercise as a therapeutic modality in the relief of stress. Adv Cardiovasc Disc 18:231, 1976.
13. Scherlis S (chairman): Report of the Committee on Stress, Strain, and Heart Disease. American Heart Association, Special Report. Circulation 55:825A, 1977.
14. Vickery DM, and Fries JF: Take Care of Yourself. A Consumer's Guide to Medical Care. Reading, Mass, Addison Wesley, 1976.
15. Kavanaugh T, and Shephard RS: Maximum exercise tests on postcoronary patients. J Appl Physiol 40:611, 1976.
16. Bruce RA: The benefits of physical training for patients with coronary heart disease. In Ingelfinger FJ, Ebert RV, Finland M, and Relman AS (eds): Controversies in Internal Medicine II. Philadelphia, WB Saunders Company, 1974, pp 145–161.
17. Sagall EL: In Yu PN, and Goodwin JF (eds): Progress in Cardiology 3 and Progress in Exercise Cardiology. Philadelphia, Lea and Febiger, 1974.
18. Sagall EL: Malpractice aspects of medically prescribed exercise. Leg Med Annu: 275, 1975.
19. French AJ, and Dock W: Fatal coronary arteriosclerosis in young soldiers. JAMA 123:1233, 1944.
20. McKenzie RT: Exercise in Education and Medicine, 2nd ed. Philadelphia, WB Saunders Company, 1917.
21. Kostrubala T, Orselli RC, Bassler TS, Ganda OP, Mueller J, Felts JH, Deftos LS, Schaff SH, Cantwell SD, and Stokes J: Letters to the editor: Marathon racing and myocardial infarction. Ann Intern Med 85:389, 1976.
22. Green LH, Cohen SI, and Kurland G: Fatal myocardial infarction in marathon racing. Ann Intern Med 84:704, 1976.
23. Parry CH: An enquiry into the symptoms and causes of syncope anginosa, commonly called angina pectoris. London, Cadell and Davis, 1799, p 148.
24. Blackburn H: Disadvantages of intensive exercise therapy after myocardial infarction. In Ingelfinger FJ, Ebert RV, Finland M, and Relman AS (eds): Controversies in Internal Medicine. Philadelphia, WB Saunders Company, 1974, pp 162–172.
25. Haskell WL: Cardiovascular complications during exercise training of cardiac patients. Circulation 57:920, 1978.

Patients With Coronary Heart Disease Should Avoid Strenuous Physical Exertion

Antagonist Position

NANETTE K. WENGER, M.D.

Professor of Medicine (Cardiology), Emory University
School of Medicine; Director, Cardiac Clinics, Grady
Memorial Hospital, Atlanta, Georgia

Among the advances in the care of the coronary patient during the past decade was the documentation that many patients should, can, and do return to a normal or near-normal lifestyle after recovery from myocardial infarction. In fact, the pattern of care for the coronary patient in recent years has been characterized by an increase in physical activity liberalization, a decrease in imposed invalidism, and earlier discharge from the hospital for selected patients; however, the advantages gained from this approach may be lost if rehabilitative programming does not continue after recovery.

The concept of individualized prescriptive exercise (physical activity) training is central to this rehabilitative approach. The heterogeneity of patients with coronary artery disease and their major qualitative and quantitative differences in functional impairment require that physical activity recommendations be individualized, based on the results of exercise stress testing, and that coronary patients never perform at an activity level greater than that safely completed (without untoward signs or symptoms) at prior exercise stress testing.

Physical Activity: Appropriate and Inappropriate Expectations

Before addressing the question of "strenuous" physical exertion, the beneficial effects of physical activity, in general, for patients with coronary atherosclerotic heart disease should be noted.

139

Although no definitive evidence is available that relates a physical activity program to the prevention of coronary atherosclerotic heart disease, numerous epidemiologic studies have documented the fact that habitually physically active populations have a lower incidence of, and a lower mortality from, myocardial infarction. The critical question for the post-coronary patient — whether physical training after myocardial infarction can alter the natural history of the illness — requires further research, and prescription of physical activity solely to achieve this goal is unwarranted. Perhaps the National Exercise and Heart Disease Project, a multicenter controlled study of the effect of medically supervised, prescribed physical activity on male survivors of myocardial infarction (aged 30 to 64), will provide some data.

What, then, is a realistic goal for a cardiac conditioning program? Exercise training can improve cardiovascular performance (physical working capacity) and efficiency in many patients following myocardial infarction. The physiologic response to training, both in normal individuals and in patients with cardiovascular disease, including patients who have had a myocardial infarction, is characterized by a decrease in the resting heart rate and systolic blood pressure and by a faster return to a normal heart rate after exertion; a smaller increase in heart rate and systolic blood pressure occurs at any submaximal level of work. These two parameters, the "rate-pressure product" or so-called "double product," are major determinants of myocardial oxygen requirements. One would expect, then, that the "trained" coronary patient will have less or no angina pectoris and less or no ST-segment displacement (as an indication of myocardial ischemia) on the electrocardiogram for any specific submaximal work load than before training. This is an improvement in work efficiency, i.e., less myocardial oxygen demand for any given submaximal task.

Cardiovascular training is also associated with an increase in maximal oxygen uptake, related to an augmentation of blood supply to exercising muscles and to increased extraction of oxygen. Training may also improve myocardial function and/or myocardial oxygen supply. These are the mechanisms by which training effects an improvement in exercise tolerance and alleviates symptoms of myocardial ischemia, permitting a greater intensity and duration of occupational and recreational work, before the attainment of the patient's ischemic threshold. Many patients can not only be readily restored to their pre-infarction status, but can also achieve a level of fitness superior to that before the onset of their illness.

Exercise has not been shown to have any effect on the coronary collateral circulation. Its major effect appears to result from peripheral circulatory alterations; myocardial functional alterations may also play a role, but this premise is controversial. There are good data to confirm that the development or increase of the coronary collateral circulation, at least coronary collateral vessels of a magnitude to be angiographically detectable, is related solely to the progression of the underlying atherosclerotic disease and is not altered by exercise training. No information is available, however, about alterations of flow through existing collateral vessels or about alterations in myocardial perfusion; these parameters cannot be measured angiographically and should be evaluated by myocardial scintigraphy and other newer techniques.

Thus, the physiologic advantages of an exercise training program relate primarily to the decrease in myocardial oxygen demand, after training, for the same amount of external work. There are also a number of additional benefits. Patients who exercise, who are physically fit, feel better, have an improved self-image, have lessened anxiety and depression scores (as measured by standardized psychometric tests), and appear better able to tolerate life stresses, i.e., to achieve an improvement in the quality of life. Psychologic improvement is particularly important in that there appears to be a greater incidence of impairment in post–myocardial infarction patients owing to emotional rather than physiologic factors. Physical activity programs appear to aid patients in renouncing the sick role and in returning to a normal lifestyle, including an earlier, increased, and more successful return to work. Exercise aids in weight control, which is important for the post-coronary patient; and it may provide an incentive for cessation of cigarette smoking. Exercise is associated with a decrease in the serum triglyceride level, although its effect on the serum cholesterol level is variable; it may, therefore, exert a beneficial effect by alteration of more powerful coronary risk factors. Sufficient data are not available to evaluate the effect of physical exertion on clotting parameters (fibrinolysis, platelet aggregation, and so on). Similarly, data remain controversial regarding the effects of exercise on cardiac dysrhythmias. However, exercise is important as a modality that is "prescribed" rather than "proscribed" for the post–myocardial infarction patient, as well as for the post–aortocoronary bypass surgery patient.

Strenuous Physical Exertion

What, then, is "strenuous" physical activity? And is strenuous physical activity appropriate or inappropriate for the coronary patient? The dictionary defines strenuous as vigorously active; energetic, marked by or calling for physical energy or stamina; arduous; rigorous. However, we must be concerned with "strenuous" exertion not as an absolute, but rather as it relates to the pre-infarction activity level and the physical fitness of the patient and to the extent of residual physiologic impairment following myocardial infarction.

For the executive who, before myocardial infarction, never performed activity more demanding than swiveling in his desk chair, bicycling, tennis, or golf would represent a modest increase in cardiac work (3 to 5 mets*), and snow shoveling or skiing would constitute a considerable activity increment (6 to 7 mets). But the laborer who saws wood, digs ditches, carries heavy loads, and so on, i.e., whose occupational work level is 7 to 8+ mets, can readily jog, play basketball, canoe, and so forth. Therefore, physicians must relate and compare the activities of daily living, the vocational activi-

---

*1 met = approximately 3.5 ml O_2/kg body weight/min.

ties, and the recreational activities of their patients and must make recommendations correlating activities in one sphere with those in another. They should also be familiar with the indications, contraindications, and methodology for exercise training programs designed to enhance functional capacity and should prescribe this therapeutic modality for their patients, when appropriate, to augment both their occupational and leisure physical capabilities.

The delineation of strenuous activity must also be related to the severity of the patient's coronary disease, i.e., the degree of residual physiologic impairment. About half of all patients who sustain a myocardial infarction have an uncomplicated clinical course, i.e., one not associated with significant dysrhythmia, recurrent or persistent chest pain, congestive heart failure, or shock. Most of these patients gradually improve their myocardial function after infarction, often with little or no functional impairment. Most patients with infarction of less than five per cent of their left ventricular mass have no clinically detectable cardiac functional abnormality and no abnormality of any of the laboratory parameters designed to assess myocardial function. These patients have an excellent prognosis, as the annual survival rate for these Class I functional status individuals approximates 95 per cent. Well over 85 per cent of these "uncomplicated" patients who were employed at the time of myocardial infarction return to work eight to 12 weeks afterwards, usually to the same job; and almost 80 per cent of all myocardial infarction (complicated and uncomplicated) survivors, working at the time of infarction, return to work within the year. This return to remunerative work is indicative of their cardiac reserve.

The extent of physiologic impairment resulting from myocardial infarction relates to the amount of myocardial necrosis and scarring (and the degree of pre-existing scarring from prior myocardial infarction), to the site of the infarction (e.g., ischemia or scarring of a papillary muscle may produce mitral regurgitation), and to the amount of residual ischemic myocardium. Congestive heart failure is virtually absent in patients with angina pectoris without infarction of the myocardium, whereas most patients with greater than 20 per cent destruction of the left ventricular myocardium show evidence of congestive heart failure. Using the clinically familiar New York Heart Association functional classification enables some general concepts regarding physical activity to be presented.

Class I patients, those who remain asymptomatic at ordinary daily vocational and leisure activity levels, have minimal or no functional cardiac impairment. These patients do not manifest angina pectoris, congestive heart failure, or serious dysrhythmia. They can readily perform at work loads of 7 to 8 mets or greater. They have virtually no occupational or physical activity restrictions; and it is precisely these patients with little or no detectable alteration of cardiac performance who can and do participate in very high-level recreational physical activities, including marathon running, when properly trained.

Class II patients become symptomatic with prolonged physical and/or emotional stress and may have a 20 to 40 per cent impairment of cardiac function, but should have an occupational or recreational activity tolerance in the 5- to 6-met range. They can be expected to perform most general industrial labor. Again, these patients' symptoms may relate to ischemia, to myocardial dysfunction, or to electrical instability of the heart.

Class III individuals become symptomatic with usual daily living activities; because they have a 50 to 75 per cent impairment of cardiac function, their exercise tolerance is usually limited to the 3- to 4-met range. They are not candidates for strenuous physical activity, by any definition, unless their functional capacity can be improved by medical and/or surgical intervention. Vocationally, most desk or bench jobs are within their capabilities. Nevertheless, low-level prescriptive exercise training may be appropriate for selected patients in this category, with careful monitoring of their myocardial ischemic threshold (angina pectoris and/or ischemic ST-segment changes on the electrocardiogram), of the appearance of or increase in ventricular dysrhythmia, and of the exacerbation of congestive heart failure.

Severely impaired (80 per cent plus) Class IV patients are symptomatic at rest or with minimal activity with a functional capacity of 2 mets or less. Symptoms may include myocardial ischemia (angina pectoris), congestive heart failure, dysrhythmia, or a combination of these problems. Their vocational capabilities are extremely limited, and any strenuous activity is inappropriate for this group.

In summary, not all post–myocardial infarction patients are suitable candidates for cardiac conditioning programs, for strenuous physical activity. Clinically, patients with unstable angina, with uncontrolled hypertension or heart failure, with significant cardiac dysrhythmias (especially those rhythm disturbances that increase with exercise), or with gross cardiac enlargement are not suitable candidates for exercise training. These are generally the Class III and Class IV patients.

Additionally, not all coronary patients can improve their exercise tolerance with training, even though they have no contraindications to beginning exercise training and despite their being enrolled in and adhering to an appropriate training program. This lack of response may be the result of the development of left ventricular dysfunction or heart failure at higher levels of activity or may be due to a progression of the underlying coronary atherosclerotic heart disease during the exercise training period. Serial exercise testing during exercise training is therefore requisite to document an improvement in exercise tolerance with training and to insure maintenance of this improvement of cardiovascular functional capacity. Failure to improve cardiac performance requires that the physician carefully reassess the patient for alternate medical and/or surgical intervention.

Exercise Recommendations for Coronary Patients

Exercise recommendations for coronary patients, both after myocardial infarction and after aortocoronary bypass surgery, are designed to attain and maintain the "training effect," the improvement in cardiovascular functional capacity.

What type and level of exercise is requisite to achieve the benefits of training? How does this relate to the question of "strenuous physical exertion"? As previously mentioned, prescriptive, individualized exercise training demands that prior multilevel exercise stress testing be performed as the basis for the safety and the accuracy of exercise prescription. Exercise stress testing permits quantitative determination of the patient's functional capacity and hemodynamic response to exercise and defines the level of activity at which evidence of myocardial ischemia and/or dysrhythmias may occur.

Exercise training (cardiac conditioning) requires the imposition of a target work load, calculated as a percentage of the patient's measured physical work capacity. To achieve a training effect, patients should exercise at least two or three times weekly, preferably on non-successive days, for a 20- to 30-minute session that includes a warm-up and cool-down period and at an intensity to attain 65 to 85 per cent of the maximal heart rate safely achieved at prior exercise stress testing. Although somewhat arbitrary, these recommendations are generally considered effective. In general, the 65 to 75 per cent target heart rate is used for unsupervised, individual home programs and the 80 to 85 per cent level for supervised gymnasium programs. An increased duration and frequency of exercise can compensate fairly well for the slightly lower intensity of training in unsupervised home programs, thus attaining the same benefits without undue risk.

Exercise should be dynamic (isotonic), involving rhythmic, repetitive movements of large muscle masses, with arms and legs being trained. Isotonic exercises significantly and proportionately increase the heart rate, stroke volume, and cardiac output, with little associated change in mean arterial pressure. The sustained increase in blood flow required to meet the metabolic needs of large masses of exercising muscle thus places an increased volume load on the heart, inducing the conditioning or training effect. Isotonic activities include walking, jogging, swimming, bicycling, noncompetitive running games, rowing, and cross-country skiing.

In general, cardiac patients should avoid primarily isometric or static exercises (those causing a sustained increase in muscle tension with little change in muscle length). These exercises do not produce a stroke volume and cardiac output increase commensurate with the intensity of the activity involved, as do dynamic exercises; hence, they do not result in cardiovascular fitness. The pressor response relates to the percentage of maximal voluntary contraction of the particular muscle group involved, and thus is greater in patients with decreased muscular strength (decreased maximal voluntary contraction). The abrupt disproportionate blood pressure increase associated with isometric activity imposes a sudden, undue pressure work load, and thus an increased oxygen demand, on a potentially ischemic left ventricle and may thereby precipitate angina pectoris, life-threatening dysrhythmias, and cardiac decompensation.

Although continuous training more effectively increases endurance, interval training, at least when beginning an exercise program, is more appropriate for cardiac patients in that significant oxygen debt and high blood lactate levels can be avoided. Additionally, enjoyable recreational activities should be included, as these encourage adherence to the exercise program. Exercise, as any other therapeutic modality, must become a lifetime pattern for its effect to be maintained.

Calisthenics and walk-jog sequences, often the core components of prescriptive exercise, can readily be tailored to the above recommendations by altering the complexity, the number of repetitions, and the speed of their performance. But what of the enjoyable recreational activities?

Class I patients can readily bicycle, horseback ride, do vigorous downhill skiing, mountain climb, and play hockey, basketball, paddle ball, and touch football, all activities in the 7- to 8-met range. With training, should this be their penchant, they can expect to safely and successfully bicycle and play basketball more vigorously, cross-country ski, play handball and squash, or participate in marathon running, activities in the 8- to 10 plus-met scale.

Appropriate recreational activities for the Class II patient (5- to 6-met range) would include slower bicycling and horseback riding, canoeing, stream fishing, or ice or roller skating.

A variable dosage of many therapeutic agents — digitalis, nitrate preparations, beta-blocking drugs, and so on — is appropriate for coronary patients; similarly, a variable dosage of physical activity may be indicated, to be determined by the intensity, frequency, and duration of exercise. Critical to the attainment of a training effect is the challenge to the oxygen transport system, the percentage of maximal heart rate (as safely achieved at prior exercise stress testing) attained; thus, the well-trained and/or insignificantly impaired individual exercising at an 8-met level is operating at the same relative oxygen cost (percentage of maximal oxygen uptake) as the sedentary and/or modestly impaired patient working at a 4-met level, despite the significant difference in external work load. And it is the percentage of maximal oxygen uptake that determines for the individual patient the dose/effect relationship.

Inappropriately increasing the intensity of exercise entails an undue risk of developing manifestations of myocardial ischemia; and excessive prolongation of exercise duration or increase in exercise frequency appears to increase the risk of orthopedic and other complications.

As with other therapeutic modalities, the physician must periodically assess the effect of the exercise program. Failure of the patient to achieve the target heart rate at peak exercise is an indication for increasing the work level. Imposition of a systematically upgraded exercise "dosage" will cause an improvement in functional capacity. Similarly, an excessive heart rate response to a given level of activity or the occurrence of adverse signs or symptoms demands a lessening of the increments in work level.

The proper approach, then, is not to question whether strenuous physical exertion is appropriate or inappropriate for coronary heart disease patients, but rather to identify the beneficial and safe absolute work load indicated for each individual coronary patient at a specific stage in recovery and rehabilitation. This concept maximizes the benefits of exercise training without the imposition of undue hazard.

Summary

Substantial benefits can accrue when individualized, prescriptive physical activity is incorporated into the plan of care for selected patients after myocardial infarction. Favorable responses include an improved functional capacity and work performance, decreased symptoms of myocardial ischemia, reduced psychologic impairment, and an enhanced return to vocational and leisure activities.

Comment

There are few areas in cardiology that appear to bring out as much vehemence as does the controversy over the benefit or lack of benefit of exercise in the management of coronary heart disease. Much of this relates to the fact that the amount of hard data on this subject is still relatively small.

It seems fair to state that there is no strong evidence today that exercise prolongs survival in patients who have coronary heart disease when compared with appropriate randomized controls. A multicenter cooperative study under the auspices of the Rehabilitation Services Administration of HEW is currently undertaking such research, and it is hoped that the results will be known shortly. In the interim, it would seem that if one can join a supervised exercise program and enjoys the type of physical activity involved, the evidence would seem to favor participation within the exercise prescription limits defined by Dr. Wenger. On the other hand, there are potential problems related to the use of strenuous physical exertion in an unsupervised fashion where cardiopulmonary resuscitation, should it prove necessary, is impossible or unlikely. Dr. Burchell has outlined some of these, including a medicolegal one.

It is my practice to advise patients to be physically active within the limits of noncompetitive sports and at a level of activity that does not produce detectable symptoms. The physical and psychological benefits would seem to outweigh the risks of a rare, harmful outcome. I do not recommend jogging or severe strenuous physical exertion for patients with known coronary heart disease. I do encourage my patients to engage in level walking to the fullest extent possible and to participate in noncompetitive sports that they enjoy, such as golf or swimming. Until such time as prolongation of life is demonstrated by controlled studies, this seems to be a prudent compromise between those who would promote a sedentary lifestyle in the coronary patient out of fear that exercise may precipitate a myocardial infarct or sudden death and those who would have him engage in competitive marathon running.

ELLIOT RAPAPORT, M.D.

147

Seven

Does Coronary Vein Bypass Graft Surgery Prolong Life in Patients with Chronic, Stable Angina Pectoris?

CORONARY VEIN BYPASS GRAFT SURGERY PROLONGS
LIFE IN PATIENTS WITH CHRONIC, STABLE ANGINA
PECTORIS
  Nicholas T. Kouchoukos, M.D.

WILL CORONARY VEIN BYPASS GRAFTING PROLONG
LIFE IN PATIENTS WITH CHRONIC, STABLE ANGINA
PECTORIS?
  Henry D. McIntosh, M.D.

COMMENT

Coronary Vein Bypass Graft Surgery Prolongs Life in Patients with Chronic, Stable Angina Pectoris

NICHOLAS T. KOUCHOUKOS, M.D.

Professor of Surgery, Division of Cardiovascular and
Thoracic Surgery, Department of Surgery, University of
Alabama School of Medicine, University of Alabama
Medical Center, Birmingham, Alabama

The decision to recommend coronary bypass grafting procedures for patients with angina pectoris requires knowledge of the risks of operation and the effects of the procedures on altering the natural history of the disease, particularly when comparing the results with conventional medical therapy. Considerable data have been accumulated in both retrospective and prospective studies that demonstrate rather conclusively that bypass grafting is more effective than medical therapy for relief of angina pectoris in the early years after diagnosis. As yet incompletely answered are the questions of whether coronary bypass grafting reduces the incidence of cardiac-related complications or enhances survival in patients with coronary artery disease.

A number of studies on the natural history of patients with coronary artery disease studied angiographically have defined categories of patients with differing degrees of coronary atherosclerosis and left ventricular dysfunction who are at varying degrees of risk of death from myocardial infarction or other cardiac-related causes. Currently, several prospective trials comparing medical and surgical therapy in subgroups of patients with coronary artery disease are in progress, but the definitive results of most of these studies are not yet available. Until these results are known, retrospective analysis of comparable subgroups of patients with coronary atherosclerosis managed with and without operation permits some assessment of the relative effectiveness of these two methods of therapy and allows some

151

conclusions to be drawn regarding therapy for individual patients. These conclusions may be modified as new information accumulates.

Comparison of Medical and Surgical Therapy

Since the extent of the coronary atherosclerotic process and the severity of left ventricular dysfunction are the major determinants of survival following diagnosis, subgroups of patients with left main coronary artery disease, three-vessel, two-vessel, and one-vessel disease, and varying degrees of left ventricular dysfunction managed surgically and medically will be examined.

LEFT MAIN CORONARY ARTERY DISEASE

Studies on the natural history of patients with atherosclerotic disease of the left main coronary artery have documented the relatively unfavorable prognosis of this subgroup.[1] The five-year mortality rates are high (greater than 40 per cent) in patients with more than two other vessels involved (the majority of patients), even in the presence of normal ventriculograms (45 per cent). Recent studies comparing surgical and medical therapy in comparable patients with greater than 50 per cent stenosis of the left main coronary artery have consistently demonstrated improved survival in the surgically treated patients (Fig. 1).[2-4] The study of Takaro et al.[3] represents a prospective randomized trial of these two forms of therapy. The other two studies are retrospective, comparing surgically treated patients with patients considered candidates for operation by anatomic and hemodynamic criteria but managed nonoperatively. Statistically significant differences in

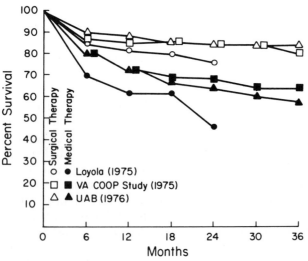

Figure 1. Actuarial survival of surgically and medically treated patients with greater than 50 per cent stenosis of the left main coronary artery. Data of Talano[2] (Loyola) and Oberman[4] (UAB) are from retrospective studies; data of Takaro[3] (VA Cooperative Study) are from a prospective randomized study. Differences in survival between surgical and medical therapy were statistically significant in all three series between 12 and 24 months following diagnosis.

survival rates have been demonstrated in all three studies in the first two years following diagnosis. While comparison of patients from different centers may be criticized on the basis of nonuniformity of medical and surgical therapy, the survival curves from all three centers for both types of therapy are strikingly similar. Thus, in this subgroup, surgical therapy is associated with a higher survival rate in the two to three years following diagnosis.

THREE-VESSEL DISEASE

Data regarding long-term survival of patients with three-vessel disease randomly allocated to surgical and medical therapy are not presently available. Retrospective analyses comparing medical and surgical therapy in patients in this subgroup have demonstrated enhanced survival in the surgically treated groups (Fig. 2).[5, 6] In our own series of 434 patients treated surgically and 97 patients considered suitable candidates for operation but managed medically, statistically significant (p < 0.05) differences in survival rates were observed at 36 and 61 months. The patients in the two groups were comparable with respect to age, sex, presence of hypertension, elevated serum cholesterol, symptoms of cardiac failure, and electrocardiographic evidence of previous myocardial infarction. Similar and statistically significant differences in survival rates at 36 months were noted in the series reported from the Cleveland Clinic Foundation.[5] Actuarial survival data of a large group of surgically treated patients with three-vessel disease reported by Stiles et al.[7] are also shown in Figure 2. The similarity of the survival curves for the three surgically treated and the two medically treated groups is apparent.

TWO-VESSEL DISEASE

Retrospective comparisons of surgical and medical therapy in patients with two-vessel disease are shown in Figure 3. In our series of 317 patients having bypass grafting and 86 patients managed nonsurgically, a statistically significant difference in survival rates was observed at 43 months. The patients in these two groups were also comparable with regard to age, sex, and coronary risk factors. In the series from the Cleveland Clinic Foundation, a statistically significant difference in survival rates was present at 24 months.[5] The survival data of 446 patients treated surgically by Stiles et al.[7] are also shown in Figure 3. Again, the similarity of the survival curves from different centers for large numbers of surgically treated patients and for patients considered as candidates for operation but managed medically is noted.

ONE-VESSEL DISEASE

With the possible exception of patients with occlusive lesions confined to the proximal left anterior descending coronary artery, bypass grafting has not been shown to enhance survival of patients with occlusive disease con-

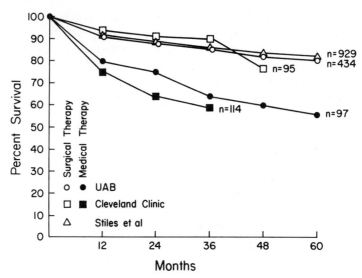

Figure 2. Actuarial survival of surgically and medically treated patients with three-vessel disease (retrospective studies). Patients in the medically treated groups met anatomic and hemodynamic criteria for bypass grafting. Differences in survival in the UAB[6] and Cleveland Clinic Foundation[5] series were statistically significant at 36 months. Also shown for comparison are the 929 surgically treated patients of Stiles et al.[7]

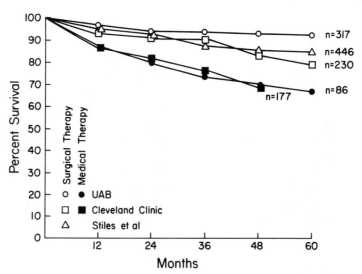

Figure 3. Actuarial survival of surgically and medically treated patients with two-vessel disease (retrospective studies). Patients in the medically treated groups met anatomic and hemodynamic criteria for bypass grafting. Differences in survival in the UAB[6] and Cleveland Clinic Foundation[5] series were statistically significant at 43 and 24 months, respectively. Also shown for comparison are the 446 surgically treated patients of Stiles et al.[7]

fined to one of the major coronary arterial systems.[5] Sheldon et al.,[5] comparing 82 surgically treated and 69 medically treated patients with occlusive disease of the anterior descending coronary artery, demonstrated a statistically significant difference ($p < 0.0001$) in survival rates three years following diagnosis (97 per cent vs. 84 per cent). However, the suitability for operation of all patients in the medically treated group was not established. In our own experience with 29 surgically and 24 medically treated patients with stable angina who were similar with regard to age, sex, duration of angina, incidence of previous myocardial infarction, and symptoms of congestive failure, as well as suitability for operation, no statistically significant differences in survival rates were noted in the follow-up period (mean of 42 months for the surgically treated and 54 months for the medically treated patients).[8]

MULTIPLE-VESSEL DISEASE WITH IMPAIRED LEFT VENTRICULAR FUNCTION

Patients with multiple-vessel disease and evidence of severe impairment of left ventricular function (cardiomegaly, symptoms of congestive failure, diffuse left ventricular contractile abnormalities, and depressed ejection fraction) have an unfavorable prognosis when managed nonsurgically.[6, 9] Although bypass grafting procedures in patients of this type were initially associated with high in-hospital mortality, improvements in operative technique and postoperative care have resulted in a substantial reduction in the operative risk. Recent comparisons of patients of this type managed with and without operation have demonstrated improved survival in the three to six years following diagnosis for the former group (Fig. 4).[6, 10, 11] While survival following operation was poorer in these patients than in surgically treated patients with normal ventricular function, as noted in the series of Manley et al. (Fig. 4B),[10] survival was greater in all categories of patients with left ventricular dysfunction managed surgically, and these differences were statistically significant at six years.

Summary and Conclusions

From these analyses we conclude that survival in several subgroups of patients with coronary atherosclerosis and angina pectoris is enhanced by coronary bypass grafting. This includes patients with greater than 50 per cent stenosis of the left main coronary artery, patients with three-vessel disease, and probably patients with two-vessel disease who have normal or only moderately impaired left ventricular function and in whom there are no major contraindications to operation. Inherent in this conclusion are the assumptions that in-hospital mortality rates are low (less than 2 to 3 per cent) and that the incidence of cardiac-related complications, especially perioperative infarction, is less than 5 to 10 per cent. This is of particular importance in those subgroups in which the annual mortality rates with

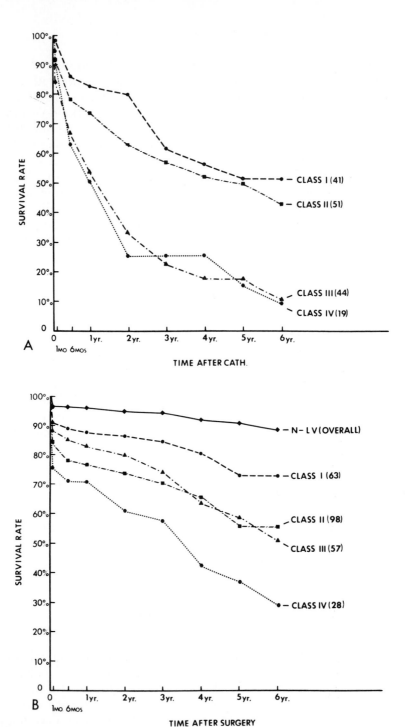

Figure 4. (A) Actuarial survival of medically treated patients with coronary atherosclerosis and varying degrees of left ventricular dysfunction [moderate (Class I) to severe (Class IV)]. (B) Actuarial survival of surgically treated patients with similar degrees of left ventricular dysfunction. Survival rates were significantly greater (p < 0.01) in the surgically treated patients in all classes at six years. N = survival of patients with normal left ventricular function. (From Manley JC, King JF, Zeft HJ, and Johnson, WD: The "bad" left ventricle: Results of coronary surgery and effect on late survival. J Thorac Cardiovasc Surg 72:841–848, 1976. Reproduced by permission.)

156

nonsurgical treatment are relatively low (i.e., two-vessel disease). Survival of patients with multiple-vessel disease and moderate or severe impairment of left ventricular function is also improved when compared with patients managed nonoperatively, despite higher operative and late mortality rates than for patients with normal or minimally impaired left venticular function. Survival is not improved by surgical therapy in patients with single-vessel disease of the right or circumflex arteries in the three to five years following diagnosis. The data with regard to the anterior descending artery are, in our opinion, inconclusive at present. Continuing evaluation of the patients described above and analysis of data from the prospective randomized trials may identify more discrete subsets of patients who will or will not benefit from bypass grafting. Until these data become available, the conclusions above appear warranted.

References

1. Lim JS, Proudfit WL, and Sones FM Jr: Left main coronary arterial obstruction: long-term follow-up of 141 nonsurgical cases. Am J Cardiol 36:131, 1975.
2. Talano JV, Scanlon PJ, Meadow WR, Kahn M, Pifarre R, and Gunnar RM: Influence of surgery on survival in 145 patients with left main coronary artery disease. Circulation 52(Suppl 1):I-1–105, 1975.
3. Takaro T, Hultgren HN, Lipton MJ, and Detre KM, and Participants in the Study Group: The VA cooperative randomized study of surgery for coronary arterial occlusive disease. II. Subgroup with significant left main lesions. Circulation 54(Suppl III):III-107–117, 1976.
4. Oberman A, Kouchoukos NT, Harrell RR, Holt JH Jr, Russell RO Jr, and Rackley CE: Surgical versus medical treatment in disease of the left main coronary artery. Lancet 2:591–594, 1976.
5. Sheldon WC, Rincon G, Pichard AD, Razavi M, Cheanvechai C, and Loop FD: Surgical treatment of coronary artery disease: pure graft operations, with a study of 741 patients followed 3–7 yrs. Progr Cardiovasc Dis 18:237–252, 1975.
6. Kouchoukos NT, Oberman A, and Karp RB: Results of surgery for disabling angina pectoris. Cardiovas Clin 8/2:157, 1977.
7. Stiles QR, Lindesmith GG, Tucker BL, Hughes RK, and Meyer BW: Long-term follow-up of patients with coronary artery bypass grafts. Circulation 54(Suppl III):III-32–34, 1976.
8. Kouchoukos NT, Oberman A, Russell RO Jr, and Jones WB: Surgical versus medical treatment for occlusive disease confined to the left anterior descending coronary artery. Am J Cardiol 35:836–842, 1975.
9. Bruschke AVG, Proudfit WL, and Sones FM Jr: Progress study of 590 consecutive nonsurgical cases of coronary disease followed 5–9 years. II. Ventriculographic and other correlations. Circulation 47:1154, 1973.
10. Manley JC, King JF, Zeft HK, and Johnson WD: The "bad" left ventricle: results of coronary surgery and effect on late survival. J Thorac Cardiovasc Surg 72:841–848, 1976.
11. Steele P, Vogel R, Anderson J, Pappas G, and Frischknecht J: Results of medical and surgical treatment of patients with coronary disease and left ventricular dysfunction. Am J Cardiol 39:286, 1977.

Will Coronary Vein Bypass Grafting Prolong Life in Patients with Chronic, Stable Angina Pectoris?

HENRY D. McINTOSH, M.D.

Adjunct Professor of Medicine, Baylor College of
Medicine, Houston, Texas; Clinical Professor of Medicine,
The University of Florida School of Medicine, Gainesville,
Florida; Cardiology Section, Watson Clinic, Lakeland,
Florida.

Recent reports indicate that deaths due to coronary heart disease (CHD) are declining in this country (Fig. 1). Despite these encouraging observations, CHD continues to be the leading cause of death. In 1975, 30.9 per cent of the 642.3 deaths per 100,000 U.S. population were due to CHD; about one quarter were in patients less than 65 years of age. It was predicted that more than 640,000 persons would die in 1976 from this condition. It is not surprising that great interest would be generated by any procedure that might reduce such an enormous death rate. Aortocoronary bypass grafting (ACBG) has been lauded as such a procedure.

Although carried out for the first time in 1964, it was not until three years later that Favaloro at the Cleveland Clinic demonstrated that the ACBG procedure could be performed on large numbers of patients with a low rate of operative mortality and a high incidence of relief of pain. When postoperative studies demonstrated patent grafts bypassing significant obstructions and perfusing ischemic or potentially ischemic myocardium, enthusiasm for the procedure mounted; scientific skepticism and inquisitiveness was frequently abandoned by surgeons and cardiologists alike who became enthusiastic devotees of the procedure. It was assumed by many that the life of the patient afflicted by CHD would most surely be prolonged by the addition of new blood flow to the native circulation.

In 1970, Morris et al.[1] reported a total in-hospital mortality rate of 8.7 per

158

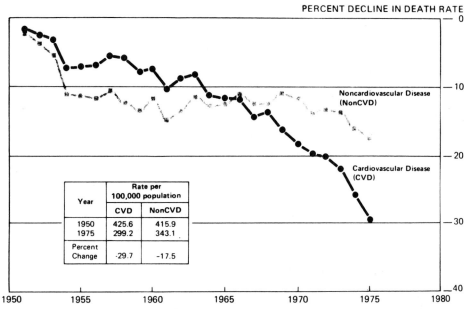

PERCENT DECLINE IN DEATH RATE

Year	Rate per 100,000 population	
	CVD	NonCVD
1950	425.6	415.9
1975	299.2	343.1
Percent Change	-29.7	-17.5

*Age adjusted to United States population in 1940.

Figure 1.   Per cent decline in death rates° since 1950 for cardiovascular and noncardiovascular disease in the United States.

cent "despite almost no exclusion of very ill or bad-risk patients as operative candidates"; they predicted that "only time and actuarial studies will provide undisputed truth of the efficacy of the distal coronary bypass."

The operative mortality declined further, and enthusiasm for the procedure increased. The procedure was adopted in many centers for the treatment not only of symptomatic CHD, i.e., ischemic heart disease (IHD), but also for people without symptoms who, for one reason or another, were found by selective arteriography to have stenosis of one or more coronary arteries. It was furthermore concluded by many investigators that it would be unethical to deny such potential benefits to patients who might constitute a control group.

No registry was established to record the frequency or the results of ACBG. Therefore, how many ACBG's have been carried out in this country is unknown. It has been estimated that over the last decade more than 300,000 such procedures may have been performed; as many 80,000 to 100,000 procedures may have been carried out in 1977 alone. The ACBG has been reported to be the most commonly performed surgical procedure in a number of cities.

If a therapy is to be useful, it should prevent or modify the clinical manifestations of the disease in question. As regards IHD, these include:
1.   Acute myocardial infarction
2.   Serious arrhythmias or conduction abnormalities

3. Congestive heart failure
4. Premature death
   a. Sudden
   b. Nonsudden
5. Pain of myocardial ischemia

What is known from this experience with approximately 300,000 ACBG's over a period of a decade about the role of this procedure in preventing or favorably modifying these clinical manifestations?

Beginning with the early reports, the efficacy of ACBG was compared to studies of patients whose coronary anatomy and pathologic involvement had been defined by selective coronary arteriography. There are five such studies (Fig. 2).

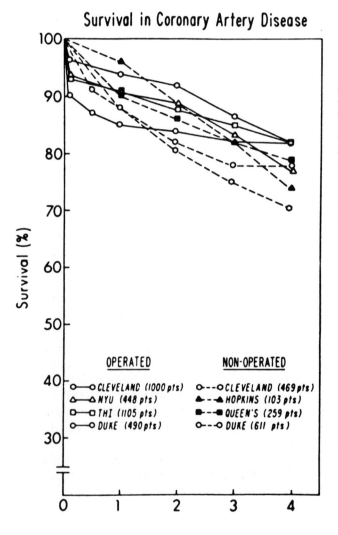

Survival in Coronary Artery Disease

OPERATED	NON-OPERATED
o—o CLEVELAND (1000 pts)	o---o CLEVELAND (469 pts)
△—△ NYU (448 pts)	▲--▲ HOPKINS (103 pts)
□—□ THI (1105 pts)	■--■ QUEEN'S (259 pts)
o—o DUKE (490 pts)	o---o DUKE (611 pts)

Figure 2. Recorded are the mortality data of three of the studies of the natural history of nonoperated patients with CHD that are frequently used for a control population against which to compare the results of surgery [Cleveland,[5] Hopkins,[2] and Queens[7]]. These studies were initiated and essentially completed in the 1960's. In addition, the survival data of three large series of patients who were operated without controls in the early 1970's [Cleveland, New York University, and the Texas Heart Institute] are recorded. Finally, data of patients operated and not operated at Duke University Medical Center but followed simultaneously and compared by computer matching techniques are recorded. (From Rosati RA, Mittler BS, Behar VS, Lee KL, McNeer JF, and Margolis JR: Does coronary surgery prolong life in comparison with medical management? Postgrad Med J 52:479, 1976.)

1A.   Friesinger et al.[2] reported the mortality from IHD in relation to the extent of atherosclerotic involvement determined angiographically in 224 patients followed two to nine years. This group was selected from 350 patients who were studied by coronary arteriography at Johns Hopkins from 1960 to 1967. One hundred twenty-six patients were excluded because they had unsatisfactory studies, evidence of primary myocardial or valvular disease, or because they received a coronary vascular surgical procedure. Of the remaining 224 patients, 121 were considered not to have CHD. Of the 103 patients with CHD, those with severe disease involving at least two coronary arteries had an annual mortality rate of 10 per cent; those with mild disease had an annual attrition rate of only one per cent.

1B.   Humphries et al.[3] extended the follow-up of the above patients for five to 12 years. The group with mild disease had no significant mortality rate. The group with moderate CHD experienced an accelerated deterioration between the sixth and ninth years; the overall mortality rate was about 50 per cent. After 10 years, 50 per cent of the patients with severe atherosclerosis had died.

2.   In 1973, Bruschke et al.[4] reported the five-year survival of 590 non–surgically treated patients studied angiographically at the Cleveland Clinic from January 1963 through July 1965. All patients had a 50 per cent or greater obstruction of a major coronary vessel. These 590 patients were consecutively studied, except for the exclusion of 17 patients lost to follow-up and an unspecified number of patients in whom a surgical procedure was done. Owing to the selection for surgery of a relatively high proportion of patients with single-vessel disease and normal left ventricular function, a relatively high proportion of high-risk patients was, from the arteriographic standpoint, delegated to the medical group. This study has been used as the control for a number of groups of operated patients, one of which was reported from the Texas Heart Institute (Fig. 3).

3.   The experience at the Cleveland Clinic was re-evaluated by Webster et al.[5] They included in this study only patients with an 80 to 100 per cent occlusion of a major coronary artery. Four hundred sixty-nine patients were collected from 1960 through 1965 and followed from six to 11 years. Although the severity of the disease and the duration of the follow-up of patients in this and the former study differed, when the mortality rate was "annualized," it was surprisingly similar for the two series. The annual mortality rate for those with single-vessel disease was 2.9 per cent and 3.3 per cent, respectively; for those with three-vessel disease, it was 10.4 per cent and 10.5 per cent per year, respectively.

4.   Oberman et al.[6] reported 301 patients studied at the University of Alabama between 1965 and 1970 and followed for a mean of 22 months. Fifty-five patients were extracted for surgery, leaving 246 patients with a greater than 50 per cent obstruction of the lumen of one or more major coronary arteries. In this study, the mortality rate for those with single-vessel disease was one per cent, and for three-vessel disease, 15 per cent.

5.   Burggraf and Parker,[7] from 1964 to the early 1970's, followed 259 of 490 patients with significant coronary artery disease who were not operated; the other 231 patients were operated. Seven additional patients with critical

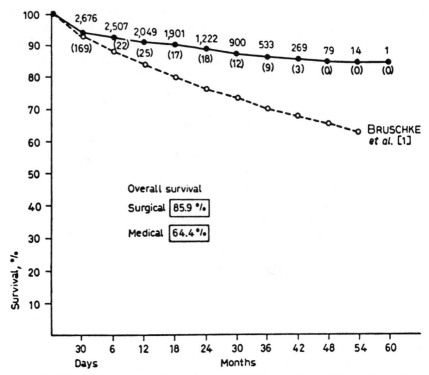

Figure 3. Survival of patients who underwent ACBG at the Texas Heart Institute from 1969 through 1974 is compared to the survival studied at the Cleveland Clinic from January 1963 through July 1965 and treated for five years medically. (From Reul GJ Jr, Cooley DA, Wukasch DC, Kyger ER III, Sandiford FM, Hallman GL, and Norman JC: Long-term survival following coronary artery bypass. Analysis of 4,522 consecutive patients. Arch Surg *110*:1419, 1975.)

stenosis of the left main coronary artery were analyzed separately. The annual mortality rate for those with single-vessel disease was 1.6 per cent, and for those with triple-vessel disease, 9 per cent.

Each of these studies was initiated in the early or mid 1960's; apparently only a few patients in any of the studies were followed after 1970. In the early and mid 1960's, only a few centers were actively involved in studying and treating patients with suspected CHD. It is reasonable to believe that many, if not most, of the patients were referred by physicians or that the patients themselves came to one of the four centers because of the severity of their symptoms. Those who, after coronary arteriography, were found not to have CHD were excluded. Those patients with CHD probably represented extensive disease. During the follow-up of several of the groups, from time to time, patients were extracted for the surgery of the day. Thus, there most likely remained the residual of patients who might be anticipated to do poorly by any therapy in vogue at the time.

One additional study has frequently served as a control to determine the benefits of ACBG. In 1974, Reeves et al.[8] reported survival data based on the previously discussed studies of Friesinger et al.,[2] Oberman et al.,[6] and three additional studies that were reported in abstract form only! Although the survival data were calculated for 995 patients, the details apparently available to the author defining the clinical, anatomical, and functional characteristics of over half of the patients were most brief. The data were included in abstracts of "300 words or less." Despite this glaring deficiency, it was concluded that the annual mortality rate for those with single-vessel disease was 2.2 per cent, and for those with triple-vessel disease, 11.4 per cent.

But the natural history of the population of patients with CHD from which patients for ACBG were selected was undergoing a striking and gratifying change. The natural history of CHD in the 1970's differs greatly from the natural history of the population from which the control groups were selected in the 1960's.

IHD reached the peak incidence of death in the U.S. in 1963. From 1950 to that date the mortality rate increased by 19 per cent. From 1963 to 1973, the age-specific death rate of subjects from 35 to 74 years old decreased by 18.4 per cent (Fig. 4). The incidence of death decreased by five per cent even for those 75 years of age. In 1975, for the first time in several years, there were less than one million deaths from cardiovascular causes (Fig. 5). The life expectancy for the average male in the U.S. increased between 1971 and 1974 by one year. It has recently been reported to have increased by three years.

Clearly, several identifiable trends have been proceeding in parallel over the last decade or more. The medical management of IHD has changed. New modes of therapy have been introduced. These include coronary care units, lidocaine, propranolol, potent diuretics, life-support systems, and so forth. The general public has become more aware of the recognized risk factors: smoking, hypertension, diet, obesity, and physical inactivity, and the public has done something about them.

Other less easily identifiable and understandable changes have occurred.[9, 10] For example, the frequency and severity of the atherosclerotic process affecting the coronary arteries of young adult males appear to have decreased. In 1953, Enos reported observations of the coronary vessels of 300 U.S. soldiers killed in the Korean conflict; 73 per cent had some degree of atherosclerosis of the coronary arteries. Fifteen per cent had over 50 per cent luminal narrowing as judged by gross examination. Eighteen years later, McNamara examined the hearts of 105 U.S. soldiers killed in the Viet Nam conflict; only 45 per cent had any evidence of atherosclerosis, and of this group only five per cent had evidence of severe coronary atherosclerosis. In only one case was any degree of stenosis observed. Both groups consisted of young male combat troops killed in action with a mean age of 22.1 years and an identical age range. The only difference was that they were separated in time by 18 years.

In light of these observations, can the thoughtful physician determine the role of ACBG in reducing the incidence or severity of the clinical manifestations of IHD, especially that of premature death, by comparing today's results of surgery with controls studied in the 1960's? Such a comparison may be of little value in light of the significant improvement in the natural history of IHD. Before recommending ACBG, should not one consider the hazards that may be produced by the procedure? Should not one consider the complications that may result from the procedure? What complications have been associated with ACBG?

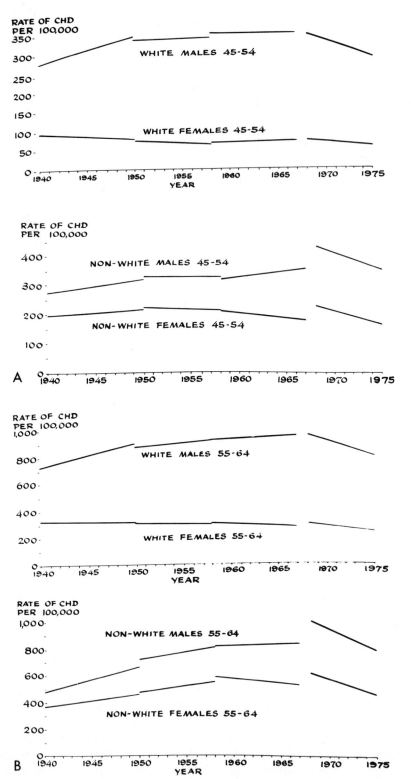

Figure 4. Trend of U.S. mortality from CHD by age, sex, and race, 1940–1975. Persons ages 45 to 54 are represented in graphs A and those between 55 and 64 years are represented in graphs B.

164

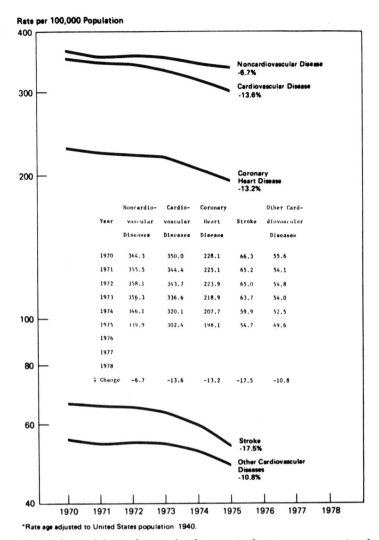

Figure 5. Death rates° for cardiovascular diseases (and major components) and noncardiovascular disease, United States 1970–1975.

1. Although small, there is an operative mortality associated with ACBG. Furthermore, mortality and morbidity are associated with coronary arteriography, which must precede ACBG.

2. An ACBG may produce a perioperative myocardial infarction. Some of the earlier reports have indicated the incidence, determined by Q waves alone, to be as frequent as one in two patients. Q waves demonstrate only transmural myocardial infarctions, and not all of those. A new transmural myocardial infarction that is electrically opposite to a previous one may, owing to the cancellation of opposing electrical forces, result in the disappearance of a previously demonstrated Q wave. Subendocardial infarctions are equally serious and may be demonstrated by less diagnostic ECG changes,

appropriate elevations of serum enzymes, or radionuclide imaging. A number of studies have demonstrated that perioperative subendocardial infarctions are almost as frequent, if not as frequent, as perioperative transmural infarctions.

Although it has been suggested that surgically induced infarcts are "controlled" infarcts and are reasonably well tolerated, most critical investigators challenge this opinion. Mundth and Austen[11] concluded "that although some patients may be benefited in terms of relief of angina pectoris by postoperative infarction, the occurrence of an infarct probably has a definitely adverse effect on the long-term functional results and longevity." It is gratifying that there is evidence that attention to the details of surgical technique can significantly reduce the incidence of perioperative myocardial infarction.

3.   There is evidence that the progression of the atherosclerotic process is accelerated in the grafted native vessels. This most commonly occurs in the segment proximal to the site of an anastomosis (Fig. 6). There is evidence to suggest that occlusion of the segment facilitates the patency of the graft — but it does not insure patency of the graft. Graft closure and proximal-segment closure can lead to catastrophic events. Closure of the proximal segment, even if the graft remains patent, particularly in the left anterior descending coronary artery, can result in the loss of important septal branches and/or sources of collateral flow.

4.   Although long-term, up to five years, graft patency is good, one in three or less grafts do occlude. The longer-term fate of the graft is unknown. There are increasing reports that the graft participates in the atherosclerotic process, particularly in patients with elevated lipids.

5.   There is increasing evidence that as a result of perioperative infarctions, acceleration of the disease in the native circulation, and/or graft closure, ventricular function may deteriorate.

Despite these complications, will ACBG reduce the incidence of acute myocardial infarction, serious and/or recurring arrhythmias, congestive heart failure, or premature death?

It is clear that evidence that such occur cannot be obtained from uncontrolled studies or from studies in which the control population was treated and followed during the decade prior to that in which the surgery was performed. Answers to such questions can be obtained only from carefully controlled studies, ideally randomized studies.

Despite over 350,000 patients receiving an ACBG during the last decade, only 1248 patients were randomized to a "surgery" or "no surgery" group. These patients are embraced by six studies:

1. *Stable angina*
    a.   Guinn and Mathur[12] randomized 116 patients at the Houston V.A. Hospital and followed them for a mean of 34 months.
    b.   Kloster et al.,[13] at the University of Oregon, randomized 95 patients and followed them for a mean of 30 months.
    c.   The V.A. Cooperative Group[14] randomized 596 patients and followed them for a mean of 36 months.
    d.   The V.A. Cooperative Group[15] randomized 113 symptomatic patients with critical stenosis of the left main coronary artery and followed them for a mean of 30 months.

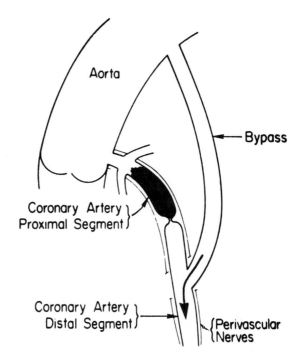

Figure 6. Progression of the atherosclerotic process is accelerated in the grafted native vessels in many patients. This most commonly occurs in the segment proximal to the site of the anastomosis. Although not shown in this sketch, it may well occlude important septal branches.

Labels in figure: Aorta; Bypass; Coronary Artery Proximal Segment; Coronary Artery Distal Segment; Perivascular Nerves

2. *Unstable angina*
   a. The NHLBI Cooperative Group[16] randomized 288 patients and followed them for a mean of 24 months.
   b. Selden et al.[17] randomized 40 patients and followed them for only four months.

None of these studies demonstrated that ACBG will reduce the incidence of myocardial infarction, serious and/or recurrent arrhythmias, or congestive heart failure. These studies indicate that ACBG will postpone premature death only in symptomatic patients with stenosis of the left main coronary artery.

The quality of surgery for the V.A. Cooperative Study of stable angina in patients without left main disease has been criticized. Only a few operated cases were reported from some of the V.A. Hospitals. It was postulated, apparently incorrectly, that in some cases the surgeons performing these operations had only limited experience with the procedure. It has been pointed out, however, that the surgeons performed an ACBG on many more patients in their own V.A. Hospital and in affiliated university and/or community hospitals than were included in this study. The operative mortality rates for surgeons in the V.A. Study appear comparable to the mortality rates reported at the time of study from other centers throughout the country. It has been stated that the veteran, operated on in a Veteran's Administration Hospital, might not be as "well motivated" to comply with instructions and to return to a state of good health as would the more affluent private patient. If valid, this criticism would have to be applied to those veterans managed without surgery. It has been said that by projecting the survival lines of the operated and nonoperated patients in the V.A. Study to four and five years, surgery can be demonstrated to be superior to nonsurgical management. Such reasoning is not impressive. But if it is accepted that such will be the case, or if in a year or so it is demonstrated to be the case, is it reasonable to undertake, on a large scale, a form of therapy that might prolong the lives of a few who are fortunate enough to survive four or five years? Would it be reasonable to initiate surgery for prolongation of life if these are the only data that support the concept that can be marshalled after experience with over 300,000 procedures over a 10-year period?

The criticism of the surgical group in the V.A. Cooperative Study could be valid. Even if it is, the study serves a useful purpose. It indicates that 87 per cent of 310 medical patients survived the three years. This group of patients included 59 per cent with a history of a previous myocardial infarction, 50 per cent with a history of angina for more than 25 months, and 51 per cent with triple-vessel disease, of whom 85 per cent had abnormally contracting ventricles. Only four per cent had single-vessel disease with a normally contracting ventricle. Certainly, the mortality rate for this group is much less than would have been predicted based on studies carried out in the 1960's of the natural history of unoperative coronary artery disease.

Because of the difficulties in conducting randomized studies, the Duke Medical Center utilized a different approach to determine if ACBG prolonged life. A computer program was developed that permitted the storage of pertinent historical data referable to physical findings, laboratory observations, and therapeutic programs of individual patients; 110 items of information were stored.[18] In 1974, they reported the results of a follow-up of 781 consecutively evaluated patients with coronary artery disease; 402 were treated medically and 379 surgically. There was a significant difference between the groups of patients in only a few of the parameters. At two years after zero time, the survival rate was the same in the medically treated (83 per cent) and in the surgically treated (85 per cent) group (see Figure 2). The Duke group subsequently concluded that "ACBG does not prolong life in comparison to medical management over a span of two to five years. There may be certain higher-risk patients whose lives may be prolonged by the procedure, however." They have reported that the combination of a total occlusion of the right coronary artery and a subtotal occlusion (< 70 per cent) of the left anterior descending artery may be improved by ACBG. The three-year survival rate for those who had received ACBG was 88 per cent, as compared with 68 per cent for the control group.

Using the same computer matching technique, the Duke group evaluated the difference in survival rates between complete and incomplete revascularization in 392 consecutive patients. Complete revascularization was defined as having been accomplished if all major arteries with a greater than 70 per cent occlusion received a bypass graft. Incomplete revascularization resulted when such an artery with such a stenosis did not receive a graft. There were 186 completely revascularized patients and 206 incompletely revascularized patients. These two groups were compared over a 24-month period. There was no difference in survival or relief of pain that could be correlated with the completeness of the revascularization program.

There are now reports of uncontrolled series of patients that have a very low operative mortality and have few deaths over several years of follow-up. The survival of patients in such groups has been compared with that expected from the population at large of age-matched subjects determined by actuarial tables. The survival of such operated patients is said to be even better than the survival of the medically treated group reported by the V.A. Cooperative Group — 87 per cent survived for three years. What is the composition of such groups of patients? How may patients were asymptomatic? How many of the patients had triple-vessel disease? Fifty-one per cent of the entire V.A. Study had such extensive involvement, and of these, 85 per cent had abnormally contracting patterns of the left ventricle.

It has been demonstrated that the greatly decreased operative mortality reported by some groups may well be the result of a preselection of fewer patients with left ventricular dysfunction. Conley et al.[19] showed that the decline in the operative mortality rate in their institution from 8.8 per cent in patients undergoing elective ACBG before January 1, 1975 to 5.4 per cent for subsequent patients was associated with a two- to three-fold decrease in the prevalence of left ventricular dysfunction. The reduced mortality was dependent primarily on the selection of patients for surgery who would most likely survive. The reduced operative mortality does not reflect solely the improvement of the skill of the surgical team. These investigators showed that within a fixed time period operative mortality varies widely, depending primarily upon the pathologic and physiologic characteristics of patients undergoing operation. Patients selected to contribute little to the operative mortality of a series may be expected to have a good and long survival.

Although there are no data that support the concept that ACBG reduces the incidence of myocardial infarction, serious arrhythmias, congestive heart failure, or premature death (except in small subsets of patients), there are ample data to support the use of the procedure for the relief of the pain of myocardial ischemia that is refractory to medical management. It is generally accepted that following ACBG, symptoms are relieved and the quality of life is improved *for a time* in up to 90 per cent of the patients; at least 75 per cent of the patients are initially free of symptoms. Such gratifying results have been observed not only in patients with stable angina, but in those with unstable angina and left main coronary artery disease as well. The symptomatic improvement is so marked that the operated patients frequently require less medication compared with those who are not operated.

But as has been pointed out, even after a decade of experience, there are still many uncertainties regarding the long-term effects of ACBG. A major cause for concern is that for many patients, the initial gratifying results may not persist and the physician may well be faced with the need for more compulsive medical management. Therefore, it appears to be prudent to be certain that the patient who has persisting angina and is considered for ACBG is truly refractory to medical management. Unfortunately, many patients are referred for surgery with only elementary efforts to control the symptoms of the disease.

These cautions are not intended to oppose the use of ACBG for the purpose of improving the quality of life in many patients with CHD. The quality of life is frequently more important that the quantity of life. The "potentially harmful effects of surgery, including even myocardial infarction, may be outweighed by the relief of angina experienced by patients who are severely incapacitated and have not responded satisfactorily to an intensive medical regimen."[20]

It has been disappointing that despite the significant initial clinical improvement in the relief of pain, rehabilitation benefits as a result of ACBG appear to be few. In one study, although 90 per cent of the patients had symptomatic improvement and relief of angina, only 50 per cent returned to work. Based on the retirement practices of the population at large, the observed retirement rate of patients following ACBG was increased 7.5 times above that of the total population for those under 55 years of age and 11.3 times for those above that age. Heart surgery, unfortunately, is viewed by many employers as being serious and carrying risks for the employee's future ability to function. Data regarding ACBG that have been cited from the literature do not reassure the employer that the productivity or the life expectancy of his employee will be prolonged except in selected subsets of patients. With an aging population and a greater-than-desired unemployed work force, the employer may be happy to grant early retirement. The physician must assume some or much of the responsibility for this poor work record. The physician may influence the patient not to return to stressful working conditions despite successful surgery.

The physician recommending ACBG to a patient who is not refractory to intensive medical management may do his patient a disservice, particularly in view of the lack of evidence that life will be prolonged, except in well-defined subsets of patients, and in view of the complications. These include, as has been stated, a small but definite operative mortality, the possibility of a perioperative myocardial infarction, acceleration of the progression of the disease in the native circulation, graft closure, deterioration of ventricular function, and the possibility that the initial gratifying relief of pain may be short-lived.

Finally, the prudent physician should consider carefully the economic burden that is attached to ACBG. The total cost is in the range of ten thousand to fifteen thousand dollars. This is so despite the fact that in a large number of centers a cardiologist will do four or more coronary arteriograms in a day while his collaborating surgical team may do as many or more ACBG's. It has been estimated that the cost of ACBG and related therapeutic and diagnostic supporting services for the entire country in 1977 approached one billion dollars. This is over two and a half times the total budget of the National Heart, Lung, and Blood Institute.

As far as managing the individual patient, it seems reasonable that the patient with stable angina should be admonished to attain and/or maintain a body weight that is determined to be that weight with minimal evidence of excessive adipose tissue. This can be determined by measuring the skin fold thickness lateral to the umbilicus, over the triceps, and in the infrascapular region. The sum at these sites should approach 30 to 50 millimeters, possibly 10 millimeters more for the female. The patient should be admonished to avoid smoking, and the cholesterol level should be maintained close to 200 to 220 milligrams per cent by diet and, if necessary, by drugs. The blood pressure should be controlled by avoiding excessive salt and, if necessary, by pharmacologic agents. A physical reconditioning or physical maintenance program should be initiated. The level of exercise can best be determined by stress testing with ECG monitoring.

If pain or ectopy is frequent, beta blockers in sufficient doses to maintain a resting pulse at 60 beats per minute or below may be beneficial. If the pain is frequent, long-acting nitrates are also indicated, as is the liberal use of *fresh* nitroglycerin. An effort should be made to control ectopy by additional pharmacologic agents.

If the patient continues to have symptoms of ischemia or if ischemic changes are demonstrated by stress testing on at least two occasions without drugs known to cause a false-positive test, then it is unlikely that the patient can be maintained without pain. This is particularly true if the ischemic changes occur during testing at low heart rates or after a short duration of exercise. A consideration of surgery is indicated under such circumstances, and coronary arteriography should be performed.

The heart rate and/or duration of exercise at which the appearance of ischemia is an indication for the decision to consider surgery depends on the age of the patient, the frequency of symptoms, and other factors. A detailed discussion of this decision-making process is beyond the scope of this article. Suffice it to say that it is individualized and that no firm rules have been established.

At the present time, there is no evidence that such a therapeutic approach will prevent or postpone the clinical manifestations of IHD. But likewise, as has been indicated, at the present time there is no evidence that surgery will prevent the occurrence of the clinical manifestations of IHD, including premature death, except in selected subsets of symptomatic patients. Therefore, the indication for surgery appears to be for the relief of pain. Patients with critical stenosis of the left main coronary artery and other subsets of patients whose lives may be prolonged by ACBG will rarely become asymptomatic on the program outlined above. Therefore, such patients will be included among those who are studied by coronary arteriography shortly after the institution of therapy. Such patients may remain asymptomatic for a while but will become symptomatic, despite medical management, and at that time they should be studied. By following such a protocol, the few patients who will benefit from surgery by a prolongation of life will be detected and studied. In our judgment, it is not necessary to study large numbers of patients in order to find a few patients who might benefit from surgery. Such patients will be identified by their refractiveness to a strictly medical type of management.

If ACBG is to be used, and indeed in many patients it is indicated, it should be in conjunction with such a major medical effort as outlined. CHD is a progressive disease; it is an epidemic disease, and thus its causes are multiple. Its prevention and treatment is therefore multifactorial. It is possible that by combining surgery with maximum medical management and modification of lifestyle, premature death from CHD may be postponed. In my judgment, this should be the goal of future investigation.

It must be realized that after a decade of experience, the data available in the literature do not support the concept that ACBG is the solution to the pathologic process of CHD. No data have been forthcoming for "actuarial studies that provide the undisputed truth of the efficacy of the distal coronary bypass."[1] Randomized studies are difficult, but they are not unethical and they are not impossible. They should be instituted, and those existing programs should be supported and encouraged. A second best but apparently satisfactory approach is that of matching cases through a computerized medical information system. In view of the current lack of proof of the efficacy of ACBG, it may be unethical in the late 1970's not to match operated patients with controls. Similarly, the efficacy of such an all-out therapeutic program without surgery should be evaluated by appropriately designed studies.

In summary, there is little evidence that ACBG will prolong the life of patients with chronic stable angina pectoris, except in selective subsets of patients. These include the symptomatic patients with left main coronary artery disease and patients with total occlusion of the right coronary artery and a greater than 70 per cent but less than total occlusion of the left anterior descending artery. There are no data that the procedure favorably affects the asymptomatic patient, even the patient with left main coronary artery disease. It is possible that other subsets of patients will be identified in the future, and the prudent physician should keep an open mind and evaluate future published data without bias or preconceived ideas.

Furthermore, there is no evidence that the procedure will prevent the development of an acute myocardial infarction, serious arrhythmias, or congestive heart failure. It is effective, for a time, in relieving the pain of angina that is refractory to medical management. The procedure may be associated with a number of early and/or late complications. These may include

1. a small but definite surgical mortality;
2. a high incidence, in many of even the "best" centers, of perioperative myocardial infarction;
3. an unpredictable acceleration of the atherosclerotic disease in the grafted vessel;
4. a closure of one in three or fewer grafts;
5. as a result of perioperative myocardial infarction, graft closure, and/or progression of the disease in the native circulation, a deterioration of ventricular function; and
6. recurrence of severe angina pectoris after a period of gratifying improvement.

Furthermore, the procedure does not appear to be an advantage in maintaining employment of the patient.

Therefore, the prudent physician will use caution and be certain that the patient is indeed resistant to medical management before recommending the procedure. Such a caution is indicated in view of the great cost to the patient or to the third-party carrier. The prudent physician will, however, maintain an open mind and be prepared to accept that the procedure can prolong·life in a larger percentage of patients should future well-controlled studies demonstrate that such occurs.

Acknowledgements
1. I gratefully acknowledge the untiring assistance of Ms. Virginia Richardson in the preparation of this manuscript.
2. The experience and opportunity to review the literature regarding ACBG was made possible in part by support of the National Heart, Lung, and Blood Vessel Research and Demonstration Center, Baylor College of Medicine, Houston, Texas, a grant-supported research project of National Heart, Lung, and Blood Institute, National Institutes of Health, Grant No. HL-17269.

References

1. Morris GC, Howell JF, Crawford ES, Reul GJ, Chapman DW, Beazley HL, Winters WL, and Peterson PK: The distal coronary bypass. Ann Surg *172*:652, 1970.
2. Friesinger GC, Page EE, and Ross RS: Prognostic significance of coronary arteriography. Trans Assoc A Physicians *83*:78, 1970.
3. Humphries JO, Kuller L, Ross RS, Friesinger GC, and Page EE: Natural history of ischemic heart disease in relation to arteriographic findings: A twelve year study of 224 patients. Circulation *49*:489, 1974.
4. Bruschke AV, Proudfit WL, and Sones FM Jr: Progress study of 590 consecutive nonsurgical cases of coronary artery disease followed 5–9 years. I. Arteriographic correlations. Circulation *47*:1147, 1973.
5. Webster JS, Moberg C, and Rincon G: Natural history of severe proximal coronary artery disease as documented by coronary cineangiography. Am J Cardiol *33*:195, 1974.
6. Oberman A, Jones WB, Riley CP, Reeves TJ, Sheffield LD, and Turner ME: Natural history of coronary artery disease. Bull NY Acad Med *48*:1109, 1972.
7. Burggraf GW, and Parker JO: Prognosis in coronary artery disease: Angiographic, hemodynamic and clinical factors. Circulation *51*:146, 1975.
8. Reeves TJ, Oberman A, Jones WB, and Sheffield LT: Natural history of angina pectoris. Am J Cardiol *33*:423, 1974.
9. McIntosh HD, and Garcia JA: The first decade of aortocoronary bypass grafting . . . 1967–1977: A review. Circulation *57*:405, 1978.
10. McIntosh HD, Wright KE Jr, and Wray NP: Indications for saphenous vein aortocoronary bypass surgery. Athero Rev *1*:183, 1976.
11. Mundth ED, and Austen WG: Surgical measures for coronary heart disease. N Engl J Med *293*:13 (Part 1), 75 (Part 2), and 124 (Part 3), 1975.
12. Guinn GA, and Mathur VS: Surgical versus medical treatment for stable angina pectoris: Prospective randomized study with one to four year follow-up. Ann Thorac Surg *22*:524, 1976.
13. Kloster FE, Kremkau EL, Rahimtoola SH, Ritzmann LW, Griswold HE, Neill WA, Rosh J, and Starr A: Prospective randomized study of coronary bypass surgery for chronic stable angina. Cardiovasc Clin *8*(2):145, 1977.
14. Murphy ML, Hultgren HN, Detre K, Thomson J, and Takaro T: Treatment of chronic stable angina. N Engl J Med *297*:621, 1977.
15. Takaro T, Hultgren HN, Lipton MJ, and Detre KM: The VA cooperative randomized study of surgery for coronary occlusive disease. II. Subgroup with significant left main lesions. Circulation *54*(Suppl III):III107, 1976.
16. Scheidt S: Unstable angina: Medical management or surgery. Cardiovasc Med *2*:541, 1977.
17. Selden R, Neill WA, Ritzmann LW, Okies JE, and Anderson RP: Medical versus surgical therapy for acute coronary insufficiency. N Engl J Med *293*:1329, 1975.

18. McNeer JF, Starmer CF, Bartel AG, Behar VS, Kong Y, Peter RH, and Rosati RA: The nature of treatment selection in coronary artery disease: experience with medical and surgical treatment of a chronic disease. Circulation 49:606, 1974.
19. Conley MJ, Wechsler AS, Anderson RW, Oldham HN, Sabiston DC, and Rosati RA: The relationship of patient selection to prognosis following aortocoronary bypass. Circulation 55:158, 1977.
20. Auchuff SC, Griffith LSC, Conti CR, Humphries JO, Brawley RK, Gott VL, and Ross RS: The "angina-producing" myocardial segment. An approach to the interpretation of results of coronary bypass surgery. Am J Cardiol 36:723, 1975.

Comment

A decade after original studies and after many hundreds of thousands of coronary vein bypass graft operations, the question as to whether this procedure prolongs life in patients with chronic stable angina pectoris remains controversial. As emphasized by McIntosh, the problem is complicated by the fact that today's patient with angina pectoris appears distinctly less at risk from death when managed medically compared to his counterpart of one or two decades ago. Consequently, those studies that compare present-day surgical mortality with earlier arteriographic natural history studies initiated in the 1960's are misleading. The situation is further complicated by the fact that surgical management is continuing to improve as well, so that the immediate surgical mortality is well under five per cent in almost all centers, and the late mortality is about two per cent per year.

It has been said that something, to be significant, should be significant. If a decade after many studies have been performed to determine if surgery prolongs survival, such studies are inconclusive, it seems reasonable to conclude that even if a difference is demonstrated, it is not likely to alter management radically. It is clear that there are certain subgroups of patients with coronary artery disease, primarily left main coronary artery disease, that are surgical problems. It is also clear that there are certain other subgroups, such as patients with single-vessel right coronary disease, that are medical problems. It is possible that, with experience, additional surgical subgroups of patients will be defined. The Veterans Administration Cooperative Study, which at the end of four years showed no difference in survival between the randomized medical and surgical patients, has accumulated some data to suggest that a difference between medical and surgical survival may be emerging in patients with three-vessel disease and abnormal left ventricular function, favoring surgical management.

Today, what is the appropriate position for the prudent clinician? In my judgment, once left main disease is reasonably excluded, the patient should be managed initially with medical therapy. It is important, however, that this therapy be holistic in the sense of total involvement of the patient in an overall effort that includes not only modification of existing risk factors, modification of his job and life situation to avoid psychological and physical stresses, but also careful management with both adrenergic and beta-blocking agents such as propranolol and long-acting nitrates throughout the day. Under these circumstances, if the patient's angina is well controlled and he is able to continue with an adequate quality of life, it would seem that this is appropriate management. Should such management fail, or should angina later worsen, one can always have subsequent recourse to surgery.

ELLIOT RAPAPORT, M.D.

175

Eight

Is Unstable Angina an Indication for Immediate Coronary Arteriography and Subsequent Coronary Bypass Graft Surgery Where Anatomically Indicated?

IMPENDING MYOCARDIAL INFARCTION—A CONDITION FAVORING SURGICAL THERAPY

> *W. Dudley Johnson, M.D., and John C. Manley, M.D.*

UNSTABLE ANGINA IS NOT AN INDICATION FOR IMMEDIATE CORONARY VEIN BYPASS GRAFT SURGERY

> *C. Richard Conti, M.D.*

COMMENT

Impending Myocardial Infarction — A Condition Favoring Surgical Therapy

W. DUDLEY JOHNSON, M.D.

Associate Clinical Professor of Surgery, Department of
Thoracic and Cardiovascular Surgery, The Medical
College of Wisconsin, Milwaukee, Wisconsin

JOHN C. MANLEY, M.D.

Director, Cardiac Rehabilitation and Exercise Stress
Laboratory, St. Luke's Hospital; Associate Clinical
Professor of Medicine, The Medical College of Wisconsin,
Milwaukee, Wisconsin

The impending myocardial infarction syndrome has been reported for decades, yet cardiologists still cannot agree on a definition or optimal therapy. From the very advent of bypass surgery, patients with unstable or progressive symptoms were felt to be more urgent candidates for surgery. The rationale for the vigorous surgical approach was based on the assumption that obstructed coronary arteries were causing acute or progressive ischemia with a corresponding increase in symptoms. Bypass surgery would immediately relieve the ischemia and should also relieve symptoms. Not only would the bypass produce immediate relief, but effective grafting would produce lasting relief that would be independent of further deterioration or change in the atherosclerotic lesions. The grafting would work by reestablishing coronary perfusion. In contrast, medical therapy, both then and now, principally relieves symptoms by depressing function. It seemed much more desirable to improve health by restoring physiology rather than by depressing it, and the early surgical efforts were made with this goal in mind. This report is based on a series of 424 patients operated on by three different surgeons* from 1971 through 1975. The patients were catheterized and have been followed by Dr. Manley and his associates.

---

*Dr. James Auer, Dr. Alfred Tector, and Dr. W. Dudley Johnson.

179

Patients with unstable angina are divided into two series. Group A (121 patients) includes those who have progressive angina. This means angina of increasing frequency and/or severity, which is either an acceleration of chronic stable angina or is angina of recent onset. Group B (60 patients) includes those with the "intermediate coronary syndrome," which is characterized by the following conditions: (1) recurrent episodes of angina at rest or of prolonged nature (over 15 minutes); (2) poor or no relief with nitrates; (3) ischemic ST-T changes, often with arrhythmias; and (4) absence of enzyme elevation or new Q waves. In all groups angiographic confirmation of 75 per cent or greater obstruction in one or more coronary arteries is, of course, essential. Group C (243 patients) consists of patients demographically matched to Groups A and B in terms of sex, previous myocardial infarction, congestive heart failure, hypertension, and other data shown in Tables 1 and 2, but with stable angina.

Methods of Management of the Patient with Unstable Angina

Patients with unstable pain are admitted to the hospital and are usually observed in the coronary care unit. Vigorous medical therapy is pursued, including the liberal use of nitrates, propranolol, and sedation. Hypertension is also vigorously treated. Electrocardiographic evaluation and monitoring is done, and rhythm disturbances are treated. Enzyme studies are evaluated, and currently, but not during the time of this study, pyrophosphate scans are often obtained. With this course of medical therapy, the great majority of patients respond with a marked decrease in symptoms. Catheterization studies are then performed semi-electively a few days after

Table 1.   *Patient Characteristics*

	STABLE (%)	PROGRESSIVE (%)	ICS (%)
Hemodynamic			
LVEDP			
<12	58.1	57.0	60.0
12–20	34.6	34.7	31.4
>20	7.3	8.3	9.6
Angiographic			
Vessel Disease			
One	23.2	20.1	19.3
Two	36.4	35.3	33.2
Three	40.4	44.6	47.5
Main Left	12.1	21.1	21.3

(LVEDP = Left ventricular end diastolic pressure; Stable = Stable angina group; Progressive = Progressive angina group; ICS = Intermediate coronary syndrome.)

Table 2. *Patient Characteristics*

	STABLE (%)	PROGRESSIVE (%)	ICS (%)
Angiographic			
Left Ventricular Contraction			
Normal	34.0	30.8	31.3
Local Scar	43.0	46.2	45.7
Diffuse Scar	19.7	19.7	18.1
Aneurysm	3.3	3.3	4.9
Ejection Fraction			
>0.50	36.2	32.4	34.1
0.35–0.50	40.3	45.3	41.7
<0.35	23.5	22.3	24.2

admission. In patients with prolonged spells of pain, despite therapy, or with sustained ECG changes, catheterization is performed at a time when an operating room (and surgeon) are available. If the patient continues to have difficulty during the catheterization, or deteriorates, he can be taken directly to surgery from the catheterization laboratory. The use of a balloon pump to relieve pain is almost never needed. Once the diagnostic evaluation is done, the patient goes to surgery as promptly as necessary and can be placed on cardiopulmonary bypass within minutes. With these precautions, there has been no mortality in the catheterization laboratory or in any patient with unstable angina transported between the catheterization laboratory and surgery. Preoperative use of balloon assist has nearly always been reserved for patients with major hemodynamic problems such as acute mitral insufficiency, shock, or acute ventricular septal defect.

Surgical Management

Most patients with unstable angina are anesthetized with little difficulty, and no unusual measures are required. Arrest or deterioration with induction has become a rare event, but if patients do deteriorate, they can be on heart-lung bypass in eight to ten minutes. During the period of this study, cardioplegic solutions were not used, but standard intermittent anoxic arrest was employed. The most critically stenotic artery was always grafted first. Since most patients remained stable, one or both mammary arteries were commonly used. All arteries with major disease were grafted. As is our usual practice in all revascularization procedures, when an unusually large artery was critically stenosed (left main, large LAD), we inserted two separate grafts into the distal artery. Recognizing the fact that a small number of grafts close, doubly bypassing large arteries helps reduce the chances of infarct related to closure of a single graft. In these patients, dis-

Table 3. *Surgical Mortality*

GROUP	NUMBER	PER CENT
Stable Angina	5/243	2.1
Unstable Angina Progressive	3/121	2.5
Intermediate Syndrome	2/60	3.3

ease so diffuse as to contraindicate surgery was identified. Approximately 20 per cent of the patients had ejection fractions under 35 per cent. Standard bypass techniques were employed using hemodilution. Postoperative management was similar to that for all other patients.

The surgical mortality rate was similar in all three groups and varied from 2.1 to 3.3 per cent (Table 3). Perioperative infarcts were defined by new Q waves. The infarct rate was higher in Group B, the intermediate syndrome, and was 6.6 per cent (Table 4). This could be explained in part as due to the difficulty in clinically differentiating this group from acute infarct patients.

Angiographic studies after surgery were not done routinely, but usually for a clinical suspicion of difficulty. In studying mostly symptomatic patients, one would anticipate that graft patency rates would be less than if the entire group were studied. The average number of bypasses per patient was over three in all three groups. Patency rates from 83 to 86 per cent were similar in the three groups and not different from our overall experience. Sixty-one to 64 per cent of the patients had all grafts open and less than five per cent in each group had all grafts closed (Table 5).

Relief of pain was dramatic in most patients and has continued. The results in all three groups were virtually identical (Table 6). Over 90 per cent in each group were relieved totally or in part from their pain and have continued with this pain relief for years.

Long-term survival studies have extended into the fourth and fifth year. Stable angina (Group C) patients have a yearly mortality rate of 1.8 per cent,

Table 4. *Perioperative Myocardial Infarction*

GROUP	NUMBER	PER CENT
Stable Angina	7/243	2.9
Unstable Angina Progressive	2/121	1.7
Intermediate Syndrome	4/60	6.6

Table 5. *Graft Status*

GROUP (% STUDIED)	# GRAFTS/ # PATIENTS (1–6)	GRAFTS PATENT (%)	ALL GRAFTS OPEN (%)	ALL GRAFTS CLOSED (%)	AT LEAST 1 GRAFT OPEN (%)
Stable (38)	826/243 (3.4/PT.)	84	64	4.1	94.3
Unstable Progressive (34)	424/121 (3.5/PT.)	86	63	4.0	95.7
Intermediate Syndrome (36)	195/60 (3.3/PT.)	83	61	4.6	95.4

(PT. = Patient)

while group A and B group mortality rates are 2.0 and 4.0 per cent per year, respectively. These rates are not statistically different and are quite comparable to annual mortality rates for patients with single-vessel disease treated medically (Fig. 1).

Discussion

Patients with unstable angina can be treated surgically, with results nearly identical to patients with stable angina. Most can be controlled with medical therapy while definitive diagnostic studies are performed. These diagnostic studies themselves carry almost no risk (0 per cent in this series). The results are not only immediate, but long-lasting. Late mortality rates appear to approach the mortality rates of the general population.

In addition to improvement in the quality of life, cardiac function appears to improve with bypass surgery.[1-4] While the ejection fraction usually does not change markedly postoperatively, occasionally improvements of 30 per cent are seen (Fig. 2). In our experience, this degree of change in contractility has been observed only in patients with severe ischemia (and

Table 6. *Relief of Angina*

GROUP	IMPROVED (%)*	UNCHANGED (%)	WORSE (%)
Stable	91.6 (74)	5.6	2.8
Unstable Progressive	91.9 (75)	3.4	4.7
Intermediate Syndrome	94.7 (75)	5.3	0.0

*Figures in parentheses = total relief

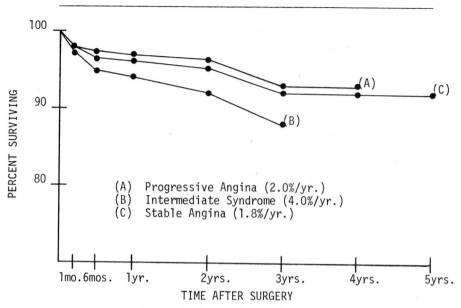

Figure 1. Actuarial survival curves.

unstable angina). Bicycle ergometry studies consistently show improvement in the ability of the heart to respond to stress after successful bypass surgery (Fig. 3). Simple stress testing often shows marked postoperative improvement. In contrast, medical therapy has shown minimal, if any, effect in improving contractility or in improving the function of the heart under stress. Nitrates and blocking agents rely on relieving symptoms by depressing the work of the heart. Symptom relief is palliative and temporary, lasting for minutes or hours.

It has been difficult to understand the pure medical approach advocated by some when the entire concept is based on suppressing the function of the organ. When a condition can be relieved by improving performance, it would seem the preferable approach. Admittedly, the results described here are from a portion of one center and do not reflect the experience of all others. It is axiomatic that bypass grafts must remain open to be effective. When centers report over 30 per cent of grafts closed and many diseased arteries not grafted, it is not surprising that results reported are different from those above. An aggressive surgical approach for nearly all patients with deteriorating symptoms can only be justified if follow-up studies validate the results. The variations in coronary disease are exceeded by the variations in surgical procedures done for it. The surgical results should be as carefully evaluated as the disease itself, and the ability of the surgical team will then be known and will rapidly become the most valuable guide in the selection of patients for surgery. When surgery is done well, the rate of relief of pain and long-term survival greatly exceeds that of any documented medical series.

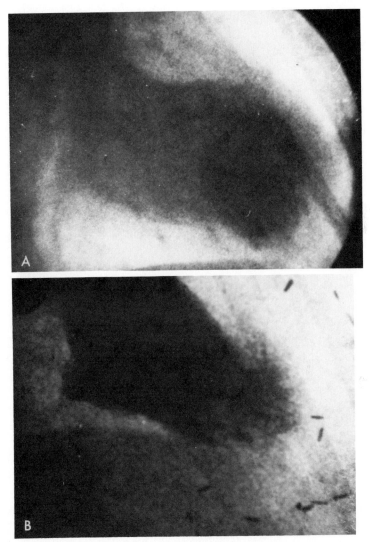

Figure 2. (A) Preoperative and (B) postoperative end-systolic phase ventriculogram of a patient with severe resting angina preoperatively. Ejection fractions usually improve moderately. Marked improvement such as this is almost exclusively seen in patients with severe ischemic pain.

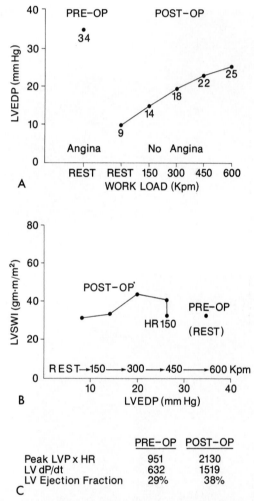

Figure 3. (A–C) Preoperative and postoperative ventricular function curves of a patient with unstable angina and two previous infarcts. The resting end-diastolic pressure of 34 mm Hg preoperatively was associated with severe pain and very low exercise tolerance. Postoperatively, the end-diastolic pressure was normal. The patient was able to do considerable work without pain. Residual postoperative dysfunction was due to myocardial damage from previous infarcts. Overall, the postoperative performance was much improved, characteristic for patients having undergone good bypass surgery.

References

1. Johnson WD, Flemma RJ, Manley JC, and Lepley D Jr: The physiologic parameters of ventricular function as affected by direct coronary surgery. J Thorac Cardiovasc Surg 60:483–490, 1970.
2. Manley JC, Johnson WD, Flemma RJ, and Lepley D Jr: Direct myocardial revascularization: Postoperative assessment of ventricular function at rest and during ergometer exercise (Abstr). Circulation 42(Suppl III):III-181, 1970.
3. Manley JC, Johnson WD, Flemma RJ, and Lepley D Jr: Objective evaluation of the effects of direct myocardial revascularization on ventricular function utilizing ergometer testing (Abstr). Am J Cardiol 26:648, 1970.
4. Manley JC, King JF, and Zeft HJ: Objective hemodynamic assessment of ventricular performance before and after coronary bypass surgery utilizing bicycle ergometry (Abstr). Circulation 52(Suppl II):II-139, 1975.

Unstable Angina Is Not an Indication for Immediate Coronary Vein Bypass Graft Surgery

C. RICHARD CONTI, M.D.

Professor of Medicine; Chief, Division of Cardiology,
University of Florida College of Medicine, Gainesville,
Florida

In this presentation I will attempt to show that vigorous medical management of patients with unstable angina is a worthwhile alternative to immediate coronary artery surgery. At the outset, I want to emphasize that I am not taking a position that coronary artery surgery in patients with unstable angina is not good at all. However, I believe it is worth considering the possibility that the emergency surgical therapy of this condition may not be necessary. In the past, *immediate* surgical mortality and morbidity of patients with obvious proximal coronary artery disease and reasonably good ventricular function have been compared with *long-term* mortality and morbidity in medically treated patients, most of whom were not studied angiographically. Many of these medically treated patients may not have been suitable surgical candidates. It is only fair to both forms of that therapy that data be analyzed in terms of in-hospital morbidity and mortality for the medical and surgical groups, preferably comparably studied patients. If it can be shown that an inordinate number of medically treated patients are not dying or having a myocardial infarction during the initial hospitalization, then a reasonable case can be made for medical management, at least in the acute stage of the illness.

The Clinical Problem

The clinical problem of what to do with a patient who presents with unstable angina pectoris still exists despite numerous publications and pre-

188

sentations on the subject. Part of the dilemma relates to confusion generated by the use of multiple terms to define this subset of patients with ischemic heart disease. For example, the term *pre-infarction angina* has come into widespread use without precise definition and has contributed to the sense of urgency about surgical therapy. It is now recognized that any given syndrome of ischemic cardiac pain and ECG changes can be identified as pre-infarction only retrospectively. Only a fraction of patients with a so-called "pre-infarction syndrome" will have a myocardial infarction or die in the immediate future. When studied prospectively, the incidence of myocardial infarction and death following unstable angina is difficult, if not impossible, to predict in an individual patient.

The problem that a physician faces when dealing with the patient with this syndrome is acute. He is not concerned with what is going to happen to the patient in the future, but rather with what is going to happen to him immediately. The physician is confronted with the dilemma, "What should I do with my patient now when he is in the coronary care unit having recurrent rest angina?" Several treatment options are available. The first is vigorous long-term medical therapy. The patient can be treated with bed rest and pharmacologic therapy in a protective environment such as a coronary care unit for a time, and then given long-term treatment at home. The second option is emergency surgical therapy. The third option is initial intense medical therapy followed by surgical therapy, either during the initial hospitalization or electively after the patient has been discharged from the hospital.

The goals of therapy of this condition are similar to those for patients with stable angina. Whichever therapy is chosen, i.e., medical or surgical, must (1) prevent death, (2) prevent myocardial infarction, (3) preserve salvageable ischemic myocardium, (4) prolong useful life, and (5) relieve the patient of pain.

Theoretically, immediate coronary artery surgery should offer great promise as a means of prevention of myocardial infarction and death, since successful surgery should provide revascularization of an area of myocardium that is at risk and correct the imbalance of myocardial oxygen supply and demand by increasing the supply. The indications for immediate coronary artery bypass graft in patients with unstable angina would be very clear if the early mortality and the incidence of myocardial infarction were high in medically treated patients or if patients' symptoms were not easily controlled after admission to the coronary care unit. Alternatively, immediate coronary artery surgery would be acceptable if the perioperative mortality and myocardial infarction rates were as low as in patients undergoing elective revascularization for stable angina.

The indications for emergency bypass surgery are not related to long-term morbidity, mortality or symptomatic status of the patient, but rather to the prevention of myocardial infarction and death in the acute stage of the illness. Improvement of symptoms by revascularization surgery is desirable, but to justify emergency procedures, a reduction of myocardial infarction and early death must be demonstrated.

Comparison of Early Mortality and Myocardial Infarction Rate in Medical and Surgical Patients

The need for emergency surgery can be established if the procedure will decrease mortality and myocardial infarction rates in patients with unstable angina. Therefore, these end points must be examined in surgically treated patients and compared with the same end points in medically treated patients. However, even this type of analysis may not be fair. All of the surgically treated patients underwent angiography and, by definition, must have proximal disease, good distal vessels, reasonably good ventricular function, and no other illness that would preclude surgery. All of the medically treated patients did not undergo angiography. Thus, the severity and extent of coronary artery disease and ventricular dysfunction remain unknown in many of the medically treated patients. In addition, many of the patients who underwent angiography were not surgical candidates because of extensive coronary artery disease and gross ventricular dysfunction. It is now quite clear that a random trial comparing the results of optimal medical and surgical therapy is necessary to answer the question precisely.

A review of the recent medical literature reveals 1950 published cases of patients with unstable angina treated medically or surgically. Since one of the questions that requires an answer for the practitioner is "What do we do with the patient now?", I have analyzed the data in terms of the in-hospital morbidity and mortality rates. If it can be shown that only a few medically treated patients die or have myocardial infarctions immediately, then a reasonable case can be made for the medical management of this condition, at least in the acute stages of the illness. Table 1 summarizes the in-hospital morbidity and mortality rates in patients receiving medical therapy. The last column indicates the percentage of complication, i.e., death or nonfatal myocardial infarc-

Table 1. *Unstable Angina. Medical Therapy: In-Hospital Morbidity and Mortality Rates*

		PATIENTS	DEATHS	MYOCARDIAL INFARCTION	% COMPLICATION
Krauss	1972	107	1	6	7
Gazes	1973	140	17	8	18
Scanlon	1973	22	6	13	86
Fischl	1973	20	0	0	0.0
Goodin	1973	11	0	0	0.0
Master	1974	18	0	5	28
Bertolasi	1974	40	6	?	15
Conti	1975	80	2	7	11.2
Bender	1975	35	0	1	3.7
Selden	1975	19	0	0	0.0
Hultgren	1977	66	3	4	10.6
TOTAL		558	35 (6.2%)	44 (7.8%)	14.0%

Table 2. *Unstable Angina. Surgical Therapy:*
In-Hospital Morbidity and Mortality Rates

		PATIENTS	DEATHS	MYOCARDIAL INFARCTION	% COMPLICATION
Favaloro	1971	18	2	1	16.6
Lambert	1971	52	3	2	9.6
Flemma	1972	80	2	?	3
Scanlon	1973	48	6	10	33
Conti	1973	50	11	2	26
Traad	1973	60	4	8	25
Segal	1973	17	3	3	35
Fischl	1973	14	1	1	14
Cheanvechai	1973	63	4	6	15.8
Wisoff	1973	26	2	2	15.3
Goodin	1973	30	4	1	16.6
Bonchek	1974	55	3	6	16.3
Bolooki	1974	25	0	4	16
Bertolasi	1974	57	4	?	7
Conti	1975	70	3	15	25.7
Bender	1975	53	0	3	5.5
Selden	1975	21	1	3	19
Hatcher	1975	100	5	16	21.0
Schroeder	1976	81	7	13	24.6
Geha	1976	48	1	2	6.2
Vogel	1976	70	1	6	10
Seybold-Epting	1976	302	20	23	14.2
Hultgren	1977	52	1	8	17.3
TOTAL		1392	88 (6.3%)	135 (9.6%)	15.9%

tion, occurring during hospitalization. Although there are obvious differences, the majority of the studies show that the incidence of total complication is less than 20 per cent in hospital. The average in-hospital mortality rate was 6.2 per cent and the incidence of myocardial infarction 7.8 per cent in these medically treated patients.

Table 2 summarizes the reports of surgically treated patients during the same period of time, analyzed in the same manner. Again, it is important to point out that most reports show a less than 20 per cent complication rate in hospital. The mortality rate for surgically treated patients was 6.3 per cent, and the incidence of myocardial infarction was 9.6 per cent. These reports fail to support the hypothesis that immediate coronary artery surgery is better than medical therapy if early mortality and myocardial infarction rates are used as end points.

Optimal Medical Therapy

Acute medical therapy needs to be individualized to each patient's needs, but the common goal is relief of pain. Current optimal medical therapy for patients with unstable angina should be aggressive and consist of the following: (1) admission to a CCU; (2) bed rest; (3) sublingual nitroglycerin as necessary; (3) beta blockade with propranolol, with the dosage adjusted to pharmacologically effective levels to reduce myocardial oxygen consumption and possibly redirect coronary flow to ischemic areas; (5) long-acting nitrates, e.g., isosorbide dinitrate and/or nitrol ointment; (6) analgesia and sedation if required; (7) digitalis and diuretics if clinically indicated; and (8) anticoagulation with heparin during the acute phase of the illness.

Plotnick and Conti have reported 36 patients with unstable angina who were studied hemodynamically and angiographically and then treated with optimal medical therapy. All of these patients were admitted to a coronary care unit because their chest pain syndrome was suspected to be myocardial infarction. After hemodynamic study, these patients were divided into two groups based on their operability. Patients were considered operable if three criteria were met: (1) greater than 70 per cent reduction in lumen diameter of a major proximal coronary artery, (2) patent distal coronary artery greater than 1.5 mm in diameter, and (3) acceptable ventricular performance. Twenty-one patients were considered operable but were treated medically because of physician's preference.

Table 3 summarizes the early incidence of nonfatal myocardial infarction and death in these 36 patients. Of the 21 patients considered to be operable (Group I), there were two hospital deaths, and of the nonoperable patients (Group II), there was one hospital death. Only one patient (Group II) sustained an in-hospital myocardial infarction. It is important to point out that of these 36 patients treated medically, only 21 can be compared to surgically treated patients, since the other 15 were not surgical candidates and might be considered to have a worse prognosis.

Indications for Surgery

My current indications for surgery in patients with unstable angina are as follows: (1) urgent surgery may be performed in patients with this syndrome who are discovered to have left main coronary artery disease or patients whose symptoms (pain or life-threatening arrhythmias) are uncontrolled by vigorous medical means; (2) elective surgery can be performed in patients

Table 3. *Early Morbidity and Mortality Rates of 36 Medically Treated Patients with Unstable Angina*

		DEATHS	MYOCARDIAL INFARCTION	% COMPLICATION
Group I	21	2 (9.5%)	0 (0%)	9.5%
Group II	15	1 (6.6%)	1 (6.6%)	13.2%
TOTAL	36	3 (8.3%)	1 (2.7%)	11.0%

with multiple-vessel disease at a time convenient to all concerned, especially if there is a return of symptoms and the patient is not satisfied with his lifestyle.

Summary

In summary, the incidence of myocardial infarction and death with unstable angina remains difficult to predict in individual patients. A review of current medical literature, as well as personal experience with medically treated patients, indicates that (1) early mortality and morbidity rates are not as high as once thought; (2) the incidence of myocardial infarction is slightly greater with surgery than with medical therapy; (3) there is no significant difference in the immediate mortality rate; and (4) clinical experience indicates that the majority of patients with unstable angina, when treated vigorously with pharmacologic agents, have a marked reduction, if not total relief, of their anginal syndrome at least for the short-term period.

Observations suggest that the indication for surgery in patients with unstable angina may be the same as that for patients with stable angina; that is, the relief of symptoms, since it has not been shown that myocardial infarction or death was prevented by early surgery. In addition, evidence has indicated that it is not necessary to operate on these patients on an emergency basis, since early mortality and morbidity rates in the medically treated patients are quite low. In addition, the low early mortality and morbidity with medical therapy permit a delay of surgery, which may reduce the risk of surgery in patients with persistent, active myocardial ischemia or undetected evolving myocardial infarction.

References

1. Krauss KR, Hutter AM Jr, and De Sanctis RW: Acute coronary insufficiency. Course and follow-up. Arch Intern Med 129:808, 1972.
2. Gazes PC, Mobley EM Jr, Faris HM Jr, et al: Preinfarctional (unstable) angina — a prospective study — ten year follow-up. Circulation 48:331, 1973.
3. Scanlon PJ, Nemickas R, Moran JF, et al: Accelerated angina pectoris. Clinical, hemodynamic, arteriographic, and therapeutic experience in 85 patients. Circulation 47:19, 1973.
4. Fischl SJ, Herman MV, and Gorlin R: The intermediate coronary syndrome: clinical, angiographic and therapeutic aspects. N Engl J Med 288:1193, 1973.
5. Goodin RR, Inglesby TV, Lansing AM, et al: Preinfarction angina pectoris. A surgical emergency. J Thorac Cardiovasc Surg 66:934, 1973.
6. Master AM, and Jaffe HL: Propranolol vs saphenous vein graft bypass for impending infarction (preinfarction syndrome). Am Heart J 87:321, 1974.
7. Bertolasi CA, Trongé JE, Carreno CA, et al: Unstable angina — prospective and randomized study of its evolution, with and without surgery. Am J Cardiol 33:201, 1974.
8. Conti CR, Gilbert JB, Hodges M, et al: Unstable angina pectoris — randomized study of surgical vs medical therapy. Am J Cardiol 35:129, 1975.
9. Bender HW Jr, Fisher RD, Faulkner SL, et al: Unstable coronary artery disease: comparison of medical and surgical treatment. Ann Thorac Surg 19:521, 1975.

10. Selden R, Neill WA, Ritzmann LW, et al: Medical versus surgical therapy for acute coronary insufficiency. A randomized study. N Engl J Med 293:1329, 1975.
11. Hultgren HN, Pfeifer JF, Angell WW, et al: Unstable angina: comparison of medical and surgical management. Am J Cardiol 39:734, 1977.
12. Favaloro RG, Effler DB, Cheanvechai C, et al: Acute coronary insufficiency (impending myocardial infarction and myocardial infarction): surgical treatment by the saphenous vein graft technique. Am J Cardiol 28:598, 1971.
13. Lambert CJ, Adam M, Geisler GF, et al: Emergency myocardial revascularization for impending infarctions and arrhythmias. J Thorac Cardiovasc Surg 62:522, 1971.
14. Flemma RJ, Johnson WD, Tector AJ, et al: Surgical treatment of preinfarction angina. Arch Intern Med 129:828, 1972.
15. Conti CR, Brawley RK, Griffith LS, et al: Unstable angina pectoris: morbidity and mortality in 57 consecutive patients evaluated angiographically. Am J Cardiol 32:745, 1973.
16. Traad EA, Larsen PB, Gentsch TO, et al: Surgical management of the preinfarction syndrome. Ann Thorac Surg 16:261, 1973.
17. Segal BL, Likoff W, van den Broek H, et al: Saphenous vein bypass surgery for impending myocardial infarction. JAMA 223:767, 1973.
18. Cheanvechai C, Effler DB, Loop FD, et al: Emergency myocardial revascularization. Am J Cardiol 32:901, 1973.
19. Wisoff BG, Kolker P, Hartstein ML, et al: Surgical approach to impending myocardial infarction. J Thorac Cardiovasc Surg 65:534, 1973.
20. Boncheck LI, Rahimtoola SH, Anderson RP, et al: Late results following emergency saphenous vein bypass grafting for unstable angina. Circulation 50:972, 1974.
21. Bolooki H, Sommer L, Kaiser GA, et al: Long-term follow-up in patients receiving emergency revascularization for immediate coronary syndrome. J Thorac Cardiovasc Surg 68:90, 1974.
22. Hatcher CR, Jones EL, King SB, Gray BT, and Malley TN: Surgical treatment of unstable angina. Ann Surg 180:754, 1975.
23. Schroeder JS, Hu M, and Lamb I: The effect of coronary artery bypass on survival for unstable angina. Am J Cardiol 37:170, 1976.
24. Geha AS, Baue AE, Krone RJ, et al: Surgical treatment of unstable angina by saphenous vein and internal mammary artery bypass grafting. J Thorac Cardiovasc Surg 71:348, 1976.
25. Vogel JHK, McFadden RB, Love J, et al: Surgical treatment in unstable angina. Adv Cardiol 17:134, 1976.
26. Seybold-Epting W, Oglietti J, Wukasch DC, et al: Early and late results after surgical treatment of preinfarction angina. Ann Thorac Surg 21:97, 1976.
27. Plotnick G, and Conti CR: Unstable angina: angiography, morbidity and mortality of medically treated patients. Circulation 51(Suppl II):II-89, 1975.

Comment

The issues raised in this controversy are in many ways analogous to those expressed in the preceding one on stable angina pectoris. There is no question that surgical management of unstable angina pectoris is accomplished at a relatively low operative risk and results in an improved outlook in terms of lessened or eliminated symptoms. The improvement in the quality of life and the incidence of symptomatic improvement is greater than with medical management. On the other hand, surgery probably does increase the incidence of early myocardial infarction compared with medical management.

The big question is whether surgical management improves overall long-term survival. If one excludes left main coronary artery disease, the latest report of the National Cooperative Multicenter Study using randomized controls would suggest that there is no significant difference between the survival of those patients treated medically compared with those treated surgically. Unstable angina, like stable angina pectoris, has undergone a dramatic change in terms of the outlook of the patient managed medically. Using the vigorous therapeutic approach outlined by Conti, the overwhelming majority of patients hospitalized for unstable angina pectoris will respond with marked attenuation of their symptoms and will generally either become asymptomatic or stabilize with a picture of controlled, chronic, stable angina pectoris. Thus, part of the confusion that has surrounded the problem of unstable angina has been the fear that this illness foretold a catastrophic outcome as suggested by the natural history studies performed in past decades. However, with modern medical treatment of unstable angina, we now appreciate that overall survival appears to be quite comparable to that for stable angina pectoris. The survival statistic for medical survivors in the National Cooperative Program at the end of two years was 91 per cent, a figure quite comparable to the Veterans Administration survival statistic for stable angina pectoris.

In light of the above, it is my view that patients with unstable angina should be hospitalized in the CCU and vigorously treated over the ensuing 48 hours with propranolol, nitrates, and correction to the extent possible of any causes identified as either increasing myocardial oxygen demand or decreasing myocardial blood flow. With this kind of therapy, if the instability disappears and the patient calms down, he is ambulated after a week and then managed as any patient with chronic stable angina pectoris. If, however, the patient is still having episodes of rest pain or pain with minimal exertion associated with ECG changes, coronary arteriography is performed, and if there are demonstrable operable lesions, surgery is carried out.

ELLIOT RAPAPORT, M.D.

195

Nine

Should Anticoagulants Be Used During Hospitalization for Unstable Angina?

ANTICOAGULANTS SHOULD BE USED DURING
HOSPITALIZATION FOR UNSTABLE ANGINA
> *James J. Morris, Jr., M.D.*

THE FAILURE OF ANTICOAGULANT THERAPY IN
PATIENTS HOSPITALIZED WITH UNSTABLE ANGINA
> *David A. Rytand, M.D.*

COMMENT

Anticoagulants Should Be Used During Hospitalization for Unstable Angina

JAMES J. MORRIS, JR., M.D.

Professor of Medicine, Division of Cardiology, Department of Medicine, Duke University Medical Center, Durham, North Carolina

To rationally advise the routine use of anticoagulation during the hospital phase of unstable angina, it would be important to (1) clearly define the clinical syndrome, (2) understand the natural history of the condition, (3) know the pathophysiology, (4) know the effects, adverse and favorable, of the available anticoagulants, and (5) unequivocally demonstrate in controlled clinical trials the efficacy of this treatment mode. It is obvious to any student of coronary artery disease that these data are not available in sufficient clarity to permit "the scientific basis" for resolving this question. In complex clinical syndromes, one must frequently resort to empiric trials and to rationalization of available information and arrive at a decision. Given the information available, I believe there are enough inferential data at hand that do justify the position that short-term anticoagulation should be employed in patients with the unstable anginal syndrome. This review will attempt to highlight a few of the considerations in that decision.

Definition of Unstable Angina

The definition of unstable angina pectoris has changed from a simplistic approach to a more defined set of criteria with the passage of time. Initial reports were most often of patients who were hospitalized because the chest pain syndrome suggested the possibility that myocardial infarction might occur. Most current definitions define the type of chest pain and the time frame over which these changes occur and require electrocardiographic changes, and many include angiographic proof of obstructive coronary artery disease. There are four types of chest pain syndromes: (1) appearance of new angina pectoris, (2) definite change in the pattern of stable angina, (3) appearance of angina at rest, and (4) the intermediate syndrome — pain more prolonged and less responsive to the usual factors that relieve angina (rest, nitroglycerin). Many patients may show several of these patterns. Most definitions include a requirement that the pain pattern be present for a finite period of time, generally days to weeks. Transient and reversible ST- and T-wave changes coincident with the pain have sharpened the diagnostic accuracy of the definition. Most current definitions also include a 36- to 48-hour period of time from the diagnosis to evaluate serial enzyme and ECG changes to exclude recent myocardial infarction. Despite these rather rigid criteria of definite types of pain patterns, a necessary time frame over which they develop, and reversible electrocardiographic changes during pain, almost all series in which coronary arteriography has been utilized as part of the definition have shown that a small percentage of such patients have normal arteriograms.[1-6] These patients will have a very different natural history from those with fixed obstructive lesions and are important to recognize. It is also becoming clear that more and more patients are showing transient and reversible "spastic" lesions in their coronary arteries with electrocardiographic and clinical patterns that will indicate Prinzmetal's variant form of angina. Although it could be argued that they should be included in the unstable angina population, it would seem advisable to consider them as a separate diagnostic category until it becomes clear that their natural history would make it mandatory to consider them therapeutically as part of the unstable group.

Thus, a workable definition would appear to be

1. Change in anginal pattern over a finite time period (days to weeks)

    a. Newly developing angina pectoris
    b. Change in a stable anginal pattern
    c. Angina occurring at rest
    d. Intermediate syndrome

2. Exclusion of recent myocardial infarction over a 36- to 48-hour period by serial enzyme and electrocardiographic observation

3. Documented and reversible ST- and T-wave changes with the chest pain syndrome.

This definition will include a small number of patients who will subsequently be found to have normal coronary arteries, some who have the subsequent demonstration of spastic lesions in their coronary arteries, and also a small group who have sustained a recent myocardial infarction, but this should provide a homogeneous enough subset of patients to consider the question of acute anticoagulation. For natural history studies or for the consideration for more aggressive treatment modalities, coronary arteriography should be added as a requisite to this definition.

Natural History

Since our major concern is whether or not to recommend anticoagulation for the *acute* phase of the unstable anginal syndrome, a review of the available information regarding the acute natural history of this condition would be appropriate, and purposely we will avoid the quagmire of the question of long-term anticoagulation. Two qualifying remarks should be recognized in the study of the acute natural history of unstable angina pectoris. First, a relatively constant definition of the syndrome has only evolved in recent years, and thus a review of the literature shows a rather mixed experience in the natural history of this condition. Second, newer diagnostic and therapeutic modalities influence the practice of medicine. The advent of coronary care units, access to more precise and rapidly available enzyme analysis methods (isoenzymes of CPK and LDH), the capability to readily perform coronary arteriography, and the availability of additional therapeutic measures (propranolol and coronary artery bypass grafting) have had a very profound effect on the natural history of unstable angina pectoris as reviewed in the medical literature. As a general trend, it appears evident that the morbidity and mortality have decreased over the period of time during which clinical experience has been reported. Whether this is due to a real improvement in management or to bringing under attention patients in an earlier and less critical stage of the illness is unclear.

A search of the medical literature reveals a relatively large number of reports of short-term follow-up in patients with the unstable anginal syndrome. Despite the variability of the diagnosis and the variability of the methods in which the studies are compiled, one can readily see that the appearance of the unstable pattern in angina pectoris does imply a potential for morbid and mortal events in the next few months. Table 1 shows six studies in which specific series were collected and in which anticoagulants were not administered. Many larger series are available, but the use of anticoagulants is not broken down, and also selection in some of these was done after other patients had been selected for surgical treatment of the

Table 1. *Unstable Angina — Medical Treatment,
No Anticoagulants Used*

| | | | NO. OF | EARLY COMPLICATIONS — 3 MONTHS | |
AUTHOR	REFERENCE	YEAR	PATIENTS	*Myocardial Infarction*	*Death*
Beamish	10	1960	15	80%	60%
Wood	11	1961	50	22%	30%
Vakil	12	1964	156	24%	49%
Gazes	13	1973	49	10%	29%
Duncan	14	1976	251	10%	3%
Hultgren	6	1977	66	6%	6%°

°Less than one month.

unstable anginal syndrome. It is clear that from 1960 to 1977, the rate of subsequent infarction and death in the early months after the diagnosis of unstable angina pectoris fell. Perhaps the most broadly representative series is that of Duncan,[14] which is a follow-up report of Fulton's original series.[15] This study is a prospective study of all patients in the city of Edinburgh with the onset of new angina or worsening chest pain who were seen by a group of general practitioners and subsequently referred for further study. Of the 251 patients with unstable angina, only 85 were judged to have conditions severe enough to warrant hospitalization. This is probably the best attempt at a true population study and gives what amounts to the minimal risk. Other series have been collected after admission to the hospital or on referral to a cardiologist or after coronary arteriography, and these studies show higher risk figures. The former is probably the picture seen in the community; the other studies reflect more the experience once the patient has been admitted or has come under more intensive study. It seems fair to conclude, however, that unstable angina is not the severe prognostic sign of impending infarction or death that it was initially believed to be, but it does carry a risk of subsequent infarction of somewhere in the range of 10 to 30 per cent and a mortality risk of three to 20 per cent in the subsequent three months. This risk seems to depend on whether one is considering all patients or those whose conditions are severe enough to require hospitalization. Several authors have commented that it is possible to further subdivide the unstable angina population into other subgroups: those with persistent pain after hospital admission; those with persistent ECG changes; those with prolonged pain (coronary insufficiency); and those with angiographic proof of multiple-vessel disease — all have been reported to show higher risk than the overall population.

Although anticoagulants have been purported to be of help in this condition, there are few clinical trials directly comparing the use of anticoagulation in a series of patients with unstable angina. Table 2 lists the three available trials where "control" and treated groups were compared. Beamish[10] used as a "control" 15 patients who "were selected in part by the

Table 2.   *"Controlled" Trials of Anticoagulation in Unstable Angina*

AUTHOR	REFERENCE	YEAR	GROUPS	MYOCARDIAL INFARCTION*	DEATH*
Beamish	10	1960	Control	(12/15) 80%	(9/15) 60%
			Treated	(2/85) 2%	(0/85) 0%
Wood	11	1961	Control	(11/50) 22%	(8/50) 16%
			Treated	(3/100) 3%	(2/100) 2%
Vakil	12	1964	Control	(77/156) 49%	(37/156) 24%
			Treated	(69/190) 36%	(18/190) 10%
Combined			Control	(100/221) 45%	(54/221) 24%
			Treated	(74/375) 19%	(20/375) 5%

*Within 3 months

patient and in part by the chance unavailability of hospital accommodations." These "controls" were compared to hospitalized and treated patients. Wood[11] embarked on a controlled trial, but when an advantage was seen in the first 40 randomized patients favoring anticoagulation, the remaining 30 controls were "in the control group not chosen at random" but because anticoagulation was undesirable. Vakil[12] in his control group gives no report as to how treated and control groups were selected; certainly they were not randomized. Although all these studies fail to live up to or in fact even partially satisfy the criteria for a controlled clinical trial, they are the only studies in the medical literature that purport to directly address the problem of whether anticoagulation of patients with pre-infarction is helpful. All show that the treated groups have a low rate of myocardial infarction (45 per cent versus 19 per cent) and a lower death rate (24 per cent versus 5 per cent) in the three months after diagnosis. It should be noted that these myocardial infarction and mortality rates in the control groups are not as low as current figures reported in the 1970's. Clearly, these studies do not settle the question but leave one only with a clinical suggestion of improvement.

Pathophysiology

The exact pathologic process that produces the change from an asymptomatic patient or a patient with chronic stable angina to the patient with an unstable anginal pattern is unclear in the vast majority of patients. External factors may provoke this change, and treatment of these conditions is appropriate. Examples of this are anemia, blood loss, hyperthyroidism, and arrhythmias. In most patients, a readily identifiable cause is not apparent. The most widely held explanation is an acute alteration of blood flow to a given area of myocardium, whether by obstruction or redistribution. Because it has been suspected that this obstruction is caused by thrombosis or platelet aggregation, anticoagulation has been advocated. In acute myocardial infarction there is still considerable debate among qualified students as to the role of thrombosis. Ridolfi and Hutchins[16] state, "The present study strongly suggests that intimal ulcerations, erosions or ruptures of atheromatous plaques provide a nidus for occlusive coronary artery thrombosis which precipitates the overwhelming majority of myocardial infarctions." They studied 494 myocardial infarctions greater than 3 cm and could find vascular lesions with thrombus formation on a nidus of focal endothelial injury or disruption in 93 per cent of the arterial lesions that were associated with a recent (less than four weeks) myocardial infarction. Baroldi,[17] among others,[18] holds the opposite position: "The classic concept of the primary role of the thrombus still deserves serious consideration. Presently, however, a substantial body of knowledge supports the concept of a secondary genesis of the thrombus." Studies designed to elucidate the role of thrombosis by administration of labeled fibrinogen in the early phases of myocardial infarction have given conflicting results.

It is fair to conclude that the important question of the primacy of thrombosis in the development of a myocardial infarction is not clear, and it is equally clear that there is a growing body of information that places in some patients an important role for functional alterations (spasm) in the genesis of cardiac pain and/or myocardial infarction.[8, 9] Given the possibility that a thrombus is not the primary event, is there evidence that secondary thrombosis is important? In a controlled dog study[19] using administration of large doses of heparin prior to coronary ligation, it was possible to show that this resulted in significant improvement as reflected by epicardial electrocardiographic findings, preserved myocardial tissue (by pathologic studies), and myocardial creatine phosphokinase changes. Thus, there resides a theoretical and experimental body of data that might make anticoagulation beneficial in impending infarction.

Anticoagulation

In a certain percentage of patients with the unstable anginal syndrome, myocardial infarction and death appear early in the syndrome, and they rapidly diminish in frequency in the subsequent days and weeks. For purposes of this discussion, it is assumed that rapid anticoagulation is desired and that heparin is the agent of choice, and that anticoagulation is being considered for the hospital phase of the unstable anginal patient. Coumadin and Coumadin-like drugs by their nature are far too slow in onset to be of practical value. It should be pointed out that in the "controlled clinical trials" reported in Table 2, in which anticoagulation was purported to be beneficial, all patients were initially heparinized, and at some later point Coumadin was administered.

There are four reasons why heparin might be considered to be beneficial in the unstable angina patient: (1) If some undefined portion of the patients with unstable angina do develop thrombosis as the primary precipitating event, heparin has the potential to prevent this. (2) If thrombosis is a secondary but aggravating event, heparin has the potential to minimize the effects of the infarction. (3) Heparin has diverse biological and biochemical effects.[19] Some of the effects reported are: blood-to-tissue oxygen transfer; antilipemic, antihistaminic, antiserotonin, antiplatelet lysis, antihemolytic, antiproteolytic enzyme (anti-ribonuclease, anti–acid phosphatase, anti-glucuronidase, anti-fumarase, anti-elastase, anti-hyaluronidase); pain relief; reduction of edema; antimicrothrombi, anti-inflammatory, antithrombus, and antifibrin extension, anticomplement and ionic binding of calcium, potassium, and sodium ions. If any of these effects are important in the undefined steps that proceed from a chronic atheromatous lesion in a coronary artery to the clinical syndrome of myocardial infarction, heparin may be beneficial even though it is not acting as an anticoagulant. (4) Bed rest and inactivity can induce venous thrombosis, and this may lead to pulmonary emboli. In myocardial infarction not only may venous thrombosis and pulmonary emboli occur, but systemic embolization may also occur. It is clear that heparin can prevent this.[20]

In using heparin there are two broad treatment outlines — large doses for treatment of a known clotting disorder and low-dose heparin as a prophylactic measure. Treatment of pulmonary embolism requires large or conventional doses of heparin. In the prophylactic use of heparin in treating thromboembolism, it has already been shown in surgical patients, obstetric patients, or patients who have had a myocardial infarction[21, 22] that heparin is clearly effective in low doses, i.e., 5000 units subcutaneously twice a day. As one considers the patient population with unstable angina, they will be hospitalized and treated with bed rest, and a certain proportion will develop myocardial infarction. It is certainly clear that in patients at bed rest with myocardial infarction, heparin therapy reduces thromboembolic risk whether one assesses fibrinogen uptake in the venous system, clinical phlebothrombosis, documented pulmonary embolization, or postmortem data. It is estimated that these events can be reduced by 70 per cent with either conventional or low-dose heparin. In the multicenter trial in postsurgical patients, low-dose heparin has clearly been shown to significantly reduce thrombosis and pulmonary embolization. It is speculative, but likely, that low-dose heparin would reduce venous thrombosis and emboli in those patients with unstable angina who are hospitalized but never do develop a clinical myocardial infarction.

One principal reason for not heparinizing unstable angina patients is the potential for complications — the major ones being hemorrhagic complications. Low-dose heparin does not carry any significant hemorrhagic risk even in a surgical patient. In the use of heparin intravenously in full therapeutic doses, there is a very definite risk. The risk of a major bleeding episode is somewhat predictable. Pitney[23] studied 114 patients receiving heparin and could clearly divide patients into those at low risk for hemorrhagic complications — those with normal hemostatic systems — (risk 7.6 per cent), and those at high risk (50 per cent) with defective hemostatic mechanisms, especially those with uremia and thrombocytopenia. Salzman[24] studied 100 patients being heparinized and defined a higher-risk group of patients that consisted of those with recent surgery, thrombocytopenia, uremia, or prior bleeding tendencies and those receiving intramuscular injections or receiving concurrent administration of platelet-active drugs. Such patients had a 25 per cent risk of major bleeding, whereas those with none of these had an incidence of 10 per cent.

In summary, heparin can be given in low doses with virtually no risk and will clearly be beneficial in those patients who develop myocardial infarction by reducing venous thrombosis and its subsequent complications. It is probably true, but not proven, that low-dose heparin will also reduce the risk of venous thrombosis and embolization in patients who are confined at bed rest with unstable angina but who do not proceed to a myocardial infarction. If heparin is to be used for its other possible actions, i.e., preventing or minimizing the effects of myocardial infarction, no data exist comparing low-dose to regular heparin treatment, i.e., no positive or negative evidence has been presented.

Conclusions

Having carried out a brief review of the major considerations regarding unstable angina pectoris, certain generalizations seem worthy of emphasis.

Definition. Patients with unstable angina pectoris are those with the abrupt onset of new anginal pain, those with abrupt changes in the pattern of stable angina or rest angina, and those with more prolonged pain or pain unresponsive to nitroglycerin. During hospitalization, enzyme studies should exclude recent myocardial infarction, and reversible ST- and T-wave changes should be demonstrated during pain.

Natural History. Recent studies have shown that with prompt attention and medical treatment (bed rest, nitrates, analgesics, beta blockers), the risk of subsequent progression to myocardial infarction and death in the next three months in patients with unstable angina is lower than previously suggested and approximates a risk of about 10 per cent for a myocardial infarction and a mortality rate of 10 to 15 per cent. Patients with new angina or those with prompt relief of the syndrome on medical management seem to be at a lower risk than those with repeated and/or refractory pain in the hospital, and those with coronary insufficiency seem to be at a higher risk.

Controlled Clinical Trials. No truly adequate trials of anticoagulation exist. Three studies reported in the literature, all with unusually high infarction rates and mortality rates, compare anticoagulation and untreated patients, and each tends to favor anticoagulant treatment.

Pathophysiology. The precise mechanism whereby the unstable anginal pattern appears and what produces the final event that results in myocardial infarction are unknown in the majority of patients. Even the very basic question of whether thrombosis is a necessary primary event is still unclear.

Anticoagulation. Heparinization is the only rapid enough mode of anticoagulant treatment currently available in a practical form. Even in selected patients, however, it carries a risk of a major bleeding event when used in full therapeutic doses in approximately 10 per cent of patients. Heparinization in low doses has been shown to be remarkably effective in preventing venous thrombosis and its sequelae in patients with known myocardial infarction and can be accomplished without significant side effects. Heparin has a multiplicity of effects beyond its anticoagulant action, some of which could be potentially beneficial in the unstable anginal state, i.e., antiplatelet effects, anti-edema, antiserotonin, and so on. No data exist on low-dose heparin therapy in the unstable anginal state.

Given ι⁻ relevant clinical facts — (1) beta blockade appears to influence the pain pattern favorably in unstable angina and (2) surgical intervention may be deemed necessary in some, all, or none of the patients, depending on one's point of view — a practical clinical rationale for the use of heparin in unstable angina patients can be outlined. In patients with this syndrome who are admitted and qualify under the above definition, the risk of subsequent infarction and death appears only slightly more than the risk of a serious bleeding event if full heparinization is used. Since the definite benefit of heparin has only been suggested by poorly controlled studies and the risk of major bleeding with full heparinization seems unduly high, it is difficult to recommend routine full heparinization in all patients. Low-dose heparin can be given to all patients without risk and has the advantage of clearly preventing venous thrombosis and its sequelae. Potentially, low-dose heparin could also have the same "preventive properties" as full heparinization. In those patients who are refractory to full medical treatment, including low-dose heparin, one has two options—coronary arteriography and subsequent surgery or, if one does not employ this mode of treatment, one can resort to full heparinization, since these refractory patients seem to be at a higher risk for subsequent cardiovascular events. In the event that one employs arteriography, those patients deemed surgically amenable will be treated in that fashion, and those not surgically treated will be found to have either no coronary disease or extensive disease or badly damaged ventricles, and full heparinization can be employed in this latter group.

What is obviously required are further observations of the effects of heparin, especially low-dose heparin, in the unstable angina population. Whether this type of study can in fact be carried out in a meaningful and practical way is debatable. Short of this, the above recommendations seek to capitalize on the known clinical benefits and to weigh side effects against potential benefits in that segment of the unstable angina population that is at most risk for serious cardiovascular events.

References

1. Fischl SJ, Herman MV, and Gorlin R: The intermediate coronary syndrome—clinical, angiographic and therapeutic aspects. N Engl J Med 288:1193, 1973.
2. Scanlon PJ, Nemickas R, Moran JF, Talano JV, Amirparviz F, and Pifarre R: Accelerated angina pectoris—clinical, hemodynamic, arteriographic, and therapeutic experience in 85 patients. Circulation 47:19, 1973.
3. Conti CR, Brawley RK, Griffith LSC, Pitt B, Humphries JO, Gott VL, and Ross RS: Unstable angina pectoris: morbidity and mortality in 57 consecutive patients evaluated angiographically. Am J Cardiol 32:745. 1973.
4. Day LJ, Thibault GE, and Sowton E: Acute coronary insufficiency—review of 46 patients. Br Heart J 39:363. 1977.
5. Bertolasi CA, Trongé JE, Riccitelli MA, Villamayor RM, and Zuffardi E: Natural history of unstable angina with medical or surgical therapy. Chest 70:596, 1976.
6. Hultgren HN, Pfeifer JF, Angell WW, Lipton MJ, and Bilisoly J: Unstable angina: comparison of medical and surgical management. Am J Cardiol 39:734, 1977.
7. Maseri A, Pesola A, Marzilli M, Severi S, Parodi O, L'Abbate A, Ballestra AM, Maltinti G., De Nes DM, and Biagini A: Coronary vasospasm in angina pectoris. Lancet 1(8014):713, 1977.
8. Oliva PB, and Breckinridge JC: Arteriographic evidence of coronary arterial spasm in acute myocardial infarction. Circulation 56:366, 1977.
9. Oliva PB, Potts DE, and Pluss RG: Coronary arterial spasm in Prinzmetal angina. N Engl J Med 288:745, 1973.
10. Beamish RE. and Storrie VM: Impending myocardial infarction—recognition and management. Circulation 21:1107, 1960.
11. Wood P: Acute and subacute coronary insufficiency. Br Med J 5242:1779, 1961.
12. Vakil RJ: Preinfarction syndrome—management and follow-up. Am J Cardiol 14:55, 1964.
13. Gazes PC, Mobley EM Jr, Faris HM Jr, Duncan RC, and Humphries GB: Preinfarctional (unstable) angina—a prospective study—ten year follow-up. Circulation 48:331, 1973.

14. Duncan B, Fulton M, Morrison SL, Lutz W, Donald KW, Kerr F, Kirby BJ, Julian DG, and
    Oliver MF: Prognosis of new and worsening angina pectoris. Br Med J 1:981, 1976.
15. Fulton M, Lutz W, Donald KW, Kirby BJ, Duncan B, Morrison SL, Kerr F, Julian DG, and
    Oliver MF: Natural history of unstable angina. Lancet 1:860, 1972.
16. Ridolfi RL, and Hutchins GM: The relationship between coronary artery lesions and myo-
    cardial infarcts: ulceration of atherosclerotic plaques precipitating coronary thrombo-
    sis. Am Heart J 93:468, 1977.
17. Baroldi G: Coronary thrombosis: facts and beliefs. Am Heart J 91:683, 1976.
18. Roberts WC, and Ferrans VJ: The role of thrombosis in the etiology of atherosclerosis (a
    positive one) and in precipitating fatal ischemic heart disease (a negative one). Semi-
    nars in Thrombosis and Hemostasis 2:123, 1976.
19. Saliba MJ Jr, Covell JW, and Bloor CM: Effects of heparin in large doses on the extent of
    myocardial ischemia after acute coronary occlusion in the dog. Am J Cardiol 37:599,
    1976.
20. Kakkar VV, and Thomas DP: Heparin—Chemistry and Clinical Usage. International Hep-
    arin Symposium. New York, Academic Press, 1976.
21. Steffensen KA: Coronary occlusion treated with small doses of heparin. Acta Med Scand
    186:519, 1969.
22. Emerson PA, and Marks P: Preventing thromboembolism after myocardial infarction: ef-
    fect of low-dose heparin or smoking. Br Med J 1:18, 1977.
23. Pitney WR, Pettit JE, and Armstrong L: Control of heparin therapy. Br Med J 4:139, 1970.
24. Salzman EW, Deykin D, Shapiro RM, and Rosenberg R: Management of heparin therapy:
    controlled prospective trial. N Engl J Med 292:1046, 1975.

The Failure of Anticoagulant Therapy in Patients Hospitalized With Unstable Angina

DAVID A. RYTAND, M.D.

Arthur L. Bloomfield Professor of Medicine, Emeritus,
Stanford University School of Medicine, Stanford,
California; Chief, Division of Cardiology, Santa Clara
Valley Medical Center, San Jose, California

Years of clinical trials in patients with acute myocardial infarction have failed to demonstrate any reduction in deaths by the use of anticoagulants.[1] Furthermore, administration of these agents for angina pectoris has virtually disappeared as the popularity of "bypass" surgery has increased. Proponents of anticoagulant therapy for ischemic disease of the heart now attempt merely to reduce the morbidity of thromboembolic disease, even though this approach has not lowered fatality rates.

Current use of anticoagulants for patients with acute infarction varies widely in a number of large academic hospitals.[2] They are prescribed only for "poor-risk" and other similar patients in most American or British hospitals, but more frequently in European centers. Long-term use after infarction follows a comparable pattern, with less administration in British and American hospitals. Anticoagulants were used for "pre-infarction angina" in about half of all the hospitals that responded to a questionnaire.[2]

Methods of anticoagulant therapy during acute infarction vary widely: low-dose or high-dose heparin alone, oral agents alone, or both.[2] Thromboembolic complications occurred in one to five per cent of patients whether or not anticoagulants were used.[2]

The variable definition of unstable angina, from stable angina to acute infarction, and the persistent controversy over the use of anticoagulants for coronary artery disease, underscore the absurdity of using these agents in patients with unstable angina pectoris. Perhaps something can be learned by reviewing the relevant studies, although comparing the reports is difficult because of variable population of patients.

First, do anticoagulants prevent the development of myocardial infarction in patients with unstable angina? As a "baseline," there is a report of 158 patients with unstable angina in which less than 10 per cent of the patients received anticoagulants.[3, 4] Only 20 (13 per cent) of these had early infarction. In a second study of pre-infarction or unstable angina, 91 of 140 patients (65 per cent) received "warfarin and/or heparin."[5] Infarcts occurred in 29 patients; 15 (51 per cent) were treated with anticoagulants. In a series of patients with accelerated angina pectoris, "most" of whom received "heparin and/or coumarin agents," early infarction occurred in 13 of 22 (59 per cent) unoperated patients.[6]

Theoretically, heparin rather than oral agents is indicated in unstable angina because of its rapidity of action. In 60 episodes of acute coronary insufficiency in patients who received warfarin alone or with heparin, there were two cardiac infarcts during the first 10 days of treatment, six more episodes of acute coronary insufficiency, one pulmonary infarct, and one sudden death. Heparin was "without any demonstrable positive value," and may even have been harmful.[7] Heparin might be harmful in this setting if it induces ventricular arrhythmias by elevating free fatty acids in the plasma. An increased incidence of ventricular tachycardia after acute infarction in patients treated with heparin has been both confirmed[8] and denied.[9]

Low-dose heparin has received attention recently. In a randomized study of "medical patients suspected of having myocardial infarction" (unstable angina?), a final diagnosis of infarction was made in 14 of 38 (37 per cent) patients treated with low-dose heparin and in 13 of 40 (33 per cent) controls.[10] In patients undergoing elective "major" surgery, myocardial infarction allegedly was the cause of death at necropsy in seven of 53 patients (13 per cent) who had received heparin and in 13 of 72 (18 per cent) controls.[11] Low-dose heparin was not effective in patients undergoing surgery during an active thrombotic process.[12] If unstable angina is caused by the development of a coronary thrombus, low-dose heparin, by analogy, may be inadequate in spite of its rapid onset of action.

Thus, anticoagulant therapy is ineffective in the prevention of infarcts in patients with unstable angina pectoris or otherwise at risk. Could anticoagulants be beneficial to these patients on some other basis, by preventing venous thromboembolism or by inhibiting the occurrence or growth of coronary arterial or intracardiac thrombi? As there is no direct evidence of those actions, we must examine reports on acute infarction for analogies.

Studies of patients with acute cardiac infarcts almost unanimously show a reduced incidence of venous thrombi detected by ^{125}I-labeled fibrinogen from a control mean of 24 per cent (range 14 to 34 per cent) to eight per cent (range zero to 23 per cent) with either low-dose or high-dose heparin, whether or not warfarin was co-administered. One of these studies, however, reported improvement only in patients with congestive heart failure, while an opposite, but not statistically significant, change occurred in those without heart failure.[13] This latter finding was not confirmed in another study, in which the apparent efficacy of low-dose heparin was nearly equalled by cigarette smoking![14] Nevertheless, the clinical importance of prevention of venous thrombosis detected by ^{125}I-labeled fibrinogen requires clarification. So far, there is "no solid evidence that the incidence of pulmonary embolus had been lowered."[15]

Details on what actually occurs in the coronary arteries during unstable angina are unclear. Furthermore, the old concept of coronary thrombus as the proximate cause of cardiac infarction has come under scrutiny. A coronary thrombus is present in virtually all cases of transmural infarction only when sought assiduously by the pathologist.[16] Erhardt and his colleagues found the incorporation of ^{125}I-labeled fibrinogen to be identical in the coronary arterial thrombi of two groups of patients who died after acute myocardial infarction, whether or not heparin and oral anticoagulants had been administered.[17, 18]

Finally, a mural thrombus may occur in the left ventricle after infarction despite the use of anticoagulants.[19]

Conclusions

My own clinical impressions agree with the reports cited above. Anticoagulant therapy has been of no value in the prevention of death during acute myocardial infarction or in the prevention of infarcts in patients with unstable angina pectoris. These agents inhibit neither mural thrombus of the left ventricle nor the incorporation of fibrinogen within fresh coronary arterial thrombi. While they may inhibit venous thrombosis as judged by modern methods, this benefit is not clearly important clinically. Specific studies with low-dose heparin in patients with unstable angina have not been found; other methods of anticoagulant therapy are equally hazardous. In summary, anticoagulant therapy should not divert attention from more successful methods of management. Anticoagulants are not indicated for patients hospitalized with unstable angina pectoris.

References

1. Wessler EE, et al: Coumarin therapy in acute myocardial infarction: a Hobson's choice. Arch Intern Med 134:774–779, 1974.
2. Bassan MM, and Rogel S: Current practice in the use of anticoagulants for ischemic heart disease: a survey of 200 hospitals. Heart Lung 5:742–746, 1976.
3. Heng M-K, et al: Prognosis in unstable angina. Br Heart J 38:921–925, 1976.
4. Norris RM: Personal communication, February 25, 1977.
5. Gazes PC, et al: Preinfarctional (unstable) angina — a prospective study — ten year follow-up. Circulation 48:331–337, 1973.
6. Scanlon PJ, et al: Accelerated angina pectoris. Clinical, hemodynamic, arteriographic, and therapeutic experience in 85 patients. Circulation 47:19–26, 1973.
7. Michaels L: Heparin administration in acute coronary insufficiency. Its value in the initial stages of treatment. JAMA 221:1235–1239, 1972.
8. Warlow C, et al: A double-blind trial of low doses of subcutaneous heparin in the prevention of deep-vein thrombosis after myocardial infarction. Lancet 2:934–936, 1973.
9. Russo JV, et al: Heparin and ventricular arrhythmias after myocardial infarction. Lancet 2:1271–1275, 1970.
10. Gallus AS, et al: Small subcutaneous doses of heparin in prevention of venous thrombosis. N Engl J Med 288:545–551, 1973.
11. Kakkar VV, et al: Prevention of fatal postoperative pulmonary embolism by low doses of heparin. An international multicentre trial. Lancet 2:45–51, 1975.
12. Wessler S: Prevention of venous thromboembolism by low-dose heparin. A 1976 status report. Mod Concepts Cardiovasc Dis 45:105–109, 1976.

13. Habersberger PG, et al: Venous thromboses in myocardial infarction: comparison in heparin dosage. Br Heart J 35:538–542, 1973.
14. Emerson PA, and Marks P: Preventing thromboembolism after myocardial infarction: effect of low-dose heparin or smoking. Br Med J 1:18–20, 1977.
15. Le Quesne LP: Diagnosis and prevention of postoperative deep-vein thrombosis. Annu Rev Med 26:63–74, 1975.
16. Davies MJ, et al: Pathology of acute myocardial infarction with particular reference to occlusive coronary thrombi. Br Heart J 38:659–664, 1976.
17. Erhardt LR, et al: Incorporation of ^{125}I-labelled fibrinogen into coronary arterial thrombi in acute myocardial infarction in man. Lancet 1:387–390, 1973.
18. Erhardt LR, et al: Formation of coronary arterial thrombi in relation to onset of necrosis in acute myocardial infarction in man. A clinical and autoradiographic study. Am Heart J 91:592–598, 1976.
19. McDonald GSA, and McCaughey WTE: Mural thrombosis and myocardial infarction. J Irish Med Assoc 67:173–176, 1974.

Comment

Some of the comments on the earlier controversy concerning the role of surgery in unstable angina are equally applicable to this one. The evaluation of any therapeutic modality requires concurrent controls and clear definition of the condition being scrutinized. The early studies quoted by Dr. Morris showing the benefits of anticoagulants in unstable angina were carried out without an attempt to really divide patients into subgroups according to the different types of unstable angina that we recognize today, such as de novo angina, Prinzmetal's or variant angina, worsening or crescendo effort angina, spontaneous or rest angina, chest pain at rest during the first few days or weeks following acute myocardial infarction, and the so-called intermediate syndrome, or acute coronary insufficiency. Furthermore, mortality and subsequent myocardial infarction in both controls and treated patients were at a rate that is not seen today in the management of patients with unstable angina. As Morris correctly points out, the institution of modern management of the patient with unstable angina, including hospitalization in the coronary care unit, large doses of propranolol and nitrates, and coronary arteriography with subsequent coronary surgery if medical management fails in the early period, have combined to lower mortality significantly in patients with unstable angina. Under these circumstances, the conclusions regarding use of anticoagulation in earlier studies are of dubious applicability.

It is of interest that in the multicenter randomized trial of medical versus surgical management of unstable angina currently sponsored by the National Heart, Lung, and Blood Institute, no stipulations were made in the medically treated group of patients as to whether they should or should not receive anticoagulation. Coincidentally, it is my understanding that roughly half of the centers have utilized heparin during the acute phase of hospitalization for unstable angina and the other half have not. The data breakdown on anticoagulation to date suggests that mortality among the medically treated group of patients is unaffected by the use of anticoagulants.

It should be emphasized that Dr. Morris concludes by not advocating large doses of heparin for all patients with unstable angina. Rather, he suggests that low-dose heparin in this situation carries an extremely low risk to the patient. Furthermore, it has been demonstrated to be of benefit under certain other circumstances, as he details. Thus, he concludes that its use has a rationale with minimal risk, but he does not propose that the evidence conclusively indicates that it will either prevent subsequent myocardial infarction or decrease mortality.

I share Dr. Morris' general viewpoint. It seems to me that there is increasing evidence to suggest that spasm may be playing a role in some

213

patients with unstable angina above and beyond the usual Prinzmetal's or variant angina case. Under these circumstances, there undoubtedly must be decreased velocity of flow in the coronary circulation to the ischemic region, and anticoagulation may be of some benefit in helping to reduce the development of thrombi or propagation of existing ones. Since these patients are already hospitalized on the coronary care unit with an indwelling intravenous line, I favor the addition of small doses of heparin in the absence of a history of any bleeding diathesis or any other obvious contraindications. This approach may be purely empirical at this point, but it seems to be a rational one.

ELLIOT RAPAPORT, M.D.

Ten

Should Cardiac Imaging Be a Routine Procedure in Diagnosis of Acute Myocardial Infarction?

MYOCARDIAL IMAGING SHOULD BE A ROUTINE
PROCEDURE IN DIAGNOSIS OF ACUTE MYOCARDIAL
INFARCTION

    Bertram Pitt, M.D.

CARDIAC IMAGING SHOULD NOT BE A ROUTINE
PROCEDURE IN DIAGNOSIS OF ACUTE MYOCARDIAL
INFARCTION

    Noble O. Fowler, M.D., and Robert J. Adolph, M.D.

COMMENT

Myocardial Imaging Should Be a Routine Procedure in Diagnosis of Acute Myocardial Infarction

BERTRAM PITT, M.D.

Professor of Internal Medicine, University of Michigan
Medical School, Ann Arbor, Michigan

Myocardial imaging with radioactive tracers is playing an expanding role in evaluating patients with ischemic heart disease.[1-3] The three techniques that have been most useful are: (1) "cold-spot" imaging with thallium-201 (^{201}Tl); (2) evaluation of left ventricular function by isotope angiography and multiple gated cardiac blood pool imaging (MUGA); and (3) infarct avid imaging with tracers such as technetium-99m pyrophosphate (^{99m}Tc-PYP). Although experience with these techniques is still relatively limited, myocardial imaging may become routine in many clinical situations within the coronary care unit.

In a patient admitted to the CCU with atypical chest pain and an electrocardiogram that reveals left bundle branch block, myocardial infarction may be diagnosed in most instances by serial electrocardiographic and serum enzyme studies. However, if the serum enzyme levels are inconclusive or the onset of chest pain occurred several days prior to admission, serum enzymes may not be of diagnostic value. Myocardial infarction may be diagnosed in such a patient by finding a defect in ^{201}Tl uptake.

Thallium-201 is taken up by the myocardium in proportion to blood flow in the presence of an active sodium potassium ATPase transport system.[4] Areas of myocardial ischemia or infarction fail to take up the tracers. These areas are called "cold spots." Almost 100 per cent of transmural and nontransmural infarctions can be detected independently of the electrocardiogram by this method if the patient is imaged within the first six hours

217

after the onset of symptoms.[5] After that time the sensitivity of detection of nontransmural infarctions decreases, so that after 24 hours, approximately only 75 per cent will be detected.

Myocardial infarction may also be diagnosed independently of the electrocardiogram by finding an area of focal akinesis on a gated cardiac blood pool image.[6] However, while both ^{201}Tl myocardial imaging and gated cardiac blood pool imaging are sensitive techniques for detecting infarction, they do not distinguish acute from old infarction. Both techniques may yield a positive diagnosis immediately after onset of infarction and may remain positive indefinitely.

Another approach to the diagnosis of myocardial infarction is infarct avid scanning with ^{99m}Tc-PYP.[7] This radiopharmaceutical is normally taken up by bone. In patients with acute myocardial infarction, there is discrete uptake of tracer within the area of infarction. The uptake of tracer depends upon the extent of myocardial damage, blood flow to the infarcted region, and time from onset of damage. The mechanism of uptake of this radiopharmaceutical by the infarcted tissue is controversial, but it is probably related to deposition of calcium within the infarcted region and/or to formation of complexes with the damaged myocardial protein.

In contrast to ^{201}Tl myocardial imaging and gated cardiac blood pool imaging, which may be positive in both acute and old infarction, a positive infarct avid image with ^{99m}Tc-PYP suggests only acute myocardial damage from approximately 12 to 48 hours to seven to ten days. If ^{99m}Tc-PYP is injected 24 to 72 hours after the onset of symptoms, almost 100 per cent of transmural and most nontransmural infarctions can be detected.[8] However, imaging sooner than 24 hours and after 10 to 14 days will result in a relatively low sensitivity for detection of acute infarction; so the clinical utility of this technique is somewhat limited.

False-positive diagnosis of infarction must also be considered when imaging with ^{99m}Tc-PYP. Patients with ventricular aneurysms, calcific valvular heart disease, cardiomyopathy, and those undergoing external countershock may have myocardial uptake of PYP. Positive ^{99m}Tc-PYP images may also appear in approximately 25 per cent of patients who have unstable angina pectoris without other evidence of infarction. Whether a positive ^{99m}Tc-PYP image in such a patient represents a false-positive diagnosis of infarction or the detection of subclinical myocardial damage has not been determined.

The use of one or a combination of myocardial imaging techniques in the patient with atypical chest pain and left bundle branch block is justifiable, since the finding of a negative study for infarction could allow early CCU discharge and concentration on other potential causes of chest pain. The finding of a positive ^{201}Tl image, gated cardiac blood pool image, or ^{99m}Tc-PYP image would suggest the presence of myocardial infarction and ischemic heart disease as the probable etiology for the patient's left bundle branch block, possibly avoiding subsequent coronary arteriography to determine whether the patient's symptoms and an abnormal electrocardiogram resulted from ischemic heart disease.

Estimation of Infarct Size

The role of myocardial imaging techniques in diagnosing myocardial infarction in a patient with typical chest pain and electrocardiographic and serum enzyme evidence of infarction is less certain; but tracer techniques may become routine even in this situation in order to determine *extent* of myocardial damage.

Estimation of myocardial damage by electrocardiography is poor, so reliance has been placed upon creatine phosphokinase (CPK) release to determine infarct size and acute damage. Long-term prognosis, however, is determined by the total extent of myocardial damage,[9] not just acute damage. For example, in a patient with chest pain admitted to the CCU with a history of an extensive anterior transmural infarction two years prior to admission, serial electrocardiograms and CPK determinations may reveal evidence of an acute nontransmural infarction with an infarct size of approximately 10 g. On the basis of the CPK data alone, one might conclude that the prognosis would be good. The total myocardial damage, however, may be extensive and the prognosis poor. The extent of total myocardial damage may be estimated from the gated cardiac blood pool image by determining the percentage of the left ventricle that is akinetic and by determining left ventricular ejection fraction. These indices appear to be a better prognostic indicator than acute CPK release alone.[10]

The extent of myocardial damage may also be estimated by ^{201}Tl myocardial imaging or ^{99m}Tc-PYP imaging; but the correlation of actual infarct size by either of these two techniques is, at best, only fair. The clinical introduction of tomographic gamma imaging should allow excellent correlation of infarct size and total viable myocardium by the tracers.

Serial Imaging with Thallium-201

Myocardial imaging with radioactive tracers may also be useful in evaluating patients within the first few hours after the onset of chest pain. The electrocardiogram and serum enzymes may not be of value in the early hours after the onset of symptoms. Although the appearance of a tracer defect on a resting ^{201}Tl myocardial image could be due to myocardial ischemia or acute or old myocardial infarction, recent studies suggest that these conditions can be differentiated by serial ^{201}Tl imaging.[11] The finding of an initial ^{201}Tl myocardial defect that is no longer present on re-imaging two to three hours later suggests transient myocardial ischemia. An initial ^{201}Tl defect that is enlarging or changing size on re-imaging two to three hours later suggests acute myocardial infarction. An initial resting perfusion defect that is unchanged on the re-perfusion image suggests the possibility of an old infarct. An initially normal ^{201}Tl image in a patient with chest pain and a normal image two to three hours later suggests that the patient's symptoms are not due to acute myocardial infarction, but possibly to chest pain of noncardiac origin. Availability of this information within the early hours after onset of chest pain may be helpful in instituting therapy and selecting further diagnostic studies.

Exercise Testing with Thallium-201

Myocardial imaging with ^{201}Tl may also be used to assess patients admitted to the CCU with chest pain in whom the diagnosis of infarction has been ruled out by serial electrocardiography, serum enzymes or myocardial imaging. Exercise ^{201}Tl myocardial imaging may help to determine if the patient's symptoms are due to ischemic heart disease.[12] When injected intravenously at the peak of exercise, ^{201}Tl will detect myocardial ischemia independently of the electrocardiogram. This technique is more sensitive than standard exercise electrocardiography in detecting anatomic coronary artery disease. It is particularly useful for patients in whom the resting electrocardiogram is abnormal owing to an interventricular conduction defect, left ventricular hypertrophy, and/or digitalis effect.

Evaluating Surgery

In patients with unstable or stable angina pectoris who subsequently go on to coronary artery bypass graft surgery, tracer techniques may be helpful in evaluating the effects of surgery. Performance of a ^{99m}Tc-PYP image preoperatively and postoperatively in a patient undergoing coronary artery bypass graft surgery appears to be a sensitive means of detecting perioperative myocardial infarction.[13] Similarly, comparison of preoperative and postoperative ^{201}Tl myocardial images and/or gated cardiac blood pool images allows detection of perioperative infarction.[14] These techniques appear twice as sensitive as standard electrocardiography in detecting perioperative infarctions.

Comparison of preoperative and postoperative exercise ^{201}Tl myocardial images and multiple gated cardiac blood pool imaging allows a noninvasive determination of whether the surgery was successful. In a patient who is symptomatically improved by surgery and who preoperatively had a normal resting ^{201}Tl myocardial image but who developed a tracer defect and decreased left ventricular ejection fraction on exercise, a normal exercise ^{201}Tl myocardial image and an increase in myocardial performance after exercise postoperatively suggests that relief of the patient's symptoms was due to improved myocardial perfusion. On the other hand, in a patient with similar symptomatic improvement, the appearance of a new ^{201}Tl myocardial defect on the resting postoperative image and a new abnormality of regional myocardial wall motion suggest relief of the patient's symptoms through infarction of the previously ischemic area rather than by improvement in perfusion. The routine use of these techniques preoperatively and postoperatively, therefore, can to a large extent eliminate the need for postoperative coronary arteriography.

Other Therapeutic Uses of Myocardial Imaging

Radioactive tracer techniques may also be used to assess other therapeutic interventions. Left ventricular ejection fraction and regional myocardial wall motion determined by gated cardiac blood pool imaging correlate with standard contrast left ventriculography.[15-17] With current imaging techniques, the cardiac cycle can be divided into 56 frames of data and the images shown in a cine format similar to contrast cineangiography. Each frame of data is the composite of several beats sufficient to achieve statistical reliability. The effect of pharmacological interventions can be easily assessed at the bedside noninvasively with this technique. Perhaps much of the current hemodynamic monitoring by balloon flotation catheters could be replaced by the noninvasive determination of left ventricular volume and ejection fraction by multiple gated cardiac blood pool imaging.

Gated cardiac blood pool imaging may be particularly suitable for evaluating patients with cardiogenic shock from massive left ventricular damage. The ^{201}Tl myocardial image will show a large defect in the left ventricle and the gated cardiac blood pool image a low left ventricular ejection fraction. In patients with cardiogenic shock and electrocardiographic evidence of an acute inferior myocardial infarction, the ^{201}Tl myocardial image will, however, reveal no defect or only a small defect in tracer uptake in the left ventricle. The left anterior oblique gated cardiac blood pool image in such a situation may reveal a small, well-functioning left ventricle but a large, poorly contracting right ventricle, suggesting massive right ventricular infarction.[18] Recognition of such patients is important, since in comparison with patients suffering massive left ventricular damage, their prognosis is excellent if the cause of the cardiogenic shock is promptly recognized and the patient is treated with plasma volume expansion.

Radioactive tracer techniques are also of value for the patient with cardiogenic shock and appearance of a new, loud systolic murmur. The differential diagnosis in such a patient between rupture of a papillary muscle or an interventricular septal defect can be made easily at the bedside by oxygen sampling through a balloon flotation catheter, but it is occasionally useful to have a confirming diagnosis. Injection of ^{99m}Tc through the lumen of a Swan-Ganz catheter in the left anterior oblique projection will reveal simultaneous filling of both the right and left ventricles in the patient with rupture of the interventricular septum; while in the patient with rupture of a papillary muscle or severe papillary muscle dysfunction, filling of the right ventricle will be delayed.

More important in the evaluation of such a patient is the extent of myocardial infarction and degree of left ventricular dysfunction. In a patient with severe pulmonary congestion and cardiogenic shock due to rupture of a papillary muscle, the gated cardiac blood pool image may reveal a relatively small, well-contracting left ventricle, suggesting that the site, rather than the extent, of myocardial infarction is responsible for the patient's symptoms. Prognosis in such a patient is excellent if surgery will correct the defect.

In other patients with an identical clinical presentation, the left ventricle will be dilated and the left ventricular ejection fraction markedly reduced. Prognosis in such a patient is poor even with surgery, since the patient's symptoms are to a large degree due to the extent of the infarction, which cannot be altered by closure of the septal defect or by mitral valve replacement.

Gated cardiac blood pool imaging may also be used in the patient referred to the CCU with recurrent or intractable congestive heart failure and a history of prior myocardial infarction.[19, 20] The critical question is whether a localized left ventricular aneurysm could be detected and the patient should be considered for surgery, or whether the patient has an ischemic cardiomyopathy with diffuse left ventricular hypokinesis. The finding of a discrete left ventricular aneurysm in such a patient is an indication for cardiac catheterization and selective coronary arteriography in consideration of surgery.

After surgery, the gated cardiac blood pool image may be useful in providing objective evaluation of the surgical procedure. In the patient with diffuse left ventricular hypokinesis, we would tend to continue medical therapy and avoid the risks and expense of cardiac catheterization, since prognosis is poor even if surgery is attempted.

Summary

Experience with myocardial imaging by radioactive tracers is still limited, and the cost effectiveness of the technique is largely unknown. It appears likely, however, on the basis of our initial experience and that of others, that these imaging techniques will become an integral part of the diagnostic approach in every CCU, and possibly for almost every patient with suspected or proven ischemic heart disease.

References

1. Pitt B, and Strauss HW: Cardiovascular nuclear medicine. Sem Nucl Med 7:3–6, 1977.
2. Pitt B, and Strauss HW: Myocardial perfusion imaging and gated cardiac blood pool scanning: clinical application. Am J Cardiol 38:739–746, 1976.
3. Pitt B, and Strauss HW: Myocardial imaging in the non-invasive evaluation of patients with suspected ischemic heart disease. Am J Cardiol 37:797–806, 1976.
4. Strauss HW and Pitt B: Thallium-201 as a myocardial imaging agent. Sem Nucl Med 7:49–58, 1977.
5. Wackers FJTh, Busemann Sokole E, Samson G, et al: Value and limitations of thallium-201 scintigraphy in the acute phase of myocardial infarction. N Engl J Med 295:1–5, 1976.

6. Rigo P, Murray M, Taylor DR, et al: Left ventricular function in acute myocardial infarction evaluated by gated scintigraphy. Circulation 50:678–684, 1974.
7. Parkey RW, Bonte FJ, Meyer SL, et al: A new method for radionuclide imaging of acute myocardial infarction in humans. Circulation 50:540–546, 1974.
8. Willerson JT, Parkey RW, Bonte RJ, et al: Acute subendocardial myocardial infarction in patients: its detection by technetium-99m stannous pyrophosphate myocardial scintigrams. Circulation 51:436–441, 1975.
9. Sobel BE, Breshahan GF, Shell WE, et al: Estimation of infarct size in man and its relation to prognosis. Circulation 46:640–646, 1972.
10. Schulze RA Jr, Strauss HW, and Pitt B: Sudden death in the year following myocardial infarction: Relation to late hospital phase VPC's and left ventricular ejection fraction. Am J Med 62:192–199, 1977.
11. Pond M, Rehn T, Burrow R, et al: Early detection of myocardial infarction by serial thallium-201 imaging. Circulation 56(Suppl III):III-230, 1977.
12. Bailey IK, Griffith LSC, Rouleau J, et al: Thallium-201 myocardial perfusion imaging at rest and exercise: comparative sensitivity to electrocardiography in coronary artery disease. Circulation 55:79–87, 1977.
13. Platt MR, Parkey RW, Willerson JT, et al: Technetium stannous pyrophosphate myocardial scintigrams in the recognition of myocardial infarction in patients undergoing coronary artery revascularization. Ann Thorac Surg 21:311–317, 1976.
14. Cohen H, Rouleau J, Griffith L, et al: Myocardial perfusion and wall motion pre- and post coronary bypass surgery. Circulation 52(Suppl II):II-170, 1975.
15. Strauss HW, Zaret BL, Hurley P, et al: A scintiphotographic method for measuring left ventricular ejection fraction in man without cardiac catheterization. Am J Cardiol 28:575–580, 1971.
16. Zaret BL, Strauss HW, Hurley PJ, et al: A noninvasive scintiphotographic method for detecting regional ventricular dysfunction in man. N Engl J Med 284:1165–1170, 1971.
17. Pitt B, and Strauss HW: Current concepts: Evaluation of ventricular function by radioisotopic technics. N Engl J Med 296:1097–1099, 1977.
18. Rigo P, Murray M, Taylor DR, et al: Right ventricular dysfunction detected by gated scintiphotography in patients with acute inferior myocardial infarction. Circulation 52:268–274, 1975.
19. Rigo P, Murray M, Strauss HW, et al: Scintiphotographic evaluation of patients with suspected left ventricular aneurysm. Circulation 50:985–991, 1971.
20. Rigo P, Strauss HW, and Pitt B: The combined use of gated cardiac blood pool scanning and myocardial imaging with potassium-43 in the evaluation of patients with myocardial infarction. Radiology 115:387–391, 1975.

Cardiac Imaging Should Not Be a Routine Procedure in Diagnosis of Acute Myocardial Infarction

NOBLE O. FOWLER, M.D.

ROBERT J. ADOLPH, M.D.

Division of Cardiology, Department of Medicine,
University of Cincinnati College of Medicine, Cincinnati,
Ohio

We believe that cardiac imaging should not be a routine procedure in acute myocardial infarction. In defending this position, we would like to consider several questions:

1. What are the potential advantages of myocardial scintigraphy in the diagnosis and management of patients with acute myocardial infarction?

2. In practical terms, what are the sensitivity and specificity of cardioselective radionuclides in identification, localization, and quantification of cardiac infarction?

3. Does scintigraphy have a cost/benefit ratio that justifies its routine application in patients with acute myocardial infarction?

A variety of radiopharmaceuticals that are analogs of potassium and are so-called negative imaging agents have been used to identify infarcted myocardium. These radionuclides accumulate in normal myocardium but not in acutely ischemic or infarcted myocardium or in scarred or fibrotic tissue that represents remote infarction. The area of decreased or absent uptake of radionuclide is referred to as a "cold spot," negative image, or scintigraphic defect.

Earlier studies used intravenously administered radioactive potassium and rubidium, but image quality was poor. Image quality was better with cesium-129, but its unavailability precluded wide acceptance. More recently, thallium-201 (^{201}Tl) has been the negative imaging agent of choice. Studies with ^{201}Tl in patients with acute infarction have been useful in confirming diagnoses.

The introduction of so-called positive imaging agents such as technetium-99m–labeled pyrophosphate (^{99m}Tc-PYP) or glucoheptonate has been followed by their wide application in diagnosis. These radionuclides accumulate in acutely infarcted myocardium, but not in normal muscle. The area of increased uptake is called a "hot spot," or positive image.

Recognition of Myocardial Infarction

In the routine clinical recognition of acute myocardial infarction, three criteria are used: electrocardiographic changes, clinical history, and serial changes of the serum enzymes. The electrocardiogram cannot diagnose myocardial infarction in all instances of acute infarction, especially when the infarction is nontransmural. The size and location of the infarct determine whether pathologic Q waves will appear and, to some extent, whether ST- and T-wave changes can be recognized. The value of the electrocardiogram also depends on its form before the infarction. When infarctions have occurred previously or when there is a left bundle branch block, a right ventricular electronic pacemaker, pre-excitation syndrome, or advanced left ventricular hypertophy, the value of the electrocardiogram in the recognition of infarction is impaired. The electrocardiogram is of diagnostic value in no more than 80 per cent of acute anterior infarctions, and in a smaller percentage of acute inferior infarctions if one requires pathologic Q waves for the diagnosis. However, serial ST- and T-wave changes can be recognized in a larger percentage of acute infarctions.

While clinical history may not be a diagnostic tool for infarction, it usually calls attention to the need for diagnostic studies. An acute infarction, especially in unconscious or incoherent patients, may be suggested by the onset of hemiplegia, cardiac rhythm disturbances, or unexplained heart failure. Even in alert individuals, the symptoms of acute infarction are absent or difficult to recognize in at least 20 per cent of instances.

In specific diagnoses, characteristic changes in serum enzymes are much more sensitive. Probably only a very minor infarction would escape diagnosis with careful evaluation of serial changes in enzymes. When MB fraction of creatine phosphokinase (CPK) is determined, we can expect a much more specific diagnosis of infarction than was formerly possible, since this enzyme fraction is virtually limited to the myocardium.

Therefore, with history, electrocardiograms, and serial serum CPK enzyme studies, acute infarction of as little as 1 gram of myocardium or less should be recognizable.[1] It is difficult to believe that the diagnosis by myocardial scanning will offer improved sensitivity. Pitt has suggested that earlier diagnosis is possible with thallium scintigraphy than with CPK enzyme determinations. Since the elevation of CPK enzymes usually occurs within eight to 12 hours after the acute infarction, the time gain, although real, would be small.

Identification of infarction by scintigraphy with ^{201}Tl is said to be quite sensitive. However, only a few blind studies have confirmed this. In fact, the criteria for acute infarction in reported correlative studies rest on clinical criteria; that is, history, electrocardiographic changes, and abnormal serum enzyme levels. It is generally agreed that infarctions exceeding 10 per cent of left ventricular mass are easily identified. There is no convincing evidence that small infarctions can be identified with certainty using ^{201}Tl, particularly if the infarction involves the left ventricular apex, which normally has decreased uptake, or the inferior wall, where heart borders are usually obscured by uptake in abdominal viscera, or if the infarction is nontransmural. We need data concerning the sensitivity of the scan in the detection of small infarcts that might be recognized readily on the basis of history and serial MB/CPK enzyme changes.

Clearly, we also need a controlled clinical trial to compare these various methods of diagnosis of infarction in order to determine their merits in terms of specificity and sensitivity. But this question is aside from an analysis of the practical value of myocardial imaging. We believe that myocardial scintigraphy with ^{201}Tl is of confirmatory value in the diagnosis of acute infarction. As a primary diagnostic aid, it should have value in idenitfying old infarctions when clinical criteria are often not met. The value of ^{201}Tl imaging in conjunction with graded exercise electrocardiography to clarify suspected false positive ECG stress tests is unquestioned, but this application is not germane to our thesis. Its merits in quantification of infarct size and in diagnosis of acute infarction in patients with electrocardiographic abnormalities that impair recognition of diagnostic electrocardiographic changes are discussed below.

With ^{99m}Tc-PYP, recognition of infarction is uncertain during the first 24 hours after the onset of chest pain and after one week in the majority of patients. Within these time constraints, its sensitivity as a diagnostic test is high for both transmural and subendocardial infarctions. Its specificity is another matter. In a significant number of patients, a so-called 2+ diffuse pattern is found, a pattern that is nondiagnostic and could represent residual myocardial blood pool. False positive scintigrams are also reported in pericarditis and in cardiac valvular calcification.

The value of both ^{201}Tl and ^{99m}Tc-PYP is questionable in the patient with unstable angina for differentiation of acute infarction from transient ischemia. A defect seen with ^{201}Tl may represent inadequate perfusion with or without ischemia, recent infarction, or old infarction. Localized uptake of ^{99m}Tc-PYP probably represents acute infarction, but whether an ischemic area takes up the radionuclide is still unresolved.

Location of Myocardial Infarction

Pitt writes that myocardial imaging may be useful in determining the site of a myocardial infarction and points out that the electrocardiographic correlation with the anatomic site of the infarction is only fair. He states that ^{201}Tl imaging and gated myocardial blood pool scans show excellent correlation with the results of left ventricular angiograms. We have no quarrel with this statement. We do question whether location of the infarct is important for patient management or prognosis.

Quantification of Infarct Size

The potential for accurate infarct sizing is recognized by the National Heart, Lung, and Blood Institute, which has supported research in this area by several investigators. However, quantification of infarct size by myocardial scintigraphy remains an investigative venture. The accuracy of imaging procedures has not been demonstrated by careful correlation with postmortem findings. In our experience, reasonable estimates are possible with ^{201}Tl, but consistently accurate quantification requires minimizing subjective bias by objective grading criteria or by development of computer processing. Two-dimensional single-view imaging requires sophisticated computer programs for infarct edge detection and algorithms that compensate for cardiac enlargement. Since ^{201}Tl is not concentrated in ischemic tissue, the infarct area may be overestimated if there is a peri-infarction ischemic zone. Thallium is probably unsuitable for quantifying subendocardial infarction. Technetium is unsuitable for quantifying inferior infarctions, since in the usual collimator projections the infarct is seen in profile. The area of anterior infarct can be measured directly, but cannot be related to left ventricular mass, which is not visualized. PYP is not a useful agent in the first 24 hours, when knowledge of infarct size is most important in determining prognosis, e.g., the probability of developing congestive heart failure and/or cardiogenic shock. Perhaps dual imaging with both a negative and a positive agent would be adequate. Probably the most quantitative approach to infarct sizing involves use of positron-emission transaxial tomography. Unfortunately, three-dimensional imaging requires a cyclotron and expensive, specially-designed computerized tomographic equipment. Only a few centers have such facilities. The wider application of three-dimensional imaging may be limited by cost.

If, indeed, techniques for accurate quantification of infarct size were available, a strong case could be made for routine imaging in acute myocardial infarction; but such techniques are not available. We believe that quantification by scintigraphy should be considered an investigative tool, to be refined and evaluated in a few centers. At most, it should be applied only to those patients with serious complications of congestive heart failure or cardiogenic shock.

Development of scintigraphic techniques for infarct quantification is an important goal. Indeed, the majority of patients who die after admission to the coronary care unit do so because of cardiac pump failure, and pump failure is clearly related to total infarct size, both old and new. Whether myocardial scintigraphy will ever allow precise evaluation of the efficacy of medical interventions purported to limit infarct size is unknown, although radionuclide techniques have theoretical advantages compared to MB/CPK measurements or ST-segment and/or QRS mapping.

Recognition of the Complications of Acute Cardiac Infarction

Pitt points out that when there is minimal left ventricular damage and a greatly dilated right ventricle, one should consider the possibility of right ventricular infarction. Plasma volume expansion may be useful therapy for shock. Other patients with heart failure, or with intractable heart failure or shock who have well-maintained left ventricular perfusion shown by a thallium scan, may be suffering from a ruptured papillary muscle or ruptured interventricular septum. If left ventricular perfusion is well maintained, the prognosis for cardiac surgery is improved.

Certainly when the patient has cardiogenic shock or acute heart failure complicating acute infarction, one would use a balloon-tipped, flow-directed catheter and observe the pulmonary arterial wedge pressure and the right heart pressures. A patient in cardiogenic shock who has normal pulmonary arterial wedge pressure should ordinarily be treated initially by plasma volume expansion, since a cause of shock may be either hypovolemia or right ventricular damage, rather than major left ventricular dysfunction. It would not be necessary to have myocardial scintigrams to make the decision to proceed with this therapy.

A patient who has a ruptured papillary muscle or interventricular septum will be diagnosed by right heart catheterization through measurement of pressures and oxygen content of blood samples obtained through a balloon-tipped flow-directed catheter. In these patients, right ventricular blood samples will show a high oxygen content when there is perforation of the interventricular septum; patients with a ruptured left ventricular papillary muscle will show elevated pulmonary wedge pressure with greatly augmented C-V waves. The patient who has one of these two conditions and has either intractable heart failure or shock will ordinarily be treated surgically regardless of what blood pool scanning and myocardial imaging show with regard to left ventricular function. While the prognosis may be more accurate with the scan information, this knowledge will not influence the therapeutic decision until more precise prognostic correlations with myocardial imaging are available.

Left Ventricular Function in Acute Infarction

In acute infarction, the value of myocardial blood pool imaging as a means of estimating left ventricular performance or as an indirect measure of infarct size has not been determined. Careful studies are needed to evaluate to what extent an abnormality reflects reversibly ischemic myocardium and whether simpler clinical findings, roentgenographic changes, and measurements of pressure and flow currently available with the Swan-Ganz catheter would not give similar indirect evidence regarding left ventricular function. A more clinically useful application of radionuclide ventriculography to measure ejection fraction and wall motion may be in follow-up evaluation of postinfarction patients. Information may be provided regarding the presence of a resectable ventricular aneurysm or diffuse hypokinesis, indicating unsuitability for coronary angiography as a prelude to coronary bypass surgery, the significance of dyspnea and fatigue in the patient evaluated for disability or work classification, and prognosis in general.

Safety of Myocardial Imaging

Myocardial imaging and blood pool scanning are fairly safe procedures. However, if these procedures are to be carried out in patients with acute infarction, optimum safety requires that a portable gamma camera be available in the coronary care unit. Otherwise, the patient may have to be transported some distance to the equipment. During this time, if resuscitative apparatus and skilled professional care are not immediately available, the patient may be subjected to undue risk. We are faced with either the high expense of additional equipment in the coronary care unit to perform these studies or an additional risk to the patient by having to move him some distance to have them carried out.

Cost of Myocardial Imaging

In the United States, the cost of medical care is increasing so rapidly that all procedures should be justified in terms of a cost/benefit ratio. With over 1000 coronary care units in the country, routine myocardial imaging in acute infarction would probably cost at least 100 million dollars for initial equipment alone. This figure does not include the additional cost of a single test, which might add 200 dollars more to the bill of each patient hospitalized with acute infarction or suspected acute infarction. The cost would be justified if material improvement in patient care, survival, and rehabilitation could be shown; but this improvement has not been demonstrated.

There is no question that myocardial imaging studies will yield pertinent information in most patients with suspected acute infarction. But how useful and how necessary is the information? There are many laboratory tests that will tell us something about patients with acute infarction. One can follow the erythrocyte sedimentation rate, which is increased; one can follow the myocardial enzymes other than MB/CPK, such as SLDH, SGOT, or SGPT; and one can show acute changes in adrenal cortical function and in serum catecholamine levels. But we can no longer afford to collect laboratory data merely because they confirm a given diagnosis. Unless laboratory tests either suggest or prove a diagnosis, help determine prognosis, or affect choice of treatment, they are of little clinical merit.

Summary

Myocardial imaging may very well have something to offer in early recognition of myocardial infarction and in determination of infarct size. It unquestionably has a place in the study of patients suspected of having infarction, but at this time its use should be largely for investigation. If infarct size can be quantified with sufficient accuracy, the effect of interventions designed to reduce or limit infarct size may be tested by experimental trial in man. So far, these investigations have either been limited to animals or have relied on indirect estimates of infarct size in man (S-T vector magnitude, myocardial CPK release).

Most patients with uncomplicated acute infarction are treated with coronary care unit monitoring, restricted activity, relief of pain, and observation for complications, regardless of location or site of the infarction and regardless of infarct size. It is doubtful that myocardial imaging will improve treatment in the majority of patients with no clinical evidence of a complication. If the patient develops a complication such as cardiogenic shock or myocardial failure, it may be useful to know the size of the infarction in planning therapy; however, in most instances the therapy would be the same regardless of infarct size. The recognition of such complications as a ruptured interventricular septum, ruptured papillary muscle, hypovolemia, or right ventricular infarction, which may lead to shock or heart failure — with good left ventricular function and small infarction — does not require myocardial imaging for optimal management. Determination of infarct size may have some value in prognosis but, again, is probably not necessary for optimal care.

In some patients, information obtained from thallium scanning and regional blood pool scanning might help in patient management. However, patients benefiting from these methods probably comprise a very small percentage of the total. In most cases, therapy and diagnosis can be satisfactory without these tests. Therefore, we believe the proponents of the routine use of these procedures must collect a careful, studied series, correlating all of these data with the results of therapy and with the ultimate outcome, in order to prove their case. In postmortem specimens, correlations with scan estimates of infarct location and size during life are needed.

Reference

1. Shell EW, Kjekshus JK, and Sobel BE: Quantitative assessment of the extent of myocardial infarction in the conscious dog by means of analysis of serial changes in serum creatine phosphokinase. J Clin Invest 50:2614, 1971.

Comment

Myocardial imaging with radioactive tracers has become an important non-invasive diagnostic procedure in cardiology. In particular, imaging techniques are being applied increasingly in the area of coronary artery disease to identify areas of the myocardium that have undergone or are undergoing necrosis, to identify areas of impaired or absent perfusion, and to evaluate left ventricular performance through isotope angiography. The question in this controversy is whether these techniques are sufficiently useful to warrant their routine use within the coronary care unit to identify the presence and the extent of acute myocardial infarction.

There appears to be little difference between Dr. Pitt's and Drs. Fowler and Adolph's respective analyses of the type of data that can be obtained with myocardial imaging. Their disagreement appears rather to be a quantitative one in terms of how often these techniques need be applied within the CCU. Drs. Fowler and Adolph state that the customary diagnostic triad of electrocardiogram, serum enzymes, and clinical history are highly sensitive diagnostic criteria in the usual patient with acute myocardial infarction, and that little alteration in management will occur as a result of any further information obtained through myocardial imaging. They do not deny its value in the occasional case in which a diagnostic dilemma may exist, although they point out that the differentiation of transient ischemia from true infarction may not be clarified by imaging. They discuss a potential hazard if the procedure is not performed within the CCU and also point out the added expense for patient care.

Dr. Pitt, on the other hand, emphasizes the particular benefit in diagnosis that may be achieved with the myocardial scintigraph when the clinical history, the electrocardiogram, or serum enzymes are equivocal or uninformative. He also points out the benefits of estimating the extent of infarct size with imaging. He further emphasizes the important information that can be gained diagnostically with serial thallium-201 scans during the first few hours. Pitt also points out the value of tracer techniques in evaluating therapeutic interventions in the complicated case.

I feel that these techniques have added a new dimension to the diagnosis and evaluation of patients with acute myocardial infarction. They need not be performed routinely in the classic patient, however. They are best used selectively, either when the diagnosis is in question or when complica-

231

tions occur where the additional information gained through cardiac imaging techniques may help in choosing appropriate management.

As methodological improvements permit increasing sensitivity and specificity with these techniques, there may well come a time when myocardial imaging becomes routine for all suspected infarct patients, particularly if its cost can be reduced.

ELLIOT RAPAPORT, M.D.

Eleven

Does Myocardial Uptake of Technetium-99m Pyrophosphate Reliably Estimate Myocardial Infarct Size?

CAN ACUTE MYOCARDIAL INFARCTS BE SIZED
ACCURATELY WITH TECHNETIUM-99M STANNOUS
PYROPHOSPHATE?

James T. Willerson, M.D.

DOES THE MYOCARDIAL UPTAKE OF TECHNETIUM-99M
PYROPHOSPHATE RELIABLY ESTIMATE INFARCT SIZE?
OPPOSING VIEW

Leon Resnekov, M.D.

COMMENT

Can Acute Myocardial Infarcts Be Sized Accurately with Technetium-99m Stannous Pyrophosphate?*

JAMES T. WILLERSON, M.D.

Professor, Department of Medicine, University of Texas
Southwestern Medical School; Director, Cardiology
Division, University of Texas Health Science Center,
Dallas, Texas

Recently, attention has focused on the development of techniques for sizing infarcts in experimental animals and in man. This emphasis is the result of the recognition that the overall size of old and new myocardial infarcts determines to a large extent the subsequent short-term clinical course in patients with acute myocardial infarcts. Page, Caulfield, and their associates and other investigators have demonstrated that when 40 per cent or more of the left ventricular muscle mass is irreversibly damaged, one may expect "power failure" complications of the acute myocardial infarction, including cardiogenic shock, the development of medically refractory left ventricular failure, and/or ventricular arrhythmias.[1-4] Thus, it is logical and indeed necessary to identify techniques and methods capable of infarct sizing in experimental animals and in man.

Ideally, these techniques should be non-invasive, easy to apply, relatively inexpensive, capable of monitoring frequent changes in the overall extent of myocardial ischemia, and usable in intensive care units and in critically ill patients, and they should be able to provide a realistic estimate of the overall extent of at least the acute region of injury. One would expect

*This work was supported in part by NIH Ischemic Heart Disease Specialized Center of Research (SCOR) Grant HL-17669 and NIH Grant HL-17777.

that such measurements would help to identify prognosis in patients early in their clinical course and that such techniques might make it possible to further determine the beneficial or detrimental influence of various physiological and pharmacological interventions in man previously shown capable of altering infarct size in experimental animals.

Infarct Sizing Techniques

Various techniques have been developed to estimate infarct size, including precordial electrocardiographic mapping and estimates of myocardial enzyme release patterns detected by serum monitoring of creatine kinase (CK) and the "myocardial-specific" isoenzyme of creatine kinase ("MB isoenzyme"). Invasive measurements have also been utilized, including angiographic measurements of left ventricular wall motion abnormalities.

Each of these techniques has limitations in identifying myocardial infarcts and estimating infarct size, among which are (1) temporal constraints and (2) several other factors, including previous myocardial infarction in the same region, the presence of certain cardiac conduction abnormalities (including, importantly, left bundle branch block), the development of marked changes in QRS axis, pericarditis, and the presence of acute inferior or nontransmural infarcts, which may make precordial mapping estimates of infarct size difficult and sometimes impossible. Moreover, coronary blood flow patterns influence the rate of enzyme release from the heart, and large experimental infarcts are underestimated in size by CK release estimates when CK samples are collected for only a relatively short time.[5] Myocardial infarcts developing during open heart surgery, including after coronary artery revascularization or cardiac valve replacement, may be difficult both to detect and size using either electrocardiographic or enzymatic techniques, since pericarditis, injury to the heart associated with pacemaker implantation, insertion of apical vents, or defibrillation following the termination of the procedure may lead to alterations in both the electrocardiogram and in CK MB enzyme release. Therefore, further means of recognizing, localizing, and sizing acute myocardial infarcts that could be utilized in addition to the more traditional approaches would be desirable.

Recently, the development of both "hot-spot" and "cold-spot" myocardial imaging techniques has made it possible to see, localize, and begin to size acute myocardial infarcts. The development of infarct sizing techniques using radionuclide approaches is an evolving art and should become more precise in the future. This report presents some of the data regarding one recently developed "hot-spot" myocardial imaging technique, technetium-99m stannous pyrophosphate (^{99m}Tc-PYP) myocardial scintigraphy.

Five years ago, Bonte et al.[6] asked if ^{99m}Tc-PYP myocardial scintigraphy could identify regions of irreversible myocardial damage after infarction and other forms of severe heart injury. This question has subsequently shaped the approach and enthusiasm at our institution for myocardial imaging in general and for acute myocardial infarct detection in particular. This question was asked because it has been recognized for some time that calcium is deposited in crystalline form in irreversibly damaged myocardial cells. Technetium-99m stannous pyrophosphate myocardial scintigrams had previously been utilized for bone imaging. It was suspected that the PYP might form a complex with calcium in irreversibly damaged myocardial cells and allow the detection of regions of severe myocardial cellular injury. The initial studies utilizing this imaging technique were performed in experimental animals with coronary artery occlusion.[6] The results were exciting, and over the past three years approximately 3500 patients have been imaged at our hospital with this myocardial imaging technique. We have found that when properly utilized, the 99mTc-PYP myocardial scintigrams identify (1) acute transmural myocardial infarcts, (2) acute nontransmural (subendocardial) myocardial infarcts, (3) the presence of perioperative myocardial infarcts following either coronary artery revascularization or valve replacement, and (4) other forms of myocardial necrosis, particularly those produced by invasive cardiac tumor, bullet wound to the heart, and cardioversion (Figs. 1 and 2).

Technetium-99m stannous pyrophosphate myocardial imaging localizes acute transmural myocardial infarcts and provides results similar to the electrocardiogram; but the localization of nontransmural myocardial infarcts with this myocardial imaging technique does not agree precisely with electrocardiographic localization of similar type lesions. This is because 99mTc-PYP uptake is ordinarily fainter and less well-localized in patients and experimental animals with nontransmural infarcts (Fig. 3).

The development of a positive 99mTc-PYP myocardial scintigram in experimental animals with coronary artery occlusion correlates temporally and topographically with calcium deposition in the area of the infarct;

NEGATIVE SCINTIGRAM

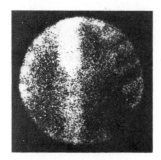 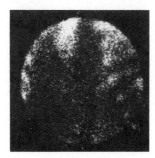 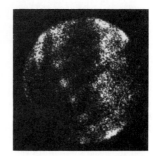

ANTERIOR　　　　　**45° LAO**　　　　**LEFT LATERAL**

Figure 1. A technetium-99m stannous pyrophosphate (99mTc-PYP) myocardial scintigram obtained from a patient with chest pain but no evidence of myocardial infarction. The imaging views obtained are identified below each panel. Note the uptake of 99mTc-PYP in skeletal structures, but the lack of increased radionuclide uptake in the heart.

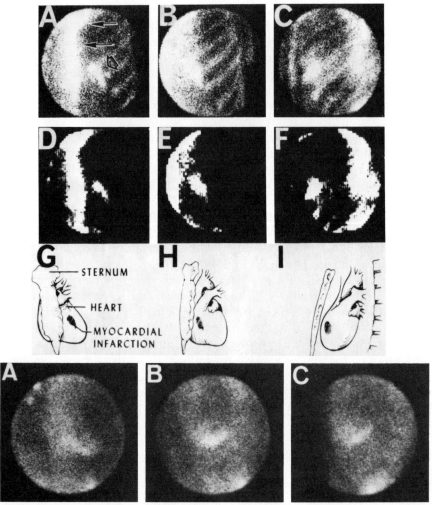

Figure 2. *Top Panel (A–I).* A 99mTc-PYP myocardial scintigram obtained from a patient with an acute anterior myocardial infarct. The top three panels (A, B, C) demonstrate non–computer-processed views in the same projections as shown in Figure 1. The open area points to the area of increased 99mTc-PYP uptake in the heart. The middle panels (D, E, F) are computer processed views of the images shown in A, B, and C. Panels G, H, and I demonstrate the artist's schematic representation of the site of the damage in each of the different imaging projections. *Bottom Panel (A–C).* A 99mTc-PYP myocardial scintigram from a patient with an acute inferior myocardial infarct. Imaging projections are the same as in Figure 1. None of the images have been computer processed.

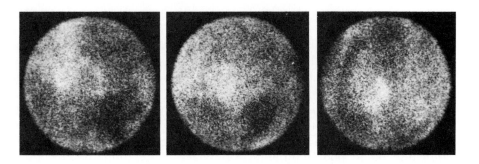

SUBENDOCARDIAL MYOCARDIAL INFARCT

DAY 4

Figure 3. A ^{99m}Tc-PYP myocardial scintigram obtained from a patient with an acute sub-endocardial infarct. The area of increased ^{99m}Tc-PYP uptake is less well localized than was true for that in the images obtained from the patients with transmural infarcts shown in Figure 2.

the resolution to a negative scan correlates temporally and topographically with resorption of calcium.[7] Buja et al. have demonstrated in experimental animals with acute myocardial infarcts that the predominant cell type taking up ^{99m}Tc-PYP is irreversibly damaged cells, but there is also some uptake of the radionuclide material in severely injured cells at the borders of myocardial infarcts that lack the classic criteria of irreversible myocardial damage. The ultimate fate of these latter cells is uncertain.[8] The resolution of this myocardial imaging technique for infarct detection purposes in experimental animals with a permanently occluded left anterior descending coronary artery is three grams; when less than three grams of severely injured myocardial tissue is present, it will not be consistently detected by this myocardial imaging approach.[5]

Imaging with ^{99m}Tc-PYP

Optimal utilization of the ^{99m}Tc-PYP myocardial imaging technique requires serial myocardial imaging during the initial six days following infarction, since an occasional patient first develops a positive image three or four days after infarction rather than 12 to 24 hours after the myocardial injury. Some patients also retain positive scintigrams several months after myocardial infarction. The reasons for persistently positive scintigrams in a subgroup of patients following acute myocardial infarction are not clear, but persistent myocardial ischemia with subsequent continued loss of small amounts of myocardial tissue and/or dystrophic cardiac calcification within the area of healing, and especially in the border zones of the myocardial infarct, could be explanations for the phenomenon.[9] It is important to emphasize that the ^{99m}Tc-PYP myocardial scintigrams become positive when myocardial necrosis or, at the very least, severe myocardial cellular injury with ultimate uncertainty in terms of potential recovery of a certain limited population of myocardial cells occurs.[8] Thus, the test would be expected to be positive in clinical or experimental circumstances that result in dead and dying myocardial cells that amount to at least three grams of myocardial necrosis, in addition to being positive in patients with acute myocardial infarcts.

When utilizing this imaging technique properly, excessive free technetium-99m pertechnetate must not be in the ^{99m}Tc-PYP to be injected. If it is, it will be incorporated into red blood cells and will produce a stable radionuclide blood pool scintigram for several hours after the injection,[10] making it impossible to determine whether there is true increased myocardial uptake of the ^{99m}Tc-PYP. The ^{99m}Tc-PYP to be injected must be tested frequently for the presence of free technetium-99m pertechnetate so that this phenomenon may be recognized.

The final important feature in the optimal utilization of the imaging technique is allowing adequate time for clearance of the radionuclide blood pool scintigram following the intravenous injection of the ^{99m}Tc-PYP. We have generally found that one to one and a half hours is adequate to insure clearance of the radionuclide blood pool and to allow determination of whether true increased myocardial uptake of the ^{99m}Tc-PYP has occurred; but in some patients two to three hours is necessary. In particular, patients with severely deranged left ventricular function and those with renal insufficiency would be expected to clear the radionuclide material somewhat more slowly than those with normal left ventricular and renal function.

Technetium-99m stannous pyrophosphate scintigraphy may be utilized to size experimental animal and human infarcts of certain types. The limitation of this imaging technique in sizing all infarcts (and this applies to other "hot-spot" and "cold-spot" myocardial imaging techniques currently in use) is a general inability to obtain three-dimensional estimates of infarct size. This will almost certainly be corrected in the future as tomographic cameras are developed that may be utilized with both positron and non–positron-emitting radionuclides and have the ability to size infarcts three dimensionally, and/or as models are developed for three-dimensional infarct reconstruction using computer techniques and multiple-imaging projections.

Two- and Three-Dimensional Approaches to Infarct Sizing

Present approaches to infarct sizing and those anticipated in the immediate future include (1) the two-dimensional projection of the entire myocardium or selected portions of the myocardium and (2) cross-sectional images obtained directly from the imaging device or by computer-aided reconstruction. Theoretically and practically, both approaches may be utilized to measure infarct size scintigraphically, but ultimately a three-dimensional or volume estimate will be mandatory for sizing infarcts when the overall extent of the infarct cannot be visualized with just two-dimensional measurement, i.e., acute inferior and nontransmural (subendocardial) infarcts.

Currently, the estimation of infarct size using ^{99m}Tc-PYP myocardial scintigraphy utilizes two-dimensional images and thus provides an area estimate of infarct size. Figure 4 demonstrates how this measurement is obtained. The area of the acute myocardial infarct is identified from the anterior, left anterior oblique, and the left lateral views of the heart of an experimental animal or patient with an acute myocardial infarct. The region of infarction is defined as that area that sequesters ^{99m}Tc-PYP and results in increased uptake of the radionuclide material. Computer processing of the infarct image aids in the definition of the infarct boundaries by eliminating some of the bone background uptake of the ^{99m}Tc-PYP. One may then manually outline the area of increased ^{99m}Tc-PYP uptake with a light pen or "joy stick;" or this may be done with the aid of a computer system utilizing any one of several different digital edge detection schemes to help determine the boundaries of the infarct.[11] Once the infarct region is defined, its area can be calculated by either manual methods using simple planimetry or automatically with computer assistance.

At our institution, the two-dimensional measurement of infarct size using area calculations provides an accurate estimate of histologic infarct weight in experimental animals with acute anterior or anterolateral myocardial infarcts (Fig. 5). When using this technique, it is important to utilize the largest projected scintigraphic area of increased ^{99m}Tc-PYP uptake for comparison with histologic infarct weight. We have found that the manual measurement of infarct size is as accurate as infarct size determined with computer assistance to detect infarct edges and to help define the boundary of the infarct.[11]

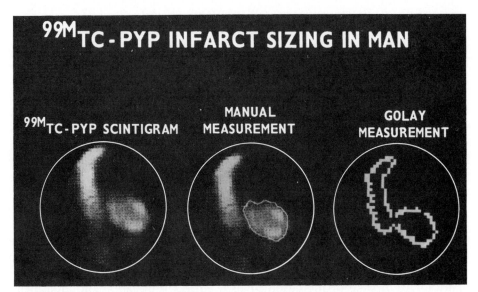

Figure 4. The technique for two-dimensional infarct sizing using computer processing of the ^{99m}Tc-PYP scintigram, a manual planimetric method (middle panel), and a computer-assisted technique for determining infarct boundaries (Golay approach) is shown. (Reproduced with permission of *Postgraduate Medicine Journal*.)

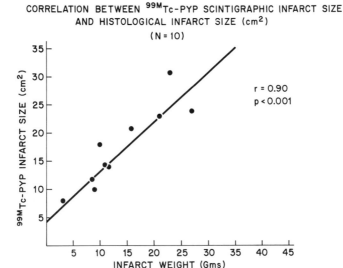

Figure 5. The significant correlation between ^{99m}Tc-PYP infarct size (area) and histologically determined infarct weight in 10 dogs with acute anterior infarcts is shown.

We have also determined that area or two-dimensional measurements of infarct size in patients with acute anterior or anterolateral infarcts allow one to separate patients who subsequently will develop left ventricular failure as a complication of their acute infarction from those who do not, i.e., those patients developing left ventricular failure as a complication of their acute infarction tend to have larger infarct sizes than those who subsequently do not (Fig. 6). It should be emphasized that these data have been obtained from experimental animals and humans with acute anterior or anterolateral infarcts; infarct size measurements in two dimensions are accurate with this type of infarction, since the overall extent of the damage can be visualized with standard imaging projections, i.e., the anterior, left anterior oblique, and left lateral projections.

However, the overall extent of acute inferior and nontransmural infarcts is not fully visualized by these imaging projections, and thus one would not expect to be able to utilize an area or two-dimensional measurement of infarct size to accurately estimate infarct size with these lesions. Instead, a three-dimensional estimate is necessary to estimate accurately the extent of the myocardial damage in experimental animals and humans with acute inferior and subendocardial infarcts.

Three-dimensional estimates of infarct size can be obtained from multiple cross-sectional slices through the myocardium; this allows a volume estimate of infarct size. Using this approach, the area of infarction would be the region that actively sequesters ^{99m}Tc-PYP (although it could also be that region of the myocardium showing abnormally reduced fatty acid or thallium-201 uptake or increased myosin antibody uptake). The area of infarction may be defined in each cross-sectional slice by planimetric or computer-assisted techniques. Subsequently, by multiplying the calculated area by the known thickness of the slice, an estimate of infarct volume for

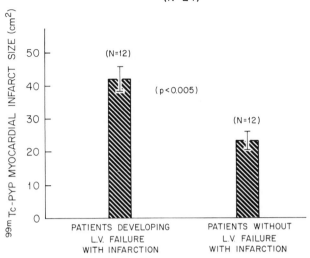

Figure 6. Patients with anterior or anterolateral infarcts developing left ventricular fail-ure have larger ⁹⁹ᵐTc-PYP infarct sizes than those patients who do not have LV failure as a complication of their infarcts. (Reproduced with permission of *Postgraduate Medicine Journal.*)

that particular cross section can be obtained. The sum of the volumes cal-culated for the individual cross-sectional slices provides an estimate of total infarct volume. Such estimates of infarct volume utilizing tomographic cam-eras are possible for a number of positron-labeled substances, including ¹¹C-labeled fatty acids.[12] Similar three-dimensional volume estimates of in-farct size should be possible utilizing ⁹⁹ᵐTc-PYP; but appropriate tomogra-phic cameras must be developed to use with non–positron-emitting radio-nuclides before this can become a reality.

An additional consideration in the optimal delineation of three-dimensional infarct size in cross-sectional slices of the myocardium is elim-ination of motion artifact, since motion may blur the scintigraphic images. This is done most simply by gating or synchronizing the collection of the image data with the cardiac cycle, as is done for defining end-diastole and end-systole for radionuclide measurement of end-diastolic and end-systolic volumes and ventricular ejection fractions. Similar gating is possible during the cardiac cycle so that motion is less of a problem in the cross-sectional determination of infarct volumes.

Since we presently lack a tomographic camera that might provide three-dimensional estimates of infarct size utilizing the ⁹⁹ᵐTc-PYP myocar-dial imaging technique, we have attempted to simulate three-dimensional reconstruction using computer-assisted techniques and making some fun-damental assumptions about the cross-sectional shape of anterior and anter-olateral infarcts in experimental animals. Lewis et al. have found that a modification of a C-shaped cross-sectional slicing technique may be used to accurately determine infarct volume in experimental animals with proximal left anterior descending coronary artery occlusion and acute anterior in-

"C-SHAPED" CROSS-SECTIONAL MODEL

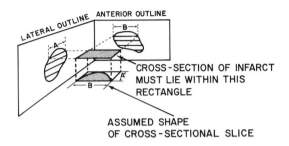

CROSS-SECTION OF INFARCT
MUST LIE WITHIN THIS
RECTANGLE

ASSUMED SHAPE
OF CROSS-SECTIONAL SLICE

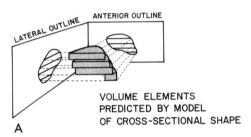

VOLUME ELEMENTS
PREDICTED BY MODEL
OF CROSS-SECTIONAL SHAPE

A

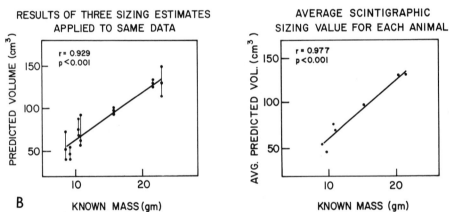

Figure 7. (A) The method for simulated three-dimensional infarct size measurements in experimental animals with anterior infarcts is shown. Details of the technique are described in reference 13 in this report. (Reproduced with permission of *Science*.) (B) The results when scintigraphic infarct volume (using the methodology shown in A) was compared to histologically determined infarct weights in seven dogs with acute anterior infarcts. Graph on the left shows the relationship obtained when three separate measurements of ^{99m}Tc-PYP infarct volumes were made in each animal and the total number of infarct volume estimates was compared to infarct weight. The graph on the right demonstrates the relationship obtained when each of the three values obtained from each animal studied were averaged and an average ^{99m}Tc-PYP infarct volume for each dog was compared with infarct weight.

farcts utilizing the ^{99m}Tc-PYP myocardial imaging technique (Fig. 7).[13] This reconstruction procedure has been obtained with a relative paucity of projections, i.e., only the anterior and left anterior oblique projections have been utilized (Fig. 7). The only prerequisite in this approach is that at least two of the projections must be orthogonal.

The approach is relatively simple, requiring only routinely used projections from ^{99m}Tc-PYP myocardial scintigraphy and access to a computer system. With this approach, the estimates of infarct size in experimental animals with anterior infarcts provided better correlation with histologic infarct weights than did our previous estimates in which only area or two-dimensional measurements of infarct size were obtained. This increase in infarct sizing accuracy was obtained without a tomographic camera and without the major cost or time limitations imposed by truly three-dimensional reconstruction techniques.

The disadvantage of our three-dimensional reconstruction technique is that fundamental assumptions must be made about the cross-sectional shape of the infarct area, and these assumptions are likely to be quite different as the infarct model is changed from anterior to inferior or nontransmural myocardial infarction. However, if similar assumptions regarding infarct size and shape can be developed that will fit the majority of acute inferior and/or nontransmural infarcts, then a similar approach might be utilized for relatively accurate estimates of infarct size in these circumstances as well. However, ultimately a tomographic camera with three-dimensional infarct sizing capability may improve the accuracy of these measurements and eliminate the potential odd experimental animal or patient whose infarct size does not conform to the general predictions that might be made.

Summary

The ^{99m}Tc-PYP imaging technique may be utilized to estimate infarct size in experimental animals and in man with acute transmural anterior or anterolateral infarcts, using two-dimensional or area estimates of infarct size. Work in progress shows that simulated three-dimensional measurements of infarct volume may also be obtained in experimental animals with acute transmural anterior infarcts. Accurate predictions of histologic infarct weight appear possible using this technique. Presently, infarct sizing for acute inferior and nontransmural infarcts remains a problem, since three-dimensional direct measurements or estimates using computer-assisted techniques are not yet possible. It seems likely that tomographic cameras will be developed that may be used with non–positron-emitting radionuclide agents; at that time, more accurate estimation of infarct size should be possible.

References

1. Page DL, Caulfield JB, Kastor JA, DeSanctis RW, and Sanders CA: Myocardial changes associated with cardiogenic shock. N Engl J Med 285:133, 1971.
2. Leinbach RC, Mundth ED, Dinsmore RE, Harthorne JW, Buckley MJ, Kantrowitz A, Austen WG, and Sanders CA: Selective coronary and left ventricular cineangiography during intraaortic balloon assist for cardiogenic shock. Am J Cardiol 26:644, 1970.
3. Willerson JT, Curry GC, Watson JT, Leshin SJ, Ecker RR, Mullins CB, Platt MR, and Sugg WL: Intraaortic balloon counterpulsation in patients in cardiogenic shock, medi-

cally refractory left ventricular failure and/or recurrent ventricular tachycardia. Am J Med 58:183, 1975.

4. Sehapayak G, Watson JT, Curry GC, Londe SP, Mullins CB, Willerson JT, and Sugg WL: The late development of intractable ventricular tachycardia following acute myocardial infarction. J Thorac Cardiovasc Surg 67:818, 1974.

5. Poliner LR, Buja LM, Parkey RW, Stokely EM, Stone MJ, Harris R, Saffer SI, Templeton GH, Bonte FJ, and Willerson JT: Comparison of different noninvasive methods of infarct sizing during experimental myocardial infarction. J Nucl Med 18:517, 1977.

6. Bonte FJ, Parkey RW, Graham KD, Moore J, and Stokely EM: A new method for radionuclide imaging of myocardial infarcts. Radiology 110:473, 1974.

7. Buja LM, Parkey RW, Dees JH, Stokely EM, Harris RA Jr, Bonte FJ, and Willerson JT: Morphologic correlates of technetium-99m stannous pyrophosphate imaging of acute myocardial infarcts in dogs. Circulation 52:596, 1975.

8. Buja LM, Tofe AJ, Kulkarni PV, Mukherjee A, Parkey RW, Francis MD, Bonte FJ, and Willerson JT: Sites and mechanisms of localization of technetium-99m phosphorus radiopharmaceuticals in acute myocardial infarcts and other tissues. J Clin Invest 60:724, 1977.

9. Buja LM, Poliner LR, Parkey RW, Pulido J, Hutcheson D, Platt MR, Mills L, Bonte FJ, and Willerson JT: Clinicopathologic findings in patients with persistently positive technetium-99m stannous pyrophosphate myocardial scintigrams and myocytolytic degeneration after acute myocardial infarction. Circulation 56:1016, 1977.

10. Stokely EM, Parkey RW, Bonte FJ, Graham KD, Stone JM, and Willerson JT: Gated blood pool imaging following technetium-99m phosphate scintigraphy. Radiology 120:433, 1976.

11. Stokely EM, Buja LM, Lewis SE, Parkey RW, Bonte FJ, Harris RA Jr, and Willerson JT: Measurement of acute myocardial infarcts in dogs with technetium-99m stannous pyrophosphate scintigrams. J Nucl Med 17:1, 1976.

12. Weiss ES, Hoffman EJ, Phelps ME, Welch MJ, Ter-Pogossian MM, and Sobel E: External detection of altered metabolism of ^{11}C labeled substrates in ischemic myocardium. Clin Res 23:383A, 1975.

13. Lewis M, Buja LM, Saffer S, Mishelevich D, Stokely E, Lewis S, Parkey R, Bonte F, and Willerson JT: Experimental infarct sizing utilizing computer processing and a three-dimensional model. Science 197:167, 1977.

Does the Myocardial Uptake of Technetium-99m Pyrophosphate Reliably Estimate Infarct Size? Opposing View*

LEON RESNEKOV, M.D.

Professor of Medicine and Joint Director, Section of
Cardiology, University of Chicago Pritzker School of
Medicine, Chicago, Illinois

In 1973, technetium-99m pyrophosphate (^{99m}Tc-PYP) scintigraphy was introduced by Bonte and coworkers as a noninvasive method for visualizing acutely infarcted myocardium. Clinical and experimental studies have confirmed the uptake of labeled PYP by the acutely damaged heart muscle.[1-4] The technique, which depends on the selective uptake of a suitable radiopharmaceutical, has an important potential use as a relatively non-invasive technique — not only for the detection, but also for the localization and quantification of myocardial infarction.

Radionuclides most intensively investigated include radioiodine, mercury 203-chlormerodrin, analogs of tetracycline, and radiomercurifluorescein. Both the radionuclides and the tracers used in early studies presented problems, largely a result of inappropriate half-lives, dosimetry, and less than ideal energy spectra. The development of technetium chelates (tetracycline, glucoheptonate, and a variety of phosphate compounds) was a major advance. In combination with sophisticated imaging equipment that was already available, myocardial imaging emerged as an important diagnostic technique clinically and as a useful experimental method for animal studies.

*Supported by NHLBI Grant HL-17648 Special Center of Research in Ischemic Heart Disease (SCOR-IHD); USPHS Center for Imaging Research Grant GM-18940; ERDA Contract E(11-1)-69; and the Chicago Heart Association

247

^{99m}Tc-PYP Uptake Mechanism

An accumulation of calcium in infarcted myocardial cells appears to have a temporal relationship with the concentration of ^{99m}Tc-PYP in this region and has led to the assumption that a hydroxyapatite complex is responsible for the chelate. However, other mechanisms may well be important, since technetium-labeled tetracycline and technetium-labeled glucoheptonate localize in necrotic myocardial tissue, yet neither is a bone-scanning agent. In contrast, phagocytosis by white cells within the infarct area has been excluded as a possible mechanism. Furthermore, local binding of the technetium atom itself may involve trans-chelation by other substances at the site of injury.

Some investigators have suggested that the principal site of uptake of ^{99m}Tc-PYP is in the mitochondria. Animal experimental studies using both rabbits and dogs show that while uptake does occur within the mitochondria, significant additional uptake is found in other subcellular and even interstitial sites.[5, 6] Whether this represents binding with denatured macromolecules remains unclear.

Use of ^{99m}Tc-PYP for Infarct Sizing

It is important not only to define infarct size but also to gauge the acutely ischemic but potentially recoverable myocardial cells if intervention therapy is to limit ischemia and myocardial necrosis. Application of ^{99m}Tc-PYP for infarct sizing can be considered under (1) animal experimental studies and (2) clinical application.

ANIMAL EXPERIMENTAL STUDIES

In general, animal investigations have used dogs. The coronary arteries have been occluded by a variety of techniques. A comparison is made of external myocardial scintigrams following an intravenous injection of ^{99m}Tc-PYP with postmortem scintigrams of the dissected heart and sometimes with multiple transmural myocardial biopsies. Botvinick[7] found good agreement between the degree of creatine kinase (CK) content of biopsy specimens and the size of infarct, based on calculations of the scintigraphic area. He also found good agreement between the weight of infarct and the area of the uptake image. Nevertheless, orientation of the camera makes it particularly difficult to determine the size of an inferior infarction. This is also a problem when imaging for infarction of the ventricular septum, demonstrating the need for imaging in multiple planes. Since the infarctions in the Botvinick study were transmural, it was not determined whether the technique is suitable for sizing nontransmural infarcts.

Other investigators have confirmed these results but, again, paid little attention to estimating the size of inferior and septal infarcts, since it was the anterior wall of the left ventricle that was necrotic. No attempt was made to study the technique in assessing nontransmural infarction.

The interpretation of the scintiscan itself is also open to question. The extent of damage must be gauged not only by the area of uptake of ^{99m}Tc-PYP, but also by the intensity of the image; but intensity of uptake is a poorer estimate of infarct size. Furthermore, the area of uptake does not appear to correlate well with either total serum CK values or their sequential changes. Zaret el al.[8] could not find any correlation between regional uptake of ^{99m}Tc-PYP and the extent of depletion of CK in the same region of the myocardium.

From the evidence presented by animal experimental studies, there is as yet no definite proof of the accuracy of sizing infarcts using ^{99m}Tc-PYP scintigraphy.

Morphological animal studies have shown that the uptake of labeled PYP, being in part flow-dependent, tends to be confined to the more peripheral segments of an acute infarct where residual perfusion is greater.[3, 9, 10] Thus, maximal uptake of the imaging agent is frequently seen in the peripheral areas of the lesion where, paradoxically, CK depletion was least; where CK depletion was most severe, namely, the center of the infarct, less uptake of ^{99m}Tc-PYP occurred. As shown by microsphere techniques, ^{99m}Tc-PYP uptake declined, as did flow. Peak overall uptake occurred with flows in the 30 to 40 per cent range of normal, and when flows were at or above normal values, uptake of the isotope decreased again. Buja[11] divided the myocardial infarct into four zones and showed that the uptake of ^{99m}Tc-PYP was high peripherally, whereas centrally the average uptake was only 1.7 times normal.

CLINICAL EXPERIENCE

There is considerable confusion regarding the use of ^{99m}Tc-PYP in a clinical setting. Important problems include determining the optimal time for undertaking the scintigraphic study. The earliest uptake in man is generally thought to be about 12 hours after myocardial infarction, but occasionally uptake may be seen at seven hours and even as early as four hours. Following the initial uptake, a progressive localization occurs for up to about three days, followed by a decline in intensity of uptake to the end of the seventh day; usually the uptake has completely faded by the fourteenth day, although occasionally a persistent positive scan remains for several months.

Equally important are the kinetics of ^{99m}Tc-PYP uptake. When used for bone scanning, some uptake by the bone occurs as early as 30 minutes following injection, but usually good quality images are not obtained for two hours. In man, myocardial imaging of infarcts seems optimal 60 to 90 minutes following injection of the isotope. Earlier imaging frequently results in a faint, diffuse pattern that might represent myocardial uptake or cardiac blood pool imaging. Walsh et al.[12] determined that there was no correlation between blood pool activity of ^{99m}Tc and the scan uptake of ^{99m}Tc-PYP in the myocardium by measurements made at least two to four hours after injecting ^{99m}Tc-

PYP intravenously in order to minimize the possibility of blood pool interference. Blood serum studies of ^{99m}Tc-PYP show a biexponential pattern of clearance from the blood. The first exponent has a relatively rapid clearance half-time of 13.6 minutes and the second, a slower half-time of 380 minutes. It is believed that the rapid first exponent represents decreasing radioactivity caused by bone uptake, while the second reflects, in the main, renal excretion of the isotope.[13] Thus, interfering blood pool images are more likely to be obtained in individuals with impaired renal function or those imaged within the first hour after injection. Since the degree of tissue attenuation varies from patient to patient, those with thin chest walls are more likely to have blood pool ^{99m}Tc-PYP images.

Willerson et al.[4, 14] reported that of 101 patients with acute myocardial infarction, 96 had positive scans. Patients were studied at about 12 hours and again at 14 days following the onset of chest pain. While good correlation was found between the electrocardiographic localization of transmural infarction and localization by ^{99m}Tc-PYP scintigraphy, nontransmural infarction was not localized as reliably. In contrast, Walsh et al.,[15] who investigated the diagnostic value of ^{99m}Tc-PYP scintigraphy in 80 patients with possible acute myocardial infarction, showed that although, as expected, transmural myocardial infarction gave positive myocardial scintiscans in a very high percentage of patients, only 56 per cent of those with nontransmural infarctions had positive scans. Forty-two per cent of those with unstable angina pectoris as a cause of their chest pain developed diagnostically positive myocardial scintiscans in the absence of any other confirmatory evidence of myocardial infarction. Furthermore, in this study the scintiscans frequently indicated more extensive areas of infarction than revealed by the electrocardiogram.

Positive ^{99m}Tc-PYP scans also appear in conditions other than myocardial infarction, including unstable angina pectoris, cardiomyopathy, breast tumors, myocardial aneurysms, rib fractures, skeletal muscle damage, calcification of heart valves, high-energy direct-current electrical shock, cardiac trauma, mitral valve prolapse, and skin lesions, and have other unknown causes, possibly even old age.

The clinical usefulness of the technique, including its sensitivity and specificity, is quoted by Wynne et al.,[16] who reviewed the data of 562 patients reported in 14 series, all of whom had suffered acute myocardial infarction. Ninety-four per cent of these scans were positive. In 14 reports of a total of 1083 patients, none of whom had evidence of acute infarction, 83 per cent of the scans were negative. Reviewing published data on patients diagnosed as having unstable angina pectoris, the same authors concluded that 77 per cent of 109 patients with unstable angina pectoris had positive scans in the absence of confirmatory evidence of myocardial infarction. Thus, using ^{99m}Tc-PYP myocardial scintigraphy for the diagnosis of myocardial infarction, the incidence of false negative scans is six per cent and false positive scans 17 per cent; the technique has an ability of correctly diagnosing acute infarction in 86 per cent of patients. These figures leave much to be desired in reliably estimating infarct size.

It is unclear whether ^{99m}Tc-PYP uptake in the myocardium occurs in ischemic and presumably reversibly damaged myocardial cells or only in necrotic tissue. As already indicated, a significant number of patients with unstable angina pectoris have positive scans. In contrast, [99m]-tetracycline seems to concentrate only in infarcted myocardium, whereas ^{99m}Tc-PYP and heptogluconate accumulate both in necrotic and ischemic tissue.

There has been no reliable report of a significant uptake of ^{99m}Tc-PYP by normal myocardium. Animal experimental studies suggest that the technique is extremely sensitive for the detection of myocardial infarction and reliably shows the presence of infarction greater than one per cent of the mass of left ventricular myocardium.[17]

Summary

In considering ^{99m}Tc-PYP scintigraphy for myocardial infarct sizing, great caution must be exercised. Is it the size of the infarct we should be concerned with, or rather the surrounding ischemic, but potentially recoverable, area? We still lack a method that will reliably differentiate necrotic myocardium damaged beyond recovery and ischemic tissue that is potentially recoverable and to which maximal therapeutic attention needs to be paid. With the goal of finding such a method, ^{99m}Tc-PYP scintigraphy can be considered only a half-way stage, both in terms of its diagnostic accuracy and particularly as a reliable measure of myocardial damage.

References

1. Fink BD, Dworkin HJ, and Lee YH: Myocardial imaging of the acute infarct. Radiology 113:449, 1974.
2. Bonte FJ, Parkey RW, Graham KD, and Moore JG: Distribution of several agents useful in imaging myocardial infarcts. J Nucl Med 16:132, 1975.
3. Buja LM, Parkey RW, Dees JH, Stokely EM, Harris RA, Bonte FJ, and Willerson JT: Morphologic correlates of technetium-99m stannous pyrophosphate imaging of acute myocardial infarcts in dogs. Circulation 52:596, 1975.
4. Willerson JT, Parkey RW, Bonte FJ, Meyer SL, Atkins JM, and Stokely EM: Technetium stannous pyrophosphate myocardial scintigrams in patients with chest pain of varying etiology. Circulation 51:1046, 1975.
5. Coleman RE, Klein MS, Ahmed SA, Weiss ES, Buchholz WM, and Sobel BE: Mechanisms contributing to myocardial accumulation of technetium-99m stannous pyrophosphate after coronary artery occlusion. Am J Cardiol 39:55, 1977.
6. Poe ND: Rationale and radiopharmaceuticals for myocardial imaging. Semin Nucl Med 7, 1977.
7. Botvinick EH, Shames D, Lappin H, Tyberg JV, Townsend R, and Parmley WW: Noninvasive quantitation of myocardial infarction with technetium-99m pyrophosphate. Circulation 52:909, 1975.
8. Zaret BL, DiCola VC, Donabedian RK, Puri S, Wolfson S, Freedman GS, and Cohen LS: Dual radionuclide study of myocardial infarction. Circulation 53:422, 1976.
9. Walsh, W, Schwartz J, Bautovich G, Booth A, Harper P, Al-Sadir J, and Resnekov L: Localization patterns of [99m]technetium-diphosphonate in experimental myocardial infarction. Clin Res 23:213A, 1975.
10. Zaret BL, DiCola VC, Donabedian RK, Puri S, Wolfson S, Freedman GS, and Cohen LS: Dual radionuclide study of myocardial infarction: relationships between myocardial uptake of potassium-43, technetium-99m stannous pyrophosphate, regional myocardial blood flow, and creatine phosphokinase depletion. Circulation 53:422, 1976.

11. Buja LM, Parkey RW, Stokely EM, Bonte FJ, and Willerson JT: Pathophysiology of technetium-99m stannous pyrophosphate and thallium-201 scintigraphy of acute anterior myocardial infarcts in dogs. J Clin Invest 57:1508, 1976.
12. Walsh W, Karunaratne B, Fill H, Harper P, and Resnekov L: Significant localization of technetium-99m pyrophosphate in patients with unstable angina pectoris. Clin Res 24:245A, 1976.
13. Krishnamurthy, GT, Huebotter RJ, Walsh CF, Taylor JR, Kehr MD, Tubis M, and Blahd WH: Kinetics of ^{99m}Tc-labeled pyrophosphate and polyphosphate in man. J Nucl Med 16:109, 1975.
14. Willerson JT, Parkey RW, Bonte FJ, Meyer SL, and Stokley EM: Acute subendocardial myocardial infarction in patients. Its detection by technetium-99m stannous pyrophosphate myocardial scintigrams. Circulation 51:436, 1975.
15. Walsh WF, Karunaratne HB, Resnekov L, Fill HR, and Harper PV: Assessment of diagnostic value of technetium-99m pyrophosphate myocardial scintigraphy in 80 patients with possible acute myocardinal infarction. Br Heart J 39:974, 1977.
16. Wynne J, Holman BL, and Lesch M: Myocardial scintigraphy by infarct-avid radiotracers. Progr Cardiovasc Dis 20:243, 1978.
17. Bruno FP, Cobb FR, Rivas F, and Goodrich JK: Evaluation of ^{99m}technetium stannous pyrophosphate as an imaging agent in acute myocardial infarction. Circulation 54:71, 1976.

Comment

There appears to be little difference in the positions taken by Drs. Willerson and Resnekov on the ability to estimate infarct size by myocardial uptake of technetium-99m pyrophosphate. Both recognize its limitations when the infarct is located inferolaterally or inferiorly. Willerson emphasizes the ability, however, to obtain an estimate of infarct area by two-dimensional analysis of the scintigram when one is dealing with anterior or anterolateral infarcts. He presents hope that a volume analysis will be even more accurate when three-dimensional imaging is accomplished. Both authors recognize the limitation of the technique when the infarct is nontransmural. Resnekov, in addition, points out that unstable angina and other miscellaneous situations in which myocardial damage may occur may be associated with positive scintigrams.

It seems to me that experimental evidence in animals suggests that one can get a semi-quantitative estimate of myocardial infarct size with this technique when the myocardial infarct is a transmural anterior or anterolateral infarction. It is not clear, however, that this estimate is necessarily more reliable in man than the semi-quantitative estimates that are currently obtained by such methods as serial CPK serum analyses and ST-segment mapping or, for that matter, from the extent of electrocardiographic changes, the peak enzyme values reached, and the clinical course of the patient. As Resnekov points out, the value of the technique as a quantitative tool lies in the hope that it might be used to help judge whether acute interventions, designed to salvage ischemic myocardial cells, are in fact successful. The critical factor, then, is not so much whether infarct weight in the experimental animal correlates with infarct area determined by technetium-99m pyrophosphate myocardial scintigrams, but whether peripheral border zone cells that are reversibly ischemic take up the isotope and whether this volume can be followed over a time to judge if infarct size is susceptible to alteration through appropriate therapeutic management.

I think at present myocardial scintigraphs during acute myocardial infarction should be used for diagnostic purposes and can be considered only semi-quantitative estimates of myocardial infarct size. At the moment I would have to conclude that although they have potential for use as a true quantitative tool, this must still be established.

ELLIOT RAPAPORT, M.D.

253

Twelve

Is Precordial ST-Segment Mapping a Practical Measure of Myocardial Ischemic Injury?

THE USE OF ELECTROCARDIOGRAPHIC PARAMETERS
TO ASSESS ALTERATIONS IN MYOCARDIAL ISCHEMIC
DAMAGE

*Peter R. Maroko, M.D.; James E. Muller, M.D.;
Robert A. Kloner, M.D., Ph.D.; and Eugene
Braunwald, M.D.*

ST-SEGMENT MAPPING IS NOT A CLINICAL TOOL

Harry A. Fozzard, M.D.

COMMENT

The Use of Electrocardiographic Parameters to Assess Alterations in Myocardial Ischemic Damage*

PETER R. MAROKO, M.D.;
JAMES E. MULLER, M.D.;
ROBERT A. KLONER, M.D., Ph.D.;
and EUGENE BRAUNWALD, M.D.

The Departments of Medicine, Deborah Heart and Lung Center,
Browns Mills, New Jersey, and Harvard Medical School and Peter
Bent Brigham Hospital, Boston, Massachusetts

The size of a myocardial infarction has been shown to be an important factor influencing the prognosis of patients who present with this condition.[1, 2] In the last decade, an intense research effort has been directed toward examining the possibility of changing the extent of myocardial necrosis after coronary artery occlusion.[3-8] It has been demonstrated that the anatomic site of the occlusion is not the sole determinant of the quantity of necrosis but that many other pharmacologic, hemodynamic, and metabolic factors can modify the necrotic process while it is still in the reversible phase, resulting in a different final extent of infarction.

The initial methods used to measure the effects of interventions that modify infarct size following a coronary artery occlusion were based either on alterations of ST-segment elevations by the interventions or on the use

*This study was supported by Contract #N01-HV-53000 under the Cardiac Diseases Branch, Division of Heart and Vascular Diseases, National Heart, Lung, and Blood Institute, NIH.

257

of ST-segment elevations occurring soon after a coronary artery occlusion as predictors of the regions of future necrosis. These techniques, although admittedly crude, were found to be extremely useful when used with a full awareness of their exact potentials and limitations. In this article we will present the experimental and clinical findings that form the basis for the use of these methods. We will describe the manner in which electrophysiologic parameters, i.e., ST-segment and QRS changes, can be successfully used to detect therapeutically induced changes in myocardial damage.

The use of ST-segment elevations to assess the appearance of reversible myocardial ischemic injury is based on the classic recognition of the association between ST-segment elevation and myocardial injury. In 1909, Eppinger and Rothberger described the appearance of ST-segment elevation following an injection of a corrosive chemical into the myocardium,[9] establishing the correlation between myocardial injury and ST-segment elevation. In 1918, Smith showed that ST-segment elevation occurred during experimental ischemic injury produced by coronary artery ligation.[10] In 1920, Pardee showed the pattern of ST-segment elevation in a patient with an acute inferior wall myocardial infarction.[11] In 1945, Rosenbaum et al. showed that additional spreading of the ST-segment elevations on the precordium indicates an extension of the infarction.[12]

Epicardial ST-Segment Mapping

Why ST-segment Mapping Is Useful

Epicardial ST-segment elevation is often a sign of severe damage in the subjacent myocardium that will eventually progress to necrosis. In addition to its usefulness as a predictor of myocardial necrosis, epicardial ST-segment mapping provides a means of assessing myocardial damage early during ischemia, when the damage is still reversible.

The reversibility of ST-segment elevations (and of the pathologic process that it represents) presents a unique advantage, since each experimental animal may serve as its own control when the effects of interventions on myocardial ischemic injury are studied. In the dog, as in man, there are large variations in the anatomic distribution of the coronary arteries and their branches, as well as in the number and caliber of intercoronary anastomoses. In a group of dogs in which the left anterior coronary artery was ligated 12 mm from its origin, it was found that the size of the infarction as determined by pathologic examination 48 hours later varied from zero to 56 per cent of the weight of the left ventricle. This wide range of variation makes it difficult (though not impossible[13]) to prove that a group of animals that receives an intervention has a decrease in infarct size as compared to controls unless the reduction in infarct size is very great or the number of animals is very large. The use of the technique of mapping epicardial ST segments obviates this problem since each dog (and each of the epicardial ST segments) serves as its own control.[4, 14]

METHODS OF EPICARDIAL ST-SEGMENT MAPPING

Recordings of epicardial ST-segment elevations to evaluate changes in myocardial ischemic injury may be performed using three different protocols, each having distinct advantages and limitations.

ST-SEGMENT CHANGES DURING SEQUENTIAL OCCLUSIONS

Occlusions of the left anterior descending coronary artery for 20 minutes or less result in no histologic damage.[15] Therefore, the effects of repetitive 20-minute coronary artery occlusions in the same dog on epicardial ST-segment elevations can be compared. It has been established that after coronary blood flow is restored, ST-segment elevations return to normal.[3, 4] Moreover, 15 minutes after a second occlusion, the location and the height of ST-segment elevations are similar to those recorded 15 minutes after a first occlusion. Thus, repetitive 20-minute occlusions result in reproducible myocardial ischemic injury as reflected in the number (NST) and the sum (ΣST) of ST-segment elevations. Because of this reproducibility, this protocol entails paired occlusions in the same animal with or without an intervention. When the NST and ΣST during occlusions without treatment are compared to NST and ΣST during occlusions with treatment, the increases or decreases in these electrocardiographic parameters are considered to reflect the increases or decreases in ischemic injury of the myocardium (Fig. 1). This experimental design is the simplest and easiest to use and, thus, in many situations may be utilized as a screening test for agents purported to modify the severity and/or extent of ischemia. This protocol, however, does not directly answer the question: What is the effect of the intervention on the ultimate amount of necrosis? Also with this protocol, only directional changes in ΣST and NST can be assessed. For example, the observation that ΣST and NST are reduced by 80 per cent is *not* an indication that the number of dying cells is decreased by 80 per cent, since the sites for the epicardial electrocardiographic recordings are chosen arbitrarily. It indicates, however, that there is a reduction in myocardial injury.

In addition, there are some interventions that cannot be evaluated using this experimental design. Those interventions that alter the ST-segment elevation independent of ischemic changes cannot, and should not, be evaluated by this method. Thus, administration of agents that alter the intracellular or extracellular electrolyte concentrations can alter ST-segment elevation[16] without altering myocardial damage. An alteration in the ST segments of electrograms recorded at a point remote from the ischemic area can indicate that the intervention alters ST segments *per se* and should not be assessed by this electrocardiographic technique. In additon to changes in electrolyte concentrations, slowing of ventricular depolarization, as indicated by QRS prolongation, may alter ST-segment elevations.[17] When the area of ischemia is extensive, focal block frequently occurs, and ST segments deviate in an opposite direction to the bizarre QRS complex (Fig. 2), according to the ventricular gradient theory.[18] Thus the deviation

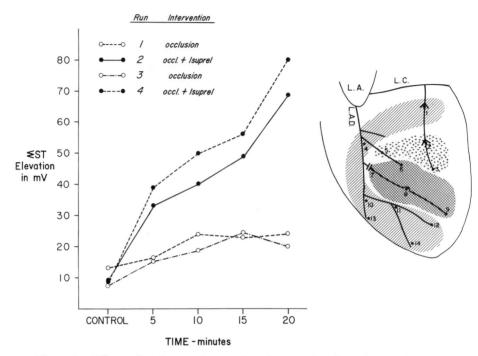

Figure 1. Effects of occlusion alone and occlusion after the infusion of isoproterenol (0.25 μg/kg/min). *(Right panel).* Cross-hatched area: area of injury after 15 minutes of occlusion. Stippled area: increase of area of injury when the occlusion was performed under the influence of isoproterenol. Lined area: area that showed no ST-segment elevation under any circumstances. *(Left panel)* ΣST in the same experiment after three simple occlusions and after two occlusions under the influence of isoproterenol. Time = minutes after occlusion.

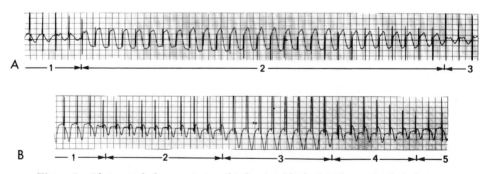

Figure 2. The spatial characteristics of infarction block. (A) The epicardial electrogram as the electrode is swept continuously from a nonischemic area (1), to the center of an ischemic area (2), to a nonischemic area (3), in a dog without infarction block. (B) A sweep from a nonischemic area (1) to the margin of the ischemic area (2), to the center of the ischemic area (3), to the opposite margin of the ischemic area (4), to a nonischemic area (5) in a dog with a localized intraventricular conduction disturbance. Note the QRS prolongation and lack of ST-segment elevation in the center of the area of ischemia.

in ST-segment elevation under these circumstances is the sum of primary (i.e., due to ischemia) and secondary (i.e., due to conduction delay) influences and ceases to be an accurate index of ischemia. The lack of recognition of focal block in the center of large ischemic regions may lead to the conclusion that in the center of the ischemic regions the ST segments show less evidence of ischemia than in the more peripheral regions of ischemic zone.[17, 19-21]

ST-Segment Changes Following a Sustained Occlusion

With this second type of protocol, the ST-segment elevations are recorded before, during, and after interventions at various intervals following a permanent coronary occlusion.[4, 22] Sudden changes in ΣST and NST may be observed at the beginning and the termination of an intervention (Fig. 3). This experimental design can be used to study the effects of interventions on myocardial damage at times later than 20 minutes after occlusion. For example, the reduction of ST-segment elevations after three hours of occlusion by the elevation of systemic blood pressure and their return to previous levels when arterial pressure returns to normal indicate the possibility of altering the fate of injured myocardial cells three hours after occlusion. This type of protocol has been used to demonstrate the effectiveness of several interventions, such as systemic hypertension and hypotension,[4, 23] isoproterenol administration,[22, 23] and intra-aortic balloon counterpulsation.[22] Since this protocol has numerous limitations, it should generally be used to evaluate interventions that have been shown to be effective by the first protocol. The limitations include: (1) the possible development of pericarditis after several hours, which alters ST-segment elevation; (2) the appearance of ventricular tachyarrhythmias in most dogs by approximately six hours after coronary occlusion. In these rhythms, in which all beats are conducted abnormally, ST-segment elevations will change secondarily to alteration in the QRS complex;[18] and finally, (3) the natural variability in the evolution of ST-segment changes following occlusion. ST-segment ele-

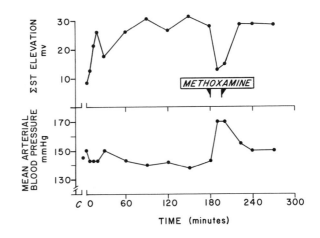

Figure 3. Influence on myocardial injury of methoxamine administered three hours after occlusion. Black bar represents infusion of methoxamine (0.015 mg/kg).

vations may remain stable for approximately three hours and decrease slowly, or if the area of ischemia is quite small, the ST segment may return to the baseline within two hours. Since the rate of resolution of ST-segment elevation is so variable, the effects of an intervention must be distinguished from changes in the natural fall in ST-segment elevations. In general, this is most easily attainable with an intervention such as isoproterenol that has an acute onset and a marked effect that disappears rapidly when the intervention is discontinued.[22, 23]

It has been argued that reduction of ST-segment elevation following an intervention does not necessarily represent a reversal of myocardial damage but may result from an acceleration of the progression from reversible injury to necrosis. If the process of necrosis is accelerated, the more rapid resolution of ST-segment elevation would be associated with an earlier appearance and a greater extent of necrosis as measured by histology, creatine kinase (CK) activity, or electrocardiographic changes. It was reported that this may occur with reperfusion;[24] however, until now, none of the pharmacologic interventions that acutely reduced ST-segment elevation caused an accelerated necrosis — in fact, these agents have actually led to smaller areas of necrosis.[25] Even reperfusion, which accelerates necrosis in the most severely ischemic myocardium, ultimately may result in less ischemic cell death in less severely ischemic myocardium.[26-28] Thus, although the possibility of faster resolution of ST-segment elevation resulting in faster and more extensive necrosis should be kept in mind, in practice its occurrence is rare. It should be emphasized that this limitation is not applicable to the first protocol (sequential occlusions), in which the development of ST-segment elevation, and not its resolution, is examined.

ST-SEGMENT CHANGES AS PREDICTORS OF NECROSIS

With this third type of protocol, the ST-segment elevations 15 minutes after coronary artery occlusion are compared with indices of necrosis 24 hours later in dogs with permanent occlusions. In contrast to the first two experimental designs, the effect of the interventions on ST-segment elevations is not analyzed. Rather, the primary end points are the signs of necrosis that develop 24 hours after occlusion (i.e., histology, CK activity, QRS changes, and so on).[4, 29-31] The ST-segment elevations are used only as indices of the degree of ischemic injury 15 minutes after occlusion at each site, which in turn predicts the amount of necrosis that will develop by 24 hours. In a control group of dogs in which the coronary artery is occluded but no intervention is applied, the predictive relationship between ST-segment elevations 15 minutes after occlusion and necrosis 24 hours later is established (Fig. 4). In the experimental group, the intervention is applied after the electrograms are recorded. If for the same level of ST-segment elevation there is less necrosis (as judged by histology, CK activity, or QRS changes), then the intervention is considered to have decreased infarct size. This type of protocol has been used to demonstrate the effects of isoproterenol,[4] propranolol,[4] hyperglycemia,[29] glucose-insulin-potassium,[29] hyaluronidase,[32] nitroglycerin,[33] hydrocortisone,[34] hyperoxia,[35] hypoxia,[36] hypoglycemia,[37] cobra venom factor,[38] and aprotinin[39, 40] (Fig. 5). The ef-

CONTROL OCCLUSION

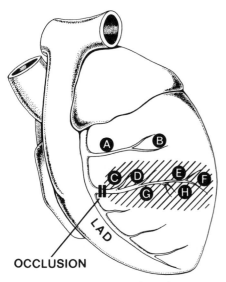

SITE	ST (mv)	CPK (I.U./mg prot.)	HISTOLOGY
A	0	33.7	NORMAL
B	0	35.3	NORMAL
C	3	14.4	ABNORMAL
D	6	8.7	ABNORMAL
E	7	8.4	ABNORMAL
F	5	9.6	ABNORMAL
G	4	23.1	ABNORMAL
H	7	10.4	ABNORMAL

● BIOPSY SITES
▨ AREA OF ST SEGMENT ELEVATION

Figure 4. The relationship of ST-segment elevation 15 minutes after occlusion and CPK activity and histological structure 24 hours later. *Left*: A schematic representation of the anterior surface of the heart and its arteries. The shaded area represents the area of ST-segment elevation 15 minutes after occlusion. The circles represent sites where biopsies were taken. (LAD = left anterior descending coronary artery.) *Right*: Comparison between ST-segment elevation 15 minutes after occlusion and CPK and histological appearance 24 hours later in the same area.

OCCLUSION + CVF

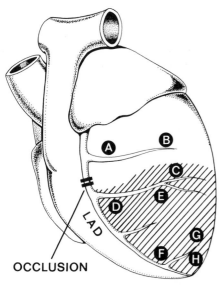

SITE	ST (mv)	CPK (I.U./mg prot.)	HISTOLOGY
A	0	37.8	NORMAL
B	0	36.0	NORMAL
C	4	16.5	ABNORMAL
D	10	15.4	ABNORMAL
E	11	26.6	NORMAL
F	8	25.0	NORMAL
G	5	24.0	NORMAL
H	12	15.8	ABNORMAL

● BIOPSY SITES
▨ AREA OF ST SEGMENT ELEVATION

Figure 5. The effect of cobra venom factor (CVF) on the relationship of ST-segment elevation (prior to CVF administration) to CPK activity and histological structure 24 hours later. *Left*: Schematic representation of the left anterior surface of the heart and its arteries. LAD = left anterior descending coronary artery; shaded area = area of ST-segment elevation 15 minutes after coronary occlusion (prior to CVF administration). *Right*: Comparison between ST-segment elevation 15 minutes after occlusion, i.e., prior to CVF administration, and CPK activity and histological structure 24 hours later.

fects of an intervention on the signs of necrosis 24 hours after occlusion are analyzed, as opposed to the first two protocols in which the effects of an intervention on myocardial injury during the early reversible phase are examined. This protocol has an advantage, therefore, over the previous two because it examines the extent of infarction when the necrotic process is complete. Another advantage is that interventions that alter the ST-segment elevations *per se*, such as the administration of a solution of glucose-insulin-potassium, can be assessed by means of this protocol. Finally, it can be used to verify that interventions that exhibit an effect on acute ischemic injury as reflected by a change in ST-segment elevation also have an effect when the size of infarction is assessed 24 hours after occlusion. It has been found that the interventions that reduce ST-segment elevations using the first two protocols also result in less necrosis for a given amount of ST-segment elevation in the third protocol.

Two criticisms have been raised concerning this third protocol. The first is that the relationship between ST-segment elevations and an index of necrosis after 24 hours, such as myocardial CK activity, is not linear;[41] and the second is that although the area of necrosis may be smaller 24 hours after occlusion, the process may not be completed at that time, and only a delay in the development of necrosis has been demonstrated. Regarding the first criticism, it is true that the "best fit" between ST-segment elevations 15 minutes after occlusion and myocardial CK activity 24 hours later is not an inverse linear relationship,[29] since most sites with ST-segment elevations higher than 7 mV will demonstrate maximum CK depletion. However, if sites are divided into those that are normal, those with moderate ST-segment elevation, and those with severe ST-segment elevation, the graded reduction in CK activity with the higher ST segments is quite apparent[29, 39] (Fig. 6). The findings in certain studies that sites with no ST-segment elevation may show marked CK depletion may be related to the occurrence of focal block. When focal block is not present, the degree of myocardial CK depression in relationship to the early ST-segment elevation between a group with an occlusion alone (control group) and one with an intervention in addition to an occlusion can be compared. If an intervention results in less CK depletion for comparable levels of ST-segment elevation, it protects the myocardium independent of the nature of the mathematical relationship between ST-segment and CK activity.

Concerning the second objection, it is possible that an intervention might only delay the necrotic process. Whether this is beneficial is unknown. However, experiments have recently been carried out in a rat model of coronary artery occlusion in which the animals were allowed to survive for three weeks. As reviewed elsewhere in this text,[42] all of the interventions that have been tested in this model, i.e., hyaluronidase,[43, 44] glucocorticoids,[4] and cobra venom factor,[44] have shown sparing of the myocardium three weeks after occlusion when the healing process is completed as they did when their effect was measured 24 hours after occlusion. In addition, when hyaluronidase was given to dogs with acute coronary occlusion, significant myocardial salvage was observed when the hearts were examined pathologically three weeks after occlusion.[13]

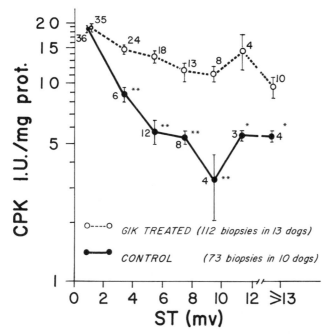

Figure 6. Comparison between ST-segment elevation 15 minutes after occlusion and logarithm of myocardial CPK values in the same sites 24 hours later in non-treated dogs, shown as the solid line, and in those treated with a GIK infusion starting 30 minutes after occlusion, shown in the broken line. The number next to each symbol represent the number of specimens at each level of ST-segment elevation. The difference between control and GIK-treated animals at any given ST-segment elevation is statistically significant (*P<0.05; **P<0.01).

CORRELATION BETWEEN EPICARDIAL ST-SEGMENT ELEVATIONS AND OTHER INDICES OF MYOCARDIAL INJURY

The ST-segment technique, when used with an awareness of its limitations, remains one of the most valuable tools in the field of modification of infarct size. When applied correctly, its reliability is demonstrated by the complete agreement between the results obtained using the ST-segment technique and the results of numerous other techniques to measure alterations in infarct size.[13, 43-47]

In a recent study in dogs, sites with ST-segment elevations 15 minutes following coronary occlusion accurately predicated the occurrence of severe ischemic injury, as determined 60 minutes after occlusion by electronmicroscopy.[48] These same sites also showed evidence of vascular damage as determined by labeling of damaged vessels with colloidal carbon black.[48] In addition, ST-segment elevation during the early phase of ischemia has been shown not only to predict accurately tissue CK depletion and histologic and ultrastructural evidence of necrosis 24 hours following occlusion in the dog,[8] but also to predict sites of gross infarction three weeks after coronary occlusion.[13]

Significant correlations have been found between epicardial ST-segment elevation and intramyocardial oxygen tension,[49, 50] regional myocardial blood flow,[51] lactate concentrations,[52] and high-energy phosphate concentrations.[52] Hearse et al.[53] showed that the tissue concentrations of ATP, creatine phosphate, and lactate were accurately predicted by epicardial ST-segment changes and that all of these indices of ischemia could be correlated with the reduction of coronary blood flow. With the use of a mass spectrometer Khuri et al. found that reduction in tissue P_{O_2} and elevation in tissue P_{CO_2} during ischemia correlated closely with local ST-segment elevation.[54]

Furthermore, in patients, ST-segment elevations in surface leads reflecting the anterior or inferior wall 48 hours following acute myocardial infarction correlate with peak SGOT activity.[55] A significant correlation has also been observed between ΣST and the area of an infarct determined by pyrophosphate nuclear scanning, although the relationship was not linear.[56]

THE RELATIONSHIP BETWEEN CHANGES IN ST-SEGMENTS ON THE EPICARDIUM AND ON THE PRECORDIUM

The concept that the precordial leads provide semidirect measurements of epicardial events was developed by Wilson and his associates[57] and then amplified by Rakita et al.[58] An attempt was made to assess whether changes in epicardial ST-segment elevation produced by an intervention could be observed in precordial leads. Interventions known to alter epicardial ST-segment elevations were found to cause similar directional changes in precordial ST-segment elevations.[23] Three consecutive 15-minute occlusions were carried out in the dogs. The first was a control occlusion without intervention. During the second occlusion isoproterenol was infused, and before the third, propranolol was administered (Fig. 7). Isoproterenol and propranolol were already known to respectively increase and decrease epicardial ST-segment elevation and to alter correspondingly the extent of the 24-hour-old infarcts as assessed by myocardial CK activity. These agents were found to alter the precordial ST-segment elevations in the same direction as on the epicardium.[4] It was observed that isoproterenol increased ΣST by 340 per cent and NST by 250 per cent—increases similar to those observed on the epicardium. In another set of experiments, it was observed that systemic hypotension induced by hemorrhage and systemic hypertension induced by methoxamine infusion resulted in ST-segment changes similar to those observed on the epicardium.[23] More recently these experiments were repeated in dogs in which epicardial and precordial ST segments were recorded simultaneously. Following a permanent coronary artery occlusion, isoproterenol was infused,[17] and ST-segment elevations recorded from both the epicardium and the precordium rose; the discontinuation of isoproterenol invariably resulted in a return to baseline of ST-segment elevations recorded both from the epicardium and the precordium. These experiments stimulated the use of precordial ST-segment elevations as an index of directional changes of myocardial injury in patients with acute myocardial infarction.

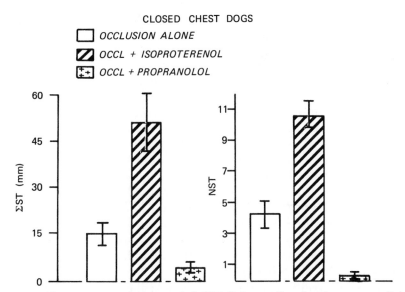

Figure 7. Changes in average precordial ΣST (*left panel*) and average precordial NST (*right panel*) 15 minutes after occlusion alone (bars at left), after occlusion during infusion of isoproterenol (middle bars), and after occlusion after adminstration of propranolol (bars at right). Brackets indicate ±1 SEM.

Use of Precordial ST-Segment Elevations in Patients with Acute Myocardial Infarction

Based on the experimental evidence of the relationship (1) between precordial and epicardial intervention-induced alterations in ST-segment elevation, and (2) between intervention-induced changes in ST-segment elevations and alterations in ultimate infarct size as judged by biochemical, histologic, and ultrastructural criteria, we have used the changes in precordial ST-segment elevations as an index of intervention-induced alterations in myocardial ischemic injury in patients with acute myocardial infarction.

The clinical relationship between precordial ST-segment elevations and the reversibility of damage to myocardial cells is best illustrated by patients with "variant" angina as described by Prinzmetal.[59] In these patients, there is a temporary occlusion of a major coronary artery, most often as a result of spasm,[60] resulting in ST-segment elevations, ventricular arrhythmias, and pain. The release of coronary spasm and subsequent abolition of ischemic injury is reflected by cessation of pain and ventricular irritability and by reduction of the ST-segment elevations. However, in patients in whom the coronary flow fails to return to previous levels, the ischemic injury progresses, and the ST segments remain elevated until a frank infarction develops.

How to use precordial ST-segment elevations to assess the effect of an intervention on myocardial ischemic injury

Patient selection. Precordial ST-segment elevations should be studied only in patients in whom it is clear that ST-segment elevation is due to an acute myocardial infarction. Specifically, patients who present with pericarditis or who develop pericarditis during the course of an acute myocardial infarction, as well as patients with ST-segment elevation secondary to ventricular aneurysms, should be excluded from the study. Similarly, patients with alterations in the serum electrolyte concentrations, as well as patients who develop a bundle branch block or a marked change in their QRS axis, and who therefore exhibit secondary changes in ST-segment elevation, should also be excluded, since the alterations in the ST-segment elevation will not necessarily be due to alterations in ischemic injury.

Since the goal of these investigations is to examine the effect of therapeutic agents on myocardial injury, optimally, patients should be entered into a study when the infarction is no more than a few hours old, when changes in ST-segment elevations are more certain to be related to ischemic injury. It is also important that the method not be used to study the effects of an intervention such as glucose-insulin-potassium, which can cause changes in the ST segment unrelated to changes in ischemic injury. Finally, patients with inferior or true posterior wall myocardial infarctions or with a nontransmural myocardial infarction cannot be studied.

Number of leads. The number of leads to be used is arbitrary, and the choice must be based on a balance between sensitivity, which is augmented with an increase in the number of leads, and the practicality of extensive recording in acutely ill patients. We have used a 35-lead precordial map to demonstrate the effectiveness of hyaluronidase in patients[61] (Fig. 8); however, a smaller number of leads was used successfully in studying propranolol, nitroglycerin, nitroprusside, and oxygen.[62-67] The disadvantage of using a reduced number of electrodes is solely the possibility of not recognizing a true change due to lack of sensitivity of the method.

Design of the protocol. Two types of protocols can be used: (1) In all patients who qualify for the study, an electrocardiographic map is obtained, and then patients are randomized into a control group and a treated group. If these groups are large enough, it may be expected that the magnitude and extent of ST-segment elevation will be similar in the two groups on the first map (prior to treatment). Then the fall in ST-segment elevation between the control group (which exhibits the natural resolution of ST-segment elevation) and the treated group are compared. This type of protocol was carried out in a study that showed that hyaluronidase induced a faster resolution in ST-segment elevation than that occurring in the control group.[61] (2) With interventions such as propranolol, nitroglycerin, and nitroprusside, which act rapidly, each patient can serve as his own control. However, in this case, repeated ST-segment maps must be carried out before treatment, and patients with unstable ST-segment elevations must be excluded.[66] In this manner, a more homogeneous group of patients is selected, and the effect of an intervention is judged within minutes of its

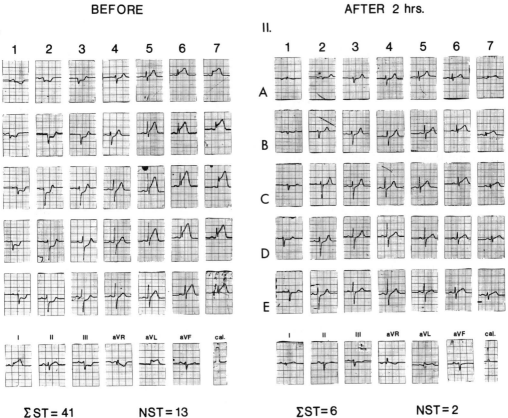

HYALURONIDASE

BEFORE   AFTER 2 hrs.

ΣST = 41   NST = 13   ΣST = 6   NST = 2

Figure 8. An example of the 35 precordial leads and the six classical electrocardiographical leads in a patient with acute lateral myocardial infarction before treatment (Panel I) and 2 hours after hyaluronidase administration (Panel II). Note the reduction in ST-segment elevations over the lateral wall (sixth and seventh columns) as well as the diminution of ST-segment depressions in the right precordial leads.

administration. If the effect of the intervention is transient, the return of ST segments toward control may be expected.[51, 52, 57-65, 67]

HOW TO INTERPRET THE RESULTS

The changes in ST-segment elevations indicate only *directional* alterations in the magnitude of ischemic injury. Thus, a faster resolution in ST-segment elevations indicates a reduction in injury, while their further elevation indicates an increase in injury. It is also important to recognize that these alterations in precordial ST-segment elevations were shown to correlate with the extent of necrosis both experimentally in the dog[8, 17, 67] and in patients in whom serum CK was shown to change in a parallel fashion.[68, 69]

Several electrocardiographic studies have linked the height of ST-segment elevations to the Killip Classification of the patient,[70] to radiologic evidence of pulmonary venous hypertension,[71] arrhythmias,[72] and sudden death.[72, 73] However, measurement of ST-segment elevation is not designed to measure infarct size or to provide a quantitative expression of the volume of myocardium salvaged. It provides data on *directional* changes in myocardial infarct size.

QRS Mapping

The classic investigations of Wilson et al.[74-76] and of Prinzmetal et al.[77-79] established experimentally the relationship between myocardial necrosis and alterations in the epicardial QRS complex. The clinical relationship between changes in the QRS complex and myocardial infarction was observed first by Pardee.[11] Later, Myers et al. established the clinico-pathologic correlations between the leads that developed Q waves and the infarcted myocardial wall.[80-84] Based on these experimental and clinical investigations, the concept of the use of the QRS complex for the diagnosis of myocardial infarction was established.

Epicardial QRS Mapping

Since alterations in the QRS complex were known to reflect the presence or absence of necrosis, an attempt was made to use this electrocardiographic parameter to assess the effectiveness of interventions in reducing infarct size. The QRS complex was not investigated as a substitute for the measurement of ST-segment elevations, since its alteration has a totally different significance. ST-segment elevations are the electrocardiographic expression of myocardial damage in its reversible phase, while the fall in R-wave voltage and the appearance of Q waves in the presence of a permanent coronary artery occlusion are the electrocardiographic expression of definitively established necrosis.

In order to assess whether the fall in R-wave voltage and the appearance of Q waves can reflect not only the extent of an infarction but also its distribution across the myocardial wall, experiments were carried out in which the fall in R-wave voltage (ΔR) and the depth of newly formed Q waves (ΔQ), occurring in leads recorded from the canine epicardium over a period of 24 hours following coronary artery occlusion, were compared to the subjacent transmural CK activity and histologic appearance.[30, 31] It was demonstrated that the sum of $\Delta R + \Delta Q$ in each site was closely related to depression of CK activity and to the degree of transmural damage (Fig. 9). It was concluded, therefore, that these changes in the QRS complex over a period of 24 hours are accurate indices of myocardial necrosis. In a second step, it was shown that interventions that have been shown by other techniques to reduce infarct size also decreased the extent of necrosis as assessed by QRS changes. When hyaluronidase and propranolol were given

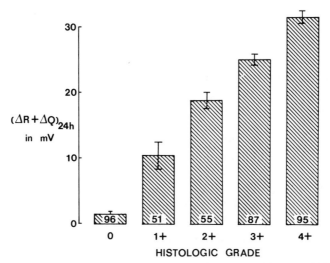

Figure 9. The relationship between Q-wave development and R-wave fall 24 hours after coronary artery occlusion [(ΔR + ΔQ)] and the extent of necrosis demonstrated histologically at the same time. Histologic grade 0 = no visible necrosis; grade 1+ = 1–25% necrosis; grade 2+ = 26–50% necrosis; grade 3+ = 51–75% necrosis; and grade 4+ = >75% necrosis.

following a coronary occlusion, they resulted in less fall in R-wave voltage and smaller Q waves after 24 hours of occlusion. Also, using this technique it was possible to demonstrate stepwise reductions in the effectiveness of hyaluronidase when its administration was delayed by 20 minutes and three, six, and nine hours following coronary artery occlusion.[31] These experiments also showed that the decrease in reversible myocardial injury (ST-segment elevations) produced by hyaluronidase or propranolol administration resulted in smaller infarcts and *not* in accelerated tissue necrosis. In addition, the QRS technique of assessing changes in infarct size was found to remain valid for as long as three weeks after coronary artery occlusion.[13]

   Therefore, it was concluded that epicardial QRS changes that occur as a consequence of a permanent coronary artery occlusion are accurate indices of the extent of myocardial infarction and can be used to assess the effect of interventions on directional changes in infarct size.

ACUTE ALTERATIONS IN THE QRS COMPLEX

   The electrocardiographic events that occur during the minutes to hours after coronary artery occlusion have been studied in both the experimental animal and in man. Although alterations in R-wave voltage several hours following a coronary artery occlusion are an accurate index of necrosis, very early after occlusion R-wave height increases. In the open-chest dog, Rakita et al.[58] observed (1) that ST-segment elevation appears within 30 to 60 seconds after coronary artery occlusion in epicardial leads from the center of the cyanotic area and (2) that the magnitude of ST-segment elevation reaches a maximum five to seven minutes after occlusion. Concomitant with this immediate elevation in the ST segment, the S wave diminishes and the R wave increases in amplitude in the same epicardial leads. Therefore, five to seven minutes after coronary artery occlusion, the epicardial electrogram from the center of the ischemic area typically demonstrates a "giant" R wave, no S wave, and an elevated ST segment. Ekmekci et al.[85] confirmed that myocardial ischemia was reflected electrocardiographically by an increase in R-wave amplitude as well as a diminution in the depth of the S wave. Furthermore, they showed that the relief of ischemia was followed immediately by a return of R- and S-wave amplitude to preligation values.

Although alterations in R-wave amplitude and S-wave depth following coronary artery occlusion have been observed consistently in the dog, they have seldom been reported in patients with severe myocardial ischemia and/or infarction. Dressler and Roesler[86] examined the electrocardiograms of patients with acute myocardial infarction obtained as early as 1.25 hours after the onset of pain, yet they noted no augmentation of R-wave voltage or diminution of S-wave amplitude when compared to electrocardiograms obtained before the clinical event. However, Prinzmetal et al.[16] noted such R- and S-wave changes in patients with the variant form of angina pectoris during episodes of chest pain; with the disappearance of ischemic pain, R- and S-wave amplitude returned to baseline levels. Madias[87] observed an increase in R-wave voltage and a diminution in S-wave depth in patients with acute myocardial infarction early after the onset of chest pain. Since this electrocardiographic phenomenon is transient and occurs early following the onset of myocardial ischemia, it has usually disappeared by the time patients with acute myocardial infarction reach a hospital.

Recently, in the dog model, we quantified this early rise in R-wave voltage and studied its utility as an index of acute myocardial ischemia and as a predictor of the extent of necrosis 24 hours later.[88, 89] It was demonstrated that the increase in R-wave voltage during the first 15 minutes after coronary artery occlusion correlates well with the fall in regional myocardial blood flow measured by the microsphere technique. Moreover, it accurately predicts subsequent depression of myocardial CK activity in subjacent transmural biopsy specimens. The use of this parameter expands the potential for electrocardiographic analysis of the reversible phase of myocardial injury in the laboratory since R-wave increase can be used in the presence of focal block — a situation in which the ST-segment elevation index cannot be utilized.

Precordial QRS Mapping

HOW TO USE PRECORDIAL QRS MAPPING

Both precordial and epicardial QRS mapping are electrocardiographic methods for detection of the final extent of necrosis. The QRS pattern can change abruptly, and following a transient ischemic episode, a Q wave may appear for only a short period of time.[89, 90] Also, as noted above, very soon after coronary artery occlusion R-wave voltage increases. However, when the evolution of R and Q waves is monitored during acute myocardial infarction, it becomes apparent that the fall in R-wave voltage and the appearance of Q waves are predictable.[91] Based on the predictability of the fall in R-wave voltage and the development of Q waves, it is possible to study whether an intervention results in more or less QRS change than occurs in a control group (Fig. 10). In a study in which this method was used, 91 patients with acute transmural myocardial infarction were randomized into control and hyaluronidase-treatment groups.[92] In the control group, the sum of the voltage of R waves (ΣR) fell by 70.9 ± 3.6 per cent ($\pm$SEM) within

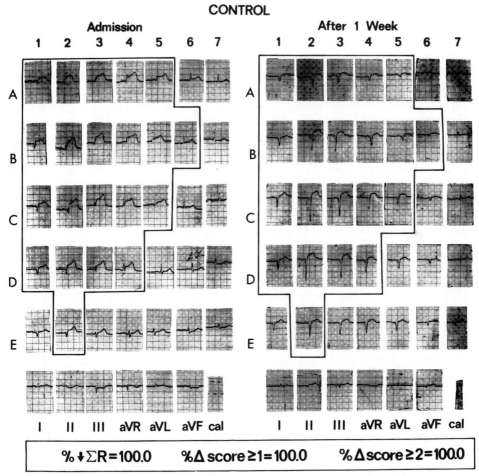

Figure 10. An example of the use of 35-lead precordial electrocardiographic mapping to evaluate the development of myocardial necrosis in a patient with an anterior myocardial infarction. The sites with ST-segment elevation ≥ 0.15mV on admission are outlined. Note the unfavorable progression from ischemic injury to necrosis with 100% loss of R-wave voltage by one week of sites within the outline.

five days. However, in the hyaluronidase-treated group ΣR fell by only 54.2±5.0 per cent (p<0.01). Thus, it was concluded that myocardial necrosis, as reflected by the fall in precordial R-wave voltage, was limited by hyaluronidase administration. These results also demonstrate that in patients with hyaluronidase-induced reduction in myocardial injury, the fall in ST-segment elevations predicts smaller infarct size rather than accelerated necrosis.

CORRELATION OF PRECORDIAL QRS ALTERATIONS TO NECROSIS

There is abundant autopsy evidence that pathologic Q waves are related to myocardial necrosis and scarring. As previously mentioned, Myers et al. described an excellent correlation between the development of Q waves in specific surface leads and the pathologic evidence of infarction in the corresponding regions of the heart.[80-84] In a similar study comparing autopsy and electrocardiographic findings in 1184 patients, Horan et al.[94] found 51 patients with Q waves >0.03 sec in leads I and V_1 to V_6. Forty-eight of these patients had autopsy evidence of infarction in the anterolateral myocardium, indicating the high specificity of Q waves in these leads for myocardial damage. Savage et al.[95] recently compared QRS changes with infarct size as measured by planimetry in 24 patients who were found to have a myocardial infarction at autopsy. A loss of R-wave voltage in V_4 to V_6 was found to indicate increasingly extensive infarction of the apex of the heart. Correlations have also been noted between precordial Q waves and ventricular performance in patients with coronary artery disease. Miller found that patients with pathologic Q waves had significantly higher left ventricular end-diastolic pressures than patients without pathologic Q waves.[96] Williams compared the location of asynergy as determined by ventriculograms with the location of transmural anterior infarction as determined by QRS analysis and concluded that the electrocardiogram can be used as an index of the location and severity of ventricular wall lesions.[97] In a similar study, Miller found that the electrocardiogram reliably predicted the presence or absence of dyssynergy in 88 per cent (108 of 123) of patients with coronary disease.[96] In patients undergoing cardiac surgery, it has been shown that precordial Q waves indicate the presence of myocardial fibrosis.[99] Awan et al. recently found a correlation coefficient of −0.87 between the number of Q waves in a 35-lead precordial map and the angiographically determined ejection fraction.[100] In addition, a correlation between the number of precordial Q waves and one-year mortality rate was found: less than 15 Q waves — nine per cent; 15 to 25 Q waves — 19 per cent; and 26 to 35 Q waves — 60 per cent. An intervention that reduces the number of Q waves appearing in a precordial map could by inference be expected to have a beneficial effect on ventricular function and mortality. Although less attention has been directed to the relationship between the loss of R-wave voltage and ventricular function, the sum of R-wave voltage in the precordial V leads has been demonstrated to correlate with the ejection fraction.[101]

Conclusions

The judicious use of these two electrocardiographic techniques (ST-segment and QRS mapping) in patients with acute myocardial infarction permits assessment of whether an intervention (1) changes the extent of reversible myocardial damage and/or (2) changes the extent of ultimate infarct size.

The main limitation of these techniques is that they can be used only in patients with transmural infarctions located on the anterior or anterolateral portions of the left ventricle. In addition, they cannot be used in patients with left bundle branch block. The ST-segment mapping technique is further limited by factors other than ischemia that may influence ST-segment elevation. Most important, these techniques do not permit the quantification of the amount of myocardium salvage — they can be used to show directional changes, i.e., to indicate whether an intervention is beneficial or detrimental or to indicate the relative efficacy of two separate interventions.

These electrocardiographic techniques have the following advantages: (1) They can be applied immediately, and hence treatment can be started without delay. This is of extreme importance in the setting of acute myocardial infarction, since the passage of time markedly reduces the quantity of myocardium that can be salvaged. (2) Each patient is his own control, and therefore, the effect of an intervention can be demonstrated in a rather small number of patients. (3) The results of an intervention on the electrocardiogram can be observed soon after its administration. (4) The techniques used are simple, inexpensive, and non-invasive and cause no discomfort to the patient.

References

1. Harnarayan C, Bennett MA, Pentecost BL, and Brewer DB: Quantitative study of infarcted myocardium in cardiogenic shock. Br Heart J 32:728, 1970.
2. Page DL, Caufield JB, Kastor JA, DeSanctis RW, and Sanders CA: Myocardial changes associated with cardiogenic shock. N Engl J Med 285:133, 1971.
3. Maroko PR, Braunwald E, Covell JW, and Ross J Jr: Factors influencing the severity of myocardial ischemia following experimental coronary occlusion (abstr). Circulation 40(Suppl III):III–140, 1969.
4. Maroko PR, Kjekshus JK, Sobel BE, Watanabe T, Covell HW, Ross, J Jr, and Braunwald E: Factors influencing infarct size following experimental coronary artery occlusions. Circulation 43:67–82, 1971.
5. Shell WE, Kjekshus JK, and Sobel BE: Quantitative assessment of the extent of myocardial infarction in the conscious dog by means of analysis of serial changes in serum creatine phosphokinase activity. J Clin Invest 50:2614–2625, 1971.
6. Redwood DR, Smith ER, and Epstein SE: Coronary artery occlusion in the conscious dog: effects of alterations in heart rate and arterial pressure on the degree of myocardial ischemia. Circulation 46:323–332, 1972.
7. Epstein SE, Kent KN, Goldstein RE, et al: Reduction of ischemic injury by nitroglycerin during acute myocardial infarction. N Engl J Med 292:29–35, 1975.
8. Maroko PR, and Braunwald E: Effects of metabolic and pharmacologic interventions on myocardial infarct size following coronary occlusion. Circulation 53(Suppl I):I–168, 1976.

9. Eppinger H, and Rothberger CJ: Zur Analyse des elecktrokardiogramms. Wien Klin Wochenschr 22:1091, 1909.
10. Smith FM: The ligation of coronary arteries with electrocardiographic study. Arch Intern Med 22:8, 1918.
11. Pardee HEB: An electrocardiographic sign of coronary artery obstruction. Arch Intern Med 26:244, 1920.
12. Rosenbaum FF, Wilson FN, and Johnston FD: Changes in precordial electrocardiogram produced by extension of anteroseptal myocardial infarction. Am Heart J 30:11–18, 1945.
13. Kloner RA, Maroko PR, and Braunwald E: Anatomic evidence for long-term reduction of infarct size by hyaluronidase (abstr). Am J Cardiol 41:393A, 1978.
14. Muller JE, Maroko PR, and Braunwald E: Precordial electrocardiographic mapping: a technique to assess the efficacy of interventions designed to limit infarct size. Circulation 57:1–18, 1978.
15. Jennings RB, Sommers HM, Herdson PR, and Kaltenbach JP: Ischemic injury of myocardium. Ann NY Acad Sci 156:61, 1969.
16. Prinzmetal M, Ekmekci A, Toyoshima H, et al: Angina pectoris. III. Demonstration of a chemical origin of ST deviation in classic angina pectoris, its variant form, early myocardial infarction, and some noncardiac conditions. Am J Cardiol 3:275, 1959.
17. Muller JE, Maroko PR, and Braunwald E: Evaluation of precordial electrocardiographic mapping as a means of assessing changes in myocardial ischemic injury. Circulation 52:16, 1975.
18. Massie E, and Walsh TJ: *Clinical Vectorcardiography and Electrocardiography.* Chicago, Yearbook Medical Publishers, 1960, pp 70–91.
19. Cohen MV, and Kirk ES: Reduction of epicardial ST segment elevation following increased myocardial ischemia: experimental and theoretical demonstration (abstr). Clin Res 22:269, 1974.
20. Holland RP, and Brooks H: Precordial and epicardial surface potentials during myocardial ischemia in the pig: a theoretical and experimental analysis of the TQ and ST segments. Circ Res 37:471, 1975.
21. Fozzard HA, and Das Gupta PS: ST segment potentials and mapping: theory and experiments. Circulation 54:533, 1976.
22. Maroko PR, Bernstein EF, Libby P, DeLaria GA, Covell JW, Ross J Jr, et al: Effects of intraaortic balloon counterpulsation on the severity of myocardial ischemic injury following acute coronary occlusion. Counterpulsation and myocardial injury. Circulation 45:1150–1159, 1972.
23. Maroko PR, Libby P, Covell JW, Sobel BE, Ross J Jr, and Braunwald E: Precordial ST segment mapping: an atraumatic method for assessing alterations in the extent of myocardial ischemic injury. The effects of pharmacologic and hemodynamic interventions. Am J Cardiol 29:223, 1972.
24. Bodenheimer MM, Banka VS, Levites R, and Helfant RH: Temporal relation of epicardial electrographic, contractile and biochemical changes after acute coronary occlusion and reperfusion. Am J Cardiol 37:486–492, 1976.
25. Maroko PR, Maclean D, and Braunwald E: Limitation of infarct size: Methods of reducing myocardial oxygen demand and extension of experimental approaches to man. *In* Mason DT (ed): *Advances in Heart Disease* Vol 1. New York, Grune and Stratton, 1977, pp 111–132.
26. Maroko PR, Libby P, Ginks WR, Bloor CM, Shell WE, Sobel BE, and Ross J Jr: Coronary artery reperfusion, I. Early effects on local myocardial function and the extent of myocardial necrosis. J Clin Invest 51:2710–2716, 1972.
27. Ginks WR, Sybers HD, Maroko PR, Covell JW, Sobel BE, and Ross J Jr: Coronary artery reperfusion. II. Reduction of myocardial infarct size at one week after coronary occlusion. J Clin Invest 51:2717–2723, 1972.
28. Kloner RA, Ganote CE, Whalen D, and Jennings RB: Effect of a transient period of ischemia on myocardial cells. II. Fine structure during the first few minutes of reflow. Am J Pathol 74:399–422, 1976.
29. Maroko PR, Libby P, Sobel BE, Bloor CM, Sybers HD, Shell WE, Covell JW, and Braunwald E: Effect of glucose-insulin-potassium infusion on myocardial infarction following experimental coronary artery occlusion. Circulation 45:1160–1175, 1972.
30. Hillis LD, Askenazi J, Braunwald E, Radvany P, Muller JE, Fishbein MC, and Maroko PR: Use of changes in the epicardial QRS complex to assess interventions which modify the extent of myocardial necrosis following coronary artery oclusion. Circulation 54:591, 1976.

31. Hillis LD, Maroko PR, Braunwald E, and Fishbein MC: Influence of the time interval between coronary artery occlusion and the administration of hyaluronidase on myocardial salvage. Circulation 54(Suppl II):II-161, 1976.
32. Maroko PR, Libby P, Bloor CM, Sobel BE, and Braunwald E: Reduction by hyaluronidase of myocardial necrosis following coronary artery occlusion. Circulation 46:430–437, 1972.
33. Hirshfeld JW Jr, Borer JS, Goldstein RE, Barrett MJ, and Epstein SE: Reduction in severity and extent of myocardial infarction when nitroglycerin and methoxamine are administered during coronary occlusion. Circulation 49:291–297, 1974.
34. Libby P, Maroko PR, Bloor CM, Sobel BE, and Braunwald E: Reduction of experimental myocardial infarct size by corticosteroid administration. J Clin Invest 52:599–607, 1973.
35. Maroko PR, Radvany P, Braunwald E, and Hale SL: Reduction of infarct size by oxygen inhalation following acute coronary occlusion. Circulation 52:360–368, 1975.
36. Radvany P, Maroko PR, and Braunwald E: Effects of hypoxemia on the extent of myocardial necrosis after experimental coronary occlusion. Am J Cardiol 35:795–800, 1975.
37. Libby P, Maroko PR, and Braunwald E: The effect of hypoglycemia on myocardial ischemic injury during acute experimental coronary artery occlusion. Circulation 51:621–626, 1975.
38. Maroko PR, Carpenter CB, Chiariello M, Fishbein MC, Radvany P, Knostman JD, and Hale SL: Reduction by cobra venom factor of myocardial necrosis following coronary artery occlusion. J Clin Invest 61:661–670, 1978.
39. Diaz PE, Fishbein MC, Davis MA, Askenazi J, and Maroko PR: Effect of the kallikrein inhibitor aprotinin on myocardial ischemic injury following coronary artery occlusion in the dog. Am J Cardiol 40:541–549, 1977.
40. Hartmann JR, Robinson JA, and Gunnar RM: Chemotactic activity in the coronary sinus after experimental myocardial infarction: effects of pharmacologic interventions on ischemic injury. Am J Cardiol 40:550–555, 1977.
41. Smith HJ, Singh BN, Norris RM, John MB, and Hurley PJ: Changes in myocardial blood flow and S-T segment elevation following coronary artery occlusion in dogs. Circ Res 36:697–705, 1975.
42. Braunwald E, and Maroko PR: Evidence to support the hypothesis that myocardial infarct size can be limited following coronary occlusion. In Rapaport E (ed): Current Controversies in Cardiovascular Disease. Philadelphia, WB Saunders Company, 1980.
43. Maclean D, Fishbein MC, Maroko PR, and Braunwald E: Hyaluronidase-induced reductions in myocardial infarct size following coronary occlusion. Science 194:199–200, 1976.
44. Maclean D, Fishbein MC, Braunwald E, and Maroko PR: Long-term preservation of ischemic myocardium after experimental coronary artery occlusion. J Clin Invest 61:541–551, 1978.
45. Pierce WS, Carter DR, McGarran MH, and Waldhauser JA: Modification of myocardial infarct volume. An Arch Surg 107:682, 1973.
46. Shatney CH, MacCarter DJ, and Lillehei RR: Effects of allopurinol, propranolol, and methylprednisolone on infarct size in experimental myocardial infarction. Am J Cardiol 37:572–579, 1976.
47. Reimer KA, Rasmussen MM, and Jennings RB: On the nature of protection by propranolol against myocardial necrosis after temporary coronary occlusion in dogs. Am J Cardiol 37:520, 1976.
48. Kloner RA, Fishbein MC, Cotran RS, Braunwald E, and Maroko PR: The effect of propranolol on microvascular injury in acute myocardial ischemia. Circulation 55:872–880, 1977.
49. Sayen JJ, Peirce G, Katcher AH, and Sheldon WF: Correlation of intramyocardial electrocardiograms with polarographic oxygen and contractility in the nonischemic and regionally ischemic left ventricle. Circ Res 9:1268–1279, 1961.
50. Angell CS, Lakatta EG, Weisfeldt MS, and Shock NW: Relationship of intramyocardial oxygen tension and epicardial ST segment changes following acute coronary artery ligation: effects of coronary perfusion pressure. Cardiovasc Res 9:12–18, 1975.
51. Kjekshus JK, Maroko PR, and Sobel BE: Distribution of myocardial injury and its relation to epicardial ST segment changes after coronary artery occlusion in the dog. Cardiovasc Res 6:490, 1972.
52. Karlsson J, Templeton GH, and Willerson JT: Relationship between epicardial S-T segment changes and myocardial metabolism during acute coronary insufficiency. Circ Res 32:725–730, 1973.

53. Hearse DJ, Opie LH, Katzeff IE, Lubbe WF, Van der Werff TJ, Peisach M, and Boulle G: Characterization of the "border zone" in acute regional ischemia in dog. Am J Cardiol 40:718–726, 1977.
54. Khuri SF, Flaherty JT, O'Riordan JB, Pitt B, Brawley RL, Donahoo JW, and Gott VL: Changes in intramyocardial ST segment voltage and gas tension with regional myocardial ischemia in the dog. Circ Res 37:455, 1975.
55. Morris GK, Hampton JR, Hayes MJ, and Mitchell JRA: Predictive value of ST segment displacement and other indices after myocardial infarction. Lancet 2:372, 1974.
56. Blomquist CG, Peshock R, Parkey RW, Bonte FJ, and Willerson JT: ST isopotential precordial surface maps in acute myocardial infarction (abstr). Circulation 52(Suppl II):II–425, 1975.
57. Wilson RN, Johnston FD, Rosenbaun FF, Erlanger H, Knostman CE, Hecht H, Cotrim N, Oliveria RM, Scarsi R, and Barker PR: The precordial electrocardiogram. Am Heart J 27:19, 1944.
58. Rakita L, Borduas JL, Rothman S, and Prinzmetal M: Studies on the mechanism of ventricular activity. XII. Early changes in the ST-T segment and QRS complex following acute coronary artery occlusion: experimental study and clinical applications. Am Heart J 48:351–372, 1954.
59. Prinzmetal M, Kennamer R, Merliss R, Wada T, and Bor N: Angina pectoris. I. Variant form of angina pectoris: preliminary report. Am J Med 27:375–388, 1959.
60. MacAlpin PN, Kattus AK, and Alvaro AB: Angina pectoris at rest with preservation of exercise capacity. Prinzmetal's variant angina. Circulation 47:946–958, 1973.
61. Maroko PR, Davidson DM, Libby P, Hagan AD, and Braunwald E: Effects of hyaluronidase administration on myocardial ischemic injury in acute infarction. A preliminary study in 24 patients. Ann Intern Med 82:516, 1975.
62. Flaherty JT, Reid PR, Taylor D, Kelly DT, Weisfeldt M, and Pitt B: Intravenous nitroglycerin in acute myocardial infarction. Circulation 51:132, 1975.
63. Come PC, Flaherty JT, Baird MG, Rouleau JR, Weisfeldt ML, Greene HL, Becker L, and Pitt B: Reversal by phenylephrine of the beneficial effects of intravenous nitroglycerin in patients with acute myocardial infarction. N Engl J Med 293:1003, 1975.
64. Borer JS, Redwood DR, Levitt B, Cagin N, Bianchi C, Vallin H, and Epstein SE: Myocardial ischemia treated with nitroglycerin plus phenylephrine. N Engl J Med 293:1008, 1975.
65. Chiariello M, Gold HK, Leinbach RC, Davis MA, and Maroko PR: Comparsion between the effects of nitroprusside and nitroglycerin on ischemic injury during acute myocardial infarction. Circulation 54:766, 1976.
66. Gold HK, Leinbach RC, and Maroko PR: Propranolol-induced reduction of signs of ischemic injury during acute myocardial infarction. Am J Cardiol 38:689, 1976.
67. Madias JE, Madias NE, and Hood WB Jr: Precordial ST segment mapping. 2. Effects of oxygen inhalation on ischemic injury in patients with acute myocardial infarction. Circulation 53:411, 1976.
68. Roberts AJ, Cipriano PR, Alonso DR, Jacobstein JG, Combs JR, Gay WA Jr: Evaluation of methods for the quantification of experimental myocardial infarction. Circulation 57:35–40, 1978.
69. Reid PR, Taylor DR, Kelly DT, Weisfeldt ML, Humphries JO, Ross RS, and Pitt B: Myocardial infarct extension detected by precordial ST segment mapping. N Engl J Med 290:123, 1974.
70. Madias JE, Venkataraman K, Hood WB Jr: Precordial ST segment mapping. 1. Clinical studies in the coronary care unit. Circulation 52:799, 1975.
71. Norris RM, Barratt-Boyes C, Heng MK, and Singh BN: Failure of ST segment elevation to predict severity of acute myocardial infarction. Br Heart J 38:85, 1976.
72. Nielson BL: ST segment in acute myocardial infarction. Prognostic importance. Circulation 48:338, 1973.
73. Kronenberg MW, Hodges M, Akiyama T, Roberts DL, Ehrich DA, Biddle TL, and Yu PN: ST segment variations after acute myocardial infarction: relationship to clinical status. Circulation 54:756, 1976.
74. Wilson FN, Macleod AG, Baker PS, Johnston FD, and Klostermeyer LL: The electrocardiogram in myocardial infarction with particular reference to the initial deflections of the ventricular complex. Heart 16:155, 1933.
75. Johnston FD, Hill IGW, and Wilson FN: The form of the electrocardiogram in experimental MI. II. The early effects produced by ligation of the anterior descending branch of the left coronary artery. Am Heart J 10:889, 1934.

76. Wilson FN, Hill IGW, and Johnston FD: The form of the electrocardiogram in experimental myocardial infarction. III. The latter effects produced by ligation of the anterior descending branch of the left coronary artery. Am Heart J 10:903, 1935.

77. Prinzmetal M, Kennamer R, and Maxwell M: Studies on the mechanism of ventricular activity. VIII. The genesis of the coronary QS wave in through-and-through infarction. Am J Med 17:610, 1954.

78. Maxwell M, Kennamer R, and Prinzmetal M: Studies on the mechanism of ventricular activity. IX. The mural-type coronary QS wave. Am J Med 17:614, 1954.

79. Shaw CM Jr, Goldman A, Kennamer R, Kimura N, Lindgren I, Maxwell MH, and Prinzmetal M: Studies on the mechanism of ventricular activity. VII. The origin of the coronary QR wave. Am J Med 16:490, 1954.

80. Myers GB, Klein HA, and Stofer BE: 1. Correlation of electrocardiographic and pathologic findings in anteroseptal infarction. Am Heart J 36:535–575, 1948.

81. Myers GB, Klein HA, and Hiratzka T: 2. Correlation of electrocardiographic and pathologic findings in large anterolateral infarcts. Am Heart J 36:838–881, 1948.

82. Myers GB, Klein HA, and Hiratzka T: 3. Correlation of electrocardiographic and pathologic findings in anteroposterior infarction. Am Heart J 37:205–236, 1949.

83. Myers GB, Klein HA, and Stofer BE: Correlation of electrocardiograph and pathologic findings in lateral infarction. Am Heart J 37:374–417, 1949.

84. Myers GB, Klein HA, and Hiratzka T: 4. Correlation of electrocardiographic and pathologic findings in infarction of the interventricular septum and right ventricle. Am Heart J 37:720–770, 1949.

85. Ekmekci A, Toyoshima H, Kwoczynski JK, Nagaya T, and Prinzmetal M: Angina pectoris. V. Giant R and receding S wave in myocardial ischemia and certain nonischemic conditions. Am J Cardiol 7:521, 1961.

86. Dressler W, and Roesler H: High T waves in the earliest stage of myocardial infarction. Am Heart J 34:627, 1947.

87. Madias JE: The earliest electrocardiographic sign of acute transmural myocardial infarction. J Electrocardiol 10:193, 1977.

88. Ribeiro LGT, Louie EK, Hillis LD, Davis MA, and Maroko PR: Early increases in R wave voltage after coronary artery occlusion: A useful index of ischemia (abstr). Clin Res 26:264A, 1978.

89. Ribeiro LGT, Louie EK, Hillis LD, Davis MA, and Maroko PR: Early augmentation of R wave voltage after coronary artery occlusion: A useful index of myocardial injury. J Electrocardiol 12:89–95, 1979.

90. Meller J, Conde CA, Donoso E, and Dack S: Transient Q waves in Prinzmetal's angina. Am J Cardiol 35:691, 1975.

91. Shugold GI: Transient QRS changes simulating myocardial infarction associated with shock and severe metabolic stress. Am Heart J 74:402, 1967.

92. Maroko PR, Hillis LD, Muller JE, Tavazzi L, Heyndrickx, GK, Ray M, Chiariello M, Distante A, Askenazi J, Salerno J, Carpentier J, Reshetnaya NI, Radvany P, Libby P, Raabe DS, Chazov EI, Bobba P, and Braunwald E: Favorable effects of hyaluronidase on electrocardiographic evidence of necrosis in patients with acute myocardial infarction. N Engl J Med 296:898, 1977.

93. Askenazi J, Maroko PR, Lesch M, and Braunwald E: Usefulness of ST segment elevations as predictors of electrocardiographic signs of necrosis in patients with acute myocardial infarction. Br Heart J 39:764, 1977.

94. Horan LG, Flowers NC, and Johnson JC: Significance of the diagnostic Q wave of myocardial infarction. Circulation 43:428, 1971.

95. Savage RM, Wagner GS, Ideker RE, Podolsky SA, and Hackel DB: Correlation of postmortem anatomic findings with electrocardiographic changes in patients with myocardial infarction: Retrospective study of patients with typical anterior and posterior infarcts. Circulation 55:279, 1977.

96. Miller RR, Bonanno J, Massumi RA, Zelis R, Mason DT, and Amsterdam EA: Usefulness of the electrocardiogram in assessment of ventricular performance and comparison with coronary arteriography (abstr). Am J Cardiol 29:281, 1972.

97. Williams RA, Cohn PF, Vokonas PS, Young E, Herman MV, and Gorlin R: Electrocardiographic, arteriographic and ventriculographic correlations in transmural myocardial infarction. Am J Cardiol 31:595, 1973.

98. Miller RR, Amsterdam EA, Bogren HG, Massumi RA, Zelis R, and Mason DT: Electrocardiographic and cineangiographic correlations in assessment of the location, nature and extent of abnormal left ventricular segmental contraction in coronary artery disease. Circulation 49:447, 1974.

99. Bodenheimer MM, Banka VS, Trout RG, Herman GA, and Helfant RH: Correlation of pathologic Q waves on the standard electrocardiogram and the epicardial electrogram of the human heart. Circulation 54:213, 1976.
100. Awan N, Miller RR, Vera Z, Janzen D, Amsterdam EA, and Mason DT: Noninvasive assessment of cardiac function and ventricular dyssynergy by precordial Q wave mapping in anterior myocardial infarction. Circulation 55:833, 1977.
101. Askenazi J, Freedman WB, Cohn PF, Braunwald E, and Parisi AF: The predictive value of the QRS complex in assessment of left ventricular function (abstr). Circulation 54(Suppl II):II–125, 1976.

ST-Segment Mapping Is Not a Clinical Tool*

HARRY A. FOZZARD, M.D.

Otho S. A. Sprague Professor, Departments of Medicine
and the Pharmacological and Physiological Sciences; Joint
Director of Cardiology, University of Chicago, Chicago, Illinois

The Clinical Challenge

ST-segment mapping is proposed as a means for monitoring myocardial infarct size in order to determine the effectiveness of various treatments that might influence infarct size. In this discussion, I wish to stipulate that the need for a monitor of infarct size is evident. Coronary heart disease is a major cause of morbidity and mortality among middle-aged Americans and Europeans. We have failed to develop an effective way to treat the underlying coronary arteriosclerosis, so that we are forced to treat complications of the disease. A major complication, leading to perhaps a quarter of the CHD deaths, is heart failure related to ischemic loss of heart muscle — usually via an acute myocardial infarction. One parameter of risk is the size of the infarcted muscle.

In the last few years, we have realized that a myocardial infarction is not simply an all-or-nothing event. In the presence of partial and fixed arteriosclerotic obstruction of coronary arteries, some factor(s) leads to development of acute ischemia. This ischemia of heart muscle is the result of an imbalance between delivery of blood and the need for oxygen or other properties provided by the coronary circulation. This ischemia can lead to irreversible and lethal cellular changes or it can be relieved. The choice of life or death for the cells is made on the basis of local conditions and probably is determined over many hours or even days.

A number of possible modes of treatment are available to reduce the size of the impending or developing infarct. These may promote the delivery of blood or nutrients to the endangered area or reduce its metabolic require-

*Supported by USPHS HL-20592-01. Additional discussion of this topic may be found in an article by H. Fozzard entitled "ST-segment potentials and mapping" in Circulation 54:533–537, 1976.

281

ments. We have a strong need to find a measure or monitor of ischemia for two reasons: to determine experimentally which therapeutic modalities are useful and to regulate the application of a potentially harmful treatment to an individual patient.

ST-segment mapping has been proposed as a valuable tool for measurement of size of the endangered zone. The method, however, has a complex physiologic mechanism that makes it unlikely to be a valuable clinical tool. I want to focus first on the physiologic problem in ST-segment mapping.

ST-Segment Mapping

ST-segment elevation has long been recognized as a sign of myocardial injury. The classical sequence of events in the local electrogram after occlusion of a coronary artery is, first, T-wave inversion, followed by ST-segment change, and finally loss of R wave and development of Q wave. T-wave change is thought to be a sign of ischemia, easily reversible. ST-segment elevation is considered a sign of injury; the muscle is not yet dead, and slow recovery is possible. Traditionally, the Q wave indicates death of muscle.

In 1971 Maroko and Braunwald first reported epicardial ST-segment mapping — systematic recording of electrograms from the epicardium overlying a region of ischemia, which was produced by ligating a branch of the left anterior descending artery of the dog heart. This technique identified the approximate extent of cardiac damage by the number of sites with ST-segment elevation. In addition, they suggested that the magnitude of elevation was proportional to the ischemia and added together the sum of all of the ST-segment elevations. They correlated this quick electrical tool for estimating infarct size with pathologic studies on specimens obtained after 24 hours and with depletion of cellular elements, especially creatine kinase. These studies have been repeated in other laboratories and should be considered to be accurate, at least in the context of their experimental design. Therefore, regardless of the conceptual criticisms to be discussed, Maroko and Braunwald have demonstrated reasons for using ST-segment mapping in their experiments. Subsequently, they have also noted that QRS changes occur in the injured zone, and the likelihood of subsequent development of the QRS changes is related to earlier ST-segment changes.

If their experiments in the open-chested dog are applicable to precordial studies in the human, it appeared possible that a technique might be available to measure the size of the injured zone in patients with acute myocardial infarction. This would permit evaluation of various proposed treatments to reduce ischemia and rescue endangered muscle. However, it is extremely important that any such technique be evaluated carefully before it is removed from the research lab. We have repeatedly discovered that clinical care is not as straightforward as laboratory experiment. Often an excellent experiment may mislead us if it is not transferable to the bedside. A misapplication of the technique could lead to serious injury to a large number of patients.

Physiologic Basis of the ECG

The electrocardiogram is a recording of the cardiac electromotive force (EMF) at some distance from the heart. This EMF derives from the excitable electrical properties of heart muscle. Cardiac cells have resting (diastolic) potentials of about −80 mV, resulting from the high concentration of intracellular K^+, relative to the extracellular K^+ concentration, and the high permeability of the membrane to K^+. Under this circumstance, the membrane potential is close to the electrochemical equilibrium potential for K^+. The high concentration of intracellular K^+ is maintained by the Na-K pump, which is sensitive to the levels of ATP in the cells. Also of importance to the resting potential is the presence of anions (negatively charged ions or molecules) that cannot easily leave the cell. The nature of these impermeant anions is not clear, but they are probably amino acids or peptides. If they are modified by hypoxia, then this would also influence the resting potential.

Cardiac cells are coupled to their neighbors by electrotonic membrane junctions. These "gap junctions" behave as if they are protoplasmic continuities between the cells, allowing movement of ions, such as K^+, or small molecules, such as polypeptides. Because the cells are connected, it is difficult under normal conditions for a standing voltage difference to exist. Therefore, all similar connected cells (e.g., ventricular muscle) assume the same resting potential. The ventricular conducting system maintains a different resting potential, but it is connected to the ventricle only at discrete points.

When brought to threshold, the cardiac cell can have an action potential. This is a sudden depolarization to inside values of about +20 mV (ventricular muscle). The action potential propagates through the ventricles rapidly because of the electrotonic connections between cells. The voltage gradients found during this period result in the QRS. Conduction of the action potential is due to "local circuit current" flow, and this concept is important to understanding the ECG.

The depolarization of the action potential due to inflow of Na^+ ions through the membrane occurs at a point along a cable-like cell and moves linearly along the cable. (This is conceptually the same as a wave front moving uniformly across a sheet.) The inflow of Na^+ obtains its EMF from the Na electrochemical gradient, which represents a battery in the simplified electrical circuit of the cardiac cell. The remainder of the circuit is completed passively in three steps. Current flows inside the cells ahead of the depolarization point or front and brings that region to threshold. Depolarization of this area in front is due to displacement of charge stored on the membrane capacity. The second phase is the (imaginary) capacity current through the membrane. The positive charges freed from the capacity on the outside of the membrane of the cells not yet excited are free to flow back to the active region. This flow of current is through the extracellular space and the surrounding tissue. The point or wave front outside the membrane where Na^+ ions are entering is thereby relatively negative and represents the sink for this extracellular current. It is the potential gradients related to the return loop that are recorded in the ECG, either precordial or epicardial.

The depolarization is rapidly propagated throughout the ventricles, and the QRS complex ends when this is complete. At this time the cells are again almost isopotential, so little current flows. Consequently the ST period is recorded as isoelectric. Gradients exist during rapid repolarization, generating the T wave.

ST-Segment Changes in Ischemia

While detailed cellular electrophysiologic studies are difficult to make under conditions simulating human myocardial infarction, certain general characteristics are clear. The cells depolarize, develop small and usually abbreviated action potentials, and finally become inexcitable.

Depolarization occurs within a few minutes in experimental coronary occlusion, because of K^+ accumulation extracellularly. This results from a net efflux of K^+ from the cells, in some way related to the failure of circulation. The most plausible explanation for this efflux is that the Na-K pump that normally balances active K^+ influx to its passive efflux is blocked in some way. As long as the cells contain a high concentration of K^+, this efflux can maintain the elevated extracellular K^+ concentration, probably for a few hours after occlusion. The duration of this phase is probably quite variable, depending on how rapidly the extracellular K^+ diffuses or is washed away. Finally the intracellular K^+ will be depleted, and the cells are depolarized even with return of normal extracellular K^+ levels.

With depolarization, the membrane excitability is reduced, as a consequence of a lower sodium conductance during the action potential. When resting membrane depolarization reaches about $-50mV$, the cells are usually inexcitable. It is possible that some excitability may remain, owing to the "slow inward current." This is a separate membrane channel from the fast Na^+ one, and current through it may be carried by both Na^+ and Ca^{++}. Its characteristic is slow conduction, and it may play a role in ventricular dysrhythmias.

During the resting period of the cardiac cycle, the ischemic zone is depolarized. Since the cells are connected by the electrotonic junctions, current will flow intracellularly from the ischemic zone toward the normal tissue. The circuit is completed by flow extracellularly from the normal region to the ischemic zone. An electrode placed over the ischemic zone results in the recording of a negative potential. This period is the TQ segment of the ECG. Its depression cannot be detected as such on the ECG, since that is an AC recording. Using the TQ segment as a reference, the ST segment appears to be elevated.

If the action potential in the ischemic zone is abbreviated, or if the area is inexcitable, then the cell becomes negative relative to the depolarized normal region during the active part of the cardiac cycle. Current then flows intracellularly into the zone and back extracellularly toward the normal region. The local electrogram now indicates positivity. This period is the ST segment, and it is elevated until repolarization is accomplished.

The clinical reading of ST-segment elevation is made by assuming that the TQ segment is isoelectric. Properly this event should be called TQ–ST–segment deviation, but for simplicity we simply call it ST-segment deviation.

This ST-segment deviation should persist as long as the cells in the ischemic zone are depolarized and/or inexcitable and as long as they are electrically connected to the healthy region. If they are metabolically improved, then the phenomenon would reverse itself. If the cells should uncouple from the normal region, then current flow would cease. Cell uncoupling is a rather poorly understood process, but it is probably related to the Ca^{++} concentration in the cells. The sick cells could uncouple in the process of dying, or they could be insulated until recovery, when they could recouple.

An important point in this discussion is that ST-segment deviation is related to external current flow and is therefore subject to the influences of the tissue external to the ischemic cells. The direction of ST-segment deviation depends on the location of the electrode. For example, subepicardial ischemia produces ST-segment elevation and subendocardial ischemia produces ST-segment depression. The physiologic process is the same, but the electrode location relative to the ischemia is different.

Errors in Interpretation of ST-Segment Deviation

We can extract certain facts from this discussion of the origin of the ST-segment deviation from which sources of error in ST-segment mapping can be derived. The first is concerned with geometry and the second with membrane events.

Fact 1 — geometric effects. The current flow that causes ST-segment deviation results from a potential difference between the normal and the ischemic areas, where the resting and/or action potentials are different. This current is greatest at the boundary of the ischemic zone. The signal at an electrode depends on its position relative to that boundary.

COROLLARY 1A. Current flow will cease if the injured cells are disconnected from the normal muscle. This means that ST-segment elevation would decrease as the result of progression of injury rather than its reduction. Indeed, the "evolution" of an infarct ECG pattern may be this process. Since the progress of ischemic injury is so variable in the human with coronary disease, in contrast to the animal with a ligated coronary artery, it will be difficult or impossible to decide if changes in ST-segments in a given lead are due to progression of damage or to its reduction because of the influence of some therapeutic agent. Since both worsening and improvement can give the same signal, it is dangerous to use the signal to monitor clinical treatment or as a measure for clinical research.

COROLLARY 1B. If the electrogram is recorded from near the source of current, it will be larger. Since the source of current in ischemia is concentrated mostly near the boundaries of the injury, then the ST segment should be most abnormal in the boundary region. Indeed, it has been reported by several investigators to be normalized in the center of a large injured region. This should be particularly true of an epicardial lead. The ST-segment elevation may be a reasonable experimental marker for the boundary of injury, at least for a period of time, but the sum of ST-segment elevation could be deceptive.

COROLLARY 1C.   The electrogram will vary in its pattern depending on its location relative to the injury. If the injury is subendocardial, the ST segment will be depressed. If it is subepicardial, the ST segment will be elevated. If we have subepicardial injury, with ST-segment elevation, and subsequently there is extension to the subendocardial region, the ST segment may normalize. A region of injury within the muscle wall, not impinging on any surface, may have no indication of ST-segment change on the surface, since all currents cancel each other. This is an oversimplified geometry of the injured region.

COROLLARY 1D.   If an electrode is at a distance, it necessarily records a smaller signal, and it integrates information over a larger region. The problem with precordial electrograms is that they are both far from the injured area and are distorted by the conductance of the noncardiac tissue between them and the source. Any change in the conductance of the extracellular return path for the cardiac EMF will alter this signal, even if the change has nothing to do with the injury process. For example, a change in hematocrit alters the conductance of blood and shunts away part of the current otherwise reflected on the surface. The effect of pericardial effusion is well recognized clinically and is the result of the same process.

The need for proximity and the ability to project surface electrograms onto the heart is the reason that apical, lateral, and inferior myocardial infarcts are not well characterized by multi-lead precordial maps. Vector recordings avoid this problem to a degree, but they are also influenced by the complex current path from the heart to the surface leads used to generate the vector.

Fact 2 — direct electrical effects.   Any factor altering the resting potential or the action potential of heart cells can alter current flow between the normal and abnormal areas.

COROLLARY 1A.   If there is an abnormal conduction pattern of excitation, then there will be an abnormal repolarization pattern. This is demonstrated clearly in bundle branch blocks, in which so-called "secondary" ST-segment changes occur. If the conduction path of excitation into the injured region is altered, we can expect consequent ST-segment changes. The appearance of blocked or delayed conduction may in itself be useful for diagnostic purposes, but it decreases the value of ST-segment mapping from the injured region. The patients with the largest injured zones, who are in greatest need of ischemia modification, are the very ones who have a high incidence of conduction delay and blockage.

COROLLARY 2B.   Any intervention that modifies the electrical properties of the injured region can change current flow independent of changes in metabolic state of the cells. Since much of the early depolarization is the result of K^+ accumulation, any intervention that slowed its efflux or that favored its wash-out would decrease ST segments. This could be an effect of hyaluronidase, quite independent of any influence on oxygen delivery. In addition, drugs such as antidysrhythmic agents may influence the action potential of the injured region by altering ion channels, again without influencing metabolic balance. Some of these drug effects may modify the excitability of the ischemic area and be valuable in that way, but not by decreasing infarct size.

COROLLARY 2C.   Any intervention that modifies the electrical properties of the normal tissue would change current flow. The simplest example of this effect is to increase the concentration of extracellular K^+ in the normal region. This depolarizes the normal cells and brings their resting potential closer to that of the injured region. This effect has been shown experimentally, and it confirms the clinical observation that patients with renal failure and hyperkalemia often do not show ST-segment changes during the course of an acute myocardial infarction. Heart rate also alters the action-potential duration of the normal cells and would bring the electrical events in the two areas closer together.

As suggested above, there may be real therapeutic benefit to this sort of treatment. The standing current reflected by the TQ-segment depression during the resting period may play an important role in precipitating ventricular dysrhythmias. Reducing the injury current may be of significant value in protecting the patient, but not necessarily by reducing the size of the injured zone.

The Value of ST-Segment Mapping

The intensive investigation into ST-segment mapping has focused our attention on a very important problem. I subscribe to the impressions that myocardial cell death is not instantaneous and that interventions might be of great value in halting the injury process. We are ignorant of the final "irreversible" step in the death of a cardiac cell from ischemia. In many patients there is probably a prolonged period of clinically manifest injury before determination of death of the cells.

It is likely that in the dog with a ligated coronary artery, the ST-segment map measures the extent and severity of K^+ accumulation. It is, therefore, a useful laboratory tool. The dramatic precordial ST-segment changes that wax and wane early in ischemic injury in the occasional patient are probably also a reflection of the same process.

In addition, the ST segment is useful in monitoring the extent of cell coupling. We have already raised the point that current flows through "gap junctions." This current flow may contribute to dysrhythmias. However, ions and small molecules may diffuse through the junction also. If the process leading to irreversible damage of the cell is a diffusible substance (such as H^+), then this "poison" may be transmitted from cell to cell, propagating cell death. The ST-segment map may be of value in investigating the uncoupling of cells and may be a monitor of agents that might facilitate uncoupling in a therapeutic manner.

Drawbacks of ST-Segment Mapping

At best, ST-segment mapping is applicable only to anterior infarcts of reasonably small size and to conditions without conduction block, dysrhythmia, or pericarditis. This greatly restricts the population in which the technique might be useful.

In addition, the ST-segment changes decline rapidly in the normal course of development of the myocardial infarct. It may be necessary to map within the first hour or so of onset of injury if it is to be a useful tool. Unfortunately, few patients arrange to have their infarcts so convenient to our study facilities.

Finally, we will be obliged to sort out the effects of any treatment on electrical properties of the membranes and surrounding conducting tissue before we can ascribe any effect on ST-segment changes to alteration in ischemia. We will need to presume the geometry of the injured region and certainly cannot handle subendocardial infarction.

If the proposed treatments to reduce infarct size, using ST-segment mapping as a monitor, were without potential harmful effects, we could tolerate this level of inaccuracy in the monitor. But this is not the case. Any agent that may drop systemic blood pressure may reduce coronary flow. Any agent that has a negative inotropic effect may dilate the heart and may reduce flow critically. Almost all of our potential treatments are double-edged swords.

Is This Argument Diagnostic Nihilism?

The concept of measuring infarct size is young, and we have only begun to focus serious scientific effort on this task. Indeed, there are promising new techniques to image the ischemic zone by measuring regional blood flow and regional metabolic events. Great advances are being made in the cellular characteristics of cardiac cell function and behavior in ischemic injury. The future is encouraging, and I feel that we can indeed develop far more reliable measurement tools than the unreliable ST-segment map.

Conclusion

The ST-segment map has many inherent faults because of its dependency on the complex geometry of the injured region of the heart and the inherent electrophysiologic properties of cardiac cells. But the greatest fault of ST-segment mapping is that it may give misleading results in the care of our patients. We cannot afford to use such a poor tool to monitor the treatment of ischemia, because the therapeutic agents we might use to decrease infarct size are potentially dangerous. We could obtain erroneous results from clinical research, but most important, we could contribute to increased cardiac damage in our patients. We have an overriding responsibility as physicians to measure accurately the effects of our interventions.

The cause is right; ischemia requires treatment to prevent cell death. The measurement tool is wrong; it is undependable in the clinical setting. The work of Maroko and Braunwald should be given great credit for focusing our attention on the task. However, we must avoid precipitous application of this technique of ST-segment mapping and support the development of a proper tool.

Comment

The interest in ST-segment mapping is heightened by the need for tools to estimate infarct size, particularly in light of the suggestion that various interventions are capable of salvaging myocardium. Progress in this area is hampered by the lack of reliable methods for judging myocardial infarct size.

Dr. Maroko has quoted experimental results in animals that suggest that under the circumstances of the studies, a correlation exists between tissue creatine kinase depletion and ST-segment mapping, which tends to validate its utility as a tool for judging infarct size. The evidence in man, however, is for the most part extrapolated from animal experiments. Dr. Fozzard presents some cogent arguments, both theoretical and practical, that tend to call into question routine use of ST-segment mapping for estimating infarct size. Succinctly stated, the major arguments are that the continued progression of injury, as well as its reduction, can lead to a return of the ST segment toward the baseline, or that even simply the extension into the subendocardium of subepicardial damage may tend to reverse the originally observed ST-segment elevation. As Dr. Maroko also appreciates, the development of pericarditis or pericardial effusion obviously invalidates the method, as does the development of abnormal conduction patterns. Furthermore, if an agent is administered that alters the extracellular potassium concentration, ST-segment changes will occur independent of its effect on infarct size. Thus, for example, ST-segment mapping is not of use in judging the ability of glucose-potassium-insulin mixtures to affect infarct size. Finally, there are limitations in its use for looking at inferior infarcts, since anterior precordial ST-segment mapping will not reflect changes in inferior myocardial damage.

These limitations clearly restrict the use of this technique. It seems to me that if one selects an intervention for which there is evidence that it has little effect on tissue conduction or local extracellular potassium concentrations and uses the technique in an experimental setting that permits direct epicardial leads, the technique can be of value in judging the effect of an intervention on infarct size. However, in the usual clinical setting, I suspect that the objections that Dr. Fozzard brings out make it a tenuous tool at best. It is possible that the addition of QRS mapping may prove more useful. Dr. Maroko does present interesting data to suggest this technique has potential, although this possibility is not addressed by Dr. Fozzard as part of this controversy.

ELLIOT RAPAPORT, M.D.

Thirteen

Is It Possible to Preserve Ischemic Myocardium in Acute Myocardial Infarction?

EVIDENCE TO SUPPORT THE HYPOTHESIS THAT
MYOCARDIAL INFARCT SIZE CAN BE LIMITED
FOLLOWING CORONARY OCCLUSION

Eugene Braunwald, M.D., and Peter A. Maroko,
M.D.

IS IT POSSIBLE TO PRESERVE ISCHEMIC MYOCARDIUM
IN ACUTE MYOCARDIAL INFARCTION? — REASONABLE
DOUBTS REGARDING POSSIBILITIES AND BENEFITS

A. James Liedtke, M.D., and Howard E. Morgan,
M.D.

COMMENT

Evidence to Support the Hypothesis That Myocardial Infarct Size Can Be Limited Following Coronary Occlusion*

EUGENE BRAUNWALD, M.D.

Hersey Professor of the Theory and Practice of Physic
(Medicine), Harvard Medical School; Physician-in-Chief,
Peter Bent Brigham Hospital, Boston, Massachusetts

PETER R. MAROKO, M.D.

Associate Professor of Medicine, Department of Medicine,
Harvard Medical School; Associate in Medicine, Peter
Bent Brigham Hospital, Boston, Massachusetts

In-hospital deaths in patients with acute myocardial infarction have resulted mainly from primary arrhythmias and from pump failure. While death due to primary arrhythmias has been markedly reduced by modern monitoring techniques and more vigorous prophylaxis and treatment, the mortality following mechanical failure manifested by cardiogenic shock and/or pulmonary edema is still very high. These syndromes have been found to be associated with larger infarctions than those exhibited by patients who succumbed to myocardial infarction but who did not die as a consequence of pump failure.[1] In addition, the prognosis for patients with larger infarcts is distinctly worse than it is for those with smaller infarcts.[2]

When myocardium becomes ischemic, its contractile function becomes seriously impaired. This depression of myocardial function may be transient if the duration of ischemia is brief, as occurs in angina pectoris; alternatively, depression of left ventricular function may be permanent if pro-

*Supported by Grants HL-20199 and HL-23140 from the National Heart, Lung, and Blood Institute

295

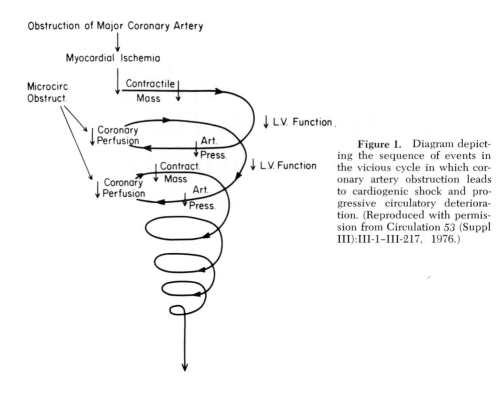

Figure 1. Diagram depicting the sequence of events in the vicious cycle in which coronary artery obstruction leads to cardiogenic shock and progressive circulatory deterioration. (Reproduced with permission from Circulation 53 (Suppl III):III-1–III-217, 1976.)

longed ischemia leads to myocardial necrosis. Hemodynamic and clinical findings of left ventricular failure become apparent when contraction ceases or is seriously impaired in 20 to 25 per cent of the left ventricle. With loss of 40 per cent or more of left ventricular myocardium, severe pump failure develops, and if this loss occurs acutely, cardiogenic shock usually supervenes.

Death from cardiogenic shock may be viewed as the end result of a vicious cycle (Fig. 1).[3] If coronary obstruction leads to an extensive area of myocardial ischemia, myocardial contractility and ventricular performance become impaired. If the impairment of the latter is severe enough, it may reduce arterial pressure and therefore coronary perfusion pressure, leading to further ischemia and extension of necrosis, until, in many instances, the patient succumbs.

Accordingly, a treatment that could limit the extent of myocardial necrosis and by this mechanism decrease the frequency of intractable cardiogenic shock and pulmonary edema would be extremely useful, not only in reducing immediate mortality, but also in leaving the patient who had suffered a coronary occlusion with more viable myocardium. Such a patient would be expected to be less likely to develop chronic heart failure and would have a greater reserve of functioning myocardium should another coronary occlusion occur.

It has long been appreciated by clinicians that factors that influence myocardial oxygen demands may aggravate or alleviate symptoms of myocardial ischemia. For example, in patients with angina and hyperthyroidism, treatment of the hypermetabolic state and the associated reduction of myocardial oxygen needs is often associated with relief of angina. Also, the reduction of myocardial oxygen needs by beta-adrenergic blockade or the development of bradycardia secondary to atrioventricular block often diminishes the severity and frequency of angina pectoris. Conversely, tachycardia, which augments myocardial oxygen needs, increases myocardial ischemia in patients with coronary artery disease.

The above-mentioned and related clinical observations suggested to us in 1967 that the ultimate size of a myocardial infarct is not irrevocably determined by the site of coronary occlusion and the patho-anatomy of the coronary vascular bed but might be modified by other factors.[4] We then proposed that when coronary occlusion occurs, the survival of a portion of the myocardium normally perfused by the obstructed vessel may well depend on the balance between the oxygen available to that segment of myocardium and its oxygen requirements and, ultimately, that left ventricular function, and perhaps even the survival of the patient with coronary occlusion, could in large measure be dependent on the balance between the oxygen supply and demand of the myocardium jeopardized by the coronary occlusion.[5-7] As we began our experimental work in 1968, we were stimulated by the report published by Cox et al.,[8] who obtained canine hearts at various time intervals following coronary occlusion and examined them by histochemical techniques. They noted an area of ischemic damage without frank necrosis during the first few hours following the coronary occlusion; the infarct expanded progressively at the expense of what they considered to be a damaged but not frankly necrotic zone.[8] Therefore, we proposed that for a finite period following cessation of coronary perfusion, a significant portion of the myocardium supplied wholly or largely by the occluded vessel remains capable of essentially full recovery or may proceed to necrosis. A principal goal of our experimental efforts has been to determine whether therapeutic interventions can increase the fraction of jeopardized, ischemic cells that ultimately survives.

Methods for Evaluating Changes in Myocardial Damage in Experimental Animals

To test the hypothesis that acute myocardial ischemic injury can be modified by interventions applied following coronary occlusion, it was necessary to develop techniques for assessing the extent and severity of ischemic damage. Our initial effort was in dogs in which electrographic ST segments were recorded from multiple epicardial sites during repeated 20-minute coronary artery occlusions.[5-7] Since all sequential electrographic recordings were made at the same epicardial sites on the same heart, the effect of the considerable variation in the distribution of the coronary arteries and in the extent of the intercoronary collaterals among different animals were eliminated, and each animal could serve as its own control. Since repetitive occlusions of 15 minutes separated by 45-minute periods of reflow resulted in reproducible elevations of ST segments,[9] an alteration in the extent and magnitude of ST-segment elevation during one of these repeated occlusions following an intervention suggests that the intervention induced a change in acute myocardial ischemic injury. Application of this technique indicated to us that many interventions, such as beta-adrenergic agonists and antagonists, cardiac glycosides, nitroglycerin, alterations in heart rate and arterial pressure, intra-aortic counterpulsation, and the inhalation of high and low concentrations of oxygen, produced striking and repeatable changes in the extent of ST-segment elevation and in the surface area of the left ventricle from which such currents of injury could be recorded. In general, an augmentation of oxygen delivery or reduction in oxygen demand reduced the current of injury, while lowering oxygen delivery or augmenting oxygen needs had the opposite effect.[3, 7] This approach is simple and quite useful as a screening procedure and provided results that have invariably been similar to those obtained by more sophisticated techniques. However, it has two inherent disadvantages: First, it is possible that the intervention being evaluated has a nonspecific effect on the ST segment that is unrelated to its effects on ischemic injury; second, it does not provide direct information concerning how any intervention alters the ultimate extent of myocardial necrosis resulting from coronary occlusion.

The 24-hour occlusion method in which early ST-segment mapping is compared to the resultant necrosis overcomes both of these limitations. As with the first method, the coronary artery is occluded, and the epicardial ST-segment map is recorded 15 minutes later; sometime thereafter the intervention is applied. However, the occlusion is maintained; the chest is closed and is re-opened 24 hours later; and transmural specimens subjacent to the sites from which epicardial electrograms had been recorded immediately following coronary occlusion are excised. The biopsied tissues are then analyzed for histologic, histochemical, and electromicroscopic evidence of necrosis and decrease of tissue creatine kinase (CK) activity. In animals that receive no intervention, there is a predictable, highly significant relationship between the height of the ST segment 15 minutes after occlusion and the tissue signs of necrosis 24 hours[7, 9-13] or four days[14] later. With this technique, the epicardial electrogram serves as a predictor of subsequent tissue viability or infarction, and the intervention being evaluated is administered *after* the ST-segment map has already been recorded. Therefore, a nonspecific effect of the intervention on the electrogram can be excluded. Studies utilizing this technique in dogs with coronary occlusion have shown that a number of interventions, such as beta-adrenergic blockers, hyaluronidase, inhalation of high concentrations of oxygen, intra-aortic balloon counterpulsation, and the infusion of a glucose-insulin-potassium mixture, significantly reduce the histologic, electron-microscopic, and biochemical (CK activity) evidence of necrosis in myocardium that is initially ischemic, as reflected in epicardial ST-segment elevation 15 minutes following coronary occlusion.[10, 11] Specifically, it was shown that in untreated control animals, myocardium subjacent to epicardial sites showing ST-segment elevation ≥ 2 mV predictably goes on to become necrotic. This progression of necrosis was interrupted by the aforementioned interventions (Figs. 2 and 3).

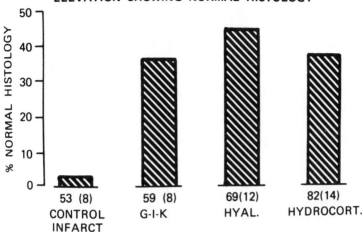

PERCENTAGE OF SPECIMENS WITH ST SEGMENT ELEVATION SHOWING NORMAL HISTOLOGY

Figure 2. Comparison of the effect of treatment on histology in areas with ST-segment elevations over 2 mV. First column: Control group; Second column: Glucose-insulin-potassium (GIK) group; Third column: Hyaluronidase group; Fourth column: Hydrocortisone group. Note that in all three treatment groups more than one-third of sites that were expected to show early signs of myocardial infarction were spared. Numbers at the bottom of each bar indicate the number of specimens in each group; the number of dogs in each group is shown in parentheses. (Reproduced with permission from Ann Intern Med 79:720–733, 1973.)

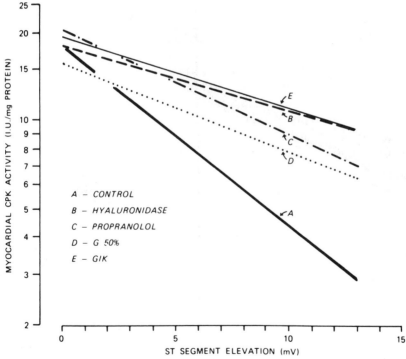

Figure 3. Relationship between ST-segment elevation 15 minutes after occlusion and log of CPK activity from the same specimens obtained 24 hours later. Line A: control group (occlusion alone) — 15 dogs, 101 biopsies. Line B: hyaluronidase (13 dogs, 94 biopsies). Line C: glucose-insulin-potassium infusion (13 dogs, 96 biopsies). All interventions started 30 minutes following coronary artery occlusion, i.e., 15 minutes after the epicardial mapping. There is a statistical difference (p < 0.01) between the slope of line A and the slopes of the other lines showing less CPK depression after treatment. (Reproduced with permission from Circulation 53(Suppl I):I-162–I-168, 1976.)

299

More recently, the influence of myocardial ischemia on intramural carbon dioxide tension ($PmCO_2$) was measured directly with a mass spectrometer in open-chest, anesthetized dogs subjected to repetitive, 10-minute coronary artery occlusions, separated by 45 minutes of reflow. The rise in $PmCO_2$ ($\triangle PmCO_2$) during the coronary artery occlusion was used as an index of ischemic injury. When propranolol, hyaluronidase, or nitroglycerin were administered individually between occlusions, $\triangle PmCO_2$ fell significantly, and the combination of the three drugs caused an even more marked decline in $\triangle PmCO_2$. In contrast, isoproterenol caused $\triangle PmCO_2$ to rise. The mass spectrometric measurement of $PmCO_2$ can be used to assess directly the efficacy of interventions to limit ischemic injury. The results of this method confirmed those obtained using electrocardiographic mapping that showed that propranolol, hyaluronidase, and nitroglycerin individually limit ischemic injury, whereas isoproterenol increases it; and that the combination of propranolol, hyaluronidase and nitroglycerin exerts a markedly beneficial effect on myocardial ischemic injury following coronary occlusion.[15]

The possibility that myocardial cells could be preserved by restoring blood flow to the obstructed vessel following a period of ischemia was considered. This approach is not only of theoretical importance, but also forms the basis for the surgical restoration of blood flow in patients with developing myocardial infarction. When coronary reperfusion was carried out three hours after occlusion, it was found that there was an immediate fall in ST-segment elevation. More importantly, CK activity and histologic appearance both 24 hours and seven days later showed preservation of extensive portions of the myocardium otherwise expected to have lost their viability.[12] In addition, ventricular function was investigated using radiopaque beads implanted in the inner third of the left ventricular wall, and the paradoxical movements of the ventricle that were present after coronary occlusion ceased or became reversed a half hour after reperfusion. Thus, not only was there a reduction in myocardial damage anatomically, but the ultimate aim of restoring viable, normally functioning myocardium was achieved.

EFFECTS OF DELAYED INTERVENTIONS

The direct clinical application of the interventions mentioned above might be limited to patients who had developed an infarct under observation or who might be treated for impending myocardial infarction, unless they could be proved to be effective when applied several hours after coronary occlusion. We observed that when hyaluronidase was given 20 minutes, three hours, or six hours after coronary occlusion, significant salvage of myocardium occurred, as reflected in less reduction in CK activity and less extensive histologic damage (compared to that in untreated dogs) for any degree of ST-segment elevation.[13] However, this effect decreased progressively as the time interval between coronary occlusion and hyaluronidase injection was increased; when administered nine hours after coronary occlusion, hyaluronidase had no detectable effect, suggesting that injury had become irreversible in all jeopardized cells by this time (Fig. 4).

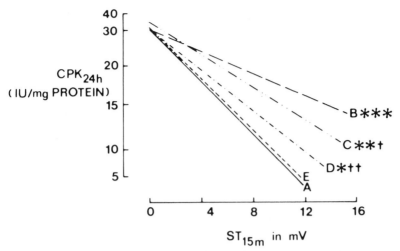

Figure 4. The relationship between ST-segment elevation 15 minutes after coronary artery occlusion (ST_{15m}) and log CK values of specimens obtained from the same sites 24 hours later. Group A (occlusion alone) (————); Group B (hyaluronidase given 20 minutes after occlusion (———); Group C (hyaluronidase given three hours after occlusion)(—··—··—); Group D (hyaluronidase given six hours after occlusion (-.-.-.); Group E (hyaluronidase given nine hours after occlusion (-------). Note that for any ST_{15m}, hyaluronidase given 20 minutes, three hours, or six hours after occlusion results in significantly greater myocardial CK activity; in contrast, hyaluronidase administered nine hours after occlusion has no such effect. (* = $p < 0.025$, ** = $p < 0.025$, *** = $p < 0.0005$ in comparison to control; † = $p < 0.025$, †† = $p < 0.0005$ in comparison to hyaluronidase at 20 minutes). (Reproduced with permission from Circ Res *41*:26–31, 1977.)

These techniques have provided interesting and, we believe, important results, but their value is limited by the fact that, as has been reviewed elsewhere,[9] ST-segment elevation recorded 15 minutes following coronary occlusion, even prior to the intervention, may not be entirely specific for myocardial ischemia. Changes in local electrolyte concentrations, particularly of potassium, in the ischemic area, in the normal tissue, and in the extracellular fluid can markedly alter the height of the ST segment. Pericarditis and intraventricular conduction defects, as well as several commonly used cardiac drugs, including the cardiac glycosides, are also known to affect the ST segment. Although these limitations can be largely controlled in experimental investigations, these considerations nevertheless prompted us to search for a technique that is entirely *independent* of changes in the ST segment and that could assess the efficacy of an intervention in reducing acute ischemic myocardial damage. It was demonstrated that the relationship between regional myocardial blood flow, measured by the radioactive microsphere technique 15 minutes after coronary occlusion, and myocardial CK activity at the same sites 24 hours later, could also be used to assess the effect of an intervention on myocardial salvage, and that favorable interventions altered this relationship so that the degree of myocardial damage as reflected in reduction of myocardial CK activity was reduced.[16] For example, in untreated dogs, sites with severe ischemia (transmural regional myocardial blood flow <15 ml/min/100 g) 15 minutes following occlusion exhibited transmural CK activity of 7.6 ± 0.6 IU/mg protein 24 hours later. In dogs given hyaluronidase 20 minutes after occlusion, sites with comparable low flows had CK activities that were significantly higher (13.1 ± 1.8 IU/mg protein). The evidence for myocardial salvage determined by several independent techniques, i.e., relating either the ST-segment or the regional myocardial blood flow measurement 15 minutes after occlusion to the evidence of necrosis as reflected in the histologic and electron-microscopic appearance, as well as in CK activity of the myocardium 24 hours later, is complementary. The results of any one of these experiments corroborate and strengthen the conclusions derived from the others.

ANATOMIC STUDIES

Perhaps the most persuasive evidence that infarct size can be limited following coronary occlusion comes from direct measurements of the infarcts themselves. We have used a rat model of coronary artery occlusion[17] to quantify infarctions directly both by serial histologic sections and by measuring total CK activity of the left ventricle. A standard-size infarct is produced in the left ventricles of Sprague-Dawley rats by occluding the left coronary artery 1 to 2 mm from its origin. The animals are sacrificed either 48 hours or 21 days after occlusion.

For the enzymatic studies, the CK activity of the homogenized whole left ventricle is measured, and infarct size is determined by comparing left ventricular CK in occluded rats with that in control (unoccluded) rats. For the histologic measurement of infarct size, the left ventricles are sectioned into slices in a plane parallel to the atrioventricular groove. Paraffin-embedded sections are prepared from each slice, stained with hematoxylin and eosin, projected onto a screen, and planimetered to determine the cross-sectional area of the entire left ventricle and of the infarcted myocardium. The effects of an intervention are determined by comparing infarct size in treated and untreated rats with coronary occlusion. Using this model we have observed that a variety of interventions administered *after* the coronary occlusion resulted in reduction of infarct size. Of greatest importance, we feel, is the finding that the beneficial effects of these interventions persist for 21 days after the coronary occlusion, at a time when the infarct is completely healed, comparable to a six-week-old infarct in man. This finding indicates that the limitation of infarct size observed 24 to 48 hours following coronary occlusion signifies permanent salvage of tissue, not simply delayed necrosis.

The usefulness of this method may be illustrated by presenting the actual values in the hyaluronidase-treated rats[17] (Fig. 5). When the animals were sacrificed 48 hours after coronary artery ligation, CK activity in the sham-operated rats averaged 12.7 ± 0.3 IU/mg of protein and in coronary-occluded rats 7.6 ± 0.2 IU/mg protein (p<0.0005). Taking into account the residual CK activity in the infarcted tissue, this difference between the two groups indicates that these untreated rats were left with 50.3 ± 2.2 per cent of their normal left ventricular myocardium. In hyaluronidase-treated rats, CK activity was 10.4 ± 0.4 IU/mg protein, corresponding to 76.4 ± 4.1 per

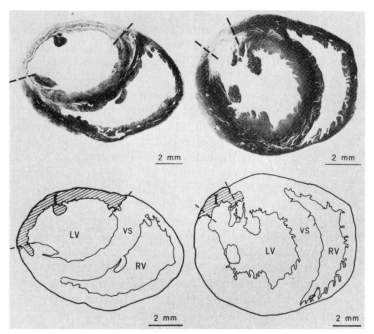

Figure 5. Histologic sections (upper panels) and diagrams (lower panels) of transverse slices of hearts of rats killed 21 days after occlusion of the left main coronary artery without (left side) and with (right side) hyaluronidase treatment: LV = left ventricle; RV = right ventricle; VS = ventricular septum; and I = infarcted myocardium. The borders of the infarctions are shown by the interrupted lines and their areas by the shaded portions of the diagrams. Note that in the rat with an occlusion alone, the infarction involved 54.1 per cent of the endocardial circumference of the left ventricle, whereas in the hyaluronidase-treated rat, it involved only 20.1 per cent. (Reproduced with permission from Science *194*:199, 1976.)

cent of the normal left ventricular myocardium. The difference in infarct size between the untreated rats and the treated rats was highly significant ($p<0.0005$) and indicated that treatment with hyaluronidase resulted in a 52.0 ± 8.1 per cent increase in the amount of preserved myocardium compared to that in the untreated rats. When infarct size was assessed histologically 48 hours after occlusion, the hyaluronidase-treated rats had 39.6 ± 7.9 per cent more viable myocardium than did the untreated controls. In the rats sacrificed 21 days after the occlusion, using the histologic method, hyaluronidase reduced the fraction of the infarcted left ventricle by an average of 36.4 ± 6.8 per cent ($p<0.0025$).

These studies demonstrated that: (1) The rat model can be used to quantify directly the extent of experimental myocardial infarction by two independent methods — total left ventricular CK activity and quantitative histology; (2) the model can be used to demonstrate and to quantify intervention-induced changes in infarct size; (3) hyaluronidase, an agent thought on the basis of indirect evidence to be capable of reducing expected infarct size, was shown to do so by direct means, and this effect was measurable; (4) the beneficial effects of hyaluronidase were apparent not only 48 hours after occlusion, but also 21 days after occlusion, when healing is complete; and (5) this drug did not appear to interfere with normal

scar formation. Following these studies with hyaluronidase, we have observed that a variety of other interventions, including beta-adrenergic
blocking agents, pentobarbital, large doses of glucocorticoids, cobra-venom
factor (an anti-inflammatory agent), ibuprofen (a nonsteroidal anti-inflammatory drug), and reserpine, all resulted in significant reductions of infarct
size.[18]

The conclusions derived from these experiments in the rat have been
amply confirmed in other species in which the effects of a variety of interventions have shown that infarct size can be reduced by direct measurement of the mass of necrotic myocardium. For example, in experiments in
the baboon in which the coronary artery was reversibly occluded for varying periods, histologic examination revealed that reperfusion carried out
within four hours after occlusion resulted in substantial salvage of myocardium and that the extent of this salvage varied inversely with the duration
of the occlusion.[19] Lucchesi and his associates[20] have studied in the dog the
effects of the dimethyl quaternary analogue of propranolol, a non–beta-
blocking drug that reduces myocardial contractility and oxygen consumption. Myocardial infarction was produced by occlusion of the left circumflex
coronary artery for 60 minutes, followed by reperfusion and measurement
of infarct volume 24 hours later, using nitro-blue tetrazolium, a dye that
stains normal but not necrotic myocardium. In untreated (control) animals,
the infarcts averaged 23.8 ± 3.2 per cent of the volume of the left ventricle,
while in treated dogs they were reduced to only 2.3 ± 0.8 per cent.[20] Similarly, Ginks et al. compared the large infarcts produced by a permanent
occlusion of the left anterior descending coronary artery with those in dogs
treated by a combination of propranolol, hypothermia, and intra-aortic balloon counterpulsation followed by release of the occlusion after three
hours. In the untreated control dogs with coronary occlusion, large infarcts
were always present on gross examination after one week. In four of six
treated dogs there was no gross infarction, and histologic changes were
minimal.[21] Hirschfeld and collaborators[22] studied the effects of a five-hour
infusion of the combination of nitroglycerin and methoxamine in closed-
chest sedated dogs subjected to coronary artery occlusion. Of the 16 untreated
control dogs, six died and the other 10 developed transmural infarcts. In contrast, of the 15 treated dogs, three died and two developed transmural infarcts;
six had only patchy subendocardial hemorrhage and four had no gross infarcts
at all.[22]

In several studies the effects of interventions on infarct size resulting
from permanent occlusions were evaluated. Shatney et al. demonstrated by
means of nitro-blue tetrazolium staining six hours after occlusion that both
propranolol and methylprednisolone administered 15 minutes after coronary occlusion resulted in reduction of infarct size.[23] Using a similar experimental design, Pierce et al. showed that propranolol administered one hour
following coronary occlusion reduced the volume of myocardial infarcts by
34 per cent.[24] Ergin and associates[14] observed that ligation of the first major
branch of the left circumflex coronary artery resulted in infarcts averaging
18.5 ± 4.4 per cent of left ventricular weight determined four days later.
Pretreatment with propranolol reduced this significantly to 10.5 ± 2.2 per

cent.[20] Rasmussen et al.[25] ligated the proximal portion of the left circumflex coronary artery, sacrificed the dog 24 hours later, and expressed necrosis as a percentage of the posterior papillary muscle. The necrotic zone averaged 85 ± 2 per cent in untreated dogs, 52 ± 4 per cent in animals pretreated with propranolol, and 71 ± 3 per cent in dogs treated with propranolol three hours following the occlusion.[25] Kloner et al.[26] sacrificed dogs three weeks following occlusion of the left anterior descending coronary artery. Viable and necrotic tissue could be easily distinguished, and infarct size was measured by planimetry of 1-cm slices. In untreated dogs the infarcts averaged 23.2 ± 2.0 per cent of the left ventricle, and in dogs treated with hyaluronidase following occlusion the infarcts were reduced to 9.0 ± 2.8 per cent (p<0.001).[26] Miura and associates found that the administration of propranolol begun before occlusion of the left anterior descending coronary artery reduced gross infarct size by an average of 53 per cent; dogs receiving propranolol three hours after coronary occlusion developed infarcts that, on the average, were 28 per cent smaller than in untreated control dogs subjected to a similar coronary occlusion.[27]

Clinical Observations

One of the most formidable barriers to the clinical application of the information that has been obtained in the laboratory is the lack of a suitable technique for assessing the efficacy, or lack thereof, of these interventions in patients. At present, myocardial ischemic injury in the clinical setting can be assessed by the following methods: (1) radionuclide scintigraphy by imaging of the myocardium after injecting an infarct-avid radionuclide; (2) release of enzymes from the injured myocardium (CK release and disappearance curves); and (3) precordial ST-segment and QRS mapping. The application of the radionuclide techniques has great potential, but their use for monitoring *changes* in the extent of an ischemic zone awaits the development of cameras having higher resolution and the availability of agents that can specifically identify injured cells and that can be used serially. The CK release and disappearance curves offer the possibility of predicting "infarct size" following at least seven hours of sampling (i.e., at least 10 hours from the onset of pain), and they are therefore of less value in studies carried out in the early hours of ischemia when the number of reversibly injured cells is maximal. Nonetheless, this technique, in which the "predicted" and "observed" infarct sizes are similar in control patients, has demonstrated that in patients with acute myocardial infarction and hypertension, administration of the vasodilator trimethaphan resulted in smaller-than-predicted observed infarcts;[28] prednisone was shown to have a similar salutary effect in one study,[29] but not in another.[30] On the other hand, the administration of digitalis glycosides to patients without heart failure appeared to result in observed infarcts that were larger than predicted.[31]

The experimental foundation for the use of ST-segment elevations recorded from multiple precordial leads was established in experiments in dogs with coronary artery occlusion with simultaneously recorded epicardial and precordial maps; these confirmed the presence of a close relationship between *changes* in epicardial and precordial ST-segment elevations.[10, 32] Interventions that caused an increase or decrease in epicardial ST-segment elevations produced similar directional changes in precordial maps.

The clinical relationship between precordial ST-segment elevation and the reversible damage to myocardial cells is well illustrated by patients with Prinzmetal's "variant" angina. In these patients, there is a temporary occlusion of a major coronary artery, most often as a result of spasm. The release of coronary spasm and subsequent abolition of ischemic injury is reflected by cessation of pain and ventricular irritability and abolition of the ST-segment elevation. However, in patients in whom the coronary flow fails to return to normal, the ischemic injury progresses and the ST segments remain elevated until a frank infarction, characterized electrocardiographically by the development in the surface electrocardiogram of Q waves and loss of R-wave potential.

A 35-lead electrode blanket was devised to record precordial maps from patients with acute infarction.[32] The precordial ST-segment mapping technique has been successfully used in patients to show that several interventions reduce precordial ST-segment elevations more rapidly than occurs in untreated controls, suggesting that these interventions effectively reduce myocardial injury while it is still in the reversible phase. These interventions include propranolol, hyaluronidase, nitroglycerin, and the inhalation of high concentrations of oxygen.[3, 9, 32] However, we have already commented upon the lack of specificity of this measurement. Therefore, there has been considerable interest in finding a non-invasive marker of myocardial viability. One such measure that is readily available clinically is the QRS complex. A reduction in the electromotive force of the epicardial R wave within four hours of experimental coronary occlusion was first demonstrated by Frank Wilson and his associates. Later it was observed that a reduction in epicardial R-wave voltage was found at sites in which ischemia produced a mixture of viable and necrotic myocardium, as determined by histologic study.

To apply this method clinically, we have proposed the use of the precordial ST segment as a predictor of the ultimate fate of the tissue, in a manner analogous to the use of the epicardial ST segment in the experimental animal. This precordial ST segment, recorded soon after the clinical event, may then be compared to the changes in the QRS complex that occur subsequently, such as the development or deepening of Q waves and the reduction of R waves;[33] these changes in the QRS complex could then be employed in a manner analogous to the alterations in CK activity or histologic appearance of the myocardium subjacent to the epicardial electrode in the experimental animal.

Experiments in our laboratory have confirmed the presence of a very close correlation between changes in the QRS complex of epicardial leads and both myocardial CK activity and histologic evidence of necrosis.[34] In these experiments, unipolar electrograms recorded from epicardial sites in open-chest dogs were analyzed for ST-segment elevation 15 minutes following coronary occlusion and for changes in Q and R waves 24 hours later. Transmural myocardial specimens were obtained 24 hours after occlusion from the same sites at which the ECGs had been recorded. Both in untreated control dogs with coronary occlusion and in dogs treated with hyaluronidase or propranolol, the development of Q waves, the fall in R waves, and their combination ($\Delta R + \Delta Q$) at 24 hours correlated well with the final depression of myocardial CK activity.[13, 34] In addition, $\Delta R + \Delta Q$ correlated well with the extent of necrosis present on histologic examination. Similar results have been obtained by other investigators.[14] From these investigations we have concluded that (1) the depth of Q-wave development and extent of the fall in R-wave voltage 24 hours after occlusion accurately reflect myocardial necrosis as measured by myocardial CK activity and by histologic appearance; (2) ST-segment elevations 15 minutes after occlusion predict subsequent changes in Q and R waves; and (3) the effectiveness of hyaluronidase and propranolol, agents shown by a variety of other techniques (including direct anatomic measurements of infarct size) to reduce myocardial necrosis following coronary artery occlusion, can be detected by a diminution in the changes in QRS morphology (i.e., less Q-wave development and smaller fall in R-wave voltage).

This method of electrocardiographic mapping has been adapted for clinical use by utilizing the ST-segment elevation in the precordial leads when the patient is first admitted to the coronary care unit as a predictor of the ultimate fate of the myocardium, in a manner analogous to the use of the epicardial ST segment in the experimental animal. The evolution of the QRS complex in those leads that demonstrate initial ST-segment elevation is then compared in control and treated groups of patients. These precordial QRS changes can be used as indices of necrosis in place of the analysis of changes in CK activity and histologic appearance of myocardial specimens.

Thus, this type of electrocardiographic analysis, while not capable of expressing the mass of infarcted myocardium or of salvaged myocardium in quantitative terms, would appear to be (1) capable of predicting the surface representation of the extent of necrosis to be expected when much of the myocardial injury is still in a reversible phase, i.e., at a time of ST-segment elevation, prior to the completion of evolution of the QRS complex; (2) capable of assessing the surface representation of the extent of necrosis that ultimately develops in any given patient or group of patients, as reflected by the changes in the QRS complexes that do develop; (3) capable of being applied immediately, so as not to delay therapy; (4) safe and atraumatic; and (5) simple to apply, easy to interpret, and inexpensive.

The effects of hyaluronidase have been assessed using this technique.[35] We randomized 91 patients with anterior infarctions into control (45 patients) or to hyaluronidase-treated (46 patients) groups. A 35-lead precordial electrocardiogram was recorded on admission and again seven days later. Hyaluronidase was administered intravenously after the first electrocardiogram and every six hours for 48 hours (Fig. 6). The sum of R-wave voltages of vulnerable sites fell more in the control group than in the hyaluronidase-

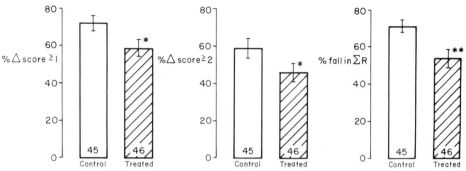

Figure 6. Changes in scores for ST-segment elevation in hyaluronidase-treated and control groups. *Left panel* shows the percentage of precordial sites with ST-segment elevations ≥0.15 mV on the admission electrocardiogram with at least minor changes in QRS complex, i.e., a score of 1 or more, in the tracing recorded on the seventh day. Numbers in the columns represent the number of patients in each group. Bars represent ± 1 SEM. The 45 control patients had 635 sites with ST-segment elevations, and the 46 hyaluronidase-treated patients had 591 sites. Note that the control patients had significantly more sites in which the QRS morphology changed at least slightly, i.e., a score of 1 or more, than the hyaluronidase-treated patients (* = p < 0.05). *Center panel* shows the percentage of precordial sites with ST-segment elevations ≥ 0.15 mV on the admission electrocardiogram with at least moderate changes in the QRS complex, i.e., a score of 2 or more, in the tracing recorded on the seventh day. In the 45 control patients the total number of vulnerable sites was 575, and in the hyaluronidase-treated patients it was 494. *Right panel* shows the percentage fall in total R-wave voltage (ΣR) in the sites with ST-segment elevation ≥ 0.15 mV on the initial electrocardiogram. Note that the controls had a significantly greater fall in R-wave voltage than the hyaluronidase-treated patients. (* = p < 0.05; ** = p < 0.01). (Reproduced by permission from N Engl J Med 296:898–903, 1977.)

treated group (70.9 ± 3.6 per cent [± 1 SEM] vs. 54.2 ± 5.0 per cent; p < 0.01). Q waves appeared in 59.3 ± 4.9 per cent of the vulnerable sites in control patients compared with 46.4 ± 4.9 per cent in hyaluronidase-treated patients (p < 0.05). Thus, the findings in this study demonstrated that hyaluronidase, when administered within the first eight hours after the onset of the clinical event, reduced the electrocardiographic evidence of myocardial necrosis in patients with acute myocardial infarction. Derrida et al.[36] have carried out a study that was virtually identical, except that they used nitroglycerin instead of hyaluronidase. They randomized 74 patients with acute myocardial infarction into control and nitroglycerin-treated groups.[36] The latter received intravenous nitroglycerin at an average rate of 51 μg/min. Using the QRS-mapping technique described above for hyaluronidase, the extent of electrocardiographic evidence of myocardial necrosis was found to be significantly reduced by nitroglycerin.

Conclusions

Experimental studies in a number of laboratories and utilizing several mammalian species — rat, dog, and baboon — have shown that several interventions are capable of reducing the quantity of myocardium that becomes necrotic following coronary occlusion. In some of these studies the intervention was applied before or simultaneously with the coronary occlusion. However, more importantly, in several investigations it was clear that significant sparing of myocardium occurred when the intervention was applied as late as six hours following the coronary occlusion. Several techniques were employed to document that tissue otherwise destined to become necrotic was salvaged. The most persuasive results came from *direct* measurements of infarct size by total tissue CK activity and histology. No comparable method for the direct measurement of myocardial salvage in man is available. However, in patients with acute myocardial infarction treated with hyaluronidase or nitroglycerin, two interventions shown to reduce infarct size in a variety of experimental preparations, the evolution of electrocardiographic signs of necrosis as reflected in the QRS complex was reduced. Intra-aortic balloon counterpulsation, as well as the administration of oxygen and propranolol, have also been shown to reduce the electrocardiographic signs of ischemic injury. These observations in patients closely resemble those made in experimental animals in which the methods of assessing necrosis are more specific since they are based on direct examination of the myocardium. Although these results in patients do not yet offer definitive proof that infarct size can be limited in man, they do offer sufficient encouragement to warrant continued clinical investigations of this important question.

References

1. Page DL, Caulfield JB, Kastor JA, DeSanctis RW, and Sanders CA: Myocardial changes associated with cardiogenic shock. N Engl J Med 285:133–137, 1971.
2. Sobel BE, Bresnahan GF, Shell WE, and Yoder RD: Estimation of infarct size in man and its relation to prognosis. Circulation 46:640–648, 1972.
3. Braunwald E (ed): Symposium on Protection of the Ischemic Myocardium. Circulation 53 (Suppl III):III-1–III-217, 1976.
4. Braunwald E: The pathogenesis and treatment of shock in myocardial infarction: topics in clinical medicine. Johns Hopkins Med J 121:421–429, 1967.
5. Maroko PR, Braunwald E, Covell JW, and Ross J Jr: Factors influencing the severity of myocardial ischemia following experimental coronary occlusion (abstr). Circulation 40(Suppl III):III-140, 1969.
6. Braunwald E, Covell JW, Maroko PR, and Ross J Jr: Effects of drugs and of counterpulsation on myocardial oxygen consumption. Circulation 40(Suppl IV):IV-220–IV-228, 1969.
7. Maroko PR, Kjekshus JK, Sobel BE, Watanabe T, Covell JW, Ross J Jr, and Braunwald E: Factors influencing infarct size following coronary artery occlusions. Circulation 43:67–82, 1971.
8. Cox JL, McLaughlin VW, Flowers NC, and Horan LG: The ischemic zone surrounding acute myocardial infarction. Its morphology as detected by dehydrogenase staining. Am Heart J 76:650–659, 1968.
9. Muller JE, Maroko PR, and Braunwald E: Precordial electrocardiographic mapping: a technique to assess the efficacy of interventions designed to limit infarct size. Circulation 57:1–18, 1978.
10. Maroko PR, and Braunwald E: Effects of metabolic and pharmacologic interventions on myocardial infarct size following coronary occlusion. Circulation 53 (Suppl I):I-162–I-168, 1976.
11. Maroko PR, Libby P, Sobel BE, Bloor CM, Sybers HD, Shell WE, Covell JW, and Braunwald E: Effect of glucose-insulin-potassium infusion on myocardial infarction following experimental coronary artery occlusion. Circulation 45:1160–1175, 1972.
12. Ginks WR, Sybers HD, Maroko PR, Covell JW, Sobel BE, and Ross J Jr: Coronary artery reperfusion. II. Reduction of myocardial infarct size at one week after coronary occlusion. J Clin Invest 51:2717–2723, 1972.
13. Hillis LD, Fishbein MC, Braunwald E, and Maroko PR: The influence of the time interval between coronary artery occlusion and the administration of hyaluronidase on salvage of ischemic myocardium in dogs. Circ Res 41:26–31, 1977.

14. Ergin MA, Dastgir G, Butt KMH, and Stuckey JH: Prolonged epicardial mapping of myocardial infarction: the effects of propranolol and intra-aortic balloon pumping following coronary artery occlusion. J Thorac Cardiovasc Surg 72:892–899, 1976.

15. Hillis LD, Khuri SF, Braunwald E, Kloner RA, Tow D, Barsamian E, and Maroko PR: Assessment of the efficacy of interventions to limit ischemic injury by direct measurement of intramural carbon dioxide tension after coronary artery occlusion in the dog. J Clin Invest 63:99–107, 1979.

16. Ribeiro LGT, Hillis LD, Louie EK, Davis MA, Maroko PR, and Braunwald E: A method for demonstrating the efficacy of interventions designed to limit infarct size following coronary occlusion: beneficial effect of hyaluronidase. Cardiovasc Res 12:334–340, 1978.

17. Maclean D, Fishbein MC, Maroko PR, and Braunwald E: Hyaluronidase-induced reductions in myocardial infarct size. Direct quantification of infarction following coronary artery occlusion in the rat. Science 194:199–200, 1976.

18. Maclean D, Fishbein MC, Braunwald E, and Maroko PR: Long-term preservation of ischemic myocardium after experimental coronary artery occlusion. J Clin Invest 61:541–555, 1978.

19. Smith GT, Soeter JR, Haston HH, and McNamara JJ: Coronary reperfusion in primates: Serial electrocardiographic and histologic assessment. J Clin Invest 54:1420–1427, 1974.

20. Lucchesi BR, Burmeister WE, Lomas TE, and Abrams GD: Ischemic changes in the canine heart as affected by the dimethyl quaternary analog of propranolol, UM-272 (SC-27761). J Pharmacol Exp Ther 199:310–328, 1976.

21. Ginks W, Ross JJ, and Sybers HD: Prevention of gross myocardial infarction in the canine heart. Arch Pathol 97:380–384, 1974.

22. Hirschfeld JW, Borer JS, Goldstein RE, Barrett MJ, and Epstein SE: Reduction in severity and extent of myocardial infarction when nitroglycerin and methoxamine are administered during coronary occlusion. Circulation 49:291–297, 1974.

23. Shatney CH, MacCarter DJ, and Lillehei RC: Effects of allopurinol, propranolol and methylprednisolone on infarct size in experimental myocardial infarctions. Am J Cardiol 37:572–580, 1976.

24. Pierce WF, Carter DR, McGarran MH, and Waldhausen JA: Modification of myocardial infarct volume: an experimental study in the dog. Arch Surg 107:682–687, 1973.

25. Rasmussen MM, Reimer KA, Kloner RA, and Jennings RB: Infarct size reduction by propranolol before and after coronary ligation in dogs. Circulation 56:794–798, 1978.

26. Kloner RA, Braunwald E, and Maroko PR: Long-term preservation of ischemic myocardium in the dog by hyaluronidase. Circulation 58:220–226, 1978.

27. Miura M, Thomas R, Ganz W, Sokol T, Shell WE, Toshimitsu T, Kwan AC, and Singh BN: The effect of delay in propranolol administration on reduction of myocardial infarct size after experimental coronary artery occlusion in dogs. Circulation 59:1148–1157, 1979.

28. Shell WE, and Sobel BE: Protection of jeopardized myocardium by ventricular afterload. N Engl J Med 291:481–486, 1974.

29. Morrison J, Reduto L, Pizzarello R, Geller K, Maley T, and Gulotta S: Modification of myocardial injury in man by corticosteroid administration. Circulation 53 (Suppl I):I-200–I-202, 1976.

30. Roberts R, DeMello V, and Sobel BE: Deleterious effects of methylprednisolone in patients with myocardial infarction. Circulation 53 (Suppl I):I-204–I-206, 1976.

31. Varonkov Y, Shell WE, Smirnov V, Gukovsky D, and Chazov EI: Augmentation of serum CPK activity by digitalis in patients with acute myocardial infarction. Circulation 55:719–727, 1977.

32. Maroko PR, Libby P, Covell JW, Sobel BE, Ross J Jr, and Braunwald E.: Precordial ST segment elevation mapping: an atraumatic method for assessing alterations in the extent of myocardial ischemic injury. Am J Cardiol 29:223–230, 1972.

33. Askenazi J, Maroko PR, Lesch M, and Braunwald E: Usefulness of ST segment elevations as predictors of electrocardiographic signs of necrosis in patients with acute myocardial infarction. Br Heart J 39:764–770, 1977.

34. Hillis LD, Askenazi J, Braunwald E, Radvany P, Muller JE, Fishbein MC, and Maroko PR: Use of changes in epicardial QRS complex to assess interventions which modify the extent of myocardial necrosis following coronary artery occlusion. Circulation 54:591–598, 1976.

35. Maroko PR, Hillis LD, Muller JE, Tavazzi L, Heyndrickx GR, Ray M, Chiariello M, Distante A, Askenazi J, Salerno J, Carpentier J, Reshetnaya NI, Radvany P, Libby P, Raabe DS, Chazov EI, Bobba P, and Braunwald E: Favorable effects of hyaluronidase on electrocardiographic evidence of necrosis in patients with acute myocardial infarction. N Engl J Med 296:898–903, 1977.

36. Derrida JP, Sal R, and Chiche P: Nitroglycerin infusion in acute myocardial infarction. N Engl J Med 297:36, 1977.

Is It Possible to Preserve Ischemic Myocardium in Acute Myocardial Infarction? Reasonable Doubts Regarding Possibilities and Benefits*

A. JAMES LIEDTKE, M.D., and
HOWARD E. MORGAN, M.D.

Departments of Medicine and Physiology
The Milton S. Hershey Medical Center
The Pennsylvania State University
Hershey, Pennsylvania

The premise upon which attempts to preserve ischemic myocardium have been based is that pump failure accounts for in-hospital deaths of most patients with ischemic heart disease and that death rate and morbidity can be reduced by preserving myocardium in the ischemic zone. Although the first portion of this premise is true and the second portion follows logically, several questions must be addressed before adopting this goal: (1) Is it possible in man to salvage ischemic myocardium that would otherwise have progressed to infarction? (2) Is the benefit to be derived from salvage of myocardium in the ischemic zone worth the risk of other complications, such as the immediate side effects of the therapy and longer-term complications, for example, life-threatening arrhythmias and severe angina? At the present time, the answers to these questions are unknown, but they are high-priority topics for both basic and clinical investigation. Salvage of ischemic myocardium in animal models has been demonstrated, but it has not been shown whether

*Work from the authors' laboratory was supported by NIH Grants HL-18258 and HL-21209

311

long-term ventricular function is significantly improved or whether the frequency of arrhythmias is increased as a result of preserving ischemic myocardium.

In attempting to understand how ischemic myocardium can be prevented from progressing to infarction, several issues must be discussed, including (1) the structural relationships of the normal and infarcted myocardium and the border zone in animal models; (2) the potential for improvement in the balance between energy production and utilization in ischemic myocardium; (3) the extension and/or healing of the infarct in animals and man; (4) techniques for quantitation of infarcted myocardium, particularly as related to evaluation of therapeutic regimens in man; and (5) the mechanism of action of therapeutic agents and the potential for both acute and delayed side effects.

Structural relationships of normal and infarcted myocardium and the border zone in animal models.   Three points need to be made in relation to this topic: (1) The lateral borders of the ischemic area are sharp and are determined largely by the size of the vascular bed of the occluded vessel and presence of preformed collaterals.[2] (2) Infarction occurs as a wave front, beginning at the subendocardium and spreading toward the epicardium. Irreversible damage to cells in the subendocardium begins after 20 to 40 minutes of ischemia. (3) The border zone, if defined as an area of damaged but potentially salvageable cells, is not static, but rather is a rim of tissue at the interface between irreversibly damaged cells and aerobic cells. The location of this zone progresses from subendocardium to subepicardium during evolution of the infarct.

The concept of protecting ischemic myocardium is based on the view that a myocardial infarct is a region of central necrosis surrounded by a substantial amount of abnormal but viable tissue.[1] The border zone is considered to be large in size and to consist of partially oxygenated cells. This arrangement is thought to last several hours before cells in the border zone are irreversibly damaged. The putative border zone is considered to be the area where treatment would have the best chance to salvage ischemic cells from irreversible injury. Such a concept of an infarct is based on gradations in histochemical, mechanical, electrophysiological, and biochemical parameters that also could have resulted from interdigitated areas of ischemic and normal myocardium with sharp borders between them. In either case, the "border zone" has been visualized as a static rather than a constantly changing boundary. For example, partial oxygenation could result from a mixture of intervals of adequate oxygen supply and inadequate oxygenation per unit time rather than a gradient of oxygen tension from the normal tissue to the center of the infarct. The fraction of time that the cells were provided adequate oxygenation would depend upon the balance between supply and demand. Recently two groups of investigators have provided evidence that the "border zone" is sharp and, at any one moment, is likely to consist of a mixture of adequately oxygenated and deoxygenated cells.[3, 4]

Barlow and Chance[3] and Williamson et al.[4] investigated oxygen gradients in the perfused rat heart by measurements of the oxygenation of cytochrome aa_3, myoglobin, and nicotinamide-adenine dinucleotide (NAD). Although the affinity of oxygen for myoglobin and cytochrome aa_3 differs by two orders of magnitude, oxygenation of these two substances decreased together, suggesting the presence of very steep oxygen gradients. A further indication of the steepness of oxygen gradients in hypoxic and ischemic myocardium was obtained by measuring NADH fluorescence from the surface of perfused rat hearts. Fluorescence was almost entirely accounted for by the reduced form of NAD, as indicated by enzymatic and chemical assays. As seen in Figure 1, photographs of the fluorescence of the surface of the heart subjected to coronary artery ligation revealed white areas of NADH fluorescence against a

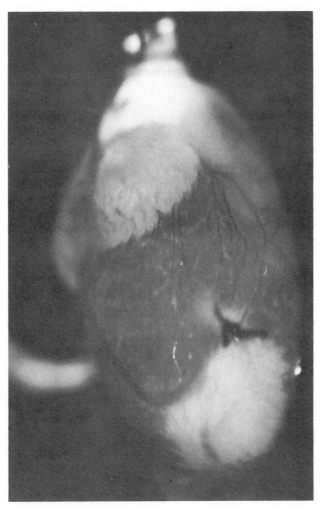

Figure 1. NADH fluorescence photography of a perfused rat heart following coronary ligation. Excitation light was provided by two xenon flash tubes with quartz envelopes for maximum transmission of the ultraviolet spectrum. Proper orientation of the two flash patterns resulted in uniform illumination of a circle with a radius of 1 inch. Colored glass filters (transmission 330 to 380 nm) were mounted in the light path between the flash tubes and the heart. Photographs were taken with a Fairchild oscilloscope camera using Kodak Royal-X Pan film. The ischemic area is near the apex, caused by ligation of a coronary artery with the black silk suture that is visible at the top of the highly fluorescent ischemic area. (From Barlow and Chance, 1976.)

darker background in which the nucleotide was more oxidized. A sharp transition between intense NADH fluorescence and little NADH fluorescence indicated that the oxygen gradient was steep. Areas of intermediate fluorescence were not observed, as would have been expected if partially oxygenated cells were present. Lack of oxygen appears to be the major factor accounting for NADH reduction, but the mechanical activity of the ischemic segment and the availability of oxidative substrates also influence the extent of NADH reduction. The tissue within the area of NADH fluorescence would be completely dependent upon anaerobic metabolism for ATP production. The surrounding area with little NADH fluorescence is likely to have sufficient oxygen to oxidize cytochrome aa_3 and thus to be able to sustain aerobic ATP production. It also is apparent that the evaluation of NADH fluorescence, as shown in Figure 1, is a static measurement. If sequential pictures of the fluorescent zone were available, they might reveal that the border was not fixed over a period of time. If this were the case, the cells that were capable of aerobic metabolism part of the time could represent cells that could be salvaged. These cells would be included in areas both with intense fluorescence and areas with little fluorescence.

Kirk and Sonnenblick[5] also have attempted to define the topography of the border zone. The tissue at risk following occlusion of the left anterior descending coronary artery (LAD) was defined by injection of different radioactive microspheres sequentially before and 10 minutes after ligation of the LAD. During the first injection, microspheres destined for the LAD were trapped while perfusion of the LAD bed was maintained at the same perfusion pressure. The technique allowed the interdigitation of normal and ischemic myocardium to be defined at one point in time. After ligation of the LAD, myocardial blood flow was normal in all parts of the nonischemic tissue, including the region immediately adjacent to the ischemic zone. Within the ischemic area, flow was reduced to a similar extent from one side of the ischemic zone to the other, although endocardial flow was less than epicardial flow. The transition between reduced and normal flow was sharp, indicating that the zone of moderately ischemic myocardium was quite small. Blood delivered to the ischemic myocardium was via preformed collaterals of the LAD rather than via small vessel connections at the border between normal and ischemic tissue. After 24 hours, the lateral limits of necrosis were determined by the anatomical distribution of the ligated artery. The transmural depth of necrosis depended largely on the status of perfusion within the ischemic zone. After 24 hours, flow in the subepicardium increased at the expense of the necrotic zone in the subendocardium. These studies, together with measurements of NADH fluorescence, indicate that at any one moment the lateral borders of the ischemic zones are sharp and determined largely by the anatomical distribution of the vessel. The lateral border may fluctuate somewhat with time, but the transmural border moves progressively outward in the first few hours after coronary artery ligation. It is within the subepicardium and mid-myocardium that cells are most likely to be salvaged.

A wave front of necrosis extending from subendocardium to subepicardium has been observed by Reimer and co-workers[6] following ligation of the circumflex artery in the dog heart (Fig. 2). These studies indicate that about half of the ischemic myocardium that is necrotic at 24 hours is dead by 40 minutes. In the mid-myocardium and subepicardium, cell death occurs more slowly. After three hours, about one third of the ischemic myocardium is still salvageable, but little such tissue remains after six hours in this model. Continuous administration of propranolol throughout the period of ischemia salvaged cells on the epicardial wave front of the developing infarct. The potential for salvage by propranolol depended upon the amount of ischemic but still viable myocardium available at the time therapy was begun. Pretreat-

PROGRESSION OF CELL
DEATH VS. TIME

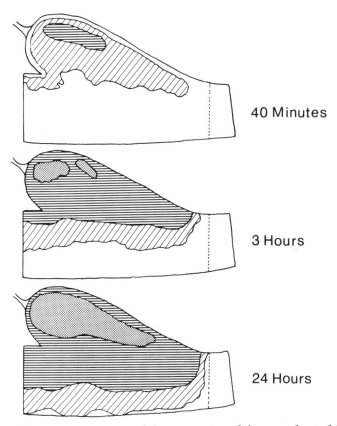

40 Minutes

3 Hours

24 Hours

Figure 2. Diagrammatic summary of the progression of the wave front of ischemic cell death (as it occurs in the posterior papillary muscle and underlying myocardium) with respect to duration of circumflex coronary occlusion. Necrosis, indicated by any of the shaded areas, occurs first in the subendocardial myocardium, and with longer durations of coronary occlusion involves progressively more of the transmural thickness of the ischemic zone. (The dashed line on the right-hand side of the diagram indicates the anatomic boundary between ischemic circumflex and non-ischemic left anterior descending coronary beds). Some additional features of the necrosis that occurs in this model are indicated on the diagram. A central area of poor perfusion with persistent coagulation necrosis (dotted areas) often develops after three or more hours of ischemia. This, as well as the hemorrhage and hyperemia indicated by horizontal lines, presumably are a reflection of microvascular necrosis. (From Reimer et al, 1977.)

ment with the drug salvaged 39 per cent of ischemic myocardium, while therapy beginning three hours after occlusion salvaged 16 per cent of the tissue at risk. The extent and progression of injury again were related to the distribution of the existing circulation and collaterals.

The concept of the border zone as a constantly changing rather than static area of jeopardized myocardium, particularly in the mid-myocardium and subepicardium, raises questions concerning the goals and effectiveness of treatment. Since the salvaged tissue will be mid-myocardium and subepicardium, contractility of this tissue of necessity will be modified by the fibrotic zone beneath it when healing is complete. Whether the contractile function that such a zone can achieve is worth the risk of arrhythmias and angina caused by the remaining ischemic myocardium is the essence of this controversy.

Potential for improvement in the balance between energy production and utilization in ischemic myocardium.   Salvageable myocardium in the ischemic zone likely consists of cells that oscillate between severe oxygen deficiency and sufficient oxygen to oxidize the terminal electron acceptors of the respiratory chain. This conclusion focuses attention on the possibility of improving energy production or decreasing energy utilization within these cells.[7] Anaerobic production of ATP is restricted to the glycolytic pathway and to substrate-level phosphorylation within the citric acid cycle. In aerobic myocardium, glycolysis accounts for approximately one per cent of total ATP production; the bulk of energy production is accounted for by oxidation of free fatty acids (approximately 80 per cent), lactate, and glucose. In hearts perfused at high rates of coronary flow with buffer gassed with N_2CO_2, the glycolytic rate increases 10-fold, but even with this degree of acceleration, energy production is only 10 per cent of that found in well-oxygenated hearts. In this situation, the glycolytic rate is restricted by accumulation of metabolites, particularly NADH, lactate, and hydrogen ions. In oxygen-deficient tissues in which coronary flow is also reduced, as in the ischemic myocardium, the glycolytic rate may be unchanged or inhibited compared with that in well-oxygenated tissue. Accumulation of NADH, lactate, and hydrogen ions, the products of the pathway, rather than lack of glucose, the substrate, accounts for glycolytic inhibition. These considerations indicate that a substantial increase in ATP production cannot be achieved in severely ischemic cells, such as those undergoing cell death within 20 to 40 minutes of circumflex coronary artery ligation in the dog. Only restoration of coronary flow that would provide oxygen and improve wash-out of metabolites would be of benefit.

ATP production in cells that oscillate between periods of anaerobic and aerobic metabolism may be improved by appropriate metabolic interventions. At the end of an anaerobic period, cytosolic and mitochondrial levels of NADH are high, tissue levels of the products of glycolysis and fatty acid activation, such as lactate, hydrogen ions, long-chain acyl CoA, and long-chain acyl carnitine, are present in large amounts, and energy levels are low. If oxygen availability increases, mitochondrial NADH can be oxidized rapidly. On the other hand, oxidation of cytosolic NADH depends on transport of reducing equivalents into the mitochondria via the malate-aspartate shuttle or on conversion of pyruvate to lactate. An increase in ATP production via glycolysis will not occur until the levels of cytosolic NADH decrease. Interventions such as provision of pyruvate and additional buffering capacity will (1) aid in reoxidation of NADH through the conversion of pyruvate to lactate; (2) provide an oxidative substrate that will not generate additional reducing equivalents in the cytosol and that bypasses the inhibited pathways of glycolysis and β-oxidation; and (3) increase intracellular pH and accelerate glycolytic rate.[8] Provision of high levels of glucose and insulin would not be expected to be as effective in increasing ATP production, since these agents would not facilitate oxidation of NADH or increase intracellular pH. However, glucose and insulin may protect ischemic myocardium in other ways, for example, by inhibiting activity of the lysosomal system or by inhibiting lipolysis in adipose tissue and thereby reducing plasma free fatty acids.

Energy utilization decreases rapidly in severely ischemic cells, apparently owing to a fall in pH and interference with the calcium cycle. Contractility is markedly reduced before ATP levels are substantially lowered. Further reduction in energy utilization by a decrease in afterload, heart rate, and inotropic state would be of benefit, particularly since the potential for increasing energy production is limited. Overall, an improvement in the energy balance of the cell, short of restoration of blood flow, must depend upon (1) improved wash-out of metabolites, (2) provision of a readily oxidizable substrate and reoxidation of cytosolic NADH, and (3) decreased ATP consumption.

Extension and/or healing of infarction in animals and man. Knowledge of the sequence of changes to be expected in healing of an infarct is extremely important in interpreting hemodynamic, electrophysiologic, and biochemical data bearing on infarct size. Since the anatomical distribution of the ligated artery appears to determine the lateral limits of the ischemic region and necrosis, lateral extension should be relatively uncommon and would involve obstruction in adjacent vascular systems, relative ischemia in the normal tissue around the ischemic zone due to ventricular dilatation and increased wall stress, or interference with collateral flow due to edema or other changes in the ischemic myocardium.[9] On the other hand, a clinical study involving serial ST-segment mapping following acute anterior transmural infarction revealed an increase in total ST-segment elevation at about six days in over 80 per cent of patients.[10] These changes were interpreted as evidence of necrosis of additional myocardium, especially since some patients had a secondary rise in serum creatine phosphokinase, pain, or congestive heart failure. On the other hand, Hutchins and Bulkley[9] investigated 76 consecutive clinically diagnosed and autopsy-proven myocardial infarcts less than 30 days old. Extension, defined as new necrosis around an infarct, was found in only 17 per cent of cases; while expansion, defined as dilatation and thinning of the area of infarction, but not complicated by additional necrosis, was present in 59 per cent of acute myocardial infarcts. This study demonstrated that expansion is a common complication of acute myocardial infarction that may account for poorer ventricular function through dilatation and may *mimic* infarct extension.

Expansion of infarction would increase the akinetic area, as estimated from ventriculograms or by other techniques. Similarly, as in the study of Reid et al.,[10] the area of electrocardiographic abnormalities would increase. It also seems possible that wash-out of myocardial proteins, such as creatine phosphokinase, would be affected by changes in myocardial dimensions. In this context, the meaning of reduced areas of abnormal QRS complexes can be questioned. If an intervention designed to protect ischemic myocardium reduces the area of Q waves, does this mean that the intervention has achieved its goal of less tissue necrosis, or alternatively, has the intervention affected only the mechanical properties and/or healing process within the necrotic zone? At this time, there appears to be no firm basis for a choice between these possibilities.

Techniques for quantitation of infarcted myocardium in man. In animals, direct pathological examination of the heart has established that interventions designed to protect ischemic myocardium can reduce infarct size following coronary artery ligation. In man, quantitation of infarct size is much more difficult, a situation that has fostered innovative techniques for its measurement. Electrocardiographic examination of ST-segment elevation and morphologic and temporal changes in QRS configuration are used most commonly. Pardee[11] first employed ST-segment elevation as an index of myocardial infarction; this measurement has remained one of the classic objective criteria in diagnosing this condition. The changing pattern of the QRS wave with time also has correlated well with irreversible myocardial damage. A progressive fall in R-wave voltage and development of a Q wave are seen most commonly. Despite the usefulness of these measurements as qualitative indices of ischemia and necrosis, they suffer from several difficulties when used to quantitate infarct size and to evaluate the effectiveness of various therapies. The electrical wave forms of both ventricular depolarization and repolarization are nonspecifically affected by several conditions other than cell necrosis. The ST segment can be influenced by sympathetic stimulation, pericarditis, changes in temperature, development of intraventricular conduction delays, and various drugs, including digitalis, quinidine, electrolytes, and modifiers of calcium efflux, such as verapamil. The QRS pattern, particularly the voltage of the R wave, is sensitive to day-to-day fluctuations in the mean QRS axis, the development of intraventricular conduction delays, and any attenuator of electrical forces, such as intervening lung tissue or fluid accumulations in the pleura or pericardial spaces, which are not uncommon occurrences in myocardial infarction. Both ST-segment and QRS wave forms are at their least sensitive electrical gain at precordial sites.

Recently, other criticisms have been discussed.[12] For example, mechanisms of ST-segment elevation involve interactions between normal and abnormal tissue, so that any factor influencing either area will alter the height of this segment, regardless of a change in the severity of myocardial ischemia. If drugs designed to protect ischemic myocardium influence normal tissue, false positive and negative responses would result that would interfere with interpretation of therapeutic effects. Second, the ST segment is uniquely sensitive to the spatial geometry of the infarct both with respect to placement of the sensing electrode on the epicardium or precordium and to placement either at the periphery of the infarcted tissue or over its epicenter.[13] For example, by precordial monitoring, an extension of injury in the subepicardium may cancel the ST-segment elevation from a concomitant epicardial injury, thus normalizing the ST segment with respect to the isoelectric line. If this type of change occurred following treatment, the therapy could be viewed as efficacious, when in fact the agent had extended the ischemic process. Even if the ST-segment elevation is taken together with the changing temporal profile of the QRS wave, interpretation is clouded by the distinction between extension and expansion of infarction and effects of therapeutic agents to reduce cell death as compared to modification of the size and electrical properties of the necrotic zone.

Serial monitoring of serum levels of creatine phosphokinase (CPK) has been proposed as a method to quantitate infarct size.[14] The enzyme is abundant in myocardium, skeletal muscle, and brain, and the MB isoenzyme is specific for the myocardium. Following myocardial infarction, CPK activity in necrotic tissue declines rapidly; a fraction of this enters the blood from which it is cleared. Another portion of the enzyme enters the myocardial lymph in which CPK activity is unstable. Integration of the curve depicting release and clearance of CPK from blood has been used to quantitate infarct size. The mathematical model used to predict infarct size is sensitive to several variables, including the fraction of CPK released from the necrotic zone, the fraction of body water in which the enzyme distributes, the amount of CPK depleted per gram of myocardium, and the rate at which CPK is cleared from plasma. Serum levels of CPK are estimated at hourly intervals for 10 hours, every two hours from 12 to 24 hours, and every four hours for the next two days. These data allow for construction of the complete time course of CPK release and disappearance, and infarct size has been derived assuming that disappearance follows a single exponential. Recently, disappearance has been found to consist of two exponential functions. When the data were analyzed on the latter basis, a higher fraction of CPK disappearing from the myocardium could be accounted for in the plasma. Effects of pharmacologic interventions, such as agents that modify the inotropic state of the heart, and pathophysiologic phenomena, such as decreased cardiac output, on the two components of the disappearance curve have not been defined, but these factors are known to modify the overall degradative rate. Determination of the complete time-activity curve allows for an estimate of infarct size and for the possibility of comparing groups of patients that are treated in different ways. In man, in whom the size of an individual infarct may vary enormously, as much as 100-fold from patient to patient, extremely large groups of randomized patients will be needed to establish the effectiveness of an intervention.

In an effort to use each patient as his own control, data obtained in the first seven hours of observation have been used to predict the shape of the complete time-activity curve for CPK in plasma. Although initial experience with this method was encouraging, further use of the method has shown that the predicted curve bears only a general relationship to the observed values, indicating that substantial deviation can occur in individual patients. Aside from the methodologic limitations, the time delay of seven hours needed for the prediction of the curve, together with the average elapsed time (eight to 10 hours) between onset of symptoms and arrival of the patient in the coronary care unit, makes salvage of myocardium unlikely. As noted above, little salvageable myocardium remained six hours after ligation of the circumflex artery in the dog.

Newer techniques employing radionuclides and other radiological techniques have been developed to assess the presence and extent of myocardial infarction. Radionuclides may distribute in either normally perfused myocardium (cold-spot imaging) or infarcted myocardium (hot-spot imaging). Agents for cold-spot imaging distribute in normal myocardium in proportion to the regional blood flow and cross cell membranes by the ion transport system. Thallium-201 can demarcate zones of normal versus restricted perfusion, particularly if images obtained at rest and during exercise are compared. The most commonly used hot-spot agent is ^{99m}Tc-pyrophosphate, which distributes in the same manner as calcium in infarcting cells. While both methods give an approximation of the area of the infarct, they lack the resolution required to define small infarcts and require mathematical modeling to determine configurations of the margin. Because of delays in incorporation and distribution in the myocardium and the half-lives of the tracers, neither can be used sequentially to monitor early changes in infarct size. Newer radiographic techniques, including radioiodine-labeled antimyosin antibody binding and emission-computerized axial tomography, have not been established as methods for determining infarct size.

Mechanism of action of therapeutic agents and the potential for acute and delayed side effects. Agents designed to protect ischemic myocardium are known to (1) decrease energy consumption, (2) increase coronary flow and oxygen delivery, (3) provide substrate for energy production, (4) facilitate wash-out of metabolic products, (5) inhibit degradative enzymes within the myocardium, (6) stabilize cellular and intracellular membranes, (7) inhibit the inflammatory reaction, (8) stabilize cardiac lysosomes, and (9) reduce edema formation.[15] At least 32 substances have been reported to have a beneficial effect on ischemic myocardium. The sheer size of the list of effects and agents points out the fact that the mechanism of cell death in ischemic myocardium is not known, and as a result, various assumptions have been made in designing therapy. This approach is, at best, descriptive and could be approved with moderate enthusiasm for carefully controlled studies in animals in which infarct size can actually be measured. However, the animal studies have not been carried out in a randomized, blind manner that allows for critical evaluation of both short-term and long-term effects of therapy. Instead, large transmural infarcts, often involving the entire free wall of the left ventricle, are compared with much smaller transmural infarcts in animals treated with the agent of current interest. Since the lateral borders of infarction appear to be determined by the anatomic size of the vascular bed, the effectiveness of the agent may be much less than appears.

In man, the empirical approach to protecting ischemic myocardium is complicated by the fact that many of the interventions may not be innocuous. Several of these agents are vasoactive and may detrimentally affect afterload, either by increasing myocardial demands or lowering perfusion pressure in various organs, including the heart. Although propranolol is one of the most promising drugs in the treatment of myocardial ischemia, its continued administration during or immediately following myocardial infarction calls attention to its dangers as a negative inotropic and chronotropic drug. One can go through almost the entire list of proposed therapeutic modalities currently being advocated for salvaging ischemic myocardium, based on animal experimentation, and raise questions as to whether there is a potential immediate hazard in their use in man with myocardial infarction.

Conclusions

The current situation in regard to protecting ischemic myocardium in animals and man appears to be as follows: (1) The mechanism of cell death in ischemic tissue is presently unknown but appears to result from an imbalance of energy production and utilization. (2) The lateral borders of the area of infarction are determined largely by the size of the vascular bed of the occluded vessel; salvageable cells are in the mid-myocardium and subepicardium. (3) Salvage of ischemic myocardium has been demonstrated in animals, although future studies should be designed to provide an evaluation of both long-term and short-term effects. (4) Methods for measuring infarct size in man are qualitative rather than quantitative; one must *hope* that a reduction in infarct size as assessed by a combination of electrocardiographic, radiologic, and biochemical techniques will be indicative of an actual decrease in cell death.

If one assumes that ischemic myocardium can be salvaged in man, the question posed earlier remains. Is the contractile function that the salvaged myocardium can achieve worth the risk of arrhythmias and angina that may be caused by this tissue? Preliminary data derived from patients resuscitated from out-of-hospital ventricular fibrillation suggest that long-term survival was significantly better if the episode was associated *with* acute myocardial infarction than if no necrosis occurred.[16] As seen in Figure 3, the mortality rate for the entire group was 30 per cent and 41 per cent at the end of years one and

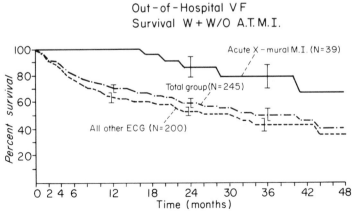

Figure 3. Survival following resuscitation from out-of-hospital ventricular fibrillation through June 1, 1974. The smaller subgroup with acute transmural myocardial infarction showed a significantly greater survival. (From Cobb et al, 1975.)

two, respectively. In those having acute transmural infarction in association with the episode, a significantly lower mortality is apparent. None of these patients died in the first 16 months and only 14 per cent were dead at the end of two years. In contrast, the two-year mortality rate in those without transmural infarction was 47 per cent. These observations suggest that old, but not recent, infarction is common in patients who develop sudden cardiac death, but that survival from this complication may be improved by eliminating viable but marginally ischemic cells by fresh infarction. Whether similar loci will be created by salvage of myocardium in the ischemic zone is unknown, but this possibility should be a deterrent to those who suggest widespread use in man of the agents designed to protect ischemic myocardium. It is clear that further work in this area in man should, at the present time, remain in the experimental realm until both the short-term and long-term effects of therapy can be evaluated.

References

1. Hood WB Jr: Modification of infarct size. In Brest AN, Wiener L, Chung EK, and Kasparian H (eds): Myocardial Infarction. Philadelphia, FA Davis Co, 1975, p 259.
2. Jennings RB, and Reimer KA: Salvage of ischemic myocardium. Mod Concepts Cardiovasc Dis 43:125, 1974.
3. Barlow CH, and Chance B: Ischemic areas in perfused rat hearts: measurement of NADH fluorescence photography. Science 193:909, 1976.
4. Williamson JR, Steenbergen C, Deleeuw G, and Barlow C: Heterogeneity of the hypoxic state in perfused rat heart. Circ Res 41:606, 1977.
5. Hirzel HO, Sonnenblick EH, and Kirk ES: Absence of a lateral border zone of intermediate creatine phosphokinase depletion surrounding a central infarct 24 hours after acute coronary occlusion in the dog. Circ Res 41:673, 1977.
6. Reimer KA, Lowe JE, Rasmussen MM, and Jennings RB: The wavefront phenomenon of ischemic cell death. 1. Myocardial infarct size vs duration of coronary occlusion in dogs. Circulation 56:786, 1977.
7. Neely JR, and Morgan HE: Relationship between carbohydrate and lipid metabolism and the energy balance of heart muscle. Ann Rev Physiol 36:1118, 1974.
8. Liedtke AJ, Nellis SH, Neely JR, and Hughes HC: Effects of treatment with pyruvate and tromethamine in experimental myocardial ischemia. Circ Res 39:378, 1976.
9. Hutchins GM, and Bulkley BH: Expansion versus extension: two different complications of acute myocardial infarction. Am J Cardiol 39:323, 1977.
10. Reid PR, Taylor DR, Kelly DT, Weisfeldt ML, Humphries JO, Ross RS, and Pitt B: Myocardial-infarct extension detected by ST-segment mapping. N Engl J Med 290:123, 1974.
11. Pardee HEB: Electrocardiographic sign of coronary artery obstruction. Arch Intern Med 26:244, 1920.
12. Fozzard HA, and DasGupta DS: ST-segment potentials and mapping. Circulation 54:533, 1976.
13. Holland RP, and Brooks H: Precordial and epicardial surface potentials during myocardial ischemia in the pig. Circ Res 37:471, 1975.
14. Shell WE, and Sobel BE: Biochemical markers of ischemic injury. Circulation 53 (Suppl I): I-98, 1976.
15. Maroko PR, and Braunwald E: Effects of metabolic and pharmacologic interventions on myocardial infarct size following coronary occlusion. Circulation 53 (Suppl I):I-162, 1976.
16. Cobb LA, Baum RS, Alvarez H 3d, and Schaffer WA: Resuscitation from out-of-hospital ventricular fibrillation: 4 years follow-up. Circulation 52 (Suppl III):III-223, 1975.

Comment

Braunwald, Maroko, and their associates proposed over a decade ago that the ischemic border surrounding a central area of myocardial infarction might be salvageable. They suggested that certain interventions, by altering the balance between myocardial oxygen demand and supply or improving the plight of the ischemic cell by other mechanisms, would salvage tissue that otherwise would go on to necrosis during an acute myocardial infarction. They and others have now accumulated impressive experimental data in a variety of animal species, using over 50 different interventions that resulted in the infarct size being less than that anticipated had the intervention been omitted. There seems little doubt, and Drs. Liedtke and Morgan do not dispute this, that the extent of myocardial necrosis, under certain experimental circumstances, can be diminished in the experimental animal.

The question remains, however, as to whether some of these interventions can be successfully applied to man during a natural myocardial infarction. The problem is complicated, since the tools primarily used to quantify infarct size in man, namely, radionuclide scintigraphs, serial serum CPK values, R-wave and ST-segment mapping, are all relatively crude. They are questionable techniques in terms of making conclusions regarding changes in infarct size in any given patient. Aside from methodological problems, observations in man are complicated by the fact that the usual patient with myocardial infarction does not enter the hospital until several hours after the onset of his infarction. Even in the experimental animal, interventions must be instituted within six hours to be beneficial, and even then this benefit is less than when the intervention is instituted earlier. Furthermore, some of the pharmacologic agents used in the experimental animal may produce significant hemodynamic alterations that might prove harmful secondarily. Finally, and perhaps most seriously, the long-term consequences from use of interventions designed to salvage ischemic myocardium in man are unknown. It is reasonable to worry that cells that survive when they would otherwise have died may be prone to chronic hypoxia and serve as the future site of life-threatening arrhythmias or post–myocardial infarction angina, or even as the site of a future myocardial infarction.

For these reasons, the use of agents designed to salvage ischemic myocardium in man must be considered experimental today. Their routine application to the patient with acute myocardial infarction is unwarranted. However, the National Heart, Lung, and Blood Institute is undertaking a large-scale clinical trial of some of the more promising of these agents. Perhaps in several years we will be in a better position to judge whether this ingenious concept will have clinical applicability.

ELLIOT RAPAPORT, M.D.

Fourteen

Has Routine Invasive Hemodynamic Monitoring in the CCU Lowered Mortality?

HEMODYNAMIC MONITORING IN THE CORONARY CARE
UNIT REDUCES MORTALITY
Kanu Chatterjee, M.B., M.R.C.P.

ROUTINE INVASIVE HEMODYNAMIC MONITORING IN
THE CCU HAS LOWERED MORTALITY: ARGUMENTS
AGAINST THE HYPOTHESIS
Arthur Selzer, M.D.

COMMENT

Hemodynamic Monitoring in the Coronary Care Unit Reduces Mortality

KANU CHATTERJEE, M.B., M.R.C.P.

Professor of Medicine; Associate Chief, Cardiovascular Division; Director, Coronary Care Unit, University of California, Moffitt Hospital, San Francisco, California

Capability of early detection of potentially life-threatening dysrhythmias and their prompt management in the present-day coronary care unit seem to have significantly reduced the mortality from primary dysrhythmias in patients with acute myocardial infarction. As a result, pump failure has emerged as the principal cause of death. Mortality from pump failure is also directly related to its severity. While the infarct size is the major determinant of the severity of depression of cardiac function, factors other than the infarct size may also induce severe hemodynamic alterations and impairment of cardiac function. For example, a strategically located but small infarct in the interventricular septum or in the papillary muscle may impose severe hemodynamic burdens by producing ventricular septal defect or mitral incompetence. Similarly, contiguous large areas of ischemic, nonfunctioning, but viable, myocardium may be responsible for severe impairment of left ventricular function even when the actual size of the infarct may be relatively smaller at the onset of the clinical syndrome of acute myocardial infarction. Severe pump failure may also be precipitated by a small, recent infarct in patients with previous infarct.

Whatever the immediate mechanism of pump failure is in patients with acute myocardial infarction, it is now well established that it is associated with a serious prognosis. The more severe the depression of cardiac function, the worse the prognosis.

Although the occurrence of left ventricular dysfunction can be suspected at the bedside by the presence of gallop sounds, reduced intensity of the first heart sound, paradoxical splitting of the second heart sound, and signs of pulmonary congestion, it has proved difficult to predict the degree

327

Table 1. *Examples of Disparity Between Clinical and Hemodynamic Findings of Left Ventricular (LV) Dysfunction Following Acute Myocardial Infarction*

CLINICAL CLASS	SYMPTOMS	ABNORMAL SIGNS	CHEST X-RAY	CARDIAC INDEX (L/MIN/M²)	LVFP (MM HG)
Uncomplicated	Nil	S_3, S_4	Prominent pulmonary veins	1.4	12
Uncomplicated	Diaphoresis Dizziness	S_3, S_4	Normal	2.2	30
Mild LV Failure	Dyspnea Diaphoresis	S_3, S_4	Normal	3.1	15
Mild LV Failure	Dyspnea	S_3, S_4	Pulmonary edema	2.1	19
Severe LV Failure	Dyspnea	S_3, S_4	Pulmonary edema	3.6	28
Severe LV Failure	Dyspnea	S_3, S_4	Prominent pulmonary veins	2.4	18
Cardiogenic Shock	Cold, clammy skin; oliguria; mental confusion	S_3, S_4	Normal	0.98	25
Cardiogenic Shock	Diaphoresis	S_3, S_4	Pulmonary edema	1.4	38

LVFP = left ventricular filling pressure

of depression of left ventricular function with useful precision. In patients with acute myocardial infarction, gallop sounds may exist in the presence of mild or very severe pump failure; paradoxical splitting of the second heart sound may be absent owing to shortening of the left ventricular ejection time because of reduced stroke volume. Significant cardiomegaly may not be present even in the presence of severe pump failure. Sustained outward movement of the left ventricular apex indicates, in most patients, reduced ejection fraction; however, the magnitude of reduction of ejection fraction cannot be precisely determined. Signs of pulmonary venous congestion may not always appear simultaneously with the elevation of pulmonary venous pressure. In Table 1, hemodynamic and radiologic findings, along with the symptoms and physical signs, in a selected group of patients with recent myocardial infarction are shown. Although all patients had gallop sounds suggesting left ventricular dysfunction, radiologic and hemodynamic findings were widely different. Thus, disparity frequently exists between hemodynamic and clinical findings of left ventricular dysfunction.

Non-invasive investigative tools such as echocardiography and radionuclide imaging techniques are being increasingly used to evaluate left ventricular function. Although such investigations undoubtedly provide useful information, changes in left ventricular function during therapeutic interventions cannot be detected easily, reliably, or repeatedly in acutely ill patients. Therefore, despite their potentials, these techniques cannot be used presently for management of acutely ill cardiac patients.

Direct hemodynamic measurements allow relatively accurate assessment of left ventricular function and provide sensitive prognostic indices for patients with acute myocardial infarction. Determinations of specific hemodynamic deficits in individual patients are essential for the diagnosis of hemodynamic subsets and, thus, for delivery of rational therapy to the patients. Evaluation of any therapy can also be done readily, and therefore possible changes can be promptly instituted, if necessary.

Of the various direct methods available for the assessment of left ventricular function in acutely ill cardiac patients, the relationship between left ventricular stroke volume or stroke work index and left ventricular filling pressure appears to be the most practical, safe, and sensitive. With the introduction of balloon-tipped, flow-directed catheters,[1-3] left ventricular filling pressure (pulmonary artery end-diastolic or pulmonary capillary wedge pressures), right ventricular filling pressure (right atrial pressures), and cardiac output (thermodilution) can be measured at the bedside reliably, repeatedly, and safely without the use of fluoroscopy and with little discomfort to the patient. Through the determination of heart rate and blood pressure concurrently, both of which are routinely monitored in the coronary care unit, several hemodynamic parameters, such as stroke volume, stroke work, systemic and pulmonary vascular resistance, and so on, can be derived.

Ideally, for the evaluation of left ventricular pump function from such hemodynamic measurements, it is desirable to determine the left ventricular stroke work index (LVSWI), an index of left ventricular pump function at various levels of left ventricular filling pressure (LVFP). Also, to estimate the cardiac reserve, it is necessary to determine the response of cardiac pump function to various stresses. However, in practice, the relationship of LVSWI to LVFP, compared to normal ranges, permits reasonably accurate assessment of left ventricular function following acute infarction, and therefore rational management of such patients can be approached. Based on such hemodynamic comparisons, several subsets of acute myocardial infarction can be identified (Table 2; Figs. 1 and 2).

Besides these broad subsets, hemodynamic monitoring permits diagnosis of special complications of acute myocardial infarction. "Low output" syndrome due to acute right ventricular infarct in patients with inferior wall myocardial infarction can be easily diagnosed by hemodynamic monitoring (Fig. 3). Right ventricular free wall infarct may precipitate acute right ventricular failure associated with a marked elevation of right ventricular filling pressure; reduced right ventricular stroke output into pulmonary circulation also causes a diminished pulmonary venous return (left ventricular preload), which in turn reduces forward cardiac output. Thus, hemodynamic characteristics of acute right ventricular infarct are disproportion-

Table 2. *Hemodynamic Subsets in Acute Myocardial Infarction*

HEMODYNAMIC PARAMETERS		SUBSETS
LVFP	*LVSWI*	
Normal	Normal	Compensated
Decreased	Increased	Hyperdynamic
Decreased	Decreased	Hypovolemia
Increased	Decreased	Pump failure

LVFP = left ventricular filling pressure
LVSWI = left ventricular stroke work index

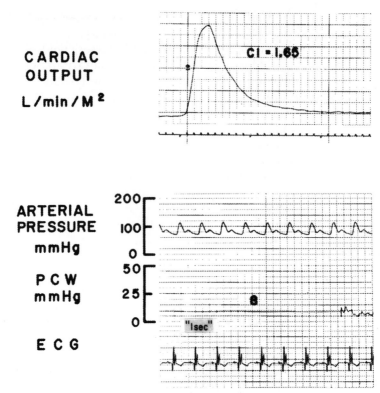

Figure 1. Hemodynamic features in a patient with hypovolemic shock. Cardiac index was markedly decreased, but pulmonary capillary wedge pressure was less than normal.

ate elevation of right ventricular filling pressure, normal or only slightly elevated left ventricular filling pressures, and low cardiac output. These patients may clinically resemble those with left ventricular pump failure; however, management of these two complications is widely different. Volume expansion, despite elevated right ventricular filling pressure, is the treatment of choice in patients with acute right ventricular infarct, whereas such treatment is contraindicated in patients with left ventricular failure.

Acute mitral regurgitation due to papillary muscle infarct and ventricular septal rupture, two serious complications of acute myocardial infarction, cannot be easily differentiated by clinical findings or by non-invasive investigations. Hemodynamic monitoring, however, allows precise diagnosis. In acute mitral regurgitation, an early (in relation to QRS complex), tall, and giant V wave in the wedge pressure tracing confirms the diagnosis (Fig. 4). In contrast, an increase in oxygen saturation in pulmonary arterial blood compared to that in right atrial blood indicates ventricular septal rupture (Fig. 5). As both conservative and surgical treatments might be different for these two complications, definitive diagnosis is mandatory. In appropriate clinical circumstances, low output syndrome due to pump failure can be differentiated by hemodynamic monitoring from other causes of low output syndrome, such as massive pulmonary embolism or cardiac tamponade.

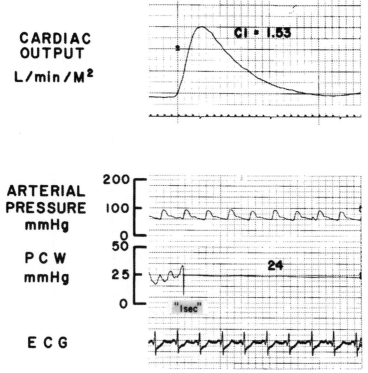

Figure 2. Hemodynamic features in a patient with cardiogenic shock. Markedly reduced cardiac index was associated with elevated pulmonary capillary wedge pressure.

ACUTE RIGHT VENTRICULAR INFARCT

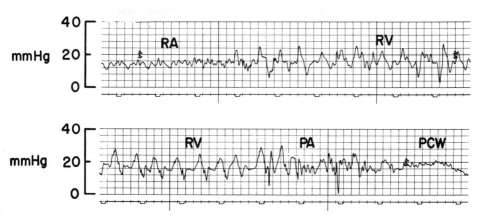

Figure 3. Disproportionate elevation of right atrial and right ventricular end-diastolic pressure compared to pulmonary capillary wedge pressure in a patient with inferior-wall myocardial infarct complicated by right ventricular free-wall infarct.

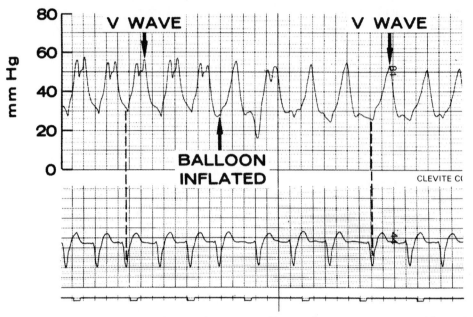

Figure 4. Giant V wave in the pulmonary capillary wedge pressure tracing, indicating severe mitral regurgitation.

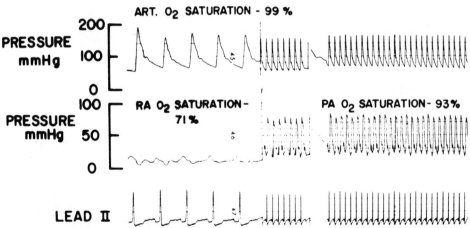

Figure 5. Higher oxygen saturation in pulmonary arterial blood compared to that in right atrial blood in a patient with recent myocardial infarction, indicating severe mitral regurgitation.

Table 3. *Suggested Therapeutic Measures in Relation to Hemodynamic Subsets*

HEMODYNAMIC SUBSETS	SUGGESTED THERAPY
Compensated	Observation
Hypovolemia	Volume expansion
Hyperdynamic	Beta-adrenergic blocking agents
Pump failure	Afterload reducing agents, diuretics, mechanical circulatory assistance

In pulmonary embolism, low cardiac output is associated with elevated right atrial, pulmonary arterial systolic, and diastolic pressures, but normal pulmonary capillary wedge pressure. In patients with cardiac tamponade, diastolic pressure in all four cardiac chambers tends to be equal. Thus, conditions associated with low output syndrome that can be diagnosed by hemodynamic monitoring with greater certainty than by clinical means can be summarized as follows: (1) hemodynamic subsets of acute myocardial infarction, (2) acute right ventricular infarct, (3) acute mitral regurgitation, (4) ventricular septal rupture, (5) acute massive pulmonary embolism, and (6) cardiac tamponade.

In patients with acute myocardial infarction, hemodynamic monitoring not only permits identification of hemodynamic subsets, but helps to provide a rational therapeutic approach (Table 3) and also to assess the effectiveness of such therapy. In patients with compensated or hyperdynamic left ventricular function, no specific therapeutic intervention is necessary except close observation for development of any complications.*

In symptomatic hypovolemic patients, intravenous fluid therapy usually improves cardiac performance. During fluid infusion, however, monitoring of ventricular filling pressures and cardiac output help to determine the optimal filling pressure. Optimal filling pressure in terms of stroke output is 14 to 18 mm Hg in most patients. Further increase in LVFP enhances the risk of precipitating pulmonary edema. In a small number of patients who initially appear hypovolemic (low cardiac output with decreased left ventricular filling pressure), maintaining optimal filling pressure is not accompanied by a significant increase in cardiac output. In such patients, concomitant "pump failure" exists, and therefore, appropriate treatment for pump failure while maintaining the optimal filling pressure should be instituted.

In recent years, therapy for pump failure complicating acute myocardial infarction has undergone a considerable change. In the past, inotropic agents and diuretics have been the only treatment available for the management of pump failure. However, in patients with severe pump failure, no sustained improvement in cardiac performance with the use of diuretics and inotropic agents alone has been demonstrated. The immediate progno-

---

*In some patients with initially compensated left ventricular function, pump failure may supervene, owing to either extension of the infarct or other complications. Hemodynamic monitoring may be useful to detect early deterioration of left ventricular function, resulting in prompt implementation of therapy.

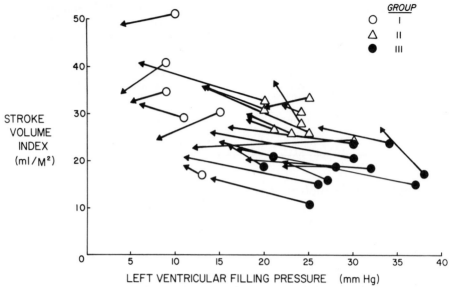

Figure 6. Influence of nitroprusside infusion in a group of patients with acute myocardial infarction. Group I represents all patients with an initial left ventricular filling pressure less than 15 mm. Hg. These patients did not have proven failure. Groups II and III have left ventricular failure with filling pressure greater than 15 mm Hg. Group II had an initial stroke work index greater than 20 gm/m². Note that in Group II and Group III patients, nitroprusside infusion produced a reduction in filling pressure, together with an increase in stroke volume. In Group I patients with a low filling pressure, however, there tended to be a reduction in stroke volume, together with a reduction in filling pressure.

sis also has not been influenced. Recently, vasodilator therapy has been shown to produce beneficial hemodynamic response in many patients with pump failure complicating myocardial infarction.[4] Even in the presence of severe pump failure with markedly reduced cardiac output but grossly elevated pulmonary venous pressure, vasodilators may improve cardiac performance (Fig. 6). A significant increase in cardiac output and a decrease in left ventricular filling pressure, the two major objectives of treatment of pump failure, can be achieved with the use of vasodilators. The hemodynamic effects of intravenous sodium nitroprusside in 43 patients with acute myocardial infarction complicated by severe left ventricular failure are summarized in Table 4.[5] All patients had frank pulmonary edema, and 17 had clinical shock. The average initial LVSWI in this group was 14 ± 1 g-m/m²; LVFP was 31 ± 1 mm Hg; and the cardiac index was 1.7 ± 0.1 L/min/m². Cardiac indices increased to an average value of 2.2 ± 0.1 L/min/m² (+29 per cent). Right atrial, pulmonary arterial, and mean arterial pressures and systemic and pulmonary vascular resistances decreased in the majority of patients. Improved left ventricular performance was indicated by an increase in stroke volume index (+32 per cent) accompanied by a decrease in LVFP (−35 per cent). Despite a reduction in arterial pressure, the stroke work index increased (+36 per cent). Improved left ventricular function, however, is usually not observed if LVFP is initially normal or low. Indeed, in such patients, vasodilator therapy may cause a reduction in stroke volume and cardiac output with a further decrease in LVFP, and also, re-

Table 4. *Hemodynamic Changes During Intravenous Vasodilator Therapy in Severe Pump Failure Complicating Acute Myocardial Infarction (N =43)**

	CONTROL	VASODILATOR	P
Heart rate (beats/min)	100 ± 2.4	99 ± 2.7	NS
Arterial pressure (mm Hg)	83 ± 1.5	73 ± 1.7	0.0005
Pulmonary arterial pressure (mm Hg)	39 ± 1.2	28 ± 1.1	0.0005
Right atrial pressure (mm Hg)	13 ± 0.8	9 ± 0.6	0.0005
Left ventricular filling pressure (mm Hg)	31 ± 1.0	20 ± 0.8	0.0005
Cardiac index (liter/min/m²)	1.7 ± 0.05	2.2 ± 0.06	0.0005
Stroke volume index (ml/m²)	17.3 ± 0.2	22.8 ± 0.8	0.0005
Stroke work index (g-m/m²)	14 ± 0.7	19 ± 0.9	0.005
Systemic vascular resistance (dyne-sec-cm^{-5})	2023 ± 112	1435 ± 65	0.0005

All values are mean ± standard error of mean.

*(From Chatterjee K, Swan HJC, Kaushik VS, Jobin G, Magnusson P, and Forrester JS: Effects of vasodilator therapy for severe pump failure in acute myocardial infarction on short-term and late prognosis. Circulation 53:797, 1976.)

flex tachycardia may be induced. Furthermore, even in patients with initially elevated LVFP, if it decreases to a very low level during vasodilator therapy, cardiac output and stroke volume may decrease. It is, therefore, essential that hemodynamics are determined before the introduction of vasodilator therapy and that changes in LVFP are constantly monitored to maintain it at optimal level. Hypotension is a potential hazard, and therefore, monitoring of arterial pressure is necessary during vasodilator therapy. The major objective of vasodilator therapy is to reduce "afterload," to facilitate left ventricular systolic ejection, and not to reduce arterial pressure. Systemic vascular resistance is the major component of the total resistance (afterload) against which the left ventricle operates as a pump. If reduction in systemic vascular resistance is proportional to the increase in cardiac output, blood pressure may not change significantly (Blood Pressure = Cardiac Output × Systemic Vascular Resistance). Indeed, in many normotensive or relatively hypotensive patients with left ventricular failure, an appreciable increase in cardiac output may be achieved without causing a significant reduction in arterial pressure. The importance of monitoring changes in systemic vascular resistance, cardiac output, and arterial pressure during vasodilator therapy in such patients cannot be overemphasized. When pump failure is precipitated by severe mitral regurgitation or ventricular septal defect, vasodilator therapy can be effectively used to retard clinical and hemodynamic deterioration that is otherwise inevitable with conventional therapy (Fig. 7). Vasodilator therapy appears to be more effective for treatment of pump failure due to mitral regurgitation than that due to ventricular septal defect. In almost all patients with mitral regurgitation, reduced systemic vascular resistance during vasodilator therapy is associated with an increased left ventricular forward stroke volume and decreased regurgitant volume and pulmonary venous pressure. In patients with ventricular septal defect, however, reduction of left-to-right shunt depends on relative changes in systemic and pulmonary vascular resistance. If systemic vascular resistance decreases relatively more than the pulmonary vascular

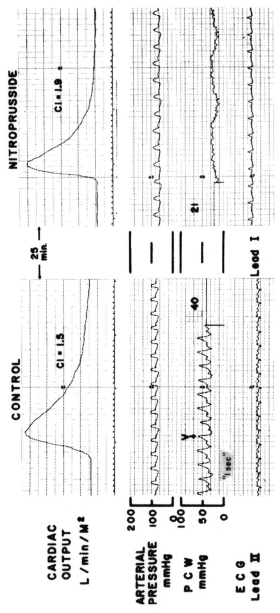

Figure 7.   Beneficial hemodynamic response of intravenous sodium nitroprusside in a patient with acute severe mitral regurgitation complicating myocardial infarction. Before nitroprusside infusion (left hand panel) cardiac output was low; mean pulmonary capillary wedge pressure and the peak magnitude of the V wave in the wedge pressure tracing were markedly elevated. During nitroprusside infusion (right-hand panel), cardiac output increased and mean pulmonary capillary wedge pressure and the V wave in the wedge pressure tracing markedly decreased.

resistance, reduction of left-to-right shunt is expected. On the other hand, if the decrease in pulmonary vascular resistance is proportionately greater than that of systemic vascular resistance, left-to-right shunt may worsen. It is apparent, therefore, that the monitoring of changes in systemic and pulmonary vascular resistance is essential when vasodilator therapy is instituted in such patients.

Another therapeutic approach for the treatment of pump failure that has shown promise is the use of circulatory assist devices such as intra-aortic balloon counterpulsation. Intra-aortic balloon counterpulsation, by systolic unloading of the left ventricle, not only reduces left ventricular systolic work and hence, myocardial oxygen consumption, but also improves cardiac output and decreases left ventricular filling pressure. During diastolic augmentation, coronary artery perfusion pressure is maintained. Beneficial hemodynamic and clinical response can be observed even in the presence of severe pump failure and cardiogenic shock. In patients with severe mitral regurgitation or ventricular septal defect, intra-aortic balloon counterpulsation may cause clinical and hemodynamic improvement, and patients can be stabilized until corrective surgery can be performed. The insertion and proper use of the intra-aortic balloon counterpulsation device, however, requires the expertise of a skilled and trained medical and surgical team; otherwise, significant and serious complications (i.e., leg ischemia, heart rupture, and so on) might be encountered. Thus, intra-aortic balloon counterpulsation is usually applied when other therapies appear to be ineffective. Constant hemodynamic and clinical assessment are therefore necessary to evaluate the response to any therapy so that prompt changes can be instituted.

Recent experience with vasodilator therapy and the use of intra-aortic balloon counterpulsation in patients with severe pump failure complicating acute myocardial infarction suggests that immediate prognosis in such patients can be improved. In patients with frank pulmonary edema, the in-hospital mortality rate with conventional therapy is 30 to 40 per cent and approaches 100 per cent when the clinical features of cardiogenic shock are present. In recent years, prognostic indices based on hemodynamics have also become available (Table 5).[6] Whether overt clinical manifestations of pump failure are present or not, these hemodynamic parameters provide a precise means of evaluating the immediate prognosis of such patients. In

Table 5. *Hemodynamic Prognostic Indices in Patients with Acute Myocardial Infarction**

LVSWI (GM/M²)	LVFP (MM HG)	HOSPITAL MORTALITY (%)
	<15	5.8
>20	>15	26
<20	>15	80

LVSWI = Left ventricular stroke work index
LVFP = Left ventricular filling pressure
*Results are based on the analysis of initial hemodynamic findings in 122 patients admitted to the Myocardial Infarction Research Unit of the Cedars of Lebanon Hospital, Los Angeles, California.

patients with LVFP of 15 mm Hg or less, in-hospital mortality is low; in patients with moderately reduced LVSWI and increased LVFP, the in-hospital mortality is approximately five times higher. In patients with severely depressed cardiac function with a LVSWI of 20 g-m/m² or less and elevated LVFP, the in-hospital mortality rate approaches 80 per cent. Recently, the influence of vasodilator therapy on in-hospital mortality in patients with severe pump failure complicating acute myocardial infarction has been investigated.[5] Forty-three patients with severe pump failure were treated with nitroprusside (40 patients) or phentolamine (three patients). Severe pump failure was defined on the basis of initial hemodynamics, i.e., initial LVSWI of 20 g-m/m² or less and LVFP greater than 15 mm Hg. Clinically, all patients had frankly pulmonary edema, and 31 of the 43 patients had cardiomegaly; 17 patients had clinical features of cardiogenic shock in addition to pulmonary edema. Besides recent myocardial infarction, 30 of the 43 patients had historical and ECG evidence of an old myocardial infarct. Vasodilators were infused continuously from four hours to 27 days, with monitoring of LVFP, arterial pressure, and cardiac output. A beneficial hemodynamic response was observed in almost all patients; cardiac output increased, while pulmonary capillary wedge pressure decreased. Nineteen of the 43 patients (44 per cent) died in the hospital, 15 with uncontrolled failure. Thus, the in-hospital mortality rate due to pump failure was 34 per cent. Most studies indicate that in the presence of severe hemodynamic depression, the in-hospital mortality rate with conventional therapy exceeds 75 per cent.[7] The mortality rate of 40 per cent or less with vasodilator therapy in this subgroup of patients suggests improvement in immediate prognosis. However, in the presence of markedly depressed cardiac function, i.e., when the stroke work index is extremely low (less than 10 g-m/m²) and the LVFP is elevated, the prognosis with vasodilator therapy remains poor. Eleven of the 43 patients had an LVSWI less than 10 g-m/m², and only two survived, giving an in-hospital mortality rate of 82 per cent. Thus, it appears that vasodilator therapy is most likely to be effective with an initial LVSWI greater than 10 g-m/m² and elevated LVFP.

Recent studies indicate that the use of intra-aortic balloon counterpulsation can improve immediate prognosis in patients with markedly depressed cardiac function complicating acute myocardial infarction. Bolooki et al.[8] have reported a 32 per cent survival rate in patients with an LVSWI less than 10 g-m/m² and a high LVFP. Further studies will be needed to evaluate the relative efficacy of vasodilator therapy and intra-aortic balloon counterpulsation for treatment of severe pump failure complicating acute myocardial infarction. At the present time, however, based on available data, a general outline for the treatment of pump failure can be formulated. If LVSWI is greater than 10 g-m/m², vasodilator therapy should be tried initially, whereas counterpulsation with or without vasodilators should be the therapy of choice for those with a stroke work index less than 10 g-m/m². It is apparent that hemodynamic monitoring is necessary to determine these subsets of pump failure in patients with acute myocardial infarction to implement this therapeutic approach.

In summary, hemodynamic monitoring allows the precise diagnosis of the severity of depression of cardiac function in patients with acute myocardial infarction. Monitoring is essential during aggressive therapy of pump failure, which appears to have improved prognosis in such patients. Serious complications during hemodynamic monitoring are rare, and the benefits far outweigh the risks.

References

1. Swan HJC, Ganz W, Forrester J, Marcus H, Diamond G, and Chonette D: Catheterization of the heart in man with the use of a flow-directed balloon-tipped catheter. N Engl J Med 283:447, 1970.
2. Forrester JS, Ganz W, Diamond G, McHugh T, Chonette D, and Swan HJC: Thermodilution cardiac output determination with a single flow-directed catheter. Am Heart J 83:306, 1972.
3. Chatterjee K, Swan HJC, Ganz W, Gray R, Loebel H, Forrester JS, and Chonette D: Use of a balloon-tipped flotation electrode catheter for cardiac monitoring. Am J Cardiol 36:56, 1975.
4. Chatterjee K, and Parmley WW: The role of vasodilator therapy in heart failure. Prog Cardiovasc Dis 19:301, 1977.
5. Chatterjee K, Swan HJC, Kaushik VS, Jobin G, Magnusson P, and Forrester JS: Effects of vasodilator therapy for severe pump failure in acute myocardial infarction on short-term and late prognosis. Circulation 53:797, 1976.
6. Chatterjee K, and Swan HJC: Hemodynamic profile in acute myocardial infarction. In Corday E, and Swan HJC (eds): Myocardial Infarction. Baltimore, Md, Williams and Wilkins, 1973, p 51.
7. Scheidt S, Wilner G, and Fillmore S: Objective hemodynamic assessment after acute myocardial infarction. Br Heart J 35:908, 1973.
8. Bolooki H, Mayorga-Corteo A, and Fried A: Hemodynamic predictions of survival during intra-aortic balloon pump (IABP) in myocardial infarction shock (abstr). Clin Res 24:210, 1976.

Routine Invasive Hemodynamic Monitoring in the CCU Has Lowered Mortality: Arguments Against the Hypothesis

ARTHUR SELZER, M.D.

Chief of Cardiology, Presbyterian Hospital, Pacific Medical
Center, San Francisco, California; Clinical Professor of
Medicine, University of California, San Francisco Medical
School; Clinical Professor of Medicine, Emeritus, Stanford
University School of Medicine, Stanford, California

Acute myocardial infarction is a short-term episode in the course of ischemic heart disease. More often than not it represents a condition independent of the underlying chronic disease of the coronary arteries, with its own natural history and prognosis. The frequency with which recovery from acute myocardial infarction is followed by years or decades of productive, often symptom-free, life illustrates this point adequately. It should be pointed out that the majority of cases of acute myocardial infarction surviving the critical initial period run a smooth and uncomplicated course and heal without treatment or any other intervention. A large number of infarcts occur without the patient's realization and are discovered later by the characteristic electrocardiographic patterns or abnormalities of wall motion, thereby showing that full recovery may occur without the customary bed rest and other components of the standard treatment. Thus, the goal of treatment is to provide the best opportunity for healing of the infarct and the protection of the patient from any influence that could interfere with smooth recovery.

Treatment of myocardial infarction is governed by the same guidelines as that for all forms of therapy: a consideration of the balance between risk and benefit. In addition, it is now important to consider the cost effective-

340

ness of therapy. Any "routine" intervention has to be justified as a form of prophylactic therapy, that is, applied for anticipated problems and not for existing problems, and not offered to many patients unnecessarily in order to prevent an undesirable event in a few. The risk-benefit equation has to be especially applied to prophylactic measures in the treatment of myocardial infarction in light of the benign course of the majority of patients who recover in response to a period of rest, without any therapy.

In defining the objectives of therapy of acute myocardial infarction, one has to consider its principal dangers: life-threatening arrhythmias, pump failure, and secondary complications. Arrhythmias coincide with the stage of ischemia and early stages of necrosis; the proneness to arrhythmias subsides gradually and promptly. Pump failure is related to the extent of myocardial damage — lesser degrees of damage often transiently bring about cardiac failure, which is self-limited and self-compensating with or without therapy. More extensive damage may produce emergent conditions, such as acute cardiac failure and cardiogenic shock, or may gradually lead to permanent impairment of cardiac function. Some of the complications cause mechanical overload (mitral regurgitation, septal perforation), which throws additional burden on the already damaged heart and may necessitate early surgical interventions.

The task of evaluation of the role of hemodynamic monitoring has to be undertaken with the above considerations in mind. In order to justify the routine use of hemodynamic monitoring, it seems reasonable to compare it to the better known and more widely used rhythm monitoring by means of the coronary care unit.

The concept of the coronary care unit revolutionized treatment of myocardial infarction. The principle of rhythm monitoring by means of continuous electrocardiographic display permitted early detection of clinically inapparent arrhythmias as well as instant recognition of life-threatening tachyarrhythmias and bradyarrhythmias. As a result, both preventive and remedial measures were greatly facilitated, reducing the incidence of serious arrhythmias and producing an almost complete salvage from previously often fatal ventricular fibrillation. Three factors supported the principle of *routine* use of coronary care unit rhythm monitoring: (1) the great frequency of arrhythmias, occurring even in otherwise uncomplicated cases; (2) the predictive value of simpler arrhythmias as harbingers of more serious ones; and (3) the time limitation inherent in recovery from cardiac arrest, which made instant recognition of it a condition for brain survival. To these factors one can add the virtual absence of risk of rhythm monitoring. The risk-benefit ratio is thus weighted toward the routine use of the coronary care unit principle, even if the cost effectiveness is suboptimal: coronary care units have been organized in every hospital, regardless of how small and how close to a larger medical center. High cost of equipment, low volume leading to inadequate experience, and often lack of fully trained manpower make many small coronary care units less than satisfactory and inefficient, while regional pooling of facilities would undoubtedly provide cheaper, more efficient, and safer units.

The success of rhythm monitoring led to the development of hemody-

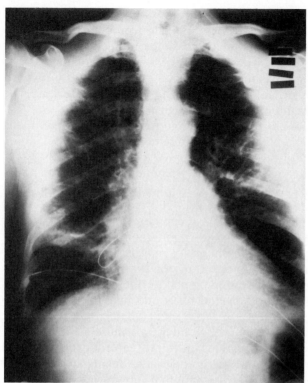

Figure 1. Radiograph of the chest of a patient who was referred to a medical center from a community hospital because of a pulmonary hemorrhage induced by placement of a flow-directed balloon-tipped catheter.

namic monitoring, which has been made possible by the introduction of flow-directed balloon-tipped catheters.[1] In addressing the problem of the effect of hemodynamic monitoring on the mortality from acute myocardial infarction, two aspects of the problem have to be considered: (1) the positive contribution of this technique in improving the therapy of myocardial infarction; and (2) the proportion of cases in which this may take place as a background for the routine use of hemodynamic monitoring in each and every case of acute myocardial infarction.

Approaching hemodynamic monitoring from the standpoint of a risk-benefit ratio, it is immediately apparent that as an invasive procedure, this technique carries a definite risk. Under the general concept of "risk," one should start with direct complications related to use of the flow-directed catheter. Complications such as pulmonary embolization,[2] pulmonary ischemic lesions,[2] rupture of a pulmonary arterial branch,[3] infection,[4] and coiling of the catheter[5] have been observed, some of them with undesirable frequency (Fig. 1). It should be emphasized that complications of diagnostic procedures are, as a rule, under-reported and underdiagnosed — real incidence is not available. Furthermore, according to the general rule of invasive procedures, the risk is inversely proportional to the case load; thus it is highly probable that complications are more likely to occur in smaller hospitals. To the "direct" risk it is necessary to add the possibility of misuse of the information obtained from the flow-directed catheter. Technical considerations in recording intracardiac and intra-arterial pressure are fraught with difficulties, e.g., identification of the source of a given pressure curve, recognition of damping, effect of various artifacts, improper setting of the zero reference point — all of which may provide the inexperienced with grossly distorted results. Thus, the safest and most effective use of the flow-directed catheter is in cardiac centers.

On the benefit side of the equation, hemodynamic monitoring provides continuous measurement of pulmonary arterial and left atrial pressures; cardiac output can also be estimated or measured by means of the Fick principle or by indicator dilution techniques, with the latter requiring specially equipped catheters. These measurements permit an accurate assessment of cardiac function and quantification of pump failure, when it develops. It should be emphasized that though they are more accurate, direct hemodynamic measurements are not the sole means of obtaining this information. Clinical estimation of cardiac function is reasonably good. Early cardiac failure produces S_3 gallop sounds, pulmonary rales, and evidence of "pulmonary congestion" in the radiographic picture; non-invasive monitoring can also be performed by serial recording of systolic time intervals.

In reviewing the potential superiority of invasive versus non-invasive evaluation of cardiac performance, it is clear that the latter gives us exact figures rather than estimates and displays them continuously, making changes easily detectable. In patients with a milder degree of cardiac failure, exact measurement has little importance; however, if pump failure is severe enough to institute specific therapy, then monitoring changes produced by the intervention are of invaluable assistance, though it is doubtful whether they are critical enough to become life-saving, except in very unusual cases.

In reviewing arguments against the *routine* use of invasive hemodynamic monitoring, it is necessary to answer the question of whether cardiac failure may develop in an unheralded manner with life-threatening implications analogous to an unexpected cardiac arrest due to ventricular fibrillation in which every second counts and time would not permit the introduction of the flow-directed catheter. A further question is: Does hemodynamic monitoring permit early detection of impending cardiac failure, therefore making it possible to prevent its progression, similar to warning arrhythmias permitting the use of measures preventing ventricular fibrillation? The answer to both questions, in our opinion, is negative. Sudden emergencies do develop in myocardial infarction associated with abrupt pump failure. In most cases, however, the time element is not as critical as in cardiac arrest. Furthermore, if a catastrophic change in the patient's condition develops with sudden pump failure, there is almost always an anatomic cause, e.g., rupture of a papillary muscle or perforation of the septum, or a physiologic reason, such as tachyarrhythmia or bradyarrhythmia. In the first case, measurements via a flow-directed catheter are usually inadequate; more complete studies involving angiocardiography are needed. In the second case, treatment or containment of the arrhythmia does not require exact knowledge of cardiac pressures. Development of these anatomic or physiologic complications of myocardial infarction also provides the reason why hemodynamic monitoring is not useful in anticipating catastrophic events: They occur, as a rule, abruptly and not gradually.

The most important point, however, in arguing against the routine use of invasive monitoring is to estimate in what proportion of cases of acute myocardial infarction can hemodynamic measurements be of any use at all.

In order to make a reasonable estimate of the proportion of cases with potential or actual benefit from hemodynamic monitoring, it is convenient to divide acute myocardial infarction into subsets according the clinical patterns and course.

1. *Uncomplicated myocardial infarction with asymptomatic course.* This group contains the largest proportion of patients with acute myocardial infarction. McNeer et al.[6] subdivided myocardial infarction into "uncomplicated" and "complicated" cases. The former category included, in the series of 522 cases, 51 per cent of the total, and 59 per cent of early survivors were in this category.

2. *Myocardial infarction complicated by recurrent arrhythmias.* While no exact figures are available, this category undoubtedly constitutes the second largest proportion of cases of acute myocardial infarction. In this category treatment is directed toward containment and prevention of arrhythmias. Hemodynamic monitoring has little relevance to the course and therapy.

The preceding two subsets of myocardial infarction account for the great majority, perhaps three fourths, of cases. Invasive hemodynamic monitoring provides no benefit to the patient in these subsets, but is associated with a risk.

3. *Myocardial infarction associated with recurrent attacks of chest pain.* In this group, a continuing ischemic process can be assumed. Even though hemodynamic abnormalities may develop in association with ischemia, the essential decision making revolves around the need for coronary arteriography and the possibility of surgical intervention. Pump failure, if present, is purely secondary; treatment is seldom required, and the knowledge of exact figures is irrelevant. This subset is relatively uncommon.

4. *Myocardial infarction with latent cardiac failure.* This category includes patients who may or may not have minor symptoms (e.g., mild dyspnea) and who on examination are found to have pulmonary rales and gallop sounds and may show radiographic evidence of "pulmonary congestion," yet remain in clinical satisfactory condition. In this category, hemodynamic monitoring confirms the clinically evident findings. In the great majority of patients aggressive therapy is not needed; mild cardiac failure may be self-correcting or may respond satisfactorily to small doses of a diuretic drug.

5. *Myocardial infarction in overt cardiac failure.* This group includes patients who are profoundly dyspneic and present with tachycardia, mild hypotension, and clear evidence of cardiac failure. Hemodynamic monitoring constitutes a valuable clinical tool that permits evaluation of the degree of pump failure, the need for various aggressive therapeutic steps, and the response to therapeutic intervention.

6. *Cardiogenic shock.* In this case, hemodynamic monitoring is mandatory.

7. *Secondary complications of myocardial infarction producing pump failure.* The principal complications include acute mitral regurgitation, perforation of the ventricular septum, and the development of ventricular aneurysm. These complications often develop abruptly and may be associated with a catastrophic change in the patient's condition. When responses to the complication present themselves as a milder degree of pump failure, hemodynamic monitoring is helpful, in a manner similar to category 5 above. Abrupt, severe deterioration often calls for immediate performance of a more comprehensive invasive study than hemodynamic monitoring; cineangiocardiography is the essential technique to determine operability of the lesion.

Thus, it is clear from the foregoing discussion that continuous hemodynamic monitoring can be of specific value in the clinical management of patients in only a small subset of myocardial infarction. Exact figures are not available, but a reasonable estimate would place the number of cases between 10 and 15 per cent.

In addressing the question of whether invasive hemodynamic monitoring can influence mortality from myocardial infarction, it should be pointed out that this would require reliable demonstration that certain life-saving interventions are not only the direct result of the information gathered from monitoring, but that the interventions would not be possible without it. Rhythm monitoring can claim such a relationship by the salvage from ventricular fibrillation. It is exceedingly difficult to provide similar evidence for hemodynamic monitoring, except by anecdotal presentation of some isolated cases. Nevertheless, the risk-benefit ratio is probably favorable for the elective, judicious use of hemodynamic monitoring in the subsets of myocardial infarction where pump failure represents a serious problem.

However, *routine* use of hemodynamic monitoring gives a strongly negative risk-benefit ratio. If for each patient in whom hemodynamic monitoring makes some (not necessarily essential) contribution one were to subject eight or nine others to an unnecessary invasive procedure associated with an appreciable risk, a case could be built to conclude that mortality from myocardial infarction is increased and not lowered.

It should be reiterated that routine use of hemodynamic monitoring in acute myocardial infarction means its utilization in every coronary care unit. Inexperience in introducing the catheter and the possibility of an inappropriate conclusion being drawn from the curves would magnify the risk and reduce the benefit. Inasmuch as the utilization of this invasive technique is primarily indicated in patients with pump failure, patients in shock, and patients with serious secondary complication of myocardial infarction, a recommendation should be considered that invasive hemodynamic monitoring should *never* be used in smaller coronary care units, but the patients in whom it is indicated be immediately transferred to a complete cardiac center where expert medical and surgical help is available.

Summary

Hemodynamic monitoring provides important information for the management of pump failure in the small subset of acute myocardial infarction in which management of heart failure represents a critical problem. Even in this group of cases, no evidence is available that it contributes to lower mortality. The routine use of invasive hemodynamic monitoring, which would involve its use in the great majority of cases for which it is not needed, is not indicated, for the risk-benefit ratio is estimated to be a strongly unfavorable one. The net effect of routine use of the flow-directed catheters in acute myocardial infarction would be an increase, rather than a decrease, of mortality.

References

1. Swan HJC, Ganz W, Forrester J, Marcus H, Diamond G, and Chonette D: Catheterization of the heart in man with use of a flow-directed balloon-tipped catheter. N Engl J Med 238:447–451, 1970.
2. Foot GA, Schabel SI, and Hodges M: Pulmonary complications of the flow-directed balloon-tipped catheter. N Engl J Med 290:927–931, 1974.
3. Chun GMH, and Ellestad MH: Perforation of the pulmonary artery by a Swan-Ganz catheter. N Engl J Med 284:1041–1042, 1971.
4. Katz JD, Cronau LH, Barash PG, and Manel SD: Pulmonary artery flow-guided catheters in the perioperative period. JAMA 237:2832–2834, 1977.
5. Lipp H, O'Donoghue H, and Resnekov L: Intracardiac knotting of a flow-directed balloon catheter. N Engl J Med 284:220, 1971.
6. McNeer JF, Wallace AG, Wagner GS, Starmer GT, and Rosati RA: The course of acute myocardial infarction. Feasibility of early discharge of the uncomplicated patient. Circulation 51:410–413, 1975.

Comment

The development of the Swan-Ganz catheter represents a major contribution to patient management, since it permits the physician to evaluate ventricular performance at the bedside. The greatest experience has been accumulated in studying and managing patients who have suffered circulatory compromise in the course of an acute myocardial infarction. The ability to measure cardiac output, ventricular filling pressures, and systemic pressures at the bedside not only allows for a hemodynamic assessment of the severity of circulatory compromise, but also permits evaluation of the effectiveness of particular therapeutic interventions. Nevertheless, it is appropriate to ask specifically whether hemodynamic monitoring in the CCU lowers mortality from acute myocardial infarction. It is clear that the average patient with a so-called completed myocardial infarct or one who has essentially no complications other than arrhythmias on entry into the CCU is overwhelmingly likely to have an uncomplicated recovery and does not need specific therapy directed toward improvement of cardiac performance. On the other hand, subsets of patients with acute myocardial infarction can be identified when pump failure is present, manifested either as shock or circulatory collapse or as pulmonary and/or systemic congestion. The use in these patients of newer therapeutic agents that influence preload, afterload, or the inotropic state of the myocardium requires hemodynamic monitoring. Decisions, whether about volume replacement, volume reduction, systemic vasodilatation, cardiac inotropic agents, or combinations of these, are made based on hemodynamic measurements, since clinical criteria under these conditions are less definitive and may even be misleading. I have seen patients under these circumstances when there has been no doubt in my mind that without hemodynamic monitoring and aggressive therapy, they would not have survived. It is also clear that mechanical lesions such as ventricular septal defect and papillary muscle rupture, which may require acute surgical intervention, may be recognized more quickly and definitively through such hemodynamic monitoring, with surgical salvage of the patient. Nevertheless, it is appropriate for Dr. Selzer to question whether routine use of such hemodynamic monitoring is, in fact, desirable, since in a number of cases the problem is clear clinically, and/or therapeutic interventions are relatively ineffective since mortality under these circumstances remains high no matter what is done.

It is my own feeling that hemodynamic monitoring should not be routine. It should be carried out when the patient with acute myocardial infarction requires a therapeutic intervention for pump failure, particularly if an initial intervention has failed to resolve the situation and repeated inter-

347

ventions are likely to be necessary. Under these circumstances, whether in fact mortality can be demonstrated to be lowered or not, one feels more confident about progressing with appropriate therapeutic agents such as nitroprusside, dobutamine, intravenous furosemide, and so on, if one is following the effects of these agents on the patient's pressures and flows.

ELLIOT RAPAPORT, M.D.

Fifteen

Can Mortality After Survival from Sudden Death Be Influenced by the Use of Membrane-Active Antiarrhythmic Drugs?

MORTALITY AFTER SURVIVAL FROM PRE-HOSPITAL
CARDIAC ARREST MIGHT BE INFLUENCED BY THE USE
OF MEMBRANE-ACTIVE ANTIARRHYTHMIC DRUGS

*Robert J. Myerburg, M.D.; Cesar Conde, M.D.;
Alvaro Mayorga-Cortes, M.D.; and Agustin
Castellanos, M.D.*

MORTALITY IN SURVIVORS OF OUT-OF-HOSPITAL
VENTRICULAR FIBRILLATION IS NOT IMPROVED
BY THE ROUTINE USE OF QUINIDINE OR PROCAINAMIDE

*Leonard A. Cobb, M.D., and Alfred P. Hallstrom,
Ph.D.*

COMMENT

Mortality After Survival from Pre-Hospital Cardiac Arrest Might Be Influenced by the Use of Membrane-Active Antiarrhythmic Drugs*

ROBERT J. MYERBURG, M.D.;
CESAR CONDE, M.D.; ALVARO
MAYORGA-CORTES, M.D.; and
AGUSTIN CASTELLANOS, M.D.

Division of Cardiology, Department of Medicine,
University of Miami School of Medicine, Miami, Florida

The magnitude of pre-hospital cardiac arrest as a public health problem has long been recognized. Estimates of the incidence of unexpected cardiac arrest as the initial manifestation of cardiovascular disease are as high as 300,000 events per year in the United States, the actual number depending in large measure upon the definition used for the time between onset of the terminal event and biologic death and for the clinical definition of "unexpected."[1]

There has been very limited progress in methods of prevention of pre-hospital cardiac arrest to the present time. Some clinical information has been accumulated regarding patients at high risk for unexpected cardiac arrest in the community, but most of these patients fall into very limited population subsets. There are relatively few patients with clearly defined clinical syndromes that can be treated on an individual basis using medical

*Supported by a grant from the National Heart, Lung, and Blood Institute, NIH, DHEW (HL-18769-04)

351

and/or surgical regimens addressed to the control or prevention of specific potentially lethal arrhythmias. Extensive epidemiologic studies have identified a group of risk factors that function individually or in conjunction with each other to identify patients at higher-than-expected risk for sudden death. Among the cardinal risk factors are cigarette smoking, hyperlipidemias, and hypertension. Unfortunately, information available to date has not clarified whether *control* of hyperlipidemias or hypertension will control their function as risk factors for sudden death; and the data on cigarette smoking are strongly suggestive of beneficial effects of stopping cigarette smoking, although not yet totally confirmed in regard to the sudden death problem.

Subgroups of patients who have survived an acute myocardial infarction have recently been reported to be at higher risk for sudden death within six months to a year following myocardial infarction than the overall post–myocardial infarction population. The population at higher risk includes those patients who had severe angina pectoris (Class III or IV) prior to the myocardial infarction, those with the hemodynamic complications of hypotension and/or congestive heart failure during the myocardial infarction, and those patients with frequent ventricular ectopic activity recorded by Holter monitor during the late in-hospital phase of convalescence from myocardial infarction.[2] Unfortunately, it has not yet been determined whether antiarrhythmic therapy in this specific subgroup of patients, who have a nearly fourfold increase in the risk of sudden death or reinfarction in the first six months after myocardial infarction, will protect individuals (or the statistical subgroup) from potentially lethal events. In this regard, however, several studies from Europe have suggested that long-term treatment of post–myocardial infarction patients with beta-adrenergic blocking agents may reduce the risk of sudden death during the first one to two years after the index myocardial infarction. However, the results of these studies are not conclusive and must await further confirmation by a large and carefully controlled study.

Despite the attention upon the epidemiologic, pathologic, and prognostic aspects of the problem of pre-hospital cardiac arrest, there have been limited significant inroads into prevention, other than the development of community-based emergency medical systems. This therapeutic activity, unfortunately responding after the fact, has a relatively low success rate — in the range of 15 per cent of the documented cases of patients surviving initial hospitalization — despite the development of highly sophisticated technical systems.

Background

Beginning approximately 10 years ago, systems have been developed that permit emergency medical intensive care to be delivered to a patient at the scene of a catastrophic medical event in the community. Such systems are more desirable than the previously developed emergency transport systems to move such victims to a fixed site for medical care because of the limited time available for successful resuscitation. Various models of effective emergency rescue systems have been developed, the key element being trained paramedical personnel who are able to perform cardiopulmonary resuscitation, telemeter electrocardiographic data to base hospital stations, and perform defibrillation, endotracheal intubation, and intravenous administration of drugs. Such mobile intensive care systems must be able to reach significant segments of a community population within four to six minutes of summons in order to achieve reasonable salvage rates. Community training programs in which citizens are taught the essentials of cardiopulmonary resuscitation on a large-scale basis serve as an adjunct to these systems with some success.

During the first three and a half years of the emergency medical rescue system program developed in the city of Miami, approximately 5000 emergency calls were received from the community. In 301 instances, ventricular fibrillation was documented electrocardiographically by telemetry to the base hospital from the site of the clinical event, and 101 of these patients (34 per cent) were defibrillated and arrived at the hospital alive. Of these, 59 patients (58 per cent) died during hospitalization, and 42 patients (42 per cent) survived and were discharged from the hospital.[3] The 101 survivors of the initial event, who were successfully resuscitated and admitted to the hospital, demonstrated a propensity toward both acute and chronic cardiac electrophysiologic instability. The *acute* instability was indicated by the fact that recurrent ventricular fibrillation or ventricular tachycardia occurred in almost 60 per cent of the group, the overwhelming majority on the first day in the hospital. The occurrence of recurrent ventricular fibrillation was a serious prognostic clue, because this event was twice as frequent in those patients who died during the index hospitalization as compared to those who surived to be discharged. The *chronic* propensity toward electrical instability is derived from the observation that among the 42 patients who survived the initial hospitalization and were discharged, there was a 28 per cent incidence of sudden death (42 per cent of total deaths) in 12.8 months average follow-up. These data are similar to data accumulated from the Seattle area.[4]

Subsequent observations from the Miami area were analyzed to determine the frequency and early prognosis of each of three mechanisms of presentation. Of a group of 128 consecutive clinical cardiac arrests in the community, in which the emergency medical rescue system arrived at the scene within four to six minutes of summons, a total of 85 of the 128 patients (66 per cent) had ventricular fibrillation as the initial telemetered event; six patients (5 per cent) had ventricular tachycardia; and 37 patients (29 per cent) had bradyarrhythmias due to high-grade heart block, slow sinus mechanisms (< 40/min), or asystole. The survival rate during initial hospitalization was best among the ventricular tachycardia patients (100 per cent), worst among the bradyarrhythmia patients (13 per cent), and intermediate among ventricular fibrillation patients (40 per cent, a figure consistent with previous experience).

Approach to Patients' Long-Term Survival

Patients who have been successfully resuscitated from pre-hospital cardiac arrest in the community and who survived the initial hospitalization constitute a unique population in which to initiate studies into the methods available to prevent pre-hospital cardiac arrest. The most important feature of this population is the occurrence of the approximately 30 per cent/year recurrent unexpected cardiac arrest rate in survivors of the initial event. Since this figure had been nearly the same both in studies from the Miami area and from the Seattle area, we designed a protocol addressed to analysis of long-term electrophysiologic instability in such patients and to therapeutic modalities directed to a possible decrease in the frequency of recurrent cardiac arrests. While we had previously accumulated data that *suggested* that coronary vein graft bypass surgery might be of value in a highly selected subgroup of these survivors,[5] our experience indicates that only a small percentage of patients are suitable for coronary bypass surgery based on the extent of disease and underlying etiology. Thus, medical approaches must be evaluated, at least for those patients who are not surgical candidates. In the design of a study related to the goals outlined above, the number of patients available from a single center was too small to allow evaluation of more than one category of drugs; and it was elected to determine the efficacy of the membrane-active category of antiarrhythmic drugs (primarily quinidine and procainamide) in suppressing arrhythmias, and perhaps in reducing mortality.

The study was divided into three segments of activity: (1) an evaluation of the frequency and severity of chronic ventricular arrhythmias in survivors of pre-hospital cardiac arrest; (2) an evaluation of the ability of the antiarrhythmic agents to suppress these arrhythmias; and (3) survival statistics.

Regarding rhythm analysis, two methods of data acquisition are being used. The first is the recording of a 24-hour Holter monitor tape once a month during long-term follow-up. The tapes are analyzed for the frequency and type of arrhythmias, using an automated scanning system that permits a direct count of the frequency of ventricular ectopic activity during the first 30 seconds of each 10-minute segment of the 24-hour tape. The extrapolated frequency of ventricular ectopic beats (ectopic beats/min) in each of the 144 10-minute segments on a tape is plotted on a histogram to determine the number of segments that are free of ventricular ectopic activity and those that have various frequencies of ventricular ectopic activity, distributed over the total 24 hours. In addition, the frequency of arrhythmias is monitored by daily telephone transmission of a 30- to 60-second rhythm strip using a telephone transmission device given to the patient and a receiving device that is operated by technical personnel during weekdays and recorded on a telephonic tape-recording system on weekends.

The ability to control ventricular ectopic activity is assessed by relating frequency of ventricular ectopic activity to blood levels of antiarrhythmic agents measured on the same day as the Holter monitor recording once a month in the long-term survivors. Blood level samples are obtained during the 60-minute period just prior to a next scheduled dose. The antiarrhythmic drug dosages are adjusted to achieve therapeutic blood levels of the study drug regardless of whether or not the patient has rhythm disturbances noted on the 24-hour Holter monitor and whether or not chronic asymptomatic arrhythmias are responding to antiarrhythmic therapy. As long as patients are able to tolerate one of the two study drugs, they are maintained on therapeutic levels of the drug (as measured by blood levels) regardless of the ability to suppress *asymptomatic* arrhythmias. If, however, rhythm disturbances become symptomatic (symptomatic of a low-output state or of episodes of sustained ventricular tachycardia), the option to change to a non-study drug is at the discretion of the patient's primary physician.

Survival data have been accumulated in a group of 29 patients followed for a total of 339 patient-months of follow-up, average 12.1 months, in the current study group and compared with the 1971–73 population of 42 patients who were followed for a total of 536 months, average follow-up 12.8 months. The 1971–73 group, while not constituting a much-preferable concurrent control group, is similar in age, functional classification, ratio of men to women, and diagnosis of underlying heart disease as the drug-monitored group currently under study. The observed and expected survival rates have been analyzed by an age-adjusted analysis, which has demonstrated that the two groups are not significantly different with respect to this variable. The intrinsically more reliable design of a concurrently controlled study is planned for the near future.

Results

Asymptomatic complex ventricular arrhythmias have been recorded in 24 of the 29 patients who entered long-term follow-up between September 1, 1975, and August 31, 1977. "Asymptomatic" refers to the absence of symptoms of inadequate cardiac output during arrhythmias or of episodes of sustained ventricular tachycardia. The definition of "complex ventricular arrhythmias" includes the following electrocardiographic patterns: (1) bursts of ventricular tachycardia; (2) frequent (> 10/hr) and/or multifocal premature ventricular beats; (3) ventricular bigeminy; and (4) couplets or salvos of ventricular ectopic depolarizations. Simple premature ventricular depolarizations, having one electrocardiographic morphology, are not included in this categorization and have been present in all patients.

As of August 31, 1977, the 29 long-term follow-up patients have been followed for an average of 12.11 months (range 1 to 24 months). Using the method of monthly Holter monitor recordings for identification of asymptomatic complex ventricular arrhythmias, all 24 patients who were positive for arrhythmias by either technique were positive on Holter monitor recordings (24 of 29, or 83 per cent). Of the first 80 tapes recorded, a total of 56 (70 per cent) were positive for asymptomatic complex ventricular arrhythmias in the 24 patients. Using the telephone transmission technique, 583 of the first 2533 telephone transmissions showed asymptomatic complex ventricular arrhythmias (23 per cent). Our experience to date demonstrates that the telephone transmission technique identifies such arrhythmias in 44 per cent of the patients, as compared to 83 per cent of the patients using the Holter monitor technique.

There has been a great deal of variability in the frequency of ventricular ectopic depolarizations (ectopic beats/min) at various times of the day on the Holter tapes of all patients having complex ventricular arrhythmias. Therefore, the analysis technique of studying 30 seconds of each 10-minute segment of the total 24-hour tape has become an indispensable part of analysis of the effect of membrane-active antiarrhythmic drugs on the arrhythmias and on survival. The number of 30-second segments of the Holter tapes free of ventricular ectopic activity in patients who have not achieved therapeutic levels of the antiarrhythmic agents has ranged from 25 per cent of the 144 segments per tape, to >80 per cent. As of this time, 17 of the 29 patients entering long-term follow-up have had asymptomatic complex ventricular arrhythmias documented on sufficient numbers of tapes to determine the effectiveness of antiarrhythmic drugs at various blood levels upon these arrhythmias. In two of the 17 patients, there is a clear relationship between achieving therapeutic levels of the antiarrhythmic drugs and the suppression of ventricular ectopic activity. For example, in one patient the number of 30-second segments *free* of ventricular ectopic depolarizations increased from 26 per cent to 90 per cent as he achieved adequate blood levels of procainamide. Neither of the two patients who responded in this way to adequate antiarrhythmic therapy had total abolition of complex ventricular rhythm disturbances. On the other hand, the majority of patients demonstrated *no* relationship between blood levels of antiarrhythmic drugs and a change in the frequency of complexity of asymptomatic ventricular arrhythmias. The failure of a clear response was observed in the remaining 15 of the 17 patients (88 per cent). For the purposes of this study, "adequate" blood levels of procainamide are considered to be 4 to 8 μg/ml, and of quinidine gluconate, 2.3 to 6 μg/ml, during the one-hour period prior to a scheduled dose.

Despite the failure of the rigid antiarrhythmic management protocol to control chronic ventricular arrhythmias, only four deaths (two sudden and two non-sudden cardiac deaths) have occurred during a cumulative 339 patient-months of post–cardiac arrest follow-up (range 1 to 24 months) as of July 31, 1977 (Fig. 1). The periods of follow-up of these four patients were three months (non-sudden death), two months (non-sudden death), three months (sudden death), and 22 months (sudden death). An additional two patients had recurrent ventricular fibrillation in the community, with successful resuscitation at three months and 11 months, respectively. The two non-sudden cardiac deaths and two sudden deaths represent a 14 per cent one-year total mortality rate and seven per cent sudden-death mortality rate.[6] This contrasts favorably to a 42 per cent total one-year mortality rate and 28 per cent sudden-death mortality rate observed in 536 patient-months of follow-up in the earlier study of survivors of pre-hospital cardiac arrest in the Miami area (Fig. 1). If the two patients who had successful resuscitation during a second cardiac arrest while in the follow-up program

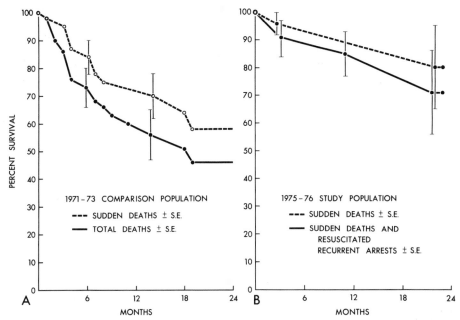

Figure 1. Survival experience among 42 long-term follow-up patients observed from 1971 to 1973 (Panel A) and 27 long-term follow-up patients entering observation between September 1, 1975 and July 31, 1977 (Panel B). The 1971–73 group were not on a controlled antiarrhythmic drug regimen (13 of 42 on no antiarrhythmic therapy), while the 1975–77 group was maintained on the blood-level–monitored membrane-active regimen outlined in the text. The 1975–77 population data were plotted for sudden deaths, as well as sudden deaths and survivors of *recurrent* cardiac arrests, as indicated in Panel B. The 1971–73 data are plotted for sudden deaths (including one recurrent cardiac arrest) and total deaths, as shown in Panel A.

are included as "sudden deaths," the resulting figures of 14 per cent sudden-death mortality and 21 per cent total mortality still compare favorably to the earlier study group. The mean age at entry into the study of the current patient population was 54 years (standard deviation ± 13 years), and that of the comparison group averaged 60 years (standard deviation ± 9 years). The differences between observed and expected deaths during the first 18 months of the study were statistically significant ($p < 0.05$) with age adjustment (using age decades) and without age adjustment. The age differences between the two groups (not statistically significant) had little impact on the difference in survival experience with the ratio of observed to expected deaths — e.g., 1/7.91 without age adjustment, and 1/7.26 with age adjustment.

Conclusions

It is clear from the present study, in addition to previous experience by others, that the majority, if not all, of the patients resuscitated from unexpected cardiac arrest in the community have complex ventricular arrhythmias, nearly all of which are asymptomatic. These arrhythmias are of the type that are generally considered to be of serious prognostic import, especially in the setting of established organic heart disease.

Our experience also suggests that these asymptomatic complex ventricular arrhythmias in this particular patient population are resistant to antiarrhythmic therapy with the commonly available membrane-active antiarrhythmic drugs using therapeutic blood levels as a measure of adequate therapy. In the majority of patients, no relationship was observed between the ability to achieve therapeutic blood levels of these drugs and the ability to suppress or significantly decrease the frequency of these arrhythmias.

Despite the failure to suppress asymptomatic complex ventricular arrhythmias in this patient population, however, the drug-treated population seems to be indicating a trend toward decreased frequency of recurrent cardiac arrest or sudden death when compared to a similar population studied previously. In the 1971–73 comparison population, lower doses of antiarrhythmic drugs were used, and approximately one third of the patients were on no antiarrhythmic therapy at all. Figure 1 shows survival curves for the 1971–73 comparison population and the 29 patients who entered long-term follow-up in the present study between September 1, 1975, and July 31, 1977. The data for the current study group (1975–76) are analyzed for observations through July 31, 1977 (the first 23 months of the study period). Although the antiarrhythmic agents are unable to suppress the complex ventricular arrhythmias, they may interfere with the function of these arrhythmias as a triggering event for potentially lethal rhythm disturbances. A dissociation between drug effect on the focus of origin of ectopic beats and the triggering of more serious arrhythmias is suggested as a hypothetical explanation for this observation. However, the absence of concurrent controls in our current experience makes us tentatively optimistic about this drug-regimen protocol and its effectiveness in preventing recurrent cardiac arrest or sudden death. We believe, at this time, that a carefully designed, concurrently controlled drug intervention study is essential to make a definitive determination regarding the effect of membrane-active antiarrhythmic drugs on mortality after survival from unexpected cardiac arrest in the community.

References

1. Myerburg RJ: Sudden death. In Hurst JW (ed): The Heart, 3rd ed. New York, McGraw-Hill Book Co, 1974, pp 585–591.
2. Moss AJ, DeCamilla J, Davis H, and Bayer L: The early posthospital phase of myocardial infarction: Prognostic stratification. Circulation 54:58, 1976.
3. Liberthson RR, Nagel EL, Hirschman JC, and Nussenfeld SR: Pre-hospital ventricular fibrillation — prognosis and follow-up. N Engl J Med 291:317, 1974.
4. Baum RS, Alvarez H, and Cobb LA: Survival after resuscitation from out-of-hospital ventricular fibrillation. Circulation 50:1231, 1974.
5. Myerburg RJ, Ghahramani A, Mallon SM, Castellanos A, and Kaiser G: Coronary revascularization in patients surviving unexpected ventricular fibrillation. Circulation 52 (Suppl III):III-219, 1975.
6. Myerburg RJ, Briese FW, Conde C, Mallon SM, Liberthson RR, and Castellanos A: Long-term antiarrhythmic therapy in survivors of pre-hospital cardiac arrest: initial 18 months' experience. JAMA 238:1261, 1977.

Mortality in Survivors of Out-of-Hospital Ventricular Fibrillation Is Not Improved by the Routine Use of Quinidine or Procainamide*

LEONARD A. COBB, M.D.

Director, Division of Cardiology, Harborview Medical Center; Professor of Medicine, University of Washington, Seattle, Washington

ALFRED P. HALLSTROM, Ph.D.

Research Assistant Professor, Department of Biostatistics, University of Washington, Seattle, Washington

> The prognosis for a patient with myocardial infarction is worse when anticoagulant drugs are given to someone else.[1]

As much as we would like to advocate the positive side of the controversy addressed in this chapter, we are skeptical of the efficacy of quinidine or procainamide in the prevention of sudden death following resuscitation from out-of-hospital ventricular fibrillation. Safe and effective agents suitable for chronic pharmacologic prophylaxis are certainly needed, but currently available drugs may be ineffective and may be poorly tolerated in many patients. There is an equally pressing need for the better identification of high-risk patients who should be given chronic prophylactic therapy.

Follow-up of patients who have been resuscitated from out-of-hospital ventricular fibrillation has helped to clarify certain aspects of the sudden

*Supported by Grant HL-18805 from The National Heart, Lung, and Blood Institute

cardiac death syndrome. Whereas sudden death most often occurs in the setting of advanced coronary atherosclerosis, we now know that sudden cardiac death is usually *not* a manifestation of *acute* myocardial infarction. It is also noteworthy that recurrences of ventricular fibrillation can be expected to develop in approximately 25 per cent of survivors during the first year following resuscitation. We have recognized in these resuscitated patients several clinical factors with significant prognostic implication for recurrent ventricular fibrillation:[2-4]

1. Gender — males
2. Age — older patients
3. Absence of acute myocardial infarction at the time of ventricular fibrillation
4. History of remote myocardial infarction prior to ventricular fibrillation
5. History of congestive heart failure prior to ventricular fibrillation
6. High-frequency, complex ventricular ectopic activity
7. Abnormal left ventricular function
8. Extensive coronary artery obstruction (angiography)

Myerburg and colleagues[5] administered quinidine and/or procainamide to a group of 16 ambulatory patients and suggested that carefully monitored therapy provided a salutary effect in preventing recurrent ventricular fibrillation. There are, however, several confounding factors in that study:

1. Historical controls were used. For a number of reasons, unintentional bias is often introduced into clinical drug trials when subjects are not randomly assigned to treatment or control groups.

2. Neither the number nor fate of resuscitated patients not enrolled in the treatment group was described. In contrast to the control group, it is possible that some patients who were resuscitated by the rescue squads were not included in the treatment group.

3. The treated patients were, on the average, several years younger than the historical controls. Most studies of sudden cardiac death have shown an average age close to that of the control patients, approximately 60 years.

4. As evidenced by the small number of non-sudden deaths, the treated patients appeared to be less seriously ill than the historical controls. Why should the administration of quinidine or procainamide protect patients from non-arrhythmic deaths?

Our observations of patients who have been resuscitated from out-of-hospital ventricular fibrillation suggest that there is no obvious protection afforded by the chronic administration of quinidine or procainamide in patients with coronary heart disease. Figure 1 shows the survival curves of 70 patients with coronary heart disease — all previously resuscitated from out-of-hospital ventricular fibrillation. The patients represented are males in whom ventricular fibrillation was not associated with acute (transmural) myocardial infarction. The rate of ventricular fibrillation or sudden death in patients who were treated with procainamide or quinidine was approximately equal to that observed in those who received no antidysrhythmic agents. Total mortality in the two groups was also comparable (Fig. 2).

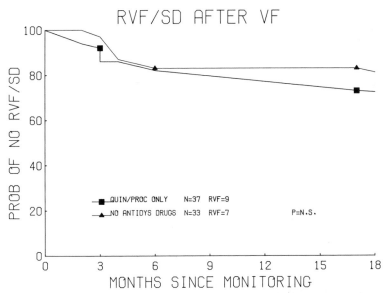

Figure 1. Survival following Holter monitoring in patients previously resuscitated from out-of-hospital ventricular fibrillation. The rate of recurrent ventricular fibrillation and/or sudden death (RVF/SD) was approximately the same in the patients who received chronic therapy with procainamide or quinidine compared to those who received no antiarrhythmic drugs. There were a total of 16 recurrences. In this analysis, deaths classified other than sudden were treated as patients lost to follow-up. All of the 70 patients were males who had experienced out-of-hospital ventricular fibrillation without co-existing *acute* myocardial infarction. All patients had coronary heart disease; patients who had undergone heart surgery were excluded from analysis.

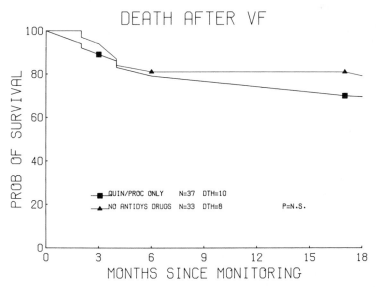

Figure 2. Survival following resuscitation from out-of-hospital ventricular fibrillation. All 18 deaths are considered. Patients are as described in Figure 1.

Table 1. *Patient Characteristics*

	GROUP I: PATIENTS ON PROCAINAMIDE/QUINIDINE	GROUP II: PATIENTS NOT ON ANTIDYSRHYTHMIC DRUGS
Number of patients	37	33
Age (years ± SD)	61.4 ± 8.8	61.4 ± 14.0
Avg. time from VF to Holter monitoring	8.3 months	9.6 months
Average follow-up from Holter monitoring	14.3 months	13.2 months
Heart volume (ml/M² ± SD)	548 (±167)	527 (±133)
No. of patients on digitalis	20 (54%)	15 (45%)
No. of patients with complex° ventricular dysrhythmias during 24-hour monitoring	28 (76%)	21 (64%)
No. of patients with history of remote myocardial infarction prior to VF	24 (65%)	7 (21%)

VF = ventricular fibrillation

° The following were classified as complex dysrhythmias: two or more successive premature ventricular depolarizations; premature ventricular depolarizations in alternate complexes or in every third complex; or multiform premature ectopics, 30 or more per half-hour interval.

However, our retrospective observations also have limitations. First, antidysrhythmic drugs were prescribed by a number of physicians in the community and were usually given with neither monitoring of drug levels nor use of standardized therapy; hence, we have not excluded the possibility that rigorously controlled antidysrhythmic therapy might have improved the outcomes. The characteristics of the two groups are shown in Table 1.

Second, there appears to have been a tendency on the part of the physicians to prescribe antidysrhythmic agents for patients who were at higher risk (patients with a history of prior myocardial infarction). However, the incidence of recurrent ventricular fibrillation (or sudden death) showed no difference with respect to treatment when patients were stratified by history of prior myocardial infarction. To test further whether this imbalance in clinical findings was masking a beneficial effect of therapy on survival time, an analysis of survival was done using as covariates: (1) history of remote myocardial infarction prior to ventricular fibrillation; (2) percentage of half-hour intervals with complex ventricular dysrhythmias during 24-hour Holter monitoring; and (3) chronic use of procainamide and/or quinidine during follow-up. The regression model of D. R. Cox was used.[6] Of the three covariates considered, history of previous myocardial infarction and extent of complex ventricular dysrhythmia, both individually and jointly, had a significant effect on the model. In contrast, the use of procainamide or quinidine therapy had no effect on the fit whatever the combination of covariates (Table 2). Because only 70 patients were studied retrospectively and since all of the possible covariates affecting recurrence could not be considered in the regression analysis, we cannot conclude from these negative results that quinidine and/or procainamide therapy has no effect in the prevention of recurrent ventricular fibrillation. However, it is clear that the effect, if any, cannot be sizable — at least when therapy is administered in the prevailing manner in the community.

We agree with Myerburg and colleagues that complex ventricular ectopic activity has been virtually impossible to eliminate in ambulatory pa-

Table 2. *Survival Regression Analysis**

COVARIATES	Univariate Significance	MULTIVARIATE ANALYSIS	
		Significance in the Full Model	Estimated Relative Hazard
Percentage of half-hour intervals with complex dysrhythmia	p<0.04	p<0.04	$\frac{50\%}{10\%}= 4.1$†
History of previous MI	p<0.07	p<0.07	$\frac{MI}{No\ MI} = 2.8$**
Chronic treatment with quinidine and/or procainamide	p>0.9	p>0.2	***

MI = myocardial infarction.
(Method of Cox DR.[6])
*70 patients described in Figure 1; survival from time of Holter monitoring.
†A patient with complex dysrhythmias in 50 per cent of monitored half-hour intervals has a probability of death at a given time (hazard) 4.1 times that for a patient with complex dysrhythmias in only 10 per cent of the monitored intervals.
**The hazard for a patient with a history of previous MI is 2.8 times that for a patient with no history of previous MI.
***Estimation of hazard not applicable since effect was not significant.

tients previously resuscitated from out-of-hospital ventricular fibrillation. However, this need not necessarily invoke a pessimistic outlook toward the feasibility of chronic pharmacologic prophylaxis against ventricular fibrillation. Ventricular ectopic activity as an isolated finding is usually benign, and a vulnerable myocardium is necessary for the emergency of ventricular fibrillation. Factors known to affect myocardial vulnerability for ventricular fibrillation include myocardial necrosis and ischemia, adrenergic stimulation, certain drugs, hypokalemia, cardiac dilatation, and others. We believe that the effective prophylaxis of ventricular fibrillation will not likely depend on reduction of ventricular ectopic activity *per se*, but rather upon the utilization of agents that reduce myocardial vulnerability. Studies with beta-adrenergic blocking agents (practolol and alprenolol) have suggested a protection from sudden death during the first year or two following acute myocardial infarction.[7, 8] These studies may well point the way to an effective prophylactic approach; however, they should not be accepted without confirmation and clarification. A large, randomized trial of propranolol in post–myocardial infarction patients in the United States is expected to begin during the coming months. If there is a salutary effect of propranolol in the prevention of sudden cardiac death, it may well be related to a reduction of myocardial vulnerability to ventricular fibrillation.[9]

It is our strong feeling that sudden cardiac death is, for many patients, a preventable disorder — or at least one that may be forestalled. However, there is a critical need for the development and testing of prophylactic regimens that are safe, tolerable, and effective. The present state of knowledge does not lead to the conclusion that quinidine or procainamide fulfill these needs. Our position in this important matter is *not* that current therapy is definitely ineffective, but rather that such therapy is of *unproven worth* and that answers can only be obtained by carefully controlled clinical trials with random allocation of patients. Such trials in high-risk patients will likely yield important information with applicability for preventive therapy in patients with coronary heart disease.

References

1. Rytand D: Anticoagulants in coronary thrombosis with myocardial infarction. Arch Intern Med 88:207–210, 1971.
2. Cobb LA, Baum RS, Alvarez H 3d, and Schaffer WA: Resuscitation from out-of-hospital ventricular fibrillation: 4 year follow-up. Circulation 52 (Suppl III):III–228, 1975.
3. Weaver WD, Lorch GS, Alvarez H, and Cobb LA: Angiographic findings and prognostic indicators in patients resuscitated from sudden cardiac death. Circulation 54:895–900, 1976.
4. Weaver WD, Cobb LA, Hallstrom AP, and Hedgecock M: Significance of ventricular dysrhythmias during ambulatory monitoring in patients resuscitated from the sudden cardiac death syndrome (abstr). Circulation 54 (Suppl II):II–172, 1976.
5. Myerburg RJ, Briese, FW, Conde C, Mallon SM, Liberthson RR, and Castellanos A: Long-term antiarrhythmic therapy in survivors of prehospital cardiac arrest: initial 18 months experience. JAMA 238:2621, 1977.
6. Cox DR: Regression models and life tables. J. Royal Stat Soc (B) 34:187–220, 1972.
7. Wilhelmsson C, Vedin JA, Wilhelmsen L, et al: Reduction of sudden deaths after myocardial infarction by treatment with alprenolol: preliminary results. Lancet 2:1157–1160, 1974.
8. Multicentre International Study: Improvement in prognosis of myocardial infarction by long-term beta-adrenoceptor blockade using practolol. Br Med J 3:735–740, 1975.
9. Verrier RL, Thompson PL, and Lown B: Ventricular vulnerability during sympathetic stimulation: role of heart rate and blood pressure. Cardiovasc Res 8:602–610, 1974.

Comment

The emergence of effective community emergency medical systems has resulted in some 15 to 30 per cent of patients with primary ventricular fibrillation outside the hospital being successfully resuscitated and discharged after initial hospitalization. Unfortunately, these patients are highly susceptible to recurrent ventricular fibrillation and death within the first one to two years after discharge. Therefore, it is important to identify measures that might be adopted to prevent recurrence of the episode.

Although coronary heart disease underlies the cause of sudden death outside the hospital in the majority of patients, the role of coronary vein bypass graft surgery in the successfully resuscitated patient is still to be determined. Only a minority of patients resuscitated have significant obstructive coronary artery disease that would normally be considered appropriate for bypass surgery. Even in this group of patients the results to date have been at best suggestive rather than dramatic in the prevention of subsequent ventricular tachyarrhythmias or death. Clinical trials with randomized controls on the utility of this approach are currently being carried out, as is a national multicenter prospective study on the ability of the beta-adrenergic blocking drug, propranolol, to prevent sudden death (or recurrent myocardial infarctions) in patients who have recovered from an acute myocardial infarction.

The controversy discussed in this chapter relates to the ability of two standard antiarrhythmic drugs, procainamide and quinidine, to prevent recurrent ventricular tachyarrhythmias. There appears to be direct conflicting evidence presented by these two noted authorities in the field. Myerburg, in his experience with these drugs in patients resuscitated from sudden death and discharged from the hospital during 1976–77, found a significant reduction in sudden and non-sudden death when compared to a group of similarly resuscitated patients in the period 1971–73 who were not given antiarrhythmic agents. Cobb challenges these results on several counts, the most serious of which is that the controls were not concurrent. Furthermore, he points out that a study of 70 aborted sudden-death patients in Seattle treated subsequently by a variety of community physicians with procainamide and quinidine showed no difference in survival compared to patients who did not receive these drugs. It should be pointed out that the Seattle study also suffered from the fact that it was not a randomized, controlled study.

One of the possible differences between these studies is in the selection of patients. It would appear that in Myerburg's study, these drugs were given to all discharged patients whether the initial bout of out-of-hospital ventricular fibrillation occurred in association with an acute myocardial infarction or not. On the other hand, Cobb's study was confined to patients in whom no evidence of myocardial infarction was present, during their after-resuscitation hospitalization. Since survivors of out-of-hospital ventricular fibrillation that was associated with myocardial infarction have a lessened chance for subsequent recurrence of ventricular fibrillation, the Seattle group may have been at more risk than the Miami group. Both of these authorities, however, agree that there appears to be no suppression of the ventricular arrhythmia, but an apparent reduction of the myocardial vulnerability or the potential of these arrhythmias to trigger a lethal rhythm disturbance.

What is prudent to recommend today while awaiting the results of more definitive, separate randomized clinical trials of both beta-adrenergic blocking drugs and coronary vein bypass surgery as preventive management for sudden death? Clearly, first and foremost, a careful search for an etiologic cause such as pulmonary embolism, sarcoid involving the heart, and so on, should be made and appropriate therapy directed to it should such a search prove fruitful. If a clear-cut myocardial infarction has occurred, I would recommend that the patient be placed on propranolol following his recovery in the hope that this beta-blocking drug will prevent recurrent infarction, ventricular tachyarrhythmia, or death. If no clear evidence of infarction has occurred, coronary arteriography should be performed after the patient recovers from the initial episode. If left main coronary artery disease or its equivalent is demonstrated, coronary vein bypass graft surgery should be carried out. In the remaining patients, whether coronary heart disease is present or not, the patient should be managed initially with quinidine. This therapy can generally be conducted without serious long-term complications (in contrast to procainamide, which is likely to produce a lupus-like syndrome), and if the therapy can be given without undue toxic effects, it is probably prudent in the hope that it may prevent a certain fraction of these fatal arrhythmias from recurring. An alternative is to use propranolol. It is well to emphasize that this recommendation is based not on any unequivocal evidence that quinidine, propranolol, or procainamide prevent recurrent sudden death, but rather on the fact that there is evidence which, while still unproven, suggests that this is probably a prudent approach to adopt while awaiting further definitive studies.

ELLIOT RAPAPORT, M.D.

Sixteen

Is M-Mode Echocardiography Useful in Coronary Artery Disease?

M-MODE ECHOCARDIOGRAPHY IS USEFUL IN PATIENTS
WITH CORONARY ARTERY DISEASE

Joseph Kisslo, M.D.

M-MODE ECHOCARDIOGRAPHY IS RARELY USEFUL
IN CORONARY ARTERY DISEASE

Nicholas J. Fortuin, M.D.

COMMENT

M-Mode Echocardiography is Useful in Patients with Coronary Artery Disease

JOSEPH A. KISSLO, M.D.
Departments of Medicine and Radiology, Duke University
Medical Center, Durham, North Carolina

Unfortunately, past arguments concerning the utility of M-mode echocardiography for the evaluation of patients with coronary artery disease have consistently centered on the suitability of this ultrasonic method for the determination of absolute quantitative descriptors of cardiac performance. Such arguments are quite narrow in their approach and serve to distract the echocardiographer from the practical advantages of the technique. To think that M-mode echocardiography should be judged solely on its ability to supply absolute quantitative information is wrong, for it (1) fails to reveal a mature understanding for the use of ultrasonic information in the basic clinical decision-making process and (2) imposes rigid standards to which very few other diagnostic imaging techniques are subject.

More important than the fact that M-mode echocardiography is useful for the evaluation of patients with coronary artery disease are the principles for how to use it effectively. Continuing clinical experience with M-mode echocardiography indicates that solutions to some critical questions involved in the assessment of these patients are available. The clinician's approach must, however, be direct and avoid the various quantitative pitfalls that have led to confusion about the proper role of M-mode echocardiography for this purpose.

Fundamentally, the clinical role of M-mode echocardiography is based upon three factors. First, there must be a sound knowledge of the characteristics of the method that define its advantages and limitations. Second,

369

the clinician must formulate a rational approach to the performance of the echocardiographic examination and the interpretation of the results. Third, there must be successful incorporation of ultrasonic data into the clinical care of patients.

Characteristics of M-Mode Echocardiography

BASIC CONTENT OF INFORMATION

Since it is currently impossible to directly visualize coronary anatomy by M-mode echocardiography, the clinician must use this technique to assess patients for the untoward effects of ischemic heart disease on the size and movements of the left ventricle. In this regard, M-mode echocardiography is like cineventriculography and judgments as to the presence of abnormalities must be made from a series of subjective or quantitative assessments of alterations in ventricular size, wall thickening, or patterns of contractility.

Figure 1 shows a schematic drawing of an ultrasonic transducer located in the third left intercostal space and angled posteriorly so that the interrogating beam intercepts the mitral valve and upper portions of the left ventricle. Using this standard approach, the septal and high posterior walls of the ventricle are usually accessible. It is therefore possible to assess ventricular chamber size (best expressed as diameter) and cyclical changes in

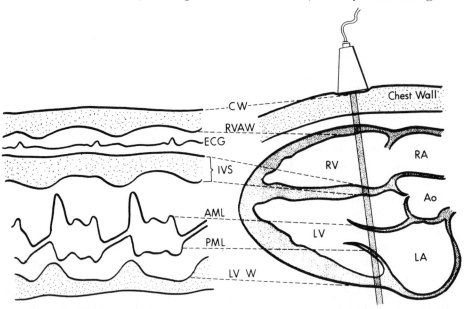

Figure 1. Schematic diagram of an M-mode transducer angled through the long axis of the left ventricle (right) and the resultant echocardiogram. The echocardiogram moves from right to left. CW = chest wall, RVAW = right ventricular anterior wall, ECG = electrocardiogram, IVS = interventricular septum, AML = anterior mitral leaflet, PML = posterior mitral leaflet, LVW = left ventricular posterior wall, RV = right ventricle, RA = right atrium, Ao = aorta, LV = left ventricle, and LA = left atrium.

the direction and amplitude of the visualized wall segments as they occur with the cardiac cycle.

For the purpose of this report, the only quantitative descriptor of left ventricular performance will be diameter. Practical experience with complex extrapolations of quantitative information of ventricular volume data or other descriptors of cardiac performance such as V_{cf} have been shown to be unreliable and are not suited for routine use.

For the most part, this uncertainty concerning quantitative descriptors is based upon four facts. First, patients with ischemic heart disease may have localized abnormalities of ventricular contractility that void the basic assumptions as to chamber morphology and geometry that provide the means for calculating ventricular volume data. An example of these erroneous assumptions will be seen later in Figures 13 and 14. Recent echocardiographic literature is filled with varying methods for this purpose that have little or no merit when applied to practical clinical situations.

Second, reliable assessment of wall motion contractility information such as V_{cf} has not been fruitful because of the previously mentioned reason and because of the fact that variable angulation of the transducer beam to the targets under examination may induce differences in rate of wall movement or timing of peak contraction. Third, quantitative descriptors concerning left ventricular performance by echocardiography have frequently been compared with those obtained by cineventriculography. There is no overwhelming reason to expect accurate correlation of information between the two techniques, since image characteristics from each method are wholly different. M-mode echocardiography provides localized cross-sectional images of the heart walls, displayed in time, while cineventriculography provides images of the left ventricular silhouette.

Fourth, search of the literature fails to reveal any meaningful, large series of patients with ischemic heart disease in whom quantitative echocardiographic information has been compared with purely clinical results over time. Thus, there is an insufficient data base to properly interpret the results of complex quantitative echocardiographic manipulations.

METHOD OF DISPLAY

The time-motion display of echocardiographic data on strip chart recorders (Fig. 2) provides a unique view of the continuous movements of the visualized cardiac structures. As such, this approach can be considered a true advantage of the technique, because it allows for the direct observation of the cyclical changes in chamber size and motion of the heart walls. The inherent importance of easy access to such information is obvious, for it allows rapid differentiation between large or small and well-contracting or poorly contracting ventricles.

IMAGE FORMATION TIME

The image formation time of M-mode echocardiography (over 1000 pulses/second) allows for successful recording of rapidly moving cardiac

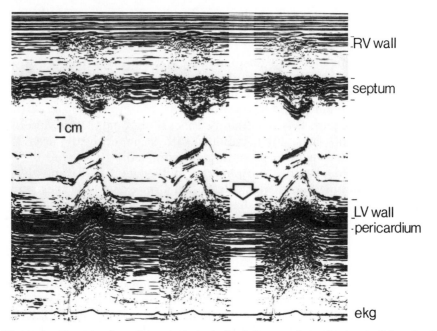

RV wall

septum

1 cm

LV wall
pericardium

ekg

Figure 2. Normal echocardiogram through the left ventricle at the level of the chordae tendineae. Note the amplitude of excursion of the septal and left ventricular posterior walls in systole. The ventricle measures approximately 5.2 cm in diastole and 3 cm in systole. By decreasing the gain of the instrument (arrow) the pericardium can be easily identified.

structures. These imaging rates are commensurate with the rapid changes of pressure within the ventricle, and at present, M-mode echocardiography is the only imaging method with such rapid cardiac image formation times. Various subtle abnormalities of wall motion in visualized portions of the heart that are not seen with other diagnostic methods may therefore be appreciated with M-mode echocardiography. The minor abnormality in septal wall motion seen later in the echogram in Figure 3 amply demonstrates this point.

IMAGE CHARACTERISTICS

The most ideal ultrasonic images are obtained when the interrogating ultrasonic beam is directed perpendicular to the target. As a result of this fact, images from the interventricular septum and posterior left ventricular wall are usually obtained, while images of the ventricular apex and inferior and anterior ventricular walls are difficult to obtain and interpret reliably.

Other factors may influence optimal image quality, including abnormal chest wall configurations, such as barrel chest or pectus excavatum; interposition of a lung between the chest wall and the heart, as with chronic lung disease; or other nonspecific factors. Experience has shown that the population of patients with ischemic heart disease is among the most difficult from which to obtain ideal echocardiographic recordings. One must keep in mind, however, that less-than-optimal ultrasonic recordings may still contain a great deal of useful information, depending upon the clinical question posed to the system. The echograms in Figures 18 and 19 exemplify this point.

ECHOCARDIOGRAPHIC TECHNIQUE

In an attempt to overcome the inability of M-mode echocardiography to provide reliable spatial information concerning the configuration of the left ventricle, the technique of sweeping the ultrasonic beam through the long axis of the left ventricle has been developed. Examples of this technique are seen later in Figures 5, 12, and 20. Despite the distortions introduced into this approach by the variable time it may take to sweep the beam through the proper arc and the constantly changing transducer-to-target distance, this method is quite useful in offering some limited idea as to ventricular spatial characteristics.

All practitioners of echocardiography would agree that a skilled ultrasonographer can obtain better-quality M-mode tracings than one with limited skill and experience. A qualified examiner is mandatory before confidence can be placed in the resultant echocardiographic information.

The additional role of the physician-echocardiographer is of fundamental importance to the issue of image quality and system operation. The physician *must be* intimately involved in the image collection process in order to obtain the most useful data. This individual must be prepared to direct and/or perform the ultrasonic procedure. Other details regarding this critical area will be addressed in more detail in a later section.

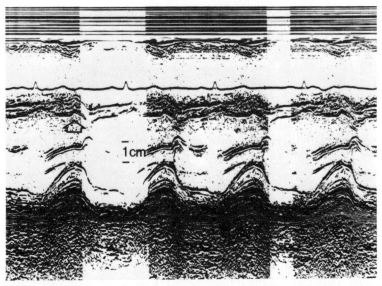

Figure 3. Echocardiogram through the level of the chordae tendineae in a patient with severe obstructive disease of the left main coronary artery. The ventricular motion is well preserved, and the size is normal (approximately 4 cm in diastole and 2.4 cm in systole). Note the minor abnormality of septal wall movement (arrow). For details, see text.

RELATIONSHIP TO OTHER IMAGING TECHNIQUES

As previously mentioned, M-mode echocardiography provides images of moving cardiac structures that are unique and different from those available from any other imaging technique. Comparisons of echocardiographic data with those obtained by common static (chest x-ray) or dynamic (fluoroscopy, angiography, or radioisotope) radiologic methods are bound to be relatively fruitless. Images from these radiologic techniques represent the heart as a silhouette and render all such comparisons limited by differences in image representation.

As a method for cardiac imaging, M-mode echocardiography is theoretically superior to that of routine chest roentgenography. Echocardiography can supply information as to relative heart chamber size, wall thickness data, and basic information concerning the movements of the cardiac valves. It further provides a well-accepted and sensitive means for the isolation of pericardial effusion.

Like M-mode echocardiography, the silhouette techniques have basic limitations. Cost factors, danger of radiation exposure, and possible morbidity from the angiographic procedures serve to limit these approaches. Furthermore, superimposition of certain heart walls over each other may obscure abnormal or normal wall motion in the resultant image.

M-mode echocardiography cannot be compared to basic electrocardiographic methods for the evaluation of ischemic heart disease. The fundamental approach to the evaluation of ischemia by resting 12-lead or exercise electrocardiography is completely different from that available with echocardiography.

When comparing M-mode echocardiography with other techniques, one should address differences and similarities of each method. In most cases these comparisons result in the conclusion that the various techniques are complementary, with each method having specific and useful purposes.

COST

Progressive reductions in the cost of standard M-mode echocardiographic equipment, coupled with increased clinical utilization, now allow for the performance of this procedure at relatively low cost. In many cases, active laboratories can deliver this service at combined laboratory and professional fees only slightly higher than that charged for a routine chest x-ray. Given this low cost, echocardiographic information is readily available on a practical clinical level.

SAFETY

In over 20 years of clinical echocardiography, no obvious untoward effects of pulsed ultrasound have been noted. Compared with other alternative imaging techniques that are based on the presence of ionizing radiation, it appears that the safety of ultrasound is considerably better. As a result, echocardiography seems well suited for both common single-time diagnostic use and serial evaluation purposes. At the present time, however, no absolute statement concerning the true biologic hazards of this method can be made.

Despite this favorable milieu, judgment would indicate that the frequent use of ultrasound should still be limited. Because it is an energy source, some biologic risk may eventually be noted.

Approach to M-Mode Echocardiography

Proper appreciation of the role of the physician-echocardiographer is critical for M-mode echocardiography to be helpful in the evaluation of patients with ischemic heart disease. The physician must interact actively in data acquisition, interpretation of results, and eventually, utilization of echocardiographic information.

DATA ACQUISITION

The questions asked of M-mode echocardiography in patients with ischemic heart disease are often complex and require a sophisticated knowledge of the functional sequelae of the disease in terms of left ventricular function. Questions regarding presence or absence of chest pain, exercise, or pharmacologically induced abnormalities and the factors involved in patient suitability for surgical intervention require that the physician direct and design the echocardiographic study to provide the most clinically useful information.

Too often, data from echocardiography in patients with ischemic heart disease are considered inadequate or meaningless because no thoughtful physician intervention was made during the data acquisition phase. Without sophisticated knowledge of echocardiographic system capabilities and limitations and a knowledge of the complexities of ischemic heart disease, routine M-mode echocardiography performed by technicians alone runs the risk of being without value.

DATA INTERPRETATION

Interpretive skills in echocardiography, particularly as they relate to the analysis of echograms from patients with suspected or proven coronary artery disease, are not easily mastered. Subtle changes in wall motion characteristics or valve movements contained in images of marginal or suboptimal quality may be quite difficult to appreciate except in the hands of an experienced individual. An observer who has mastered echocardiographic technique, is cognizant of the clinical problem at hand, and is aware of the fashion in which the data were collected is most likely to proffer the most useful interpretation.

DATA UTILIZATION

Ultimately, the clinician must be convinced that the available echocardiographic information is useful. For example, it makes no sense to find a large, dilated, and noncontractile left ventricle by echocardiography and then proceed with diagnostic cardiac catheterization in order to prove the patient inoperable for ischemic heart disease on the basis of a severe cardiomyopathy. The clinical decision against surgery could have been made after the echocardiogram.

Clinical Use of M-Mode Echocardiography

SHOULD M-MODE ECHOCARDIOGRAPHY BE USED TO DETECT CORONARY ARTERY DISEASE?

There is no evidence at the present time to suggest that routine M-mode echocardiographic examinations should be performed in patients with suspected coronary artery disease. Since experience with angiography indicates that most patients with proven coronary artery disease will have normal left ventricular function at rest, it is unlikely that the results of M-mode examinations in resting patients would be fruitful in this regard.

There are, however, several situations in which echocardiographic data are of some help. This is particularly true since there is a rapidly accumulating amount of evidence that indicates that severely ischemic myocardium will very likely have altered contractile patterns.

It is a well-accepted clinical fact that serious coronary artery disease may exist without typical angina pectoris. The echogram in Figure 3 is from a 41-year-old male with NYHA (New York Heart Association) Class III non-anginal chest pain in whom the results of graded exercise testing were inconclusive. Faced with a clinical dilemma, the referring cardiologist sought information from the echocardiogram, which showed the minor abnormality in septal wall motion. Despite the nonspecific nature of this finding, the patient underwent diagnostic cardiac catheterization, which revealed an isolated 80 per cent obstruction of the left main coronary artery. Subsequent successful aortocoronary saphenous vein bypass grafting to the left anterior descending and circumflex coronary arteries was performed. The patient is now pain-free two years postoperatively.

This clinical history should not be misinterpreted, for it does not suggest that every minor abnormality of wall motion should be interpreted as evidence for ischemic heart disease. Rather, it does indicate that when echocardiographic data are placed in a critical clinical situation, they may be used to direct the next step in the management of certain patients.

Obviously, the more severe the wall motion abnormality noted echocardiographically, the more convincing will be the likelihood it is due to coronary artery disease. The reduction in amplitude of septal wall motion in Figure 4 is much more striking than that in Figure 3. Combined with the

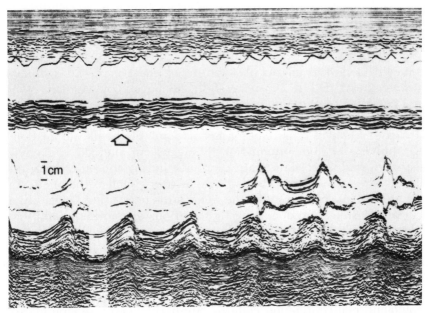

Figure 4. Echocardiogram through the level of the tips of the mitral leaflets in a patient with severe coronary artery disease. The ventricle is dilated (approximately 6.1 cm in diastole and 4.7 cm in systole), and the amplitude of septal wall motion is significantly decreased (arrow). Limits of normal ventricular size are approximately 5.5 cm in diastole and 4 cm in systole.

ventricular dilatation, these data were taken as quite suggestive of disease of the left anterior descending coronary artery in this patient with severe anginal chest pain and EKG evidence of old anteroseptal myocardial infarction. At catheterization, this patient had total occlusion of the left anterior descending coronary artery prior to the first septal perforation.

Many variable clinical situations may arise in which the detection of left ventricular asynergy by echocardiography may be helpful. Figure 5 shows an echogram of a 47-year-old individual with old anterior and diaphragmatic myocardial infarctions on EKG, Class I angina pectoris, and Class III congestive heart failure. When the transducer was directed inferiorly into the body of the left ventricle from the level of the mitral valve, an area of severe posterior wall akinesia was detected. The echocardiographic findings were particularly important in this patient with clinically suspected ventricular aneurysm because no cardiomegaly could be appreciated by chest x-ray. The combination of findings of reasonable contraction at the base of the heart, the presence of posterior wall asynergy, and the absence of significant ventricular dilatation suggested that the patient's ventricle was probably suitable for operative intervention. Cardiac catheterization was used to confirm the above findings and delineate the areas for aneurysm resection and aortocoronary saphenous vein bypass grafting.

Occasionally, the syndrome of angina pectoris may be confused with chest pain due to other causes. Echocardiography can be extraordinarily helpful in documenting the presence of other diagnostic possibilities, such as balloon mitral valve, pericarditis, or idiopathic hypertrophic subaortic stenosis (IHSS). The echogram in Figure 6, showing the typical ultrasonic findings of IHSS with resting outflow-tract obstruction, is from one such patient with a typical angina-like pattern of chest pain and symptoms of congestive heart failure unsuccessfully managed by digitalis therapy. Prompt cessation of digitalis therapy and institution of the administration of beta-blocking agents offered the patient successful symptomatic relief.

In cases such as this, careful history and physical examination will usually provide enough information to suggest an alternative diagnosis to coronary artery disease. Practical experience in this and other large referral medical centers would indicate that case histories such as the one just mentioned are not uncommon, and the echocardiogram offers a readily available means to study and document these various diagnostic possibilities.

Few data are currently available to comment specifically on the role of echocardiography in combination with graded exercise testing or pharmacologic interventions in the routine screening of patients for coronary artery disease. Early information in this regard supports the contention that the ischemic heart, when placed under physiologic stress, is much more likely to show abnormal contraction patterns. Similarly, echocardiographic studies into the reversal of abnormal resting wall motion patterns with acute afterload reduction may be helpful in predicting the successful outcome of aortocoronary saphenous vein bypass grafting in terms of potential reconstitution of normal wall contractility.

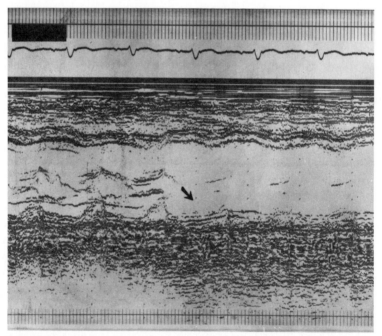

Figure 5. Echocardiogram through the level of the mitral valve leaflets (left) and body of the left ventricle (right). This patient had significant posterior-wall asynergy (arrow) due to coronary artery disease but without profound ventricular dilatation. The ventricle measures approximately 5 cm in diastole. For details, see text.

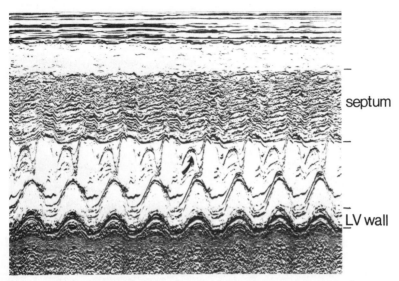

septum

LV wall

Figure 6. Echocardiogram from a patient with severe chest pain that demonstrates the typical ultrasonic feature of IHSS. There is asymmetric hypertrophy of the interventricular septum and profound abnormal systolic anterior motion of the mitral valve (arrow). For details, see text.

Thus, despite the fact that there appears to be little information to suggest that echocardiography has significant capabilities to be used as a routine diagnostic test in patients with suspected coronary disease, there are situations in which it should be used effectively. Proper interaction of the physician in the use of this technique may significantly alter the course of care in certain patients. Once data are available concerning the utility of the echocardiogram in combination with exercise testing and/or pharmacologic interventions, it is quite hopeful that the role of M-mode echocardiography can be expanded in this regard.

Is SERIAL ECHOCARDIOGRAPHY HELPFUL IN PATIENTS WITH CORONARY ARTERY DISEASE?

Since ischemic heart disease often results in clinical situations in which life-threatening circumstances exist, it is reasonable to assume that some knowledge of the functional status of the left ventricle, over time, might be helpful in the clinical decision-making process. Because echocardiography is not routinely performed on patients with coronary artery disease, very few data exist to define the role of this technique in the continuing evaluation of these patients.

The serial echocardiograms shown in Figures 7 and 8 are from a 52-year-old male who initially presented with Class II typical angina and no prior infarction. Figure 7A shows a normally contracting left ventricle at this baseline evaluation. One year later (Fig. 7B), the patient presented for admission with accelerating angina progressing to Class IV. Despite normal enzymes and an unchanged normal resting EKG, the patient's ventricle had

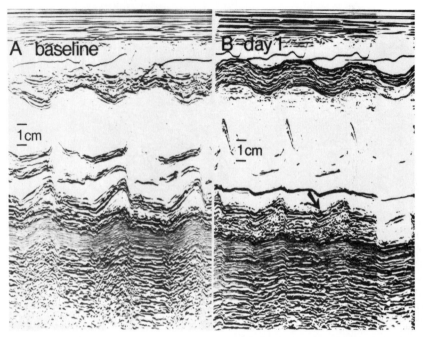

Figure 7. Serial echocardiograms on a patient with progressive ventricular dilatation and reduction in contractility. Panel A shows a normal echogram one year before admission. Admission echogram (panel B) taken with accelerating chest pain but no infarction shows increase in ventricular size and reduction in posterior wall motion (arrow).

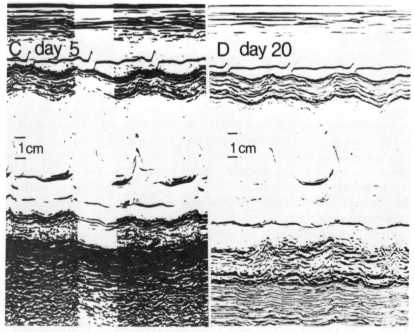

Figure 8. Completed series of echocardiograms on patient pictured in Figure 7. After frank infarction, the ventricle continues to dilate from day 5 to day 20. For details, see text.

undergone significant dilatation and reduction in contractility. EKG findings of new anterior wall myocardial infarction were noted on day three and were followed by a new posterior wall infarction on day four. Subsequent echocardiographic recordings on days five and 20 (Fig. 8) following admission revealed progressive deterioration of left ventricular contractility and increase in size.

Compare the findings in the last patient with those seen in the echograms in Figures 9 and 10 in which the baseline tracing was made on the first hospital day in the setting of acute anteriolateral wall infarction (Fig. 9) complicated by severe congestive heart failure and continuing chest pain. This echogram demonstrated that despite the significant ventricular dilatation, reasonable activity of the heart walls was observed. Clinical impressions of the patient's condition prior to the echogram had centered on the fact that the patient had sustained such a massive infarction that the prognosis was quite grave. With the stimulus of the echocardiographic findings, aggressive efforts for afterload reduction proved fruitful, as shown in the echogram one week later (Fig. 10). The ventricle was smaller and more vigorously contractile than at baseline.

Since coronary artery disease is chronic, it is obvious that serial echocardiographic tracings must be recorded in large numbers of patients over long periods of time before the utility of this approach can be judged. To date, no such data are available. Clinical experience with echocardiography in the setting of acute myocardial infarction does, however, indicate that patients with continuing ventricular dilatation and reduction in ventricular contractility do have a poor prognosis.

Should operative intervention have been considered in either of these patients early in their hospital courses? Does echocardiography reveal changes compatible with severe ischemia and predict possible impending infarction? Can we make judgments on the efficacy of medical therapy in the setting of acute infarction based on echocardiography? Continuing experimentation with the animal model suggests that echocardiography does have a role. The unfortunate fact is that suitable clinical data in patients are not yet available.

DOES ECHOCARDIOGRAPHY HELP IN DETERMINING PATIENT SUITABILITY FOR OPERATIVE INTERVENTION?

Following the logical reasoning that patients with small, well-contracting ventricles are more suitable for operative intervention than those with large, dilated, poorly contracting ventricles, it would appear that echocardiography is ideal for this purpose. Thus, the patients whose echograms appear in Figures 3, 5, 9, and 10 would have a much more favorable operative prognosis on the basis of ventricular function than those whose echograms appear in Figures 4, 7, and 8. It is obvious that consideration for surgery must be based on the clinical status of the patient in combination with the findings at cardiac catheterization and coronary arteriography.

Echocardiography may aid in selecting which patients should or should

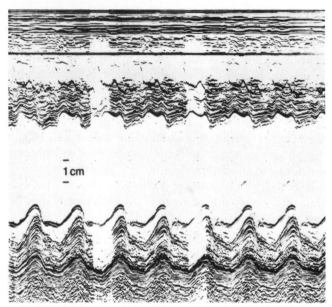

Figure 9. Baseline echocardiogram of patient with recent infarction showing significant ventricular dilatation (approximately 6.2 cm in diastole and 4.2 cm in systole). For details, see text.

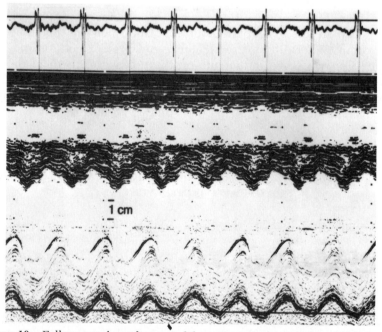

Figure 10. Follow-up echocardiogram of the patient shown in Figure 9. After aggressive efforts at afterload reduction, the ventricle has resumed normal size. The pericardium is identified by use of the "switched-gain" feature on many commercially available ultrasonoscopes. For details, see text.

not go on to coronary arteriography. Figures 11 and 12 show echograms from two patients with recent myocardial infarctions, each complicated by cardiac dilatation by chest x-ray, continuing angina, and pulmonary and peripheral venous congestion. The finding of the massive akinetic ventricle in the patient whose echogram is shown in Figure 11 indicated that no further diagnostic measures, such as cardiac catheterization, were worthwhile. In contrast, the findings of mild septal asynergy, small left ventricle, and pericardial effusion in the patient whose echogram appears in Figure 12 indicated the risks of catheterization in this acutely ill patient were worthwhile.

Admittedly, these are extreme examples at either end of the spectrum of patient suitability for operative intervention on the basis of left ventricular function. They do serve, however, to make the point that data concerning patients with coronary artery disease are readily available and that judicious use of the catheter may be enhanced by using the echocardiographic information.

To date, almost all available studies of patients with coronary artery disease have centered on complex quantitative manipulations of echocardiographic data. As previously mentioned, these manipulations are hazardous, and it is easy to see why they have had little impact on the clinical care of patients. The fallacy of this approach is demonstrated in the patient whose echogram appears in Figure 13. One might conclude that this patient had rather good left ventricular performance on the basis of the echocardiographic ejection fraction (cube method) of 70 per cent. The angiographic ejection fraction was calculated at 34 per cent (Fig. 14) and indicated the opposite impression from that in the echocardiogram. Unfortunately, the interrogating echocardiographic beam was directed through the only contractile portions of the ventricle and rendered the quantitative information erroneous.

Echocardiography is the only presently available method to easily assess the changes in ventricular wall thickness that occur with ventricular systole. Figure 15 shows an echogram of a patient with severe posterior wall asynergy but preservation of wall thickening, while Figure 16 shows an echogram of a patient with inappropriate wall thinning. Data are insufficient at the present time to comment on the functional clinical or prognostic significance of these differences. Most likely, these changes are significant.

IS ECHOCARDIOGRAPHY USEFUL IN ASSESSING THE COMPLICATIONS OF CORONARY ARTERY DISEASE?

It is a well-accepted fact that M-mode echocardiography is the most sensitive method available for detecting pericardial effusion (Fig. 12). It also allows for documentation of other complications, such as flail posterior leaflet due to chordal disruption (Fig. 17). There are no specific data to allow for absolute documentation of rupture of the ventricular septum.

Figure 18 shows an echogram of a patient admitted with history of a recent left hemiparesis. Although the EKG findings were nonspecific, serial

Text continued on page 389

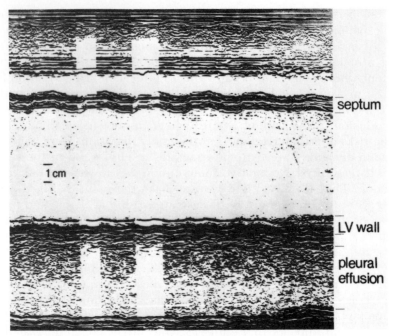

Figure 11. Echocardiogram through the left ventricle from a patient with a severe ischemic cardiomyopathy. The ventricle is barely moving in systole and is dilated. The posterior left ventricular wall is quite thin. For details, see text.

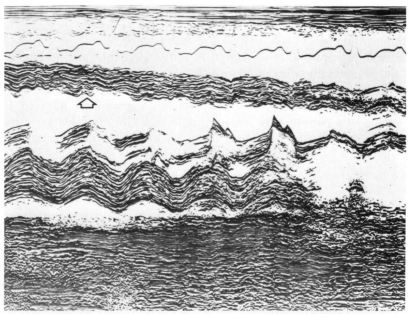

Figure 12. Echocardiographic sweep from the left ventricle (left) to the aortic root (right) showing a pericardial effusion. The ventricle is of normal size with localized decrease in contractility of the septum (arrow). The patient in this figure and in Figure 11 showed significant cardiomegaly on routine chest x-ray and had evidence of vascular congestion on physical exam. The echo allowed differentiation of the contractile nature of each patient's ventricle. For details, see text.

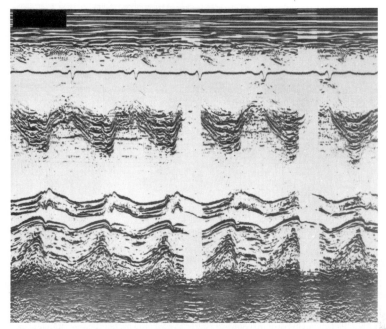

Figure 13. Echocardiogram of a patient with severe coronary artery disease through the level of the chordae tendineae showing moderate dilatation but accentuated contractility. The ventricle measures approximately 6.3 cm in diastole (250 cc³ volume by the cube method) and 4.2 cm in systole (74 cc³ volume by the cube method). Ejection fraction was calculated echocardiographically at 70 per cent. Compare these data with those obtained through angiography in Figure 14.

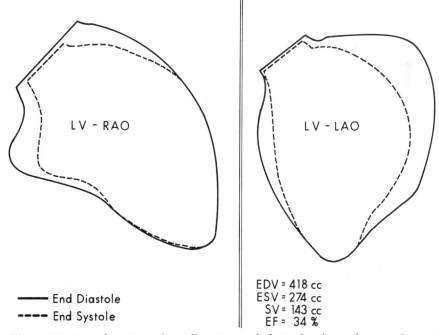

LV – RAO

LV – LAO

—— End Diastole
- - - - End Systole

EDV = 418 cc
ESV = 274 cc
SV = 143 cc
EF = 34 %

Figure 14. Traced angiographic silhouettes and derived volume data on the patient shown in Figure 13. Marked differences in derived quantitative data point out the inadequacies of echocardiography for this purpose. For details, see text.

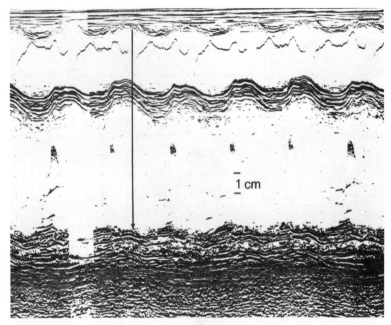

Figure 15. Echocardiogram of patient with severe coronary artery disease showing decreased systolic contractility of posterior wall (arrow). Despite significant ischemia, the wall still thickens.

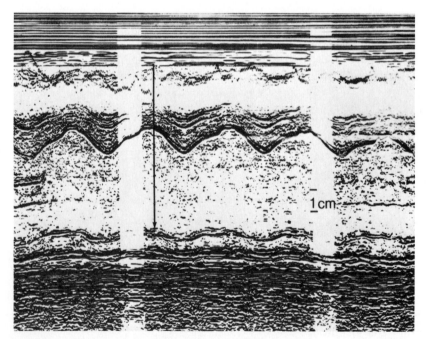

Figure 16. Echocardiogram from patient with severe coronary artery disease and posterior wall thinning with systole (arrow). For details, see text.

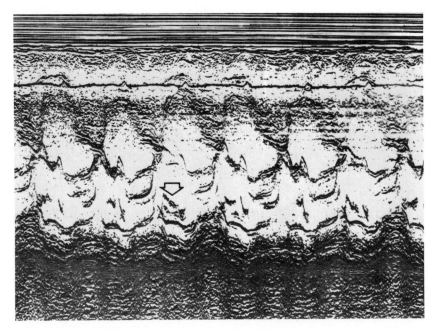

Figure 17. Echocardiogram from patient with coronary artery disease complicated by chordal disruption and flail mitral valve posterior leaflet (arrow).

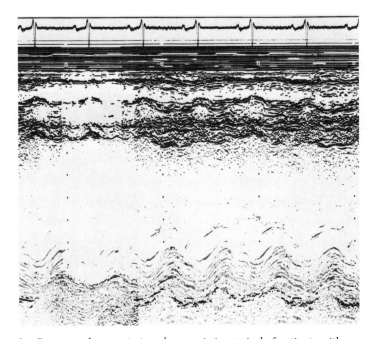

Figure 18. Poor sound transmission characteristics typical of patients with coronary artery disease showing ventricular dilatation and reduced contractility.

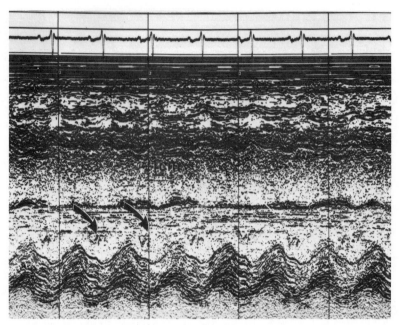

Figure 19. Echocardiogram from same patient as in Figure 18. Careful angulation of transducer into left ventricular cavity revealed oscillating target of mural thrombus (arrows). Despite poor quality of target information, the echocardiogram may still reveal useful data. For details, see text.

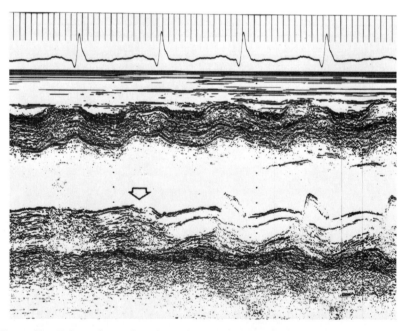

Figure 20. Echocardiographic sweep from body of the left ventricle (left) to mitral valve leaflets (right). The posterior wall is reduced in contractility and thickened (proved at autopsy to be mural thrombus). The arrow points to the area of transition between thrombus and normal myocardium. For details, see text.

enzymes did suggest the probability of recent myocardial infarction. By carefully directing the transducer deeper into the left ventricular cavity, the rapidly oscillating target of a ventricular thrombus was detected (Fig. 19). Note that the diagnostic information was available in this patient in spite of the rather poor sound transmission characteristics. The echogram of another patient, one with old myocardial infarction and organized mural thrombus (proven at autopsy), is shown in Figure 20.

Conclusions

This discussion indicates that standard M-mode echocardiography can be used effectively in the evaluation of certain patients with coronary artery disease. Although the role of the physician-echocardiographer and clinician are paramount, M-mode data do have a role in influencing patient care.

It is also obvious that there are many areas in which M-mode echocardiography may be of considerable use in the future. Large population studies concerning serial echocardiographic evaluation of patients with coronary artery disease remain to be completed. M-mode evaluation of patients undergoing graded exercise testing and/or pharmacologic intervention are incomplete. Similar effort remains in examining the importance of left ventricular wall thickening or wall thinning in these patients.

The advent of new ultrasonic techniques will, most likely, render the results of M-mode echocardiography more meaningful. Real-time, two-dimensional echocardiography, when combined with one or more simultaneous M-mode recordings, would overcome the spatial limitation of the M-mode approach when used alone. M-mode echocardiography combined with range-gated, pulsed Doppler ultrasonic methods promises to supply certain physiologic cardiac flow information not previously available. One of the more important areas for potential application of M-mode echocardiography is the possibility of using ultrasonic data to supply information regarding the differentiation of normal, ischemic, or infarcted myocardial tissue.

M-mode echocardiography, placed in its proper perspective, is most helpful in patients with ischemic heart disease. Confusion comes when too much is expected of the technique before clinical practical evaluation methods have been developed and validated. Prudent use of the results of M-mode echocardiography can supply critical information to assist in the clinical decision-making process.

M-Mode Echocardiography is Rarely Useful in Coronary Artery Disease

NICHOLAS J. FORTUIN, M.D.
Associate Professor of Medicine, The Johns Hopkins
University School of Medicine, Baltimore, Maryland

Wise clinicians have long upheld the "five-year rule" for acceptance of new diagnostic or therapeutic methodologies in clinical medicine. This rule proposes that one must wait at least five years before making final decisions on the merits of a new procedure. Many past and long-forgotten fads in cardiology, a specialty particularly susceptible to technologic gimmickry without clinical substance, attest to the wisdom of this rule. When any new technique is introduced, its virtues are often sung in such stentorian voices by developers and early disciples of the method that the potential drawbacks or limitations go relatively unheralded. Observer and patient selection bias by those with a personal investment in the method may accentuate the tendency to overemphasize positive results, with relative neglect of the negative. There is a reluctance on the part of both researchers and journal editors alike to promulgate negative results, so that positive reports often go uncontested in the literature, although there are many who may have contrary experience. Finally, all too often, techniques that are designed for research applications in selected patient groups quickly find their way into general clinical situations for which they were not intended or for which there is insufficient validation of their utility.

These general remarks are applicable to many of the uses of echocardiography. Although the technique has been in use for 25 years, and thus has long surpassed the five-year rule, many of the applications have not yet withstood the test of long-term scrutiny. In particular, the place of echocardiography in the evaluation of the patient with coronary artery disease has not been established. It is my contention that single-dimensional M-mode echocardiography has a very limited role to play in patients with acute or chronic coronary artery disease.

390

Assessment of Overall Ventricular Function by Echocardiography

Few would argue that one of the most important of the "newer" applications of echocardiography is the direct evaluation of left ventricular size and function in conditions in which the entire left ventricle can be assumed to be uniformly involved, i.e., valvular heart disease, hypertensive heart disease, or myocardial disease. This use is based on the well-documented, close relationship between the minor axis of the left ventricle measured by echocardiography and that measured by angiocardiography. Since there is a linear relationship between minor-axis dimension and overall ventricular volume, left ventricular size can be estimated by measurement of the minor ventricular axis alone. Since most of the shortening of the left ventricle during ejection occurs along the minor axis, there is a linear relationship between the percentage of minor axis shortening (%ΔD) and the percentage of overall volume change with systole (ejection fraction). Thus, it is possible to predict ejection fraction from %ΔD. Adding the dimension of time of shortening of the minor-axis dimension to the formulation allows quantitation of velocity of minor-axis or circumferential fiber shortening (mean V_{cf}). These measurements have been adequately validated by studies comparing angiographic and echocardiographic data. Clinical utility in myocardial and valvular heart disease has been established in several studies. Computer quantitation of instantaneous minor-axis dimension allows calculation of peak velocities of minor-axis shortening and lengthening, which is an important research tool in characterizing systolic and diastolic performance in various pathologic states. Each of these measurements relies on the assumption that what the narrow, "ice pick" ultrasound beam is sampling in the interventricular septum and posterior ventricular wall is a representative sample of what is occurring in other parts of the left ventricle. The single beam thus serves as a biopsy of the left ventricle at its minor axis, just below the mitral valve. The single-dimensional view is then extrapolated to the entire chamber. As noted, this extrapolation is valid in many kinds of cardiac diseases in which there is diffuse involvement of all areas of the left ventricle, but it is particularly invalid in coronary artery disease. Here the involvement is patchy, with loss of motion in one wall of the chamber compensated by over-activity of another wall. Thus, the ultrasonic biopsy may not be representative of the whole in this setting, and indices of overall ventricular function may seriously underestimate or overestimate ventricular performance, depending on whether compensating or diseased segments are sampled.

Assessment of Regional Ventricular Function in Coronary Artery Disease

It is possible to assess regional wall function with echocardiography in areas of the left ventricle that can be sampled by the ultrasonic beam. This is

ANT.
WALL

POST.
WALL

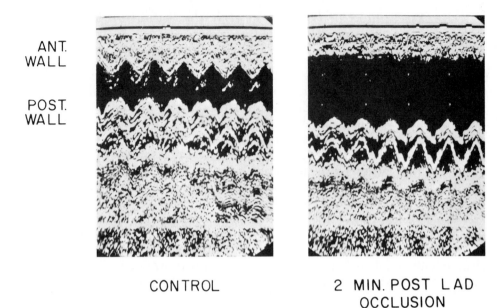

CONTROL   2 MIN. POST LAD
                                  OCCLUSION

Figure 1. Canine study obtained with transducer placed directly on the anterior wall of left ventricle. After occlusion of left anterior descending coronary artery (LAD), there is abrupt loss of movement of anterior wall (akinesis), dilatation of cavity, and hyperactivity in the posterior wall.

well illustrated in the canine study shown in Figure 1. In this example the echocardiogram shows sudden loss of endocardial motion in the anterior wall shortly after its blood supply is interrupted. Changes in endocardial wall motion, including hypokinesis, akinesis, and dyskinesis, can be described qualitatively from echocardiograms. Measurement of endocardial movement and the extent or velocity of wall thickening permit quantification of regional dysfunction. Local wall relaxation indices, such as the rate of wall thinning, may be even more sensitive and earlier indicators of local ischemic injury. Even when the ultrasonic beam does not sample an injured area of the ventricle, there may be evidence of altered cardiac function in other aspects of the echocardiogram. Gibson[1] has shown that the ventricle chronically injured by coronary artery disease displays incoordinate relaxation such that shape change of the ventricle in early diastole as assessed at the minor axis occurs before opening of the mitral valve. Detection of this abnormality requires computer analysis of ventricular minor-axis change, and so is not applicable to routine clinical use. In advanced disease, when diastolic pressure has become altered by acute or chronic injury, the mitral valve may demonstrate delayed closure. When this sign is present, however, there is usually abundant other evidence of altered cardiac performance.

Problems in Assessing Regional Left Ventricular Function

This section will consider the following reasons why echocardiographic evaluation of regional ventricular function is not yet adequate: (1) Inability to obtain echocardiographic information from large portions of the left ventricle; (2) lack of landmarks and standardization when scanning techniques are employed; (3) inability to quantify the extent of myocardial damage; (4) underestimation of motion due to movement tangential to the axial sonic beam; (5) inability to obtain diagnostic quality studies in 25 to 33 per cent of patients with coronary artery disease; and (6) lack of demonstrated cost effectiveness or clinical utility.

The major problem faced by the echocardiographer in evaluating the patient with coronary artery disease is localizing injured myocardium within the ultrasonic beam. When myocardium can be imaged, sophisticated analysis of contraction and relaxation abnormalities is possible, as noted in the previous section. Unfortunately, the echocardiographic window to the left ventricle is limited, largely because ultrasonic waves cannot be passed through the air-containing lung that surrounds the heart. In the standard transducer position adjacent to the sternum in the third to fifth left intercostal spaces, the ultrasound beam samples the upper, anterior third of the interventricular septum and a small area of the posterolateral wall of the left ventricle just beneath the mitral annulus, extending perhaps a third of the way down toward the apex. These areas are illustrated in Figure 2, which attempts to depict the complexities of left ventricular geometry viewed in three dimensions. The shaded areas of ventricular myocardium in this figure are an estimate of what can be imaged by the single-dimensional system from the standard transducer position. It must be remembered that sound waves reflected from structures within the heart will be seen by the transducer only if they are rebounded in a nearly perpendicular direction. Waves encroaching on structures at angles less or greater than 90° will be rebounded tangentially and thus will not be seen by the transducer. This means that the posteromedial, anterolateral, and anterior walls, the distal two thirds and the posterior portion of the interventricular septum, and most of the apex cannot be visualized by angulating the transducer from the standard position. These areas represent most of the ventricular myocardium and are some of the most frequently damaged by coronary artery disease.

A consideration of Figure 2 explains why it is common experience to find so little evidence of damage by echocardiography when there are obvious abnormalities seen by other techniques. For example, electrocardiographic inferior infarction resulting from right coronary occlusion produces damage in the posteromedial wall extending out to the apex. In most instances, the echocardiographer cannot find evidence of abnormal wall motion in this situation because this area is difficult to image. The same can be said for the distal septum, anterior wall, anterolateral wall, or apex, so commonly damaged in anterior descending occlusive disease. Unless there is proximal occlusion of the artery, producing proximal septal damage, little may be seen on the echocardiogram in spite of considerable damage.

Several technicians have attempted to overcome these problems by moving the transducer from the standard position up and down interspaces, laterally along the longitudinal axis of the ventricle to the apex, or to the subxiphoid area. These techniques may be useful when the left ventricle is severely damaged and dilated so that more of it is in contact with the anterior chest wall. In the normal-sized ventricle, it is difficult to find these windows that allow visualization of other areas of the heart. Even when successful, these scanning techniques suffer because of an absence of anatomic landmarks. In the standard transducer position, the mitral valve serves as an important guidepost. Keeping it partially in view lets one know that he is sampling the minor ventricular axis just below the mitral annulus and allows for reproducibility in the same patient and in different patients. Loss of this landmark during scanning from other transducer positions makes it particularly difficult to be certain what areas of the left ventricle the ultrasound beam is traversing and makes reproducibility nearly impossible. The problem is compounded by the different orientation to the chest wall that occurs as a result of variation in chest configuration, which is common in older adults.

Figure 2 also indicates the complexities inherent in this type of scanning. Consider the difficulties in imaging the anterior and posteromedial walls. In order to do this, the transducer would have to be moved laterally away from the sternal edge directly over the anterior wall, so that perpendicular beam direction is maintained. Unless the ventricle is considerably enlarged or the subject has ideal chest wall anatomy, this is usually not possible. Imaging the

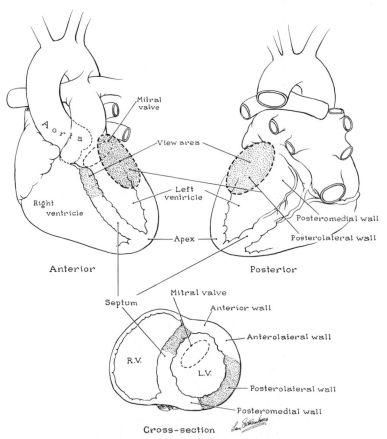

Figure 2. Three views of normal left ventricle to illustrate complexities of ventricular geometry and areas of myocardium visualized by the ultrasound beam (shaded areas) from standard transducer position. The anterior view is a coronal section in which the anterior and anterolateral walls have been removed. The posterior view looks at the heart from behind. The cross section is just beneath the mitral annulus.

anterolateral wall is even more difficult because of the frequency with which air intervenes between the chest wall and the heart in this area.

One of the most important reasons to image the left ventricle in patients with coronary artery disease is to determine the extent of regional myocardial damage or dysfunction. Even when damaged myocardium can be visualized by the single-dimensional system, it is difficult to quantify the extent of the damaged area. For example, it may be possible to scan longitudinally in one damaged area, but it will then be difficult to determine the horizontal extent of injury. It goes without saying that attempts to reconstruct damaged areas in a complex three-dimensional structure such as the left ventricle from a moving, single-dimensional view will be fraught with considerable error. Consider an ideal system, and the problems are obvious. Take a simple balloon, and mark a rectangular area on one of its walls. Now take a small pen flashlight, hold it on the opposite surface of the balloon, and angulate and move the light beam so that it impinges on the marked rectangle and yet maintains a perpendicular beam direction. It is clear that the transducer must be moved in many different locations in order to accurately outline the rectangle from a perpendicular position. Imagine how much more difficult it is to determine the extent of a damaged area in an elliptical, convoluted structure like the left ventricle, particularly when geometry has been further distorted by the damaged area.

Most echocardiographers recognize the potential for underestimation of motion that exists with this technique. This is particularly relevant to the application under discussion, for which quantitation of local wall motion is critical. Figure 3 illustrates the problem of how the ultrasound beam sees motion. When the structure being imaged is moving parallel to the axis of the sound beam, motion is faithfully reproduced, as shown in the left panel. However, when the motion is tangential (center panel) or perpendicular (right panel) to the sound beam, motion will be underestimated or not recognized at all. The interventricular system is an area where motion underestimation is common. Figure 4 shows an echocardiogram from a healthy young man in which the septum appears hypokinetic compared to the posterior wall. It is doubtful whether the septum is truly hypokinetic in this vigorous athlete, but it appears artifactually so, probably because of motion tangential to the axial beam of the sound waves.

Another major problem relates to the ability to obtain studies of diagnostic quality in patients with coronary artery disease. While some workers have reported that it is possible to image the left ventricle in a large proportion of patients with acute infarction, this has not been a universal experience, even in laboratories of high technical competence. In some very good centers, one third or more of patients with acute and chronic coronary artery disease provide unsatisfactory studies of the left ventricle. This is because of changes in chest configuration and adiposity with age that introduce more air-containing structures or fat between the transducer and the heart. These problems are compounded in acutely ill subjects, particularly those who have had recent cardiac surgery and from whom the diagnostic yield may be even poorer. One has to wonder about the clinical utility of a technique that can provide satisfactory studies in only 75 per cent or fewer patients.

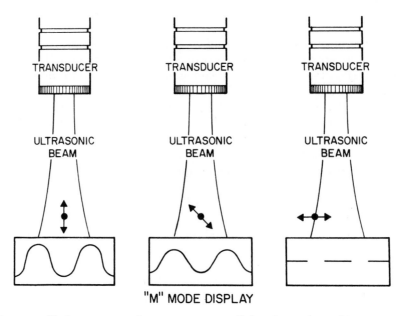

Figure 3.   Underestimation of movement not parallel to the axial sound beam. See text for discussion.

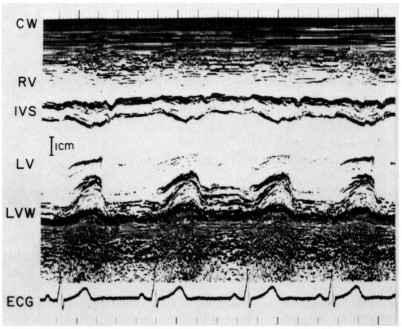

Figure 4.   Echocardiogram from healthy young athlete showing decreased movement of septum (hypokinesis) compared to posterior wall, probably resulting from septal motion tangential to the sonic beam.

There are also practical matters that merit consideration at a time when cost effectiveness of medical procedures must be rigorously scrutinized. What information are we obtaining with this technique that has a palpable benefit in patient management? Or, does this information add anything to that which is easily obtained by the experienced bedside clinician? In a large clinical practice with heavy use of and bias for echocardiography, I have yet to make a major therapeutic decision based on echocardiographic examination of the left ventricle in patients with coronary artery disease except in a few cases of ventricular aneurysm as described below. Because of the inherent limitations of this method in defining and quantifying myocardial damage, it seems to me that physical examination, chest roentgenography, enzyme curves, and electrocardiography provide a better view of the presence and extent of damage in the patient with acute infection and at a lower cost. Interrupted closure of the mitral valve is said to be a useful indication of poor prognosis in acute infarction, but it is neither a subtle nor an early sign of pump failure, which is usually obvious by other simpler evaluations (i.e., the pulse rate). Despite some published reports to the contrary, it is not possible to measure accurately cardiac output by this technique in patients with acute infarction, even when the ventricle is properly imaged. In those few patients for whom hemodynamic information may be of benefit for management, the Swan-Ganz catheter will provide important information, but echocardiography will not. In the chronic situation, there is little to be learned in the patient with angina pectoris by echocardiography. Again, bedside techniques readily allow decisions about when and how much to administer beta-blocking drugs, and one would not rely on echocardiographic assessment in the patient for whom surgery is considered. In this situation, angiographic study of the left ventricle is mandatory.

It is in the patient with chronic coronary artery disease and congestive heart failure that echocardiography may play some role. Ventricular aneurysms that produce heart failure are not subtle affairs, but can be readily diagnosed from palpation, electrocardiography, or chest roentgenogram. I have yet to find an aneurysm by echocardiography that was not obvious clinically. However, assessment of what the rest of the myocardium is doing may be aided by echocardiographic evaluation of the left ventricle. If the echo scan shows uniformly poor contractility in several areas of the ventricle, with dilatation of the cavity, the chances of finding enough viable myocardium to permit surgical resection of the aneurysm are nil, and the patient can be spared catheterization. On the other hand, when there is actively moving myocardium in uninvolved areas, the possibility of surgical therapy is excellent, and further studies can be pursued if clinically indicated.

Two-dimensional echocardiography may overcome many of the objections to the single-dimensional technique advanced here. However, early studies suggest significant problems with this method as well as in quantification and localization of regional disease.

One must also ask why there is the mania for quantification of damage and meticulous analysis of contraction abnormality in patients with coronary artery disease when as yet there is no clearly demonstrated antidote. This is not to deny the important potential research applications of infarct quantification or the possible role that echocardiography may play in this area. However, I do suggest that for the practicing physician, currently available ultrasonic technology is still not yet up to the task and is of marginal benefit to the patient with coronary artery disease.

Reference

1. Upton MT, Gibson DV, and Brown DJ: Echocardiographic assessment of abnormal left ventricular relaxation in man. Br Heart J 38:1001, 1976.

Comment

There does not appear to be too much divergence between the views expressed by Dr. Kisslo and those by Dr. Fortuin. Dr. Kisslo does not suggest that all patients with coronary artery disease require M-mode echocardiography. Rather, he points out that under certain circumstances the information provided can be highly useful.

The average patient with angina pectoris who has not suffered a prior myocardial infarction is unlikely to have impaired global function at rest, and a routine, one-dimensional echocardiogram is likely to be uninformative. With exercise, echocardiographic abnormalities reflecting impaired myocardial performance may be demonstrable. However, exercise studies are not normally performed by the usual echocardiographic laboratory because of technical difficulties. Furthermore, under these circumstances, multigated radionuclide angiography would be a more definitive procedure if, in fact, one wants to demonstrate an impaired ejection fraction in a patient with coronary artery disease during exercise that might not be apparent at rest. In the case of the patient who has had a previous myocardial infarction, this should be evident from the past history and the electrocardiogram. It might well be fortuitous if one were to demonstrate localized impaired function on the echocardiogram, and the value of this information would normally not justify the procedure under these circumstances.

I tend to agree with Dr. Fortuin that there appears to be a mania for quantifying myocardial damage and overzealous attempts to analyze *ad infinitum* minor abnormalities in contractile function when these have little clinical significance. Thus, I believe that one has to be highly selective in performing M-mode echocardiography on the average patient with coronary artery disease. If there is something unusual in the history or physical findings, such as the suggestion of a ventricular aneurysm, some question as to the diagnosis, or a case in which performance of echocardiography might be of help or used for research purposes, M-mode echocardiography may be indicated in coronary artery disease. I suspect that as we study more patients with cross-sectional echocardiography, a greater role will appear for ultrasound in the diagnosis and management of patients with coronary heart disease.

ELLIOT RAPAPORT, M.D.

Seventeen

Is Hammocking a Reliable Echocardiographic Sign of Mitral Valve Prolapse?

HAMMOCKING IS A RELIABLE ECHOCARDIOGRAPHIC
SIGN OF MITRAL VALVE PROLAPSE

    Richard L. Popp, M.D.

PANSYSTOLIC BOWING ON ECHOGRAM DOES NOT
ESTABLISH THE DIAGNOSIS OF THE MITRAL VALVE
PROLAPSE SYNDROME

    Anthony N. DeMaria, M.D., and Dean T. Mason, M.D.

COMMENT

Hammocking Is a Reliable Echocardiographic Sign of Mitral Valve Prolapse

RICHARD L. POPP, M.D.

Associate Professor of Medicine; Director, Non-Invasive
Laboratory, Cardiology Division, Stanford University
School of Medicine, Stanford, California

In the late 1960's cardiologists began to recognize both the potential of echocardiography for clinical diagnosis and the presence of mitral valve prolapse, with its associated clicks and late systolic murmurs, as a specific entity; so it was not surprising to see echocardiography applied to this newly recognized clinical situation. Interest in both the technique and the syndrome at Stanford led to Kerber's description of the echocardiographic pattern associated with patients having mid-systolic clicks and late systolic murmurs, with nearly simultaneous studies reported by Dillon et al. at Indiana University.[1, 2] Since angiograms had shown mid- and late systolic bowing of the mitral valve leaflets toward the left atrium, the reported echocardiographic findings of mid- and late systolic bowing of the mitral echoes toward the left atrium were satisfying and seemingly specific.

When trying to apply these findings to patients seen in the Stanford Non-Invasive Lab, we were surprised by two observations. First, there were some patients with mid-systolic clicks and late systolic murmurs who seemed to show bowing of the leaflets toward the left atrium immediately upon onset of systole, while many others showed a holosystolic murmur in the presence of this echocardiographic pattern and the angiographic picture of mitral valve prolapse.

Second, we found several examples of late systolic bowing of the mitral valve echogram, typical of that described in Kerber and Dillon's articles, when no clicks or murmurs could be identified.[1, 2] The majority of these ex-

403

amples were either patients in whom clicks and murmurs had been heard previously, but were not present at the time of examination, or patients in whom chest pain or arrhythmias were primary presentations and echocardiograms were being done for screening. As we tried to understand these observations by carefully studying the records of patients prospectively, we found there were some patients with intermediate forms of bowing of the mitral valve echo. Rather than the normal, gradual anterior systolic motion, there was horizontal or slightly posterior motion in early systole with an accentuation of this motion in late systole without a clear "break" point as previously described. In other patients, portions of the record showed a late systolic bowing alone, while other portions showed early systolic posterior motion. The late systolic type had the appearance of a question mark turned 90° clockwise, and we have come to call this the "question mark" pattern (Fig. 1). The early systolic posterior motion proceeds posteriorly for about 50 or 60 per cent of systole and then gradually comes anteriorly again before the mitral valve opens, resulting in a deep "U-shaped" pattern (Fig. 1). Since this looks like a hammock sagging under the weight of an echocardiographer, it has come to be known as "hammocking" or the "hammock" pattern.

Some laboratories accepted both the question mark and the hammock patterns, while others accepted only the question mark type for the diagnosis of mitral valve prolapse by echocardiography. It became clear on careful analysis of all echocardiograms going through our active laboratory that there were varying degrees of hammocking or "sagging," from very severe

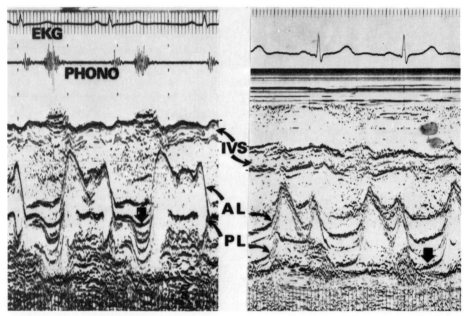

Figure 1. Echocardiograms showing late systolic or "question mark" pattern (left panel) and holosystolic or "hammock" pattern (right panel) of mitral valve prolapse. The abnormal posterior motion is indicated by short arrows. The phonocardiogram (PHONO) in the left panel shows a late systolic murmur. EKG = electrocardiogram; IVS = interventricular septum; AL = anterior mitral leaflet; PL = posterior mitral leaflet.

to very mild forms. In other patients, there was a very delicate, low-intensity echo, suggesting the pattern of late systolic prolapse in patients with very mild sagging of the dominant systolic mitral echo. Many investigators found the same problem in their own laboratories, and much work has gone on to try to define criteria for what is and what is not "hammocking" and the "question mark" pattern.

I would like to separate the following discussion into two portions. The first is addressed to the question, "Does the hammock pattern mean the same thing as the question mark pattern?" And second, "Does the hammock pattern or the question mark pattern truly mean mitral valve prolapse from an anatomic or clinical standpoint?"

As stated earlier, we have identified patients with the hammock pattern having the typical clinical syndrome of mitral valve prolapse. This includes single or multiple early and mid-systolic clicks, late systolic murmurs, holosystolic murmurs with late systolic accentuation, electrocardiographic abnormalities, arrhythmias, peculiar chest pain, some cases associated with bacterial endocarditis, and cases of life-threatening arrhythmias. We have been able to record only the echocardiographic pattern of hammocking in many patients with both the clinical and angiographic picture of mitral valve prolapse despite our experience. In other such typical cases, we may see both hammocking and the question mark pattern or an intermediate pattern of sagging during systole, as mentioned above. A very strong point in favor of considering hammocking as significant for the diagnosis of prolapse as the question mark pattern is the number of studies done using two-dimensional ultrasonic dynamic imaging devices.[3] The first reports by Sahn et al.[3] using a linear array device have been confirmed by other laboratories using electronic, phased-array instruments and mechanical sector scanners. These studies demonstrate both hammocking and question mark patterns from the same valve by sampling various portions of the valve. That is, the portion nearest the aortic root may show little or no abnormal motion, while the recording more distal toward the midportion of the leaflet gives a hammocking pattern, and the most distal portion of the leaflets gives a question mark pattern (Fig. 2). While this is not true invariably, such cases are very convincing when they are observed.

Obviously there are some problems in equating all sagging of the mitral valve echo during systole with mitral valve prolapse. In our laboratory and other laboratories, transducer position on the chest wall has been found to be an important technical point relating to the echocardiographic pattern recorded.[4] Since normal motion of the mitral annulus is both anterior toward the chest wall and also toward the cardiac apex, it is possible to place the transducer so high on the chest wall that the annulus is moving away from the transducer during systole as it moves toward the cardiac apex. Thus, the record shows net negative or echocardiographic "posterior" motion during systole in most normal people if the transducer is located high enough on the chest wall. In some patients this may be the second or third intercostal space, but this high position can be recognized by noting the inferior angulation of the transducer when recording the mitral valve. Conversely, if the transducer is located close enough to the cardiac apex or

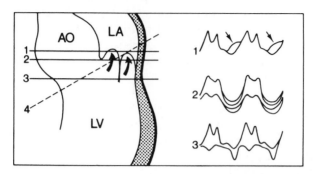

Figure 2. Diagrammatic representation of mitral valve prolapse shows the postero-superior orientation of the prolapsed leaflets. The M-mode output from line 1 demonstrates the pseudo-systolic anterior motion artifact caused by superimposition of echoes from the valve annulus and the anterior leaflet. The output from line 2 shows a multiple line sequence from the various portions of arched leaflets subtended by the beam. The echo beam at line 3 shows the pattern of prolapse demonstrated at the free edges of the leaflets. Line 4 represents the direction from which most published single crystal recordings have been obtained. Aortic root dilation (AO) is also shown. LA = left atrium; LV = left ventricle. (From Sahn DJ, Allen HD, Goldberg SJ, Friedman WF: Mitral valve prolapse in children: a problem defined by real-time cross-sectional echocardiography. Circulation 53:651–656, 1976. Used with permission.)

very low on the chest wall at the left sternal border, the exaggerated annulus motion may partially obscure late systolic or holosystolic posterior bowing of the leaflet toward the atrium. Therefore, we perform all of our studies, especially those investigating mitral valve prolapse, with the transducer in an intercostal space that allows us to record both leaflets of the mitral valve and their point of coaptation and separation when the transducer is perpendicular to the chest wall. As a further technical point, we try to visualize this closure, or "C point," and the separation, or "D point," while passing the sound beam across the A-V groove and recording both left atrium and left ventricle behind the mitral valve leaflets.

We have found a statistical association between the patterns of prolapse and the auscultatory or phonocardiographic findings associated with mitral valve prolapse when the main systolic mitral echo deviates posterior to the line between the C and D points by more than 2 mm (Fig. 3).[5] When there is minimal sagging throughout systole or mild posterior motion late in systole less than 2 mm from the C-D line, there is no correlation with these clinical findings. Typical prolapse cases may have echocardiograms with the main systolic echo deviating 3, 4, or 5 mm below the C-D line and often associated with even further posterior motion by a cascade of echoes behind the dominant one. When using these criteria, we believe hammocking is as reliable as the late systolic pattern in predicting mitral valve prolapse.

If one gives amyl nitrite to a patient with the late systolic pattern, the aggressive posterior bowing begins to occupy more and more of systole and may be converted to the holosystolic pattern in many cases[6] (Fig. 4). This is further evidence that the two patterns represent a single entity.

A second problem remains. Does the echocardiographic pattern of prolapse mean anatomic prolapse? So far we have not seen a truly normal mitral valve at surgery or autopsy in a patient with either of the patterns discussed here that fulfills the prolapse criteria of our laboratory. Neverthe-

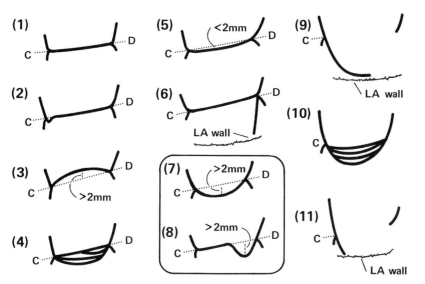

Figure 3. Diagrammatic schema used to classify echocardiographic patterns. Patterns 7 and 8 are read as echocardiographic patterns of mitral valve prolapse in our laboratory. Patterns 9, 10, and 11 were represented by too few patients to make a valid statistical statement from the study cited as reference 3. (From Markiewicz W, Stoner J, London E, Hunt S, Popp RL: Mitral valve prolapse in one hundred presumably healthy young females. Circulation 53:464–473, 1976. Used with permission.)

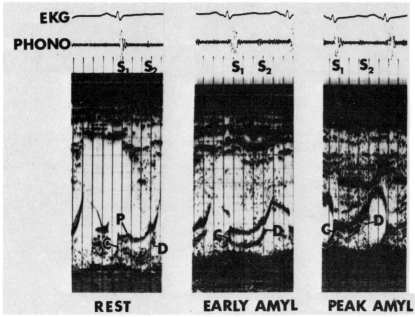

Figure 4. Echo-phono-EKG from a patient with late-systolic prolapse at rest that became holosystolic prolapse during amyl nitrite inhalation. Rest: Rest showing late-systolic pattern of prolapse. There were no consistent auscultatory phenomena. Early amyl: Same patient very early during amyl nitrite inhalation. The prolapse became holosystolic, with a hammock contour. Peak amyl: Near the peak heart rate response to amyl. The hammock pattern remains. (From Winkle RA, Goodman DJ, Popp RL: Simultaneous echocardiographic-phonocardiographic recordings at rest and during amyl nitrite administration in patients with mitral valve prolapse. Circulation 51:522–529, 1975. Used with permission.)

less, the angiocardiogram may fail to show prolapse when the echocardiogram is positive, placing the echo finding in doubt. Occasionally, the echocardiogram is negative when there is apparent prolapse on the angiogram, or even in the face of typical clinical findings. The angiocardiographic criteria of mitral valve prolapse are not well defined. If a single right anterior oblique projection is used, only a limited portion of the valve is seen in profile, and this may account for some of the disparity. But we need to know what to think of a patient with echocardiographic mitral valve prolapse without clinical or angiographic findings. We have used the semantic ploy of reporting all patients as having "echocardiographic patterns of prolapse" without saying that the patient actually has mitral valve prolapse. This allows the possibility that the pattern of prolapse could be simulated by a relatively nonredundant leaflet that goes through a series of motions under the transducer, resulting in a pattern of prolapse when anatomic and pathologic prolapse is not present.

Another way of assessing the meaning of these echocardiographic patterns is to recognize that the five to six per cent prevalence of echocardiographic prolapse in the general population is a figure that has been observed in several laboratories.[7, 8] This same incidence is found by the few autopsy studies done by pathologists specifically looking for this condition, again implying echocardiographic prolapse means anatomic prolapse.[9]

In conclusion, I would summarize by saying that marked systolic hammocking of the echocardiographic mitral valve signal means the same anatomic and physiologic prolapse indicated by the late systolic pattern. The controversy regarding the former pattern will be reduced by using fairly strict and perhaps arbitrary criteria of what is and what is not posterior motion during systole. Since both the hammock and the late systolic pattern can be seen in a single case by recording from different parts of the valve and can be interchanged under the influence of pharmacologic agents, there is no reason to believe the two patterns are different. Experience so far suggests both patterns are moderately specific for anatomic prolapse. Causes of false positivity have not been well defined, but apparently this represents little problem. Only through longitudinal follow-up will we have clear information on possible clinical significance of a predominant hammock or late systolic pattern relative to specific symptoms or long-term prognosis.

References

1. Kerber RE, Isaeff DM, and Hancock EW: Echocardiographic patterns in patients with the syndrome of systolic click and late systolic murmur. N Engl J Med 284:691–693, 1971.
2. Dillon JC, Haine CL, Chang S, and Feigenbaum H: Use of echocardiography in patients with prolapsed mitral valve. Circulation 43:503–507, 1971.
3. Sahn DJ, Allen HD, Goldberg SJ, and Friedman WF: Mitral valve prolapse in children: a problem defined by real-time cross-sectional echocardiography. Circulation 53:651–656, 1976.
4. Markiewicz W, Stoner J, London E, Hunt S, and Popp RL: Effect of transducer placement on echocardiographic mitral valve systolic motion. Eur J Cardiol 4/3:359–366, 1976.

5. Markiewicz W, Stoner J, London E, Hunt S, and Popp RL: Mitral valve prolapse in one hundred presumably healthy young females. Circulation 53:464–473, 1976.
6. Winkle RA, Goodman DJ and Popp RL: Simultaneous echocardiographic-phonocardiographic recordings at rest and during amyl nitrite administration in patients with mitral valve prolapse. Circulation 51:522–529, 1975.
7. Procacci PM, Savran SV, Schreiter SL, and Bryson AL: Prevalence of clinical mitral valve prolapse in 1169 young women. N Engl J Med 294:1086–1088, 1976.
8. Brown OR, Kloster FE, and DeMots H: Incidence of mitral valve prolapse in the asymptomatic normal (abstr). Circulation 52(Suppl II):II–77, 1975.
9. Hill DG, Davies MJ, and Braimbridge MV: The natural history and surgical management of the redundant cusp syndrome (floppy mitral valve). J Thorac Cardiovasc Surg 67:519, 1974.

Pansystolic Bowing on Echogram Does Not Establish the Diagnosis of the Mitral Valve Prolapse Syndrome*

ANTHONY N. DEMARIA, M.D.

Associate Professor of Medicine; Director, Cardiac
Non-Invasive Laboratory, University of California School
of Medicine, Davis, California; Sacramento Medical
Center, Sacramento, California

DEAN T. MASON, M.D.

Professor and Chief, Cardiovascular Medicine, University
of California School of Medicine, Davis, California;
Sacramento Medical Center, Sacramento, California

In the short interval since its recognition as a clinical entity in 1966,[1,2] the mitral valve prolapse syndrome has undergone an amazing transformation from a cardiac disorder originally believed to be infrequently encountered to one that has recently been alleged to affect up to 17 per cent of healthy females.[3,4] Accordingly, many physicians have begun to re-evaluate the sensitivity and specificity of many of the criteria utilized to diagnose the presence of the mitral valve prolapse syndrome.

One of the factors of major importance in the apparent prolific increase in the prevalence of this syndrome has been the echocardiogram. Thus, by virtue of its atraumatic nature, echocardiography has enabled the examination of mitral valve motion in a large number of asymptomatic as well as symptomatic subjects. Although the validity of all of the echocardiographic manifestations associated with mitral valve prolapse syndrome has recently come under close scrutiny, the foremost criticism has been directed to-

*Supported by grants from the Golden Empire and Central Valley California Heart Associations

ward the pattern of mitral valve motion consisting of pansystolic posterior bowing. Although the exact significance of pansystolic bowing of the mitral leaflets on echogram remains uncertain, for the purposes of this article we will attempt to support the proposition that this echographic finding is not, of itself, sufficient to establish the diagnosis of the mitral prolapse syndrome.

Are Mitral Valve Prolapse and Mitral Valve Prolapse Syndrome the Same Thing?

It is our feeling that the major factor responsible for the current confusion regarding the various echographic manifestations of mitral valve prolapse syndrome has been the failure to determine whether "mitral prolapse" and "the mitral valve prolapse syndrome" are identical entities. Thus, the data that have been critically lacking in previous considerations of the significance of various patterns of mitral valve motion on echogram have been those showing correlation of these ultrasonic findings with the appearance of symptoms and signs of cardiac dysfunction over an extended follow-up. This problem is further compounded by the fact that no "gold standard" currently exists by which to independently establish the presence of mitral valve prolapse syndrome with certainty. With this in mind, our approach to this discussion will entail a consideration of the clinical features of the mitral valve prolapse syndrome, then an analysis of the patterns of systolic mitral valve motion as recorded by ultrasound, and finally a critical appraisal of the relationship of mitral valve motion on echogram to the entity recognized as the mitral valve prolapse syndrome.

MITRAL VALVE PROLAPSE SYNDROME

The initial medical observation regarding the mitral valve prolapse syndrome was recorded in the late nineteenth century when the auscultatory findings of a mid-systolic click and late systolic murmur were described in a group of individuals who were otherwise free of signs and symptoms of cardiac disease.[5, 6] Indeed, so benign were the physical examination and subsequent clinical course associated with these auscultatory findings that it was believed that the click and murmur were of extracardiac origin and were the result of old healed pericarditis.[6] The extracardiac theory of the genesis of the auscultatory phenomena prevailed until the early 1960's, when Barlow and associates documented by cineangiography that mitral regurgitation was responsible for the systolic murmur.[7] It was not until 1966, however, that Barlow and associates[1] and Criley and co-workers[2] simultaneously recognized that the pathophysiologic basis of mitral regurgitation in these patients was unique and consisted of aneurysmal protrusion or prolapse of the mitral leaflets posteriorly into the left atrium during systole.

Almost simultaneous with the unraveling of the pathophysiology of this cardiac disorder, it was observed that patients with mid-systolic clicks and/or late systolic murmurs frequently manifested additional symptoms and signs of heart disease.[8] Thus, chest pain, arrhythmias,[9] and electrocardiographic abnormalities[8, 10] were described in a substantial proportion of patients manifesting click-murmur on auscultation, and thereby the condition was elevated to the stature of the mitral valve prolapse syndrome. Subsequently, patients were described in whom this syndrome was present in the absence of any auscultatory abnormalities, or with only a pansystolic murmur typical of the usual types of mitral regurgitation.[11, 12]

Despite the incrimination of mitral apparatus malfunction in the genesis of this disorder and the appreciation of the prevalence of additional cardiac abnormalities in these patients, the mitral valve prolapse syndrome continued to be regarded as an essentially benign condition with little therapeutic or prognostic significance. Soon, however, disquieting reports began to appear detailing the appearance of serious cardiac complications in patients with mitral valve prolapse syndrome. Thus, abnormalities of left ventricular hemodynamic function and contractile pattern were observed in patients with this disorder.[13-15] More important, major complications, including bacterial endocarditis,[16] mitral regurgitation of sufficient hemodynamic significance to warrant mitral valve surgery,[17-19] and even sudden death,[20, 21] were reported secondary to mitral valve prolapse syndrome. Although the precise frequency with which catastrophic complications of mitral valve prolapse syndrome occurs remains uncertain, the potential for such events in even a small percentage of these patients, who are typically young, asymptomatic individuals, would have major implications regarding long-term medical therapy and follow-up. Accordingly, the diagnosis of mitral valve prolapse syndrome assumed greater importance to practicing physicians.

Throughout the evolution of the mitral valve prolapse syndrome, considerable controversy and uncertainty have surrounded the question of the etiology of this disorder. Thus, although clinical signs of this condition have been observed in the setting of rheumatic[22] and congenital heart disease (especially atrial septal defect),[23, 24] evidence of such underlying disorders is present in only a small number of patients with mitral valve prolapse syndrome. In addition, although this syndrome has been documented to occasionally occur in a familial pattern,[25-27] evidence of genetic transmission is absent in most patients with clinical signs of mitral prolapse. Similarly, although mitral prolapse may occur in patients with Marfan's Syndrome[28] and has been seen in association with coronary artery disease,[29, 30] the majority of prolapse patients have been found to be free of these disorders.

Recently, attention has turned to a consideration of the role of myxomatous degeneration of the mitral leaflets as opposed to that of a primary cardiomyopathy in the etiology of mitral valve prolapse syndrome.[31] Thus, it has been emphasized that myxomatous degeneration, or replacement of the normal fibrous stroma of the mitral leaflets with acid mucopolysaccharides, has been a constant observation in all mitral prolapse patients in whom histologic examination has been performed.[31-34] Such mucoid degeneration typically results in thickened, redundant, hooded mitral leaflets with elongated chordae tendineae. However, it is possible that only those prolapse patients with substantial myxomatous degeneration have sufficient dysfunction to result in surgery or death. Conversely, the finding of abnormalities of left ventricular hemodynamic function and contraction pattern by cardiac catheterization in the majority of prolapse patients has led many investigators to conclude that this syndrome represents a primary cardiomyopathy.[13-15] However, ventricular dysfunction is far from a universal finding in prolapse patients and differs markedly both qualitatively and quantitatively from patient to patient.[35] Therefore, although an element of myocardial dysfunction may accompany mitral prolapse in many patients, it is unlikely that cardiomyopathy is an acceptable etiology for this disorder.

Recently, a unifying hypothesis for the etiology of mitral valve prolapse syndrome has been proposed based upon a functional concept of the disorder.[36] Accordingly, it has been hypothesized that mitral prolapse will occur anytime there exists a disproportion between the length of the mitral-chordal apparatus and the volume of the left ventricle. Thereby, mitral prolapse could occur in the setting of a normal left ventricular volume and excessive mitral leaflet–chordal length, such as in the presence of myxomatous degeneration, or conversely in the setting of a normal mitral valve apparatus with a particularly small left ventricle, such as idiopathic hypertrophic subaortic stenosis. In this formulation, every individual would be potentially "prolapsable" under the appropriate circumstances. Although this proposed unifying theory remains unproven, it would provide a most attractive mechanism to explain the variable clinical presentation and course of patients with stigmata of the mitral valve prolapse syndrome.

It is obvious from the foregoing discussion, therefore, that considerable uncertainty continues regarding the nature, and even the existence, of the mitral valve prolapse syndrome, and this lack of assurance may have important implications regarding the understanding of pansystolic bowing on echogram. On the one hand, it may be reasoned that the mitral valve prolapse syndrome is not a distinct disorder, but rather a collection of signs and symptoms that may be produced by a variety of heart diseases, or even physiologic phenomena in normal individuals. In this case, prognosis and therapy would be directly related to the underlying condition. Alternately, the mitral valve prolapse syndrome could be considered as a distinct clinical cardiac disorder (presumably related to myxomatous changes of the mitral apparatus), the individual features of which could be manifested in a variety of other abnormal and even normal conditions. In either event, however, it would be recognized that a group of patients do exist in whom posterior displacement of the mitral leaflets into the left atrium in systole could be accompanied by definite symptoms, such as chest pain, and serious complications, such as severe mitral regurgitation and sudden death. At issue is whether isolated pansystolic bowing of the mitral leaflets on echogram is sufficient evidence to identify this specific group of patients with an acceptable degree of sensitivity and specificity.

THE MITRAL VALVE ECHOGRAM

It was not long after the realization that the mitral regurgitation in patients with mid-systolic click–late systolic murmur was due to prolapse of the mitral leaflets into the left atrium that several investigators described the typical echocardiographic findings in such patients. Thus, Drs. Dillon[37] and Kerber[38] simultaneously reported that mitral prolapse patients exhibited a unique abnormality on echogram consisting of an abrupt posterior buckling movement in mid-systole that continued to the end of this period of the cardiac cycle (Fig. 1). This pattern of mitral motion on echogram contrasted sharply with that observed in normals, which consisted of a gradual, straight, slightly anterior movement as the left ventricle emptied and the left atrium filled in systole (Fig. 2). This abnormal pattern was observed in the vast majority of patients with mid-systolic clicks and/or late systolic murmurs, was not observed in association with any other cardiac lesion, and therefore became recognized as the echocardiographic hallmark of the mitral valve prolapse syndrome.

Soon, however, a number of patients were encountered with the classic clinical and angiographic manifestations of mitral valve prolapse syndrome in whom the characteristic abrupt mid-systolic buckling motion of the mitral leaflets could not be identified on echogram. Rather, the ultrasonic abnormality observed in these patients consisted of a continuous backward motion of the mitral leaflets throughout systole, resulting in a hammock-like configuration of these structures[11, 39] (Figs. 3 and 4). It was additionally observed that the mitral leaflets reached the nadir of posterior motion in mid-systole (Figs. 3 and 4), rather than early systole (Fig. 5), and also frequently exhibited an exaggerated amplitude of diastolic excursion as well as multiple systolic echoes (Figs. 3 and 4). Thereby, pansystolic posterior bowing of the mitral leaflets was recognized as an alternative echographic manifestation of mitral valve prolapse syndrome.

It was not long, however, until a number of investigators noted the high frequency with which patients referred for echocardiographic examination exhibited evidence of mitral valve prolapse syndrome consisting of pansystolic bowing of the mitral leaflets. Indeed, retrospective analysis of echograms in our laboratory revealed this abnormality in up to eight per cent of patients undergoing evaluation by ultrasound. Even more disturbing was the fact that pansystolic bowing of the mitral leaflets on echogram was the only manifestation of mitral valve prolapse syndrome observed in many of these individuals. Accordingly, many thoughtful investigators questioned the reliability of pansystolic hammocking on echogram in the identification of the mitral valve prolapse syndrome.

Initially, technical factors related to the performance of echocardiography were invoked to explain the relationship between pansystolic bowing on echogram and mitral valve prolapse syndrome. Thus, utilizing cross-sectional echocardiography in children with mitral prolapse, Sahn and associates[40] demonstrated that prolapse consisted of a composite superior as well as posterior motion. Accordingly, with certain positions and angulations of the ultrasonic transducer, continuous, pansystolic, backward move-

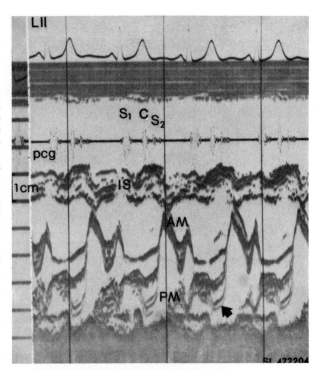

Figure 1. Shown is the mitral valve echogram obtained in a patient with the classic clinical and cineangiographic features associated with the mitral valve prolapse syndrome. The mitral leaflets move in a straight-line motion in early systole and then abruptly buckle posteriorly into the left atrium in the later portion of this period of the cardiac cycle (arrow). A phonocardiogram (pcg) demonstrates a prominent mid-systolic click (C). IS = interventricular septum; AM = anterior mitral leaflet; PM = posterior mitral leaflet.

ment of the mitral leaflets would be recorded. Thereby, in certain individuals the typical mid-systolic buckle of the mitral leaflets would be recorded with one transducer angulation, while pansystolic bowing would be recorded with another. Additionally, a relationship was demonstrated between the onset of mitral prolapse and left ventricular size, in that backward protrusion of the leaflets into the left atrium would occur earlier in systole in the presence of a small ventricular chamber. Thereby, pansystolic bowing would occur in the setting of marked reductions in ventricular volume.[41, 42] Finally, it was pointed out that the inferior motion of the mitral apparatus during systole could be sufficient to account for net movement of the mitral leaflets away from the transducer if the probe were positioned very superiorly on the chest wall and angled downward[3] and that the pattern of prolapse could appear in the presence of precardial effusion[43] (Fig. 6) or premature ventricular contractions.[44] Nevertheless, although these factors may account for the presence of pansystolic bowing in some patients, it is clear that there exist a number of patients with mitral valve prolapse syndrome in whom multiple echograms with various transducer positions yield a continuous hammocking motion as the only echographic abnormality.

In an attempt to further elucidate the relationship of the various ultrasonic patterns of systolic mitral valve motion to the presence of the mitral valve prolapse syndrome, Markiewicz and associates[3] performed echocardiograms and phonocardiograms in 100 presumably healthy females. Al-

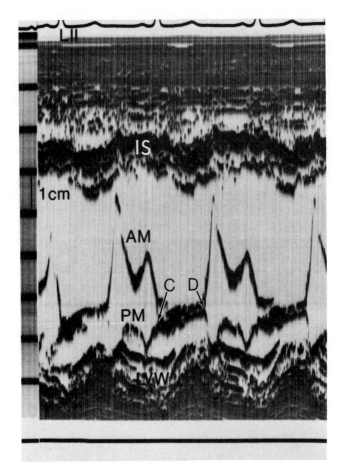

Figure 2. Mitral valve echogram in a normal subject obtained in our laboratory. Note that following the apposition of the mitral valve leaflets at the onset of systole (C), the mitral echogram exhibits a gradual straight anterior motion until the separation of the mitral leaflets at the onset of diastole (D). LVW = left ventricular posterior wall.

though, as might be expected, symptoms compatible with heart disease were present in a substantial number of the subjects who volunteered for this examination, all were judged to be "healthy" by themselves and their personal physicians. Surprisingly, 17 per cent of the females evaluated were found to have mid-systolic clicks or late systolic murmurs on phonocardiogram either at rest or after amyl nitrate inhalation. When these auscultatory findings were related to a variety of echographic patterns of systolic motion, a correlation was found to exist between a mid-systolic click–late systolic murmur and both abrupt mid-systolic buckling as well as pansystolic bowing when such sagging was at least 2 mm posterior to an imaginary line connecting the C and D points of the mitral echogram.

In regard to the ultrasound recordings, the two echographic patterns associated with the auscultatory findings of mitral prolapse were unexpectedly observed to be present even more frequently than the phonocardiographic abnormalities, that is, in 21 per cent of these presumably healthy subjects. Moreover, it is important to point out that 18 per cent of the sub-

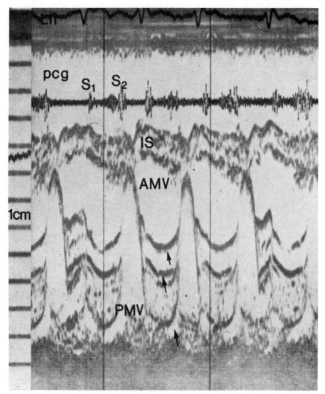

Figure 3. Mitral valve echogram obtained in a patient in whom the diagnosis of the mitral valve prolapse syndrome was based upon clinical, surgical, and pathological findings. Note that multiple systolic echoes, all of which exhibit a continuous posterior bowing motion (arrows), are recorded on echogram. Nevertheless, the phonocardiogram reveals a predominant late-systolic murmur. AMV = anterior mitral leaflet; PMV = posterior mitral leaflet.

jects exhibited pansystolic bowing of 2 mm or greater on echogram, although less than half of these females manifested auscultatory abnormalities, whereas only eight per cent of the subjects exhibited mid-systolic buckling, in whom three-fourths had auscultatory abnormalities. Thereby, pansystolic bowing on echogram was substantially more prevalent in these healthy females than mid-systolic buckling, especially in those subjects with normal phonocardiograms. Finally, another significant finding of this study was the fact that 41 per cent of the subjects with click-murmur on phonocardiogram did not manifest echographic evidence associated with mitral prolapse, while 33 per cent of individuals with characteristic echographic abnormalities were free of phonocardiographic abnormalities.

As is so often the case, therefore, the data of Dr. Markiewicz and associates raised as many questions as were answered. Thus, while it would seem unlikely that 17 per cent of otherwise healthy females have a cardiac disorder, as suggested by the phonocardiographic data, it is even more unlikely that 21 per cent have heart disease, as would be suggested by the ultrasonic findings. Particularly suspect is the significance of isolated pansystolic bowing on echogram, which was observed so frequently in the absence of

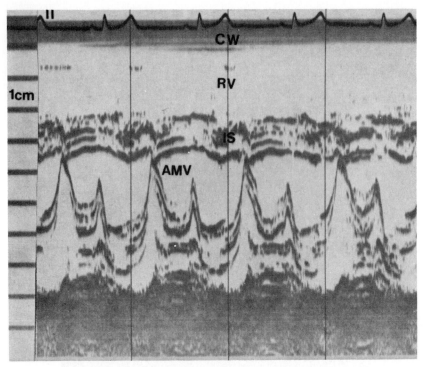

Figure 4. Mitral valve echogram obtained in a patient with the mitral valve prolapse syndrome in whom continuous pansystolic posterior hammocking is observed throughout systole. CW = chest wall; RV = right ventricle.

other evidence of cardiac abnormality. Accordingly, the reluctance of physicians to freely accept solitary pansystolic bowing on echogram as establishing the presence of a potentially fatal cardiac disease is readily understandable.

Although the concept that pansystolic posterior bowing of the mitral leaflets may be a normal echographic variant is attractive, several factors make this relatively unlikely. First, sophisticated studies of mitral motion in a canine preparation have failed to reveal any evidence of backward movement at the free edges of the mitral leaflets.[45] Second, although pansystolic bowing has been found to be unexpectedly prevalent on mitral echogram, it remains true that the vast majority of asymptomatic individuals do not exhibit this pattern of motion by ultrasound. Accordingly, the presence of pansystolic bowing on echogram would seem to warrant an explanation.

RELATIONSHIP BETWEEN MITRAL PROLAPSE AND MITRAL VALVE PROLAPSE SYNDROME

Clearly, then, a great disparity exists between those uncommon prolapse patients with symptomatic ventricular arrhythmias, congestive heart failure secondary to mitral regurgitation, or sudden death and the 18 per

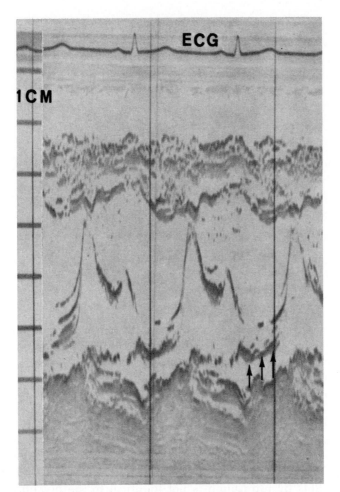

Figure 5. Mitral valve echogram obtained in an individual in whom no evidence of mitral valve prolapse syndrome could be found either by clinical evaluation or cineangiography. Note that following the apposition of the mitral valve leaflets at the onset of systole, there is a brief posterior movement that is subsequently followed by a gradual straight anterior motion throughout the duration of systole (arrows). This pattern of mitral valve motion in systole has not been found to correlate with other evidence of mitral valve prolapse syndrome in our experience.

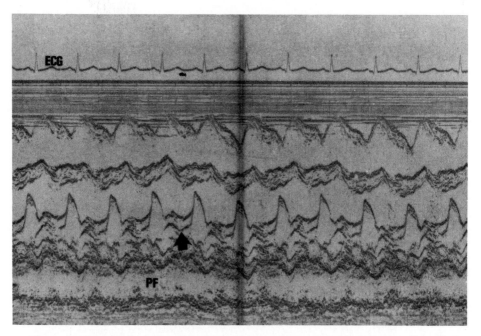

Figure 6. Mitral valve echogram obtained in a patient with a large pericardial effusion. Pericardial fluid (PF) is seen both anterior and posterior to the cardiac structures. Note that the profound posterior motion of the entire heart during systole conveys a backward motion upon the mitral valve leaflets similar to that seen in the mitral valve prolapse syndrome (arrow).

cent of presumably normal females in whom pansystolic bowing on echogram is present. Indeed, a similar disparity also exists for the less threatening but more common symptoms and auscultatory irregularities attributed to mitral valve prolapse syndrome and the high prevalence of the hammock-type ultrasonic abnormality in asymptomatic subjects. Accordingly, it would seem that, whatever its significance, mitral prolapse as exhibited by isolated pansystolic bowing on echogram does not invariably establish the existence of a cardiac disorder manifested by the clinical features and potential complications associated with the mitral valve prolapse syndrome. Stated in an alternative way, the presence of pansystolic prolapse of the mitral leaflets by ultrasound is not identical to the presence of the mitral valve prolapse syndrome.

In regard to the etiology of the mitral valve prolapse syndrome, it is possible that pansystolic bowing on echogram may be related to those physiologic or pathophysiologic states that result in prolapse by virtue of mitral apparatus–left ventricular disproportion rather than because of a distinct clinical entity. Accordingly, as previously discussed, pansystolic bowing may occur predominately in those subjects in whom mitral prolapse is functional and not associated with anatomic cardiac abnormalities. However, such a relationship is highly speculative, and it is again worthy of emphasis that certain patients with the classic clinical features of mitral prolapse manifest only pansystolic bowing on echogram.

An acceptable "gold standard" for the presence of mitral valve prolapse syndrome would provide a mechanism by which the exact relationship between pansystolic prolapse and the mitral valve prolapse syndrome could be determined. However, as is evident from the discussion above, auscultatory abnormalities appear to be as capricious in appearance as pansystolic bowing. Furthermore, studies performed by us in conjunction with other cardiovascular laboratories have revealed considerable interobserver variability in the cineangiographic diagnosis of mitral valve prolapse.[46] Even pathologic examination is not infallible, since histologic changes similar to those observed in mitral valve prolapse syndrome have been seen to occur in elderly individuals as a function of aging.[47]

The recent advent of cross-sectional or two-dimensional echocardiography has provided the ability to study the structural as well as motion characteristics of the mitral apparatus from a variety of imaging angles. Accordingly, in addition to the pattern of movement, cross-sectional echocardiography has enabled the assessment of such anatomic variables as the length and thickness of the mitral leaflets and chordae tendineae. In this regard, preliminary studies in our laboratory[48] have revealed that patients with obvious manifestations of mitral prolapse, such as both click and murmur and marked posterior mitral motion on echogram, usually manifest structural abnormalities of the mitral leaflets, such as thickening and elongation on cross-sectional echo as compared with normals. In contrast, subjects with only intermittent clicks or no abnormalities on phonocardiogram and only mild (typically pansystolic bowing) posterior motion on M-mode echogram rarely exhibited such structural changes. Thus, it is possible that cross-sectional echocardiography may provide a mechanism by which to distinguish mitral prolapse from mitral valve prolapse syndrome and to identify those patients with mitral prolapse at risk for the serious complications associated with this disorder.

Perhaps the most acceptable "gold standard" that could be applied to the recognition of the mitral valve prolapse syndrome is the eventual appearance of signs and symptoms of heart disease. Thus, if pansystolic bowing on echogram were a reliable harbinger of the ultimate development of a clinical cardiac disorder, this ultrasonic abnormality would assume great importance. Unfortunately, at the present time no data exist regarding the long-term follow-up of individuals whose only phonographic or echographic abnormality consists of pansystolic posterior hammocking on echogram. Until this information is available, the question of the precise significance of pansystolic bowing on echogram will be unanswered.

In conclusion, at the present time it does not appear justified to regard solitary pansystolic bowing on echogram as sufficient evidence to establish the diagnosis of the mitral valve prolapse syndrome. Therefore, it has been the practice in our institution to diagnose mitral valve prolapse syndrome only when isolated pansystolic bowing on echogram is accompanied by other evidence of this disorder. Although it is possible that cross-sectional echocardiography may ultimately enable the recognition of those patients with pansystolic bowing who have organic mitral disease, further data will be required before this capability can be ascertained. Ultimately, however, it is likely that the true significance of pansystolic bowing will await the results of a long-term prospective follow-up of individuals with this echographic finding.

References

1. Barlow JB, and Bosman CK: Aneurysmal protrusion of the posterior leaflet of the mitral valve. Am Heart J 71:166, 1966.
2. Criley JM, Lewis KR, Humphries JO, et al: Prolapse of the mitral valve: clinical and cineangiographic findings. Br Heart J 28:488, 1966.
3. Markiewicz W, Stoner T, London E, et al: Mitral valve prolapse in 100 presumably healthy young females. Circulation 53:464, 1976.
4. Procacci PM, Savaran SV, Schreidter SL, et al: Prevalence of clinical mitral-valve prolapse in 1169 young women. N Engl J Med 294:1086, 1976.
5. Cuffer P, and Barbillon L: Nouvelles recherches sur les bruits de galop. Arch Gen Med 1:129, 1887.
6. Gallavardin L: Pseudo-dédoublement du deuxième bruit simulant de rétrécissement mitral par bruit extracardiaque télésystolique surajoute. Lyon Med 121:409, 1913.
7. Barlow JB, Pocock WA, Marchand P, et al: The significance of late systolic murmurs. Am Heart J 66:443, 1963.
8. Hancock EW, and Cohn K: The syndrome associated with mid-systolic click and late systolic murmur. Am J Med 41:183, 1966.
9. DeMaria AN, Amsterdam EA, Vismara LA, et al: Arrhythmias in the mitral valve prolapse syndrome: prevalence, nature and frequency. Ann Intern Med 84:656, 1976.
10. Barlow JB, and Bosman CK: Aneurysmal protrusion of the posterior leaflet of the mitral valve: an auscultatory-electrocardiographic syndrome. Am Heart J 71:166, 1966.
11. DeMaria AN, King JF, Bogren HG, et al: The variable spectrum of echocardiographic manifestations of the mitral valve prolapse syndrome. Circulation 50:53, 1974.
12. Jeresaty RM: Mitral valve prolapse–click syndrome. Prog Cardiovasc Dis 15:623, 1973.
13. Liedtke AJ, Gault JH, Leaman DM, et al: Geometry of left ventricular contraction in the systolic click syndrome. Characterization of a segmental myocardial abnormality. Circulation 47:27, 1973.
14. Scampardonis G, Yang SS, Maranhao V, et al: Left ventricular abnormalities in prolapsed mitral leaflet syndrome: review of 87 cases. Circulation 48:287, 1973.
15. Gulotta SJ, Gulco L, Padmanabban V, et al: The syndrome of systolic click, murmur and mitral valve prolapse: a cardiomyopathy? Circulation 49:717, 1974.
16. Lachman AS, Bramwell-Jones DM, Lakier JB, et al: Invective endocarditis in the billowing mitral leaflet syndrome. Br Heart J 37:326, 1976.
17. Read RC, Pahl AP, and Wendt VE: Symptomatic valvular myxomatous transformation (the floppy valve syndrone): a possible forme fruste of the Marfan syndrome. Circulation 32:897, 1965.
18. McKay R, and Yacoub MH: Clinical and pathological findings in patients with "floppy" valves treated surgically. Circulation 48(Suppl III):III-63, 1973.
19. Hill DG, Davies MJ, and Braimbridge MV: The natural history and surgical management of the redundant cusp syndrome (floppy mitral valve). J Thorac Cardiovasc Surg 67:519, 1974.
20. Shappell SD, Marshall CE, Brown RE, et al: Sudden death and the familial occurrence of mid-systolic click, late systolic murmur syndrome. Circulation 48:1128, 1973.
21. Koch FAH, and Hancock EW: Ten-year follow-up of 40 patients with the mid-systolic click/late systolic murmur syndrome. Am J Cardiol 37:149, 1975.
22. Pocock WA, and Barlow JB: Etiology and electrocardiographic features of the billowing posterior mitral leaflet syndrome: analysis of a further 130 patients with a late systolic murmur or non-ejection systolic click. Am J Med 51:731, 1971.
23. Pocock WA, and Barlow JB: An association between the billowing posterior mitral leaflet syndrome in congenital heart disease, particularly atrial septal defect. Am Heart J 81:720, 1971.
24. Betriu A, Wigle ED, Felderhof CH, et al: Prolapse of the posterior leaflet of the mitral valve associated with secundum atrial septal defect. Am J Cardiol 35:363, 1975.
25. Jeresaty RM: Etiology of the mitral valve prolapse–click syndrome. Am J Cardiol 36:110, 1975.

26. Ranganathan N, Silver MD, Robinson TI, et al: Angiographic-morphologic correlation in patients with severe mitral regurgitation due to prolapse of the posterior mitral leaflet. Circulation 48:514, 1973.
27. Marshall CE, and Shappell SD: Sudden death in the ballooning posterior leaflet syndrome. Arch Pathol 98:134, 1974.
28. Brown OR, DeMots H, and Kloster FE: Prevalence of aortic root dilation and mitral valve prolapse in Marfan's syndrome. Am J Cardiol 35:124, 1975.
29. Steelman RB, White RS, Hill JC, et al: Mid-systolic clicks in arteriosclerotic heart disease: a new facet in the clinical syndrome of papillary muscle dysfunction. Circulation 44:503, 1971.
30. Cheng TO: Late systolic murmur in coronary artery disease. Chest 61:346, 1972.
31. Jeresaty RM: Etiology of the mitral valve prolapse–click syndrome. Am J Cardiol 36:110, 1975.
32. Pomerance A: Ballooning deformity (mucoid degeneration) of atrioventricular valves. Br Heart J 31:343, 1969.
33. Trent JK, Adelman AG, Wigle ED, and Silver MD: Morphology of a proposed posterior mitral valve leaflet. Am Heart J 79:539, 1970.
34. McCarthy LH, and Wolf PL: Mucoid degeneration of heart valves: "blue valve syndrome." Am J Clin Pathol 54:852, 1970.
35. DeMaris AN, Bogren H, Caudill C, et al: Evaluation of the non-valvular factors of cardiac performance, left ventricular contractile pattern, and coronary anatomy in the mitral valve prolapse syndrome. Am J Cardiol 35:132, 1975.
36. Criley JM, and Kissel GL: Prolapse of the mitral valve: The click and late systolic murmur syndrome. In Goodwin J, and Yu PF (eds): Progress in Cardiology, Vol 4. Philadelphia, Lea and Febiger, 1976, pp 23–36.
37. Dillon JC, Haine CL, Change S, et al: Use of echocardiography in patients with prolapsed mitral valve. Circulation 43:503, 1971.
38. Kerber RE, Isaeff DM, and Hancock EW: Echocardiographic patterns in patients with the syndrome of systolic click and late systolic murmur. N Engl J Med 284:691, 1971.
39. Popp RL, Brown, OR, Silverman JF, et al: Echocardiographic abnormalities in the mitral valve prolapse syndrome. Circulation 49:428, 1974.
40. Sahn DJ, Allen HD, Goldberg SJ, et al: Mitral valve prolapse in children. A problem defined by real-time cross-sectional echocardiography. Circulation 53:651, 1976.
41. Mathey DG, Decoodt PR, Allen HN, et al: The determinants of onset of mitral valve prolapse in the systolic click–late systolic murmur syndrome. Circulation 53:872, 1976.
42. Winkle RA, Goodman DJ, and Popp RL: Simultaneous echocardiographic-phonocardiographic recordings at rest and during amyl nitrite administration in patients with mitral valve prolapse. Circulation 51:522, 1975.
43. Vignola PA, Pohost GM, Curfman GD, et al: Correlation of echocardiographic and clinical findings in patients with pericardial effusion. Am J Cardiol 37:701, 1976.
44. Chandraratna PAN, Lopez JM, Littman BB, et al: Abnormal mitral valve motion during ventricular extrasystoles. An echocardiographic study. Am J Cardiol 34:783, 1974.
45. Rushmer RF, Finlayson BL, and Wash AA: Movements of the mitral valve. Circ Res 4:337, 1956.
46. DeMaria AN, Riggs K, Bogren H, et al: Observer variability in the cineangiographic diagnosis of the mitral valve prolapse syndrome. Clin Res 25:216A, 1977.
47. Pomerance A: Ageing changes in human heart valves. Br Heart J 29:222, 1967.
48. DeMaria AN, Bommer W, Weinnert L, et al: Abnormalities of cardiac structure in mitral prolapse syndrome: evaluation by cross-sectional echocardiography. Circulation 57(Suppl III):III–111, 1977.

Comment

The increasing use of echocardiography has uncovered a large asymptomatic population, particularly among young females, in whom isolated systolic posterior movement of the mitral valve is observed. This controversy deals with the significance of this finding in establishing the diagnosis of mitral valve prolapse. DeMaria and Mason have no quarrel in accepting the observation as indicating posterior bulging of the mitral valve into the left atrium, provided appropriate technical care is used (to eliminate an artifact produced by erroneous angulation of the transducer). They distinguish mitral valve prolapse, however, from the classic mitral valve prolapse syndrome and question whether this isolated echocardiographic observation has any pathologic significance. They point out that it may occur whenever there is a disproportion between the length of the chordae tendineae – mitral apparatus and the chamber size of the left ventricle and feel that the evidence to suggest the classic pathologic myxomatous degeneration of the mitral valve leading to the click-murmur syndrome should be diagnosed only when other manifestations in addition to the echocardiographic one of hammocking is observed.

Popp presents convincing evidence, however, to suggest that hammocking has the same significance echocardiographically as does the classic "question mark" pattern. He brings out the fact that one may convert the typical late systolic posterior movement into a holosystolic pattern by giving the same patient amyl nitrite, further suggesting that the patterns represent a single entity. He points out that pathologic studies specifically looking for prolapse find an incidence comparable to the five to six per cent prevalence of echocardiographic prolapse in the general population, thus suggesting that the echocardiographic evidence implies anatomic prolapse.

It is clear that the problem is complicated by the absence of what DeMaria calls a "gold standard." That is, there is currently no reliable method of independently establishing the presence or absence of prolapse of the mitral valve. Angiographic visualization may at times fail to demonstrate the presence of prolapse, despite clear-cut clinical evidence, whereas in other situations the presence of angiographic evidence has been unassociated with other manifestations.

How should the practicing physician react to an echocardiographic interpretation that mitral valve prolapse is present by virtue of hammocking of the mitral valve leaflets during systole? It seems to me that in the absence of other clinical signs or symptoms and in light of the high prevalence figure within the population as a whole, it would be best not to label the patient as having a cardiac lesion. Until such time as prospective studies demonstrate that echo-cardiographic evidences of prolapse lead to a clinical disorder, it must remain an interesting finding of dubious importance. Certainly the danger of producing iatrogenic cardiac neuroses would outweigh categorizing the patient as having a cardiac disorder at this stage of our knowledge.

ELLIOT RAPAPORT, M.D.

Eighteen

Should Prophylaxis Against Subacute Bacterial Endocarditis Be Undertaken in All Patients with Mitral Valve Prolapse?

PROPHYLAXIS AGAINST SUBACUTE BACTERIAL
ENDOCARDITIS SHOULD BE UNDERTAKEN IN ALL
PATIENTS WITH MITRAL VALVE PROLAPSE
   Pravin M. Shah, M.D.

BACTERIAL PROPHYLAXIS IN PATIENTS WITH THE
CLICK-MURMUR SYNDROME
   Melvin D. Cheitlin, M.D.

COMMENT

Prophylaxis Against Subacute Bacterial Endocarditis Should Be Undertaken in All Patients with Mitral Valve Prolapse

PRAVIN M. SHAH, M.D.

Professor of Medicine, University of California, Los Angeles; Chief, Cardiology Section, Wadsworth Veterans Administration Medical Center, Los Angeles, California

Mitral valve prolapse was essentially an unknown entity up until some 15 years ago. Virtually all apical systolic murmurs of mitral regurgitation were thought to be the result of presumed rheumatic etiology and the mid- and late systolic clicks the result of presumed pericardial adhesions. Mitral valve prolapse was first recognized by selective angiocardiography, and the term billowing mitral leaflet syndrome was introduced. The association of the non-ejection systolic clicks and billowing of the leaflets was established. Indeed, all the mid- and late systolic clicks, which vary in timing and/or intensity by physiologic and pharmacologic maneuvers, resulting in alterations in ventricular volume, are now considered to originate in the mitral valve apparatus, with a presumed diagnosis of mitral valve prolapse. The advent of echocardiography as a non-invasive diagnostic tool and its application for the diagnosis of mitral valve prolapse permitted an independent confirmation of the diagnosis in addition to the auscultatory findings. Thus, the dual non-invasive diagnostic modalities, i.e., auscultation–phonocardiography and echocardiography, led to a relatively frequent recognition of this syndrome, and the studies of population incidence have been reported. It is now the consensus that mitral valve prolapse is a rather common entity, with an incidence of approximately six per cent among women and 0.5 to 1.0 per cent among males. It might then be projected

429

that between 10 million and 20 million people in the United States alone may have this condition. The discovery of a clinical entity in such a large group has raised questions about the wide spectrum of mitral valve prolapse, bordering on one end with the normal variant and on the other with the symptomatic clinical syndrome with mitral regurgitation and/or serious arrhythmias.

Bacterial endocarditis has been reported in patients with mitral valve prolapse. It had therefore been recommended that the patients with mitral valve prolapse, just like those with congenital and acquired heart disease in whom a risk of bacterial endocarditis is reported to exist, should receive prophylactic antibiotic therapy. This recommendation preceded the current realization that the wide spectrum of the syndrome observed in the population studies is a rather frequent occurrence. If extrapolation of the incidence of the condition were accurate, approximately 10 million to 20 million people in the United States would be considered to be at risk to develop bacterial endocarditis on the basis of mitral valve prolapse. The question is therefore raised if the prophylaxis is indeed justified on such a large scale. Is the cost-benefit ratio of such an endeavor defensible? Does the risk of serious adverse reactions to the drugs used in the prophylaxis exceed the risk of endocarditis? These questions assume even greater relevance when it is appreciated that the practice of prophylactic use of antibiotics to prevent endocarditis is not based on any controlled clinical trials. The rationale for prophylactic use of antibiotics for any heart condition can thus be challenged, and the wisdom of its use in a condition with such a high prevalence may be doubted.

I defend the position that antibiotics should be used for prophylaxis against bacterial endocarditis in all patients with mitral valve prolapse diagnosed by clinical criteria and additional phonocardiographic, echocardiographic, or angiographic criteria. The basis for this stand is first outlined below:

1. Transient bacteremia with varying frequency and intensity occurs following a variety of procedures and manipulations.

2. Bacterial endocarditis has been observed following bacteremia associated with dental and other manipulations.

3. The duration, and possibly the intensity, of bacteremia is reduced with the use of antibiotics.

4. Reports of bacterial endocarditis following optimal doses of appropriate antibiotics for prophylaxis are extremely rare.

5. Experimental studies show that appropriate antibiotic administration will prevent endocarditis.

6. Patients with mitral valve prolapse have been reported to develop bacterial endocarditis.

Let us examine the above points at some length.

1. *Transient bacteremia with varying frequency and intensity occurs following a variety of procedures and manipulations.* Several studies have examined the incidence of bacteremia following different medical and surgical manipulations. The rate of transient bacteremia following dental ex-

traction varies from 60 to 90 per cent, with *Streptococcus viridans* as a common pathogen. Common daily activities such as tooth brushing and chewing hard candy or gum can also result in transient bacteremia, but the incidence is much lower. Urogenital surgery and procedures such as internal urethrotomy or external urethrotomy with dilatation, TUR, and retropubic prostatectomy with urinary infection are done fairly often. Although the list of conditions associated with transient bacteremia is a long one, the bacteremia is generally short-lived, asymptomatic, and inconsequential, except for some urologic and dental manipulations. In the evaluation of the risk of endocarditis, presence of bacteremia *per se* is perhaps less relevant than its intensity and duration. There is some experimental support that this is an important consideration.

2. *Bacterial endocarditis has been reported following bacteremia associated with dental and other manipulations.* These studies, largely in the pre-antibiotic era, report varying frequency of this occurrence. One study reported four cases among 350 "rheumatic" children undergoing dental extraction without antibiotics. Fifty-two per cent had streptococcal bacteremia, transient in all but the four children who subsequently died of endocarditis. Other studies have reported virtually no cases of endocarditis following dental procedures.

3. *The duration, and possibly the intensity, of bacteremia is reduced with the use of antibiotics.* Bacteremia has been reported to be reduced with prophylactic penicillin, although it seems likely that prophylaxis does not prevent bacteremia but may eradicate the organisms after they have entered the blood stream. The incidence of bacteremia was reduced by one half in a series of patients undergoing transurethral prostatic resection following the use of antibiotics. The bactericidal agents are much more useful in this regard than the bacteriostatic agents.

4. *Reports of bacterial endocarditis following optimal doses of appropriate antibiotics are extremely rare.* With rare exception in cases that have been reported, prophylactic doses of antibiotics were suboptimal by current standards. This observation is subject to criticism, because the incidence of endocarditis following procedures is extremely low.

5. *Experimental studies show that appropriate antibiotic administration will prevent endocarditis.* Valves traumatized by polyethylene catheter in rabbits are prone to develop vegetations and endocarditis with intravenous injections of organisms. Bactericidal agents in sufficient single or multiple doses and appropriate regimens have been shown to be effective in prevention of endocarditis, while bacteriostatic agents in single or multiple doses were unsatisfactory.

6. *Patients with mitral valve prolapse have been reported to develop bacterial endocarditis.* In one report of 10 patients, two had a non-ejection systolic click and eight had both a click and a late murmur. The auscultatory findings were intermittent in four and were inconspicuous or brought out only on postural change. Seven patients were unaware of their cardiac lesions, but three were known to have features of mitral valve prolapse. This experience is not unique, and almost every large series with follow-up data includes some patients with endocarditis. It is, however, apparent that

no single subset of patients, i.e., with or without murmurs, is more or less likely to develop endocarditis. This is an important point that needs to be stressed, since prophylaxis should be used either in *all* patients with mitral valve prolapse or in none.

A controlled trial to study the efficacy and cost-benefit ratio of prophylactic antibiotics against bacterial endocarditis has not been carried out, and may never be, owing to the large number of patients required for meaningful results, since the overall incidence is low. Although rigorous scientific discipline requires us to demand a statistically convincing study, the management of an individual patient requires exercise of judgment in the absence of hard proof. Despite advances in antibiotic therapy, bacterial endocarditis is an illness associated with high mortality. With some organisms, such as staphylococcal infections, it reaches nearly 100 per cent, whereas even with "favorable" organisms, such as streptococcal infections, it can be as high as 30 per cent. These stark observations with the best available antibiotics against known organisms give one pause to consider prophylaxis with less scientific fervor. I would take the position that if one objects to the prophylactic use of antibiotics in all the patients with mitral valve prolapse, one might as well not use it in any. Furthermore, if one were internally consistent, a recommendation of prophylaxis against bacterial endocarditis for any cardiac condition, whether congenital or acquired, would be unjustified.

In the absence of convincing scientific data, one's attitudes for or against a therapeutic approach have to be tentative and must be continually reexamined in light of new evidence. Since mitral valve prolapse is now known to be so common in the general population, a study sufficiently wide in scope to address to this question may be considered of significant public health import to justify the cost. The NIH may be persuaded to mount a multicenter study, since the long-term implications of such a study are likely to be enormous.

While awaiting such a study, I would presently recommend that a clinical diagnosis of mitral valve prolapse based on cardiac auscultation should be subjected to further objective confirmatory evidence with phonocardiography and echocardiography. Each of these tests should be carried both at rest and with provocative tests such as change in posture, the Valsalva maneuver, and amyl nitrite inhalation. Occasionally, left ventriculography may be done, if indicated for evaluation of chest pain or associated heart disease. If the evidence strongly supports the diagnosis of mitral valve prolapse, prophylactic antibiotics should definitely be used at times of dental and urologic procedures and other potential bloodstream infections. It is further stressed that if the diagnosis is suggested by only one of the above methods (auscultation, phonocardiography, echocardiography, angiocardiography), the evidence is not deemed sufficient for a definitive diagnosis, unless the abnormalities are advanced and incontrovertible. Thus, a false positive diagnosis due to subtle abnormalities is avoided by insisting on independent confirmation with two diagnostic methods.

The future directions in the prophylaxis against endocarditis are likely to consist of identification of the individual host at risk of such an occurrence, based on his immunologic response to transient bacteremia. Since the vast majority of patients with cardiac disorders undergoing dental procedures without antibiotics do not develop endocarditis despite the potential risk, the immunologic factors in the patient who develops such an infection must be relevant. The ultimate rational approach will be to identify a specific subset of patients with cardiac disease at greatest risk of developing endocarditis.

Selected References

1. Everett ED, and Hirschmann JV: Transient bacteremia and endocarditis prophylaxis. Annu Rev Med 56:61, 1977.
2. Editorial: Prophylaxis of bacterial endocarditis: faith, hope, and charitable interpretations. Lancet 1:519, 1976.
3. Pelletier LL Jr, Durack DT, and Petersdorf RG: Chemotherapy of experimental streptococcal endocarditis. IV. Further observations on prophylaxis. J Clin Invest 56:319, 1975.
4. Lachman AS, Bramwell-Jones DM, Lakier JB, Pocock WA, and Barlow JB: Infective endocarditis in the billowing mitral leaflet syndrome. Br Heart J 37:326, 1975.

Bacterial Prophylaxis in Patients with the Click-Murmur Syndrome

MELVIN D. CHEITLIN, M.D.

Professor of Medicine, University of California, San
Francisco School of Medicine; Associate Chief, Cardiology
Service, San Francisco General Hospital, San Francisco,
California

It is considered good, even required, medical practice to recommend antibacterial prophylaxis when procedures are contemplated that predispose to bacteremia and potential endocarditis in patients with cardiac lesions. Because it is known that bacterial endocarditis can develop in patients with the click-murmur or mitral valve prolapse syndrome, it would also seem reasonable to recommend antibacterial prophylaxis in these patients at the time of performing procedures, especially dental manipulations, associated with transient bacteremia.

It is the purpose of this paper to review the subject of antibacterial prophylaxis in the prevention of bacterial endocarditis, especially as it applies to patients with the click-murmur syndrome. The problem of proving the effectiveness of antibacterial prophylaxis in preventing infective endocarditis in patients with any kind of valvular lesion and the magnitude of risk of development of infective endocarditis in patients with the click-murmur syndrome are examined. I believe when the frequency of the occurrence of click-murmur syndrome in the population together with the problems arising from recommending prophylaxis in all these patients are considered, that it does more harm than good to make such a recommendation except in unusual cases.

Although infective endocarditis can be caused by fungi (*Candida, Histoplasma*), rickettsiae (Q fever), and even viruses (psittacosis), prophylaxis to prevent endocarditis is directed against bacterial invasion, and thus I will confine my discussion to bacterial endocarditis.

434

The most important conditions for the development of infective endocarditis are the following:

1. the presence of an underlying jet lesion on a generally avascular valve or on the endocardium that can predispose to bacterial invasion and colonization;

2. the presence of bacteremia — the greater the magnitude of the inoculum and the longer the duration of bacteremia, the greater the chance of invasion and development of infective endocarditis; and

3. the degree of susceptibility to infection, which is increased in patients with diseases such as leukemia and lymphoma, in patients who are receiving antimetabolite and steroid therapy, and in certain situations such as the postoperative period after heart surgery.

The central fact that supports the recommendation of antibacterial prophylaxis in preventing infective endocarditis is the demonstration that administration of appropriate antibiotics in sufficient doses and at a proper time before, during, and after the bacteremia-associated procedure can reduce markedly the magnitude and the duration of the bacteremia. In animal models, proper antibiotics given appropriately have been shown to reduce the prevalence of development of experimental endocarditis.[1]

Although it is true that endocarditis occurs most often in patients with underlying cardiac disease, in some series[2] over one third of the instances of infective endocarditis occur in patients without known underlying heart disease. Endocarditis on normal valves is more likely to occur with infection by virulent organisms such as staphylococcus and pneumococcus, which cause an acute septic condition that has been called "acute endocarditis." Infections with less virulent organisms, leading to less tissue destruction and a more subtle clinical picture, the so-called "subacute endocarditis," are more likely to occur in patients with predisposing endocardial lesions. Endocarditis can occur on previously normal valves when there is prolonged or massive bacteremia such as in IV drug abusers and in patients who have an increased susceptibility to infection as described above. In these populations, not only virulent organisms but also usually benign commensals can invade the body and cause gram-negative septicemia (*Serratia marcescens* and *Pseudomonas*) and infection with fungi (*Candida* and *Aspergillus*).

It is obvious that patients without underlying cardiac disease are not usually considered for antibacterial prophylaxis in anticipation of bacteremia-associated procedures. It is also obvious that routine recommendations for prophylaxis would be inadequate to prevent bacteremia and infection with the unusual organisms just described. Consequently, prophylaxis is possible only against organisms susceptible to the antibiotics given and in patients identifiable as being at risk of development of infective endocarditis.

Not all cardiac lesions are equally prone to development of infective endocarditis. The underlying cardiac conditions with the greatest risk of development of infective endocarditis are those diseases with lesions resulting in jet formation with subsequent intimal or endocardial damage. For this reason, aortic and mitral insufficiency and, to a much lesser extent, stenosis of these valves are the common predisposing lesions. Certain congenital lesions such as interventricular septal defect, patent ductus arteriosus, and tetralogy of Fallot are associated with a significant incidence of infective endocarditis. Less frequently, other cardiovascular lesions such as arteriovenous fistulas and ventricular and abdominal aortic aneurysms are associated with infection. Because secundum atrial septal defects are not associated with a high-velocity jet, infective endocarditis in this lesion is rare. Recently, development of infective endocarditis has been reported in patients with the click-murmur syndrome, most but not all of whom had at least a late systolic murmur of mitral insufficiency. Apparently, the murmur of mitral insufficiency is not a necessary prerequisite for infection because LeBauer et al.[3] reported development of bacterial endocarditis in a patient with a non-ejection click without a systolic murmur.

According to the present understanding of the click-murmur syndrome, the physical findings are secondary to the development of an abnormal prolapse of a portion of the mitral valve into the left atrium as the volume of the left ventricle decreases during systole. At some point, there is a sudden slippage of the mitral valve cusps as they abut on each other. The sudden checking of the prolapsing leaflet results in the non-ejection or "mid-systolic" click. If during further reduction in left ventricular volume the leaflets no longer coapt, mitral insufficiency and the late systolic murmur result. With a smaller end-diastolic volume or a more rapid ventricular contraction, the click and the mitral insufficiency occur earlier in systole. The non-ejection click and/or the mitral insufficiency murmur can be completely absent on one occasion, for instance when the patient is supine and the ventricle is relatively large, and be obviously present moments later on sitting or standing, when there is venous pooling and a smaller end-diastolic left ventricular volume. For these reasons, it is probable that mitral insufficiency is intermittently present in most patients, and therefore, most may be at some risk of development of infective endocarditis during bacteremia.

Central to the idea that antibacterial prophylaxis protects against bacterial endocarditis is the fact that bacteremia is a necessary prerequisite to its development. The clinical and experimental evidence that this is the case is excellent. Although there has been a change in the bacterial flora causing endocarditis over the years with an increase in staphylococcus and a disappearance of pneumococcus, the most common organism causing endocarditis is *Streptococcus viridans*, the common commensal in the human mouth. Consonant with this is the fact that about one fourth of the cases of subacute bacterial endocarditis have had recent dental manipulation.[4]

O'Kell and Elliot,[5] in 1935, showed that 75 per cent of people with poor dental hygiene and one third of people without pyorrhea or extensive dental caries had bacteremia with dental extraction. Lesser dental procedures such as the filling of teeth and deep scaling of dental calculus have also been shown to cause bacteremia.[4] Even such activities as rocking a tooth, brushing teeth, and using the water-pick type of apparatus now popular for dental hygiene have been associated with bacteremia. The incidence and duration of bacteremia are related to the degree of pyorrhea present in the mouth and the extent of the manipulation. For this reason, Pogrel and Welsby[6] suggested that maintenance of proper dental hygiene is important and probably more effective in preventing subacute bacterial endocarditis than prophylactic antibiotic therapy.

It has been demonstrated adequately that proper administration of antibiotics before and after dental procedures can reduce the incidence and duration of bacteremia. The effectiveness in any given antibiotic regimen in preventing detectable bacteremia depends on the timing of administration of the antibiotic, the blood level achieved, the duration of maintenance of adequate blood level of drug, and the size of the bacterial inoculum.

In addition to dental procedures, there are other procedures associated with bacteremia, usually with different types of organisms, that may not be sensitive to penicillin. Abscess formation anywhere in the body and manipulations such as sigmoidoscopy, labor and delivery, and cystoscopy in septic areas such as the genitourinary or gastrointestinal tract have all been shown to cause bacteremia. For these reasons, the recommendation to provide antibacterial prophylaxis with appropriate antibiotics during these procedures is also valid.

In the clinical situation, the value of antibiotics in preventing subacute bacterial endocarditis (SBE) has been inferred from their ability to reduce the incidence of detectable bacteremia during a procedure, and this has been equated with protection against SBE. Recently, Durack and Petersdorf[1] showed in animals that a single high dose of penicillin or single dose of benzathine penicillin one-half hour before an injection of S. viridans did not prevent colonization of the prepared rabbit aortic valve. However, administration of penicillin with streptomycin or a high initial dose of penicillin followed by lower continued doses of penicillin prevented SBE in these animals. This is the first experimental proof of the value of antibiotics in the prevention of SBE.

In clinical series, it has not been possible to prove that prophylactic antibiotic therapy can prevent bacterial endocarditis. The incidence of bacterial endocarditis is quite low and, except in the addict population, has not changed from decade to decade. Patients with valvular lesions are at greatest risk of developing SBE, and the incidence of minor valvular disease in the population is quite high. Lichtman and Master[7] noted anatomic evidence of valvular heart disease in 234 of 406 consecutive autopsies in persons 50 years or older at Mount Sinai Hospital in New York City. In many of these people, no clinical evidence of valvular disease was present during life. Considering the estimated two per cent incidence of a bicuspid aortic valve[8] (manifested by mild aortic insufficiency in many) in the general population; the large number of people with mild calcific aortic stenosis, many with mild aortic insufficiency also; and the incidence of mild mitral insufficiency from a variety of causes, ranging from arteriosclerotic heart disease with papillary muscle dysfunction to congestive heart failure and left ventricular dilatation from any cause, the number of people potentially at risk of developing subacute bacterial endocarditis is enormous. Compared to the population at risk, the apparent incidence of SBE is quite low. Since, except for rare instances, untreated SBE is fatal, it is unlikely that the true incidence of SBE is much greater than the apparent incidence. The inevitable conclusions must be that the incidence of development of SBE in the population at risk must be low indeed.

Pogrel and Welsby[6] calculated the incidence of infective endocarditis in Aberdeen, Scotland, to be on the order of 11 cases per million people per year. Because of this extremely low incidence, it has never been possible to prove the effectiveness of any antibiotic regimen in the prophylaxis of SBE in human beings.

Specifically with regard to recommending antibiotic prophylaxis for possible bacteremic exposure in patients with the click-murmur syndrome, the problem revolves around the prevalence of the abnormality or physical finding and the known incidence of development of SBE in these people. In 1973, Rizzon[9] examined 1009 young women and detected a non-ejection click or late systolic murmur in 0.33 per cent. Barlow and Pocock[10] reported an incidence of click-murmur of 1.4 per cent in 12,050 South African school children. Markiewicz et al.[11] examined 100 presumably healthy female volunteers without known heart disease, ranging from ages 17 to 35 years; 21 per cent had echocardiographic evidence of mitral valve prolapse; 17 per cent had only auscultatory evidence; and 10 per cent had both echocardiographic and auscultatory evidence. Procacci et al.,[12] in screening 1169 women, found an incidence of click-murmur syndrome of 6.3 per cent by auscultation. Brown et al.[13] in Oregon found an incidence of 6 per cent in 520 women and 0.5 per cent in 180 men by auscultation. Thus, the population with click-murmur syndrome who are "at risk" of development of SBE, and who are therefore candidates for prophylaxis when "appropriate," is indeed enormous.

There are some data concerning the incidence of SBE in patients with prolapsing mitral valves. The total number of reported cases is relatively small. In 1975, Lachman et al.[14] reported 10 patients with SBE, eight with non-ejection click and systolic murmur, and two with non-ejection click alone. Six of the 10 had *Staphylococcus albus* endocarditis, which is relatively resistant to penicillin. In their review of the literature, they found 12 clearly documented cases; thus the total number of well-documented cases of SBE with the click-murmur syndrome was 22 by 1975. In 1974 Allen, Harris, and Leatham[15] reported the follow-up of 62 patients with a late systolic murmur, 33 of whom had an associated non-ejection click for nine to 22 years (mean 13.8 years); infective endocarditis developed in five patients. Other investigators reported an incidence of infective endocarditis of one to two per cent in long-term follow-up of patients with the click-murmur syndrome. However, it is not clear in these studies whether the click-murmur came first and the infective endocarditis developed during the follow-up period or vice versa.

The click–late systolic murmur is also known to occur in certain diseases affecting the connective tissue, i.e., Marfan's disease and Ehlers-Danlos syndrome. Prolapsing mitral valve by angiocardiography and the click-murmur syndrome have also been documented as occurring in arteriosclerotic heart disease,[16] in cardiomyopathy, especially idiopathic hypertrophic subaortic stenosis, and in patients with secundum atrial septal defects. The angiocardiographic findings of prolapse in the mitral valve are common; in fact, in one series reported by Aranda et al.[17] of patients with arteriosclerotic heart disease, 32 per cent of people studied by left ventricular angiography had prolapsed mitral valves. It is estimated in a number of studies that 37 per cent of patients with secundum interatrial septal defect have prolapsed mitral valves by angiocardiography.[18] Since SBE is extremely uncommon in patients with either arteriosclerotic heart disease or interatrial septal defect, it is evident that the high prevalence of the prolapsing mitral valve in these conditions does not dispose the patient to development of SBE. Since the prevalence of click-murmur syndrome in the female adult population can approach six to 10 per cent, and the absolute number of patients with this syndrome reported to have infective endocarditis is small, the incidence of SBE in patients with click-murmur syndrome must therefore be vanishingly low.

If antibiotic prophylaxis was totally harmless, both physically and psychologically, there would be nothing wrong in recommending it in hope of preventing even the remote possibility of infective endocarditis. Unfortunately, this is not the case. The regimen of penicillin prophylaxis as presently recommended[19] consists of the intramuscular administration of 1,000,000 units aqueous penicillin and 600,000 units of procaine penicillin one half hour to one hour before the operative procedure and then 500 mg of penicillin V every six hours for two days afterwards. If bacteremia with other penicillin-resistant organisms is anticipated, recommendation for prophylaxis would also include an aminoglycoside, either streptomycin or gentamycin. All of these drugs, including penicillin, have a morbidity and even a mortality, albeit small, associated with their use.

More important is the psychologic effect of recommending prophylaxis for procedures so frequently performed, such as dental procedures, in such a large proportion of the population. At present, we try to minimize the importance of the physical finding in the asymptomatic patient without a family history of sudden death and without fixed mitral insufficiency. If a physical finding is as prevalent as reported, it is possibly better to consider it to be a variant of normal rather than a disease, especially in the asymptomatic patient. In some patients, nonspecific symptoms are common, including weakness, shortness of breath, palpitations with and without arrhythmias, faintness, chest pain almost always atypical for angina, and ST-T–wave changes on the electrocardiogram. In long-term follow-up, even when the group is preselected with bias toward the more seriously affected, ill patients, the number who remain unchanged for years varies from 65 to 90 per cent during the period of follow-up.

It is difficult to reassure a patient about a minor physical finding that will almost certainly never cause any trouble, and at the same time to counsel him/her as to the necessity for prophylaxis to prevent the possible development of SBE, which could result in a most serious and even fatal infection of the valve if not promptly recognized and treated with antibiotics for four to six weeks.

To a young person already concerned about the finding of a "cardiac abnormality" that has excited the interest of the doctor, this advice, even when meticulously explained, is more likely to create confusion and anxiety than it is to alleviate these feelings. I have seen too many previously asymptomatic patients with a mid-systolic click frightened by the possible threat of not only endocarditis but also sudden severe mitral insufficiency, sudden dangerous arrhythmias, or even sudden death. All of these problems *can* occur in patients with the click-murmur syndrome, but the incidence of serious problems, considering the prevalence of these physical findings in the population, is small indeed. It does not alleviate the anxiety to tell an asymptomatic young person who has always considered him or herself healthy that he/she has a good heart but. . . .

Because of the lack of definite clinical proof of the effectiveness of antibiotics, the inability to cover most episodes of bacteremia in the patient's life, and the extremely low incidence of infective endocarditis in people with the click-murmur syndrome, the argument for antibiotic prophylaxis in all patients with click-murmur syndrome is weak indeed. To add the fear of the possibility of infection of the heart valve when you are trying to reassure the patient about the absence of heart disease is contradictory and results in more problems than are solved for the patient in accepting his or her "abnormality" without anxiety and worry. At present, I believe it is unwise to advise prophylaxis against infective endocarditis in the vast majority of patients with the click-murmur syndrome.

References

1. Durack DT, and Petersdorf RG: Chemotherapy of experimental streptococcal endocarditis. J Clin Invest 52:592–598, 1973.
2. Lerner PI, and Weinstein L: Medical progress: infective endocarditis in the antibiotic era. N Engl J Med 274:259–266, 1966.
3. LeBauer EJ, Perloff JK, and Keliher TF: The isolated systolic click with bacterial endocarditis. Am Heart J 73:534–537, 1967.
4. Harvey WP, and Capone HA: Bacterial endocarditis related to cleaning and filling of teeth. Am J Cardiol 7:793–798, 1961.
5. O'Kell CC, and Elliott SD: Bacteremia and oral sepsis with special reference to the etiology of subacute endocarditis. Lancet 4:869, 1935.
6. Pogrel MA, and Welsby PD: The dentist and prevention of infective endocarditis. Br Dent J 139:12–16, 1975.
7. Lichtman P, and Master AM: The incidence of valvular heart disease in people over fifty and penicillin prophylaxis of bacterial endocarditis. NY State J Med 49:1693, 1949.
8. Roberts WC: The congenitally bicuspid aortic valve. A study of 85 autopsy cases. Am J Cardiol 26:72–83, 1970.
9. Rizzon P, Biasco G, Brindicci G, et al: Familial syndrome of midsystolic click and late ejection murmur. Br Heart J 35:245–259, 1973.
10. Barlow JB, and Pocock WA: The problem of nonejection systolic clicks and associated mitral systolic murmurs: emphasis on the billowing mitral leaflet syndrome. Am Heart J 90:636–655, 1975.
11. Markiewicz W, Stoner J, London E, et al: Mitral valve prolapse in one hundred presumably healthy young females. Circulation 53:464–473, 1976.
12. Procacci PM, Savram SV, Schreiter SL, and Bryson AL: Prevalence of clinical mitral-valve prolapse in 1169 young women. N Engl J Med 294:1086–1088, 1976.
13. Brown OR, Kloster FE, and DeMots H: Incidental mitral valve prolapse in the asymptomatic normal. Circulation 52(Suppl II):II-77, 1976.
14. Lachman AS, Bramwell-Jones DM, Lakier JB, Pocock WA, and Barlow JB: Infective endocarditis in the billowing mitral leaflet syndrome. Br Heart J 39:326–330, 1975.
15. Allen H, Harris A, and Leatham A: Significance and prognosis of an isolated late systolic murmur: a 9- to 22-year follow up. Br Heart J 36:525–532, 1974.
16. Steelman RB, White RS, Hill JC, Nagle JP, and Cheitlin MD: Midsystolic click in arteriosclerotic heart disease. Circulation 44:503–515, 1971.
17. Aranda JH, Befel B, Lazzara R, Embi A, and Machado H: Mitral valve prolapse and coronary artery disease. Circulation 52:245–253, 1975.
18. Betriu A, Wigle ED, Felderhof CH, and McLoughlin MJ: Prolapse of the posterior leaflet of the mitral valve associated with secundum atrial septal defect. Am J Cardiol 35:363, 1975.
19. Kaplan EL, Anthony BF, Bisno A, et al: Prevention of bacterial endocarditis. Circulation 56:139A–143A, 1977.

Comment

Both Drs. Cheitlin and Shah agree that bacterial endocarditis may occur in patients with mitral valve prolapse. The critical question is whether the prevalence of bacterial endocarditis justifies the cost and risk of routine antibiotic prophylaxis. It is clear that mitral valve prolapse is a surprisingly common anatomic abnormality among the general population. It is also clear that the incidence of bacterial endocarditis in the mitral valve prolapse syndrome is quite small. Furthermore, the risk of complications from prophylactic antibiotics in patients undergoing dental, urologic, or other procedures that lead to transient bacteremia is also quite small. Ideally, one would like to identify a particular subset of patients with mitral valve prolapse particularly at risk and/or a specific medical or dental procedure that was more likely to result in significant bacteremia. Bacterial endocarditis can occur in mitral valve prolapse even in the absence of the systolic murmur, with just the presence of the click. However, it has been our experience as well as that of others that bacterial endocarditis occurs more frequently in patients who have the mid- or late systolic murmur with or without the click. This is not totally surprising in view of the likelihood that true mitral insufficiency is presumably present whenever a murmur is present; but when only a click is heard, the valve may be prolapsing, but without mitral insufficiency. I therefore believe that the risk of bacterial infection on a prolapsed mitral valve is distinctly higher when there is a systolic murmur with or without a click than it is in patients in whom the prolapse is diagnosed either from the click alone or from echocardiographic surveys of patients, such as young women in their 20's or 30's. Consequently, it is my practice to administer antibiotic prophylaxis prior to dental and other procedures likely to produce a bacteremia in patients with mitral valve prolapse when a click-murmur syndrome is present or when a significant murmur alone is present. I do not undertake such prophylaxis when, in fact, the only evidence for diagnosis is either echocardiographic evidence of prolapse or auscultatory findings of a mid- or late systolic click.

ELLIOT RAPAPORT, M.D.

Nineteen

Should Pulmonary Arteriography Be Performed Routinely in Patients with Suspected Acute Pulmonary Emboli?

PULMONARY ARTERIOGRAPHY SHOULD BE PERFORMED
ROUTINELY IN PATIENTS WITH SUSPECTED ACUTE
PULMONARY EMBOLI

Joseph V. Messer, M.D.

PULMONARY ANGIOGRAPHY IN NOT INDICATED IN ALL
PATIENTS WITH SUSPECTED PULMONARY EMBOLISM

James E. Dalen, M.D.

COMMENT

Pulmonary Arteriography Should Be Performed Routinely in Patients with Suspected Acute Pulmonary Emboli

JOSEPH V. MESSER, M.D.

Director, Section of Cardiology; Professor of Medicine,
Rush Medical College, Rush Presbyterian–St. Luke's
Medical Center, Chicago, Illinois

Next to knowing the truth itself is to know the
direction in which it lies.

Peter Mere Latham (1789–1875)
Diseases of the Heart, Lecture XX

Pulmonary embolism is among the most misdiagnosed and mistreated conditions encountered in hospital practice. In a recent postmortem study, the frequency of false negative or missed diagnoses was 67 per cent, while positive diagnoses were incorrect in 62 per cent of the patients.[1] Numerous studies using angiographic documentation have indicated that the clinical diagnosis of pulmonary embolism is correct in about one third of patients.[2]

Numerically, pulmonary embolism is a major health problem. In a reasonable analysis based on the available data, Dalen and Alpert have estimated the incidence of symptomatic pulmonary embolism per year in the United States.[3] Their analysis, summarized in Table 1, emphasizes the importance of accurate diagnosis and appropriate therapy in determining ultimate outcome. Reported mortality rates average eight per cent in diagnosed, treated patients, but nearly four times greater, or 30 per cent, in undiagnosed, untreated patients. Unfortunately, 11 per cent of patients die

445

Table 1. *Annual Incidence of Pulmonary Embolism in the United States**

	SURVIVAL	DEATHS	TOTAL (%)
Within 1 hour		67,000	67,000 (11)
Beyond 1 hour			
Diagnosed and treated	150,000	13,000	163,000 (26)
Not diagnosed or treated	280,000	120,000	400,000 (63)
Total	430,000	200,000	630,000 (100)

*From data provided in Dalen JE, and Alpert JS: Natural history of pulmonary embolism. Prog Cardiovasc Dis 27:259–270, 1975.

within one hour, before diagnosis can be established and therapy initiated. On the basis of 630,000 symptomatic pulmonary embolic episodes annually, this condition may be the third most frequent cause of death in the United States, more common than cerebral vascular accidents and half as frequent as acute myocardial infarction.[3]

Although other authors have reported similar incidence estimates, it should be emphasized that such estimates do not include the toll resulting from unnecessary treatment of patients erroneously diagnosed on the basis of nonspecific, inaccurate criteria. Robin recently concluded that pulmonary embolism is extensively overdiagnosed and overtreated in previously normal patients, especially in previously normal women using oral contraceptives.[4] Pooled data from three recent series[4-6] reveal that 80 per cent of patients diagnosed as having pulmonary embolism by clinical findings, blood gases, and perfusion lung scanning have negative pulmonary angiograms. The application of such criteria without angiographic validation clearly results in extensive overdiagnosis and overtreatment.

The implications of these data are far-reaching. Apparently, the diagnostic criteria used by a majority of clinicians are inaccurate and in need of revision, based on recent advances in our understanding of the pathophysiology of pulmonary embolism.

Therapeutically, the results of misdiagnosis are particularly hazardous. In all but a small subgroup of patients, the primary goal of treatment is prophylaxis against recurrent thromboembolism, which occurs in approximately 50 per cent of untreated patients and is fatal in about half of these recurrences.[7] Failure to treat is a life-threatening omission. Conversely, anticoagulant therapy is costly, inconvenient, and associated with a significant incidence of mortality and major bleeding. Recent well-conducted studies have reported mortality rates as high as 2.4 per cent in short-term, fully heparinized patients and two per cent in patients on long-term oral anticoagulants.[8-10] Although these risks may be justified in patients with documented venous thromboembolism, they cannot be tolerated in the instance of false positive diagnosis.

The advent of thrombolytic therapy for major pulmonary embolism and the similarly higher risks of caval interruption and pulmonary embolectomy in selected patients accentuate the importance of accurate diagnosis in the management of patients suspected of having venous thromboembolic disease.

The clinician is thus confronted with a cruel paradox. Utilizing widely accepted, non-invasive diagnostic criteria, venous thromboembolism appears to be underdiagnosed and undertreated as judged by autopsy studies, but overdiagnosed and overtreated in surviving patients as judged by pulmonary angiographic validation. The magnitude of this paradox is illustrated in Figure 1. Were therapy for venous thromboembolism of limited utility or without significant hazard, diagnostic accuracy would be relatively unimportant. Precisely the opposite is true.

Several studies during the past decade have provided a basis for significant improvement in the management of venous thromboembolism. Although some key questions remain unanswered and the interpretation of some available data remains controversial, knowledge is now at hand to correct many deficiencies in the current management of suspected pulmonary embolism. Discussions of the most important among these deficiencies follow.

1. Failure of the clinician to incorporate recently acquired natural history and pathophysiologic knowledge into the process of decision making

The National Cooperative Trials of Thrombolytic Therapy provide previously unavailable, definitive information concerning clinical presentation, pathophysiology, therapeutic efficacy, complications, and mortality in patients with documented, quantified pulmonary embolism.[11, 12] This new knowledge has been presented in several clinical reviews that should be

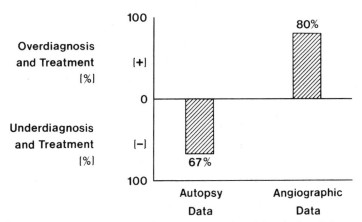

Pulmonary Embolic Disease

Accuracy of Non-Invasive Diagnostic Criteria

Figure 1. Graphic representation of the accuracy of widely employed diagnostic criteria for pulmonary embolism when judged by autopsy[1] and angiographic studies.[4-6]

familiar to all practitioners.[2, 3, 13] As frequently occurs in our understanding of disease, these pivotal studies have exposed major inaccuracies in commonly held beliefs, discrediting much of the previous literature on the pathophysiology and diagnosis of pulmonary embolism.

It is now well documented that the pathophysiologic consequences of pulmonary embolism are nonspecific derangements of circulatory and respiratory function that can be mimicked by many cardiac and pulmonary conditions. Moreover, in many patients, pulmonary embolism is clinically silent. Although reliance on nonspecific diagnostic tests frequently results in overdiagnosis and overtreatment, the clinician's index of suspicion is generally too low. Surveillance, early detection, and prophylaxis are inadequate in patients with established predisposing conditions, such as immobilization, venous disease, prior cardiovascular disease, and trauma or surgery involving the pelvis and lower extremities.

Clinically apparent thrombophlebitis, which occurs only in one third of patients, and the signs and symptoms of pulmonary infarction, which occurs only in 10 to 20 per cent of patients, too often are sought before the diagnosis of pulmonary embolism is actively pursued. Conversely, the diagnosis is erroneously excluded when the electrocardiogram, chest x-ray, and arterial blood gases fail to reveal abnormalities considered "classic" for embolism. Overestimation of mortality and recurrence rates and underestimation of the complications of anticoagulation and surgical intervention often lead to aggressive therapy even when the diagnosis of pulmonary embolism has not been clearly established.

Improvements in the management of venous thromboembolism will occur when more accurate information concerning clinical presentation, diagnostic aids, and therapy is incorporated into the practitioner's decision-making process.

2. Inadequate understanding of the accuracy and risks of available diagnostic aids

The diagnostic aids most frequently employed in evaluating suspected pulmonary embolism include history, physical examination, chest x-ray, electrocardiogram, arterial blood gases, lung scanning, and pulmonary arteriography. Data are now available concerning the sensitivity, specificity, and risk of each of these aids.[5, 6, 11, 12, 14] Because the therapy for venous thromboembolism has great value as well as significant hazard, false negativity and false positivity assume major importance, together with true positivity and true negativity, in assessing the accuracy of various diagnostic tests. Most reports have emphasized "predictive accuracy" or "probability estimates," the percentage of positive tests that are truly positive, without adequately considering the therapeutic implications of false positivity and negativity in the management of suspected pulmonary embolism.

HISTORY AND PHYSICAL EXAMINATION

History and physical findings have been mentioned in the foregoing discussion, and it is sufficient to state that neither has particular sensitivity or specificity for pulmonary embolism. As observed in the Cooperative Thrombolytic Trials, dyspnea is the most common symptom of pulmonary embolism, followed by pleuritic pain and apprehension. Rales, cough, and a loud pulmonary second sound are noted in about one half of patients, whereas tachycardia, gallops, fever, hemoptysis, pleural friction rubs, and phlebitis are more frequently absent than present in patients with documented pulmonary embolism. When present, pleural pain and hemoptysis suggest less severe pulmonary vascular obstruction, while a loud pulmonary second sound, right ventricular S_3 gallop, cyanosis, and syncope suggest massive embolism.

Because the classic clinical findings of pulmonary embolism are frequently absent or may reflect nonembolic cardiac and pulmonary disease when present, history and physical examination have minimal diagnostic accuracy. Their greatest value relates to predisposing factors and early detection of deep venous thrombosis, especially when non-invasive screening methods for this condition are employed in predisposed patients.

CHEST ROENTGENOGRAPHY AND
ELECTROCARDIOGRAPHY

Chest x-ray and electrocardiographic abnormalities have little value in diagnosing pulmonary embolism because they are highly nonspecific. The most common roentgenographic findings of pulmonary embolism are consolidation and elevation of the hemi-diaphragm, seen in about 40 per cent of patients. These changes are not specific for pulmonary embolism and are most important because they limit the value of lung scanning. The electrocardiogram, though abnormal in nearly 90 per cent of patients with pulmonary embolism, is highly nonspecific. The most common abnormality is T-wave inversion, seen in 40 per cent of patients, while less than one-third have changes of acute cor pulmonale. The primary value of electrocardiography is in differential diagnosis, since approximately seven per cent of patients admitted to the Thrombolytic Trials had a clinical presentation compatible with acute myocardial infarction. Thus, the chest x-ray and electrocardiogram have very limited diagnostic accuracy for pulmonary embolism, but are essential components of patient evaluation in order to define the value of subsequent lung scanning and to detect the presence of possible myocardial involvement.

ARTERIAL BLOOD GASES

Of all diagnostic aids employed in the evaluation of suspected pulmonary embolism, arterial blood gases are the most abused. Although originally introduced as a screening test that, when normal, tended to exclude the diagnosis, arterial blood gas measurements are commonly used to support the diagnosis when abnormal. Unfortunately, neither conclusion is reliably accurate. The arterial blood sample must be properly processed and analyzed immediately on an instrument just previously calibrated. Even when these precautions are taken, approximately 12 per cent of patients with pulmonary embolism will have arterial oxygen tensions above 80 mm Hg. Thus, arterial hypoxemia has a sensitivity for pulmonary embolism of approximately 88 per cent. Little data are available concerning its specificity, although hypoxemia is very common in many forms of cardiopulmonary disease. In fact, in a recent study of the accuracy of diagnostic tests in patients suspect for pulmonary embolism, McNeil and associates[15] found that arterial blood gases were not useful in identifying young patients with the disease (sensitivity) or in distinguishing such patients from those with other diseases (specificity). It is of interest to note that in 97 young patients with pleural pain, the mean arterial oxygen tension was *higher* in those who had pulmonary embolism than in those who did not.[15]

Considering the potential hazards of arterial entry in patients about to be anticoagulated, especially when punctured in the commonly used femoral arterial location, a strong case can be made for abandoning this relatively insensitive and highly nonspecific diagnostic test in the evaluation of patients suspect for pulmonary embolism.

PERFUSION LUNG SCANNING

Given the disappointing inaccuracy of history, physical examination, chest x-ray, electrocardiogram, and arterial blood gases, it is understandable that more useful diagnostic aids have been sought in evaluating patients with possible pulmonary embolism. Pulmonary scintigraphy, including both perfusion and ventilation scanning, is the most valuable screening tool available for the diagnosis of this condition.

The value of perfusion lung scanning was well established in the Thrombolytic Trials, in which only six per cent of the patients were unable to tolerate the procedure. Although acute respiratory and hemodynamic embarrassment has occurred in association with perfusion scanning, this procedure can be employed virtually without patient risk. Initial optimism concerning the diagnostic value of perfusion scanning has been tempered by the experience gained in the Thrombolytic Trials[5, 11, 12] and, more recently, by the excellent correlative studies of McNeil and associates.[6, 15, 16] Four-view perfusion scanning has its greatest value when completely normal in the presence of a normal chest x-ray. Under these circumstances, pulmonary embolism is essentially excluded. Only rare instances have been reported of pulmonary embolism with negative perfusion scans.

Thus, the sensitivity of perfusion lung scanning is very high, with virtually all patients with pulmonary embolism being detected by this screening technique. Conversely, however, an abnormal perfusion scan does not necessarily reflect pulmonary embolic disease. Any pre-existing lung disease may cause perfusion defects. Although such conditions are frequently apparent on chest x-ray, many are not. Furthermore, perfusion defects matched by x-ray abnormalities are not necessarily artifactual. Twenty-five per cent of patients with such defects had pulmonary emboli in McNeil's study[6] and 41 per cent of patients with pulmonary emboli had consolidation on chest x-ray in the Thrombolytic Trials.[11] Overall, pulmonary angiography is negative in 60 to 80 per cent of abnormal perfusion scans, indicating that this screening test, though sensitive, is highly nonspecific for pulmonary embolic disease and yields an unacceptably high rate of false positivity (Table 2, Criterion G).

When abnormal perfusion scans are interpreted more critically according to the anatomic subdivisions, number, and bilateral nature of defects, specificity is improved. McNeil's study compared pulmonary scintigraphy and angiography in 105 consecutive patients suspected of having pulmonary embolism from clinical findings, most commonly pleuritic chest pain or dyspnea.[6] Forty-two patients (40 per cent) had pulmonary embolism, an unusually high incidence of disease in an unselected population subjected to scanning and angiography for clinically suspected pulmonary embolism. A maximum true positivity of 81 per cent could be achieved by perfusion scanning when positivity was defined as multiple defects involving at least a lung or lobe (Table 2, Criterion D). Unfortunately, this limiting definition significantly reduces the sensitivity of perfusion scanning, since only one half of patients with pulmonary embolism demonstrate this abnormal perfusion pattern. The inclusion of at least multiple segmental defects increases the sensitivity of perfusion scanning, but decreases its specificity and diagnostic accuracy (Table 2, Criterion E). Other interpretive criterion, such as multiple segmental defects alone or single defects, segmental or greater, further impair diagnostic accuracy (Table 2, Criteria F and H).

In a similar attempt to improve the specificity of perfusion scanning in the Thrombolytic Trials, a lung-scanning panel of five experts classified scans according to high, medium, or low probability of pulmonary embolism. In addition to significant inter-interpreter disagreement on the proba-

Table 2. *Pulmonary Embolic Disease — Sensitivity, Specificity, and Diagnostic Accuracy of Lung Scanning***

LUNG SCAN ABNORMALITY	SENSI-TIVITY	SPE-CIFICITY	POSITIVITY True	POSITIVITY False	NEGATIVITY True	NEGATIVITY False	ERROR
Ventilation-Perfusion Mismatch Defects							
A. Multiple lobe or lung	56	95	95	5	59	41	28
B. Multiple lobe, lung, or segmental	88	90	93	7	83	17	11
C. Multiple segmental	31	95	91	9	48	52	43
Perfusion Defect(s)							
D. Multiple lobe or lung	52	92	81	19	74	26	24
E. Multiple lobe, lung, or segmental	86	70	66	34	88	12	24
F. Multiple segmental	33	78	50	50	64	36	40
G. Any abnormality	100	2	40	60	100	0	59
H. Single lobe, lung, or segmental	7	89	30	70	59	41	44
Combination of Criteria							
I. Criteria B and D	76	92	86	14	85	15	14
J. Criteria B and E	86	79	73	27	89	11	18

*Adapted from McNeil BJ: A diagnostic strategy using ventilation-perfusion studies in patients suspect for pulmonary embolism. J Nucl Med *17*:613–616, 1976; and McNeil BJ: Personal communication.

All values are percentages. Incidence of pulmonary embolism in patient population: 60 per cent for ventilation-perfusion scans; 40 per cent for perfusion scans and combination criteria (see text).

bility of embolism, 16 per cent of patients with high-probability perfusion scans had normal pulmonary angiograms, and 17 of 18 patients with low-probability scans had massive or submassive emboli by angiography.[5]

PERFUSION SCANNING IN SUSPECTED RECURRENT EMBOLIZATION

If perfusion scanning has limited utility in the diagnosis of suspected pulmonary embolism, its value in assessing recurrent embolization is even less secure. From several viewpoints, the precise delineation of embolic recurrence has importance equal to accurate diagnosis of the initial episode. In most instances, embolic recurrence is accepted as conclusive evidence of the failure of medical therapy and an indication for surgical intervention, the mortality and morbidity of which far exceed those of anticoagulation.

Autopsy data indicate that two thirds of cases with fatal pulmonary embolism have evidence of prior emboli occurring days or weeks before the fatal episode. In the Thrombolytic Trials, approximately one fourth of the patients had histories of one or more previous embolic episodes. In the heparin-treated group, 23 per cent were diagnosed as having recurrent embolization within the first two weeks of therapy. Although angiographic documentation was not obtained, nearly 40 per cent of these patients had inferior vena caval ligation for presumed recurrent embolization.

The reported incidence of recurrent pulmonary embolism varies considerably, from less than five per cent to nearly 50 per cent, reflecting the great difficulty encountered in clinical diagnosis. Signs and symptoms suggesting recurrence may be related to the delayed effects of an earlier embolus, its thrombotic extension, or the fragmentation and distal migration of the original embolus.[2, 13, 17] The perfusion lung scan is of little value in distinguishing these mechanisms from true embolic recurrence, and may even falsely suggest recurrence when varying rates of embolic resolution produce changes in the regional distribution of pulmonary vascular resistance.[17]

Sufficient serial scanning and angiographic observations are not available in patients suspected of having recurrent pulmonary embolization. In addition to three patients with spurious scintigraphic recurrence reported by Moser et al.,[17] 15 per cent of the patients in the Thrombolytic Trials demonstrated post-treatment worsening of the perfusion lung scan despite reduction in angiographic severity. The tendency of emboli to fragment and migrate distally was as common in patients receiving heparin as in those given urokinase.[11] Figures 2 and 3 illustrate anterior perfusion scans and pulmonary angiograms before and after treatment in a patient from the author's series demonstrating this phenomenon. The clinical presentation and perfusion scan suggested recurrent embolization, although serial angiograms revealed only dissolution of proximal large-vessel filling defects and new occlusion of distal segmental and smaller vessels. Perfusion scanning without angiographic validation would have invited the therapeutic error of unnecessary caval interruption in this seriously ill patient.

Thus, the definitive diagnosis of pulmonary embolism or of recurrent embolization cannot be made on the basis of perfusion scanning. A normal or unchanged scan virtually excludes these diagnoses. Despite these limitations, baseline perfusion scanning should be performed routinely in the assessment of patients suspect for pulmonary embolism, even when the initial chest x-ray reveals parenchymal abnormalities.

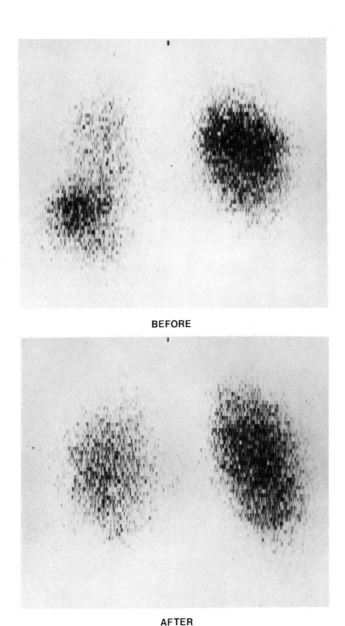

BEFORE

AFTER

Figure 2. Anterior lung scans before and after treatment was begun, suggesting recurrent embolization in association with a new clinical episode.

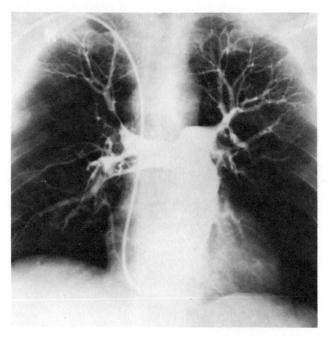

BEFORE

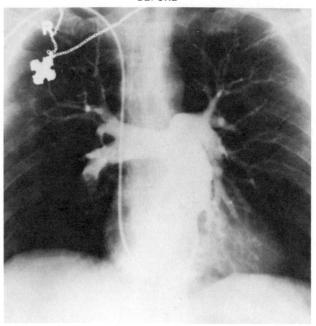

AFTER

Figure 3. Pulmonary arteriograms obtained at the times of scanning shown in Figure 2, demonstrating fragmentation of proximal emboli and distal migration in the right lower lobe. No new emboli were demonstrated.

VENTILATION SCANNING

The addition of ventilation studies to pulmonary scintigraphy has increased its specificity for pulmonary embolism. In common practice, the demonstration of impaired perfusion in a pulmonary region with intact ventilation — the so-called ventilation-perfusion mismatch — has been considered diagnostic of pulmonary embolism. Matching defects by both methods of scanning is usually assumed to reflect pulmonary parenchymal abnormalities with secondary vascular obstruction.

In the largest available series comparing pulmonary scintigraphy and pulmonary arteriography, McNeil reported that the addition of ventilation studies to perfusion scanning produced a probability estimate (percentage true positive) of 100 per cent in patients with pulmonary embolism having multiple segmental perfusion defects.[6] Patients having *both* matching and mismatching defects were excluded from McNeil's computation of true positivity.[16] Since such patterns must be dealt with in clinical practice, data from all of McNeil's subjects having multiple segmental or greater ventilation-perfusion mismatches, with or without coexisting matching defects, have been used to calculate the sensitivity, specificity, and diagnostic accuracy of ventilation-perfusion scintigraphy presented in Table 2, Criteria A to C. Clearly, the addition of ventilation studies enhances the value of pulmonary scintigraphy whenever multiple perfusion defects are observed, especially at the segmental level.

As discussed below, the predictive accuracy of diagnostic testing is influenced by the incidence of disease in the patient population studied. McNeil's total group had a 40 per cent incidence of pulmonary embolism, while the subgroup in whom ventilation scans could be obtained had a 60 per cent incidence of pulmonary embolism. When applied to a patient population whose incidence of disease is this high, ventilation-perfusion mismatched defects of multiple segmental or greater extent appeared to have a 91 to 95 per cent true positivity for pulmonary embolism (Table 2, Criteria A–C). When positivity is limited to these highly specific criteria, however, the sensitivity of pulmonary scintigraphy is decreased significantly, with only 31 per cent of ventilation-scanned patients with pulmonary embolism being detected by multiple segmental defects (Criterion C), 56 per cent by multiple lobe or lung defects (Criterion A), and 88 per cent by a combination of these scintigraphic findings (Criterion B). Although false positivity inviting unnecessary treatment occurs at a rate of five to 10 per cent, false negativity occurs at a rate of 17 to 52 per cent, inviting withholding of treatment in the absence of angiographic validation.

Only one half of patients with abnormal perfusion scans are considered candidates for ventilation studies.[6] The remainder display inadequate patient cooperation, defects too small to be resolved by ventilation techniques, or matching chest x-ray abnormalities. Approximately 20 per cent of these patients have pulmonary embolism by arteriography. Thus, when applied to McNeil's total series of 104 patients suspect for pulmonary embolism, the Criterion B combination of optimal ventilation-perfusion sensitivity and specificity applied to only 27 per cent of the total (28 of 104) and to only 67 per cent of all patients with pulmonary embolism (28 of 42).

Conversely, had the type B lung-scanning criterion been required for the diagnosis and treatment of pulmonary embolism, 16 patients would have been mistreated: Fourteen patients with pulmonary embolism would not have been treated (19 per cent false negativity), and two patients without pulmonary embolism would have received treatment (seven per cent false positivity).

When the applicability of pulmonary scintigraphy is extended by considering positive multiple lobe-lung defects in patients having perfusion scans alone and multiple lobe, lung, or segmental mismatches in those additional patients suitable for ventilation scanning, mistreatment would have occurred in 14 per cent, with 14 per cent false positives and 15 per cent false negatives (Table 2, Criterion I).

It has been stated that a normal perfusion scan virtually excludes the diagnosis of pulmonary embolism. A similar screening value has been attributed to the finding of only *matching* ventilation-perfusion defects in patients suspect for pulmonary embolism.[6] In his analysis of pulmonary scintigraphy, Robin warns that ventilation scanning should frequently reveal defects in areas of pulmonary vascular occlusion producing matching ventilation-perfusion abnormalities.[4] Thus, this pattern may lead to false negative conclusions concerning pulmonary embolism if pulmonary angiographic validation is not obtained. Robin also addresses the problem of false positivity of ventilation-perfusion scanning due largely to the poor spatial resolution of ventilation scanning. In this regard, eight of 20 patients (40 per cent) without pulmonary embolism had ventilation-perfusion mismatches (false positivity) in McNeil's series.[6]

In summary, ventilation scanning is a safe, relatively inexpensive technique for improving the predictive accuracy of pulmonary scintigraphy. The technique is applicable only to one half of patients with suspected pulmonary embolism. When rigid criteria are applied to the interpretation of ventilation-perfusion scanning, specificity for pulmonary embolism is greatly enhanced, although sensitivity decreases significantly. Depending on the criteria employed in interpretation and the incidence of disease in the population, false positive results may be anticipated in a significant percentage of patients studied. Employing specific criteria, false negative results are common, although more data are required to assess the magnitude of this problem. Ventilation-perfusion scanning is of no greater value than perfusion scanning alone in documenting true recurrence of pulmonary embolism.

PULMONARY ARTERIOGRAPHY

Pulmonary arteriography is the only definitive method available for diagnosing pulmonary embolism during life. When performed within 72 hours of the suspected embolic episode, pulmonary angiography has extremely high sensitivity, specificity, and predictive accuracy. Although autopsy correlations in close proximity to angiography are limited, available data indicate nearly 100 per cent accuracy.[5, 14, 18]

As with scintigraphy, angiographic signs of pulmonary embolism may be classified according to their diagnostic specificity. Filling defects and vessel cut-offs are the only findings generally considered reliable evidence of emboli. Less specific signs such as vessel pruning, oligemia, asymmetrical filling, and prolongation of arterial opacification are supportive of the diagnosis, but are also observed with chronic pulmonary and cardiac diseases, for which lung scanning is even less accurate.

Fortunately, equivocal angiograms are obtained in only 15 to 20 per cent of patients and are usually correctly interpreted by experienced angiographers. In the Thrombolytic Trials, for example, the angiographic panel disagreed with the angiographer performing the study in less than four per cent of cases. Interpanel disagreement was less than six per cent, compared with 67 per cent disagreement among interpreters of lung-scanning data.

The routine use of subselective contrast injection with oblique views greatly increases angiographic specificity. Magnification and subtraction angiography have similar value, but are cumbersome, technically demanding, and expensive. Wilson's recent introduction of a balloon-tipped catheter technique permitting subselective stop-flow filming with minute volumes of contrast material has virtually eliminated arteriographic inaccuracy, while increasing patient safety, especially in the presence of pulmonary hypertension.[19] In the rare instance when these approaches fail to clarify the possibility of "small-vessel" emboli, management is best guided by the presence or absence of deep venous thrombosis in the pelvis or lower extremities as determined by venography or appropriate non-invasive techniques.

Pulmonary arteriography should be performed from the arm, usually by venous cut-down. Immediate heparinization when pulmonary embolus is first suspected is not a contraindication to subsequent arteriography. The arm approach allows direct control of bleeding in anticoagulated patients, multiple subselective injections when required, and exchange of catheters without end holes and reduces the risk of ventricular arrhythmia and perforation during catheter passage through the right ventricle. The inferior vena cava and both iliac and femoral veins can be examined during the same procedure. The potential of dislodging venous thrombi through the transfemoral route is obviated, and careful hemodynamic measurements are facilitated. Hemodynamic observations are invaluable guides to assessing the pathophysiologic consequences of pulmonary embolization and the presence of pre-existing cardiopulmonary disease.

The problem of suspected recurrent pulmonary embolism deserves special emphasis in relation to pulmonary arteriography. Comparison of post-recurrence and baseline angiograms is the only method allowing reliable distinction between true and spurious recurrent embolization.[2, 3, 13, 17] The therapeutic implications of this distinction are most important.

Pulmonary arteriography is absolutely or relatively contraindicated in some patients with suspected pulmonary embolization. These conditions are listed in Table 3. Severe pulmonary hypertension is the condition most feared when pulmonary arteriography is considered essential to patient management. In occasional desperate, life-threatening situations, pulmona-

Table 3. *Contraindications to Pulmonary Arteriography*

ABSOLUTE
    Known allergic sensitivity to contrast material

RELATIVE
    Severe pulmonary hypertension
    Recent myocardial infarction
    Left bundle branch block
    Ventricular arrhythmias
    Pregnancy
    Right-sided bacterial endocarditis
    Inadequate patient cooperation

ry arteriography is required to exclude recurrent pulmonary emboli as etiologic or complicating factors in severe pulmonary hypertension prior to inferior vena caval interruption. Under these circumstances, the risk of acute right ventricular failure, systemic hypotension, cyanosis, and ventricular fibrillation can be reduced by the administration of oxygen throughout the procedure, small hand injections of contrast material with cinefluoroscopy to assure patency of the main pulmonary trunks, and full opacification of the pulmonary vasculature on an individual, subselective lobar basis. Several successful studies have been reported after placing the patient on femoral-femoral partial cardiopulmonary bypass.

The use of a temporary transvenous pacemaker can obviate the danger of precipitating complete heart block during catheterization of the pulmonary artery in patients with left bundle branch block. The hazards of fetal radiation decrease in the later stages of pregnancy, can be minimized by proper shielding, and probably constitute a lower fetal and maternal risk than unnecessary anticoagulation. The importance of other relative contraindications has not been well studied, and decisions must be made on an individual basis, weighing the hazards of arteriography against those of inappropriate therapy.

The risks of pulmonary arteriography have been significantly overestimated by most practitioners. The most important complications of arteriography are listed in Table 4, and can be divided into those related to contrast material and to right heart catheterization. The vast majority of these complications can be avoided or successfully managed by an experienced angiographic team, proper premedication, and monitoring during the procedure.

Table 4. *Complications of Pulmonary Arteriography*

Allergic reactions to contrast material
Myocardial perforation with or without pericardial tamponade
Ventricular arrhythmias
Bleeding
Atrial arrhythmias
Infection
Pyrogenic reactions

In designing the study protocol for thrombolytic agents, the Trial's Steering Committee examined the complications of over 2000 pulmonary arteriograms reported by six centers. These data, together with those reported from the Trial, are presented in Table 5. A mortality rate of less than 0.2 per cent occurred in these studies, with a morbidity rate of approximately one per cent.

From statements in the literature[4, 6, 15] and discussions with referring physicians and house staff, it is apparent that the safety record of pulmonary arteriography is not accurately incorporated into the practitioner's decision-making process.

3. Failure to appreciate that the diagnostic accuracy of screening tests is dependent on the prevalence of disease in the population under study

The prevalence of disease in a given patient population strongly influences the predictive accuracy of diagnostic tests.[21] This relationship has not received proper attention in the diagnosis of pulmonary embolism, since only limited prevalence data are available for many subgroups of the patient population. As emphasized by Robin, these circumstances lead to the unwarranted extrapolation of incidence data obtained from autopsy series, resulting in erroneous presumptions concerning the predictive accuracy of many diagnostic tests.

The Thrombolytic Trials and other recent correlative studies offer new information concerning the prevalence of pulmonary embolism in hospitalized populations.[4, 6, 15] For example, in patients suspected of having pulmonary embolism on the basis of a suitable clinical history, hypoxemia, and a positive perfusion scan, pulmonary arteriography was positive in only 17 to 40 per cent of patients.[4-6] McNeil has reported an incidence of 10 per cent in hospitalized patients over 40 years of age presenting with multiple complaints suggesting pulmonary embolism and 20 per cent in patients under 40 years of age presenting with the single symptom of pleuritic chest pain.[15] These data and estimates reported for other patient subgroups are presented in Table 6.

It is clear from these data that the prevalence of pulmonary embolism varies widely among different subgroups of the patient population. The im-

Table 5. *Mortality and Morbidity of Pulmonary Arteriography*

	NUMBER OF PULMONARY ARTERIOGRAMS PERFORMED	SERIOUS COMPLICATIONS		
		Cardiac Perforations	*Arrhythmias*	*Death*
Pre-UPET analysis°	2347	15	8	5
UPET experience†	310	1	5	0
Totals: number	2657	16	13	5
%	100	0.6	0.5	0.19

UPET = Urokinase Pulmonary Embolism Trial.
° = 20, † = 11.

Pulmonary Embolic Disease

Influence of Prevalence of Pulmonary Embolism

on Predictive Accuracy of Lung Scanning

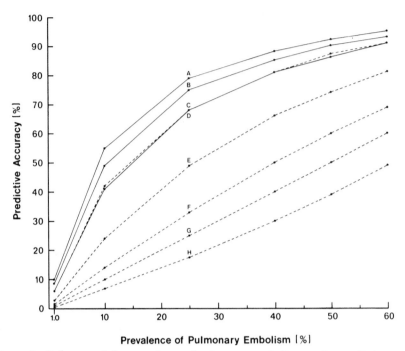

Figure 4. Influence of the prevalence of pulmonary embolism on the predictive accuracy of various abnormalities observed in lung scans. Curves A to H as identified in Table 2, calculated from the data of McNeil.[6, 16]

pact of these prevalence variations on the predictive accuracy of those abnormalities commonly observed in lung scanning is illustrated in Figure 4. Based on the incidence data available in the literature (Table 6), it would appear that the vast majority of patients suspect for pulmonary embolism derive from subgroups with a disease prevalence of one to 25 per cent. Within this broad range, the predictive accuracy (true positivity) of the most highly specific diagnostic criteria for ventilation-perfusion scanning does not exceed 80 per cent and may be as low as six per cent (Fig. 4, Criteria A and C).

The therapeutic implications of these observations cannot be overemphasized. In a patient suspect for pulmonary embolism from a population having a 25 per cent likelihood of the disease, anticoagulation based on the scintigraphic finding of multiple lobe or lung ventilation-perfusion mismatches (Table 2, Criterion A) has an 80 per cent chance of being the correct therapy (true positive test), but a 20 per cent chance of being unnecessary (false positive test). Conversely, should this criterion be required before therapy is initiated, there is a 13 per cent chance that therapy would be withheld in the presence of pulmonary embolism (false negative test). Unfortunately, the data base from which such analyses can be made is lim-

Table 6. *Incidence of Pulmonary Embolism in Various Patient Groups*

PATIENT POPULATION	INCIDENCE OF PULMONARY EMBOLISM (%)	REFERENCES
Sudden death, ages 15 to 45	0.0003	22
Abdominal-thoracic surgery	1–4	23
Hip surgery	2–12	23
Heart failure	8–15	23
Post myocardial infarction	9	23
Post mitral valve surgery	10	23
Fractures, pelvis and lower extremities	10	24
Over 40 years, multiple symptoms of pulmonary embolism	10	15
Under 40 years, pleuritic chest pain	20	15
General hospital, positive history, hypoxemia, perfusion scan	17–40	4–6
Heart failure at death	48	25

ited, and additional correlative studies of the incidence of pulmonary embolism and the sensitivity and specificity of diagnostic procedures are urgently needed.

The effect of disease prevalence influences all diagnostic tests for pulmonary embolism that lack high sensitivity and specificity. In fact, the predictive accuracy of diagnostic tests with either limited sensitivity or specificity tends to vary directly with the prevalence of disease in the population studied (Fig. 4, Criteria E–H). Confronted with this reality, advocates of screening tests often resort to more stringent criteria for positivity. Unfortunately, this does little to improve the diagnostic accuracy of a positive test in patient populations with a low prevalence of pulmonary embolism and further reduces the *sensitivity* of the test, thereby excluding patients with disease, the most serious error in the management of suspected venous thromboembolism. Of the various diagnostic procedures currently available for patients suspect for pulmonary embolism, only pulmonary arteriography, properly performed, possesses sufficient sensitivity and specificity to retain high diagnostic accuracy for all subgroups of the patient population.

4. Inadequate appreciation of the hazards of mistreatment resulting from inaccurate diagnosis in suspected pulmonary embolism

While the risks of pulmonary arteriography are overestimated by most practitioners, the risks of mistreatment of suspected pulmonary embolism have been significantly underestimated. Because the therapy for venous thromboembolism has both great value and significant hazards, accurate knowledge of the relative risks of therapeutic and diagnostic interventions is essential for optimal patient management.

As previously indicated, failure to treat venous thromboembolism is the most serious error in management of this condition, exposing the patient to a nearly fourfold greater mortality and recurrence rate than when proper therapy is instituted.[3, 26] Conversely, the risks of all forms of therapy for pulmonary embolism are sufficiently high to require definitive diagnosis before treatment is begun.

The major complications of treatment are summarized in Table 7. Although factors such as patient age, pre-existing cardiopulmonary status, care in detecting contraindications to anticoagulation, and rigid monitoring of therapy influence overall complication rates, initiation of therapy exposes many patients to a cascade of risks that must be considered in effective decision making.

ALTERATIONS IN HEMOSTASIS

As the keystone of adequate therapy, acute heparinization involves greater hazard than generally appreciated. In nine recently reported, well-conducted clinical series involving acute heparinization in more than 800 patients, fatal bleeding averaged 1.2 per cent and major hemorrhage requiring transfusion and cessation of therapy was observed in an additional 13 per cent of patients.[7-9, 11, 26-30] Complication rates in chronic oral anticoagulation are rarely reported per patient-year of therapy, although data allowing such calculations are available from the cardiac surgical literature. In two well-conducted studies, fatal bleeding rates averaged 1.2 per cent per patient-year of treatment in over 600 patients chronically anticoagulated following prosthetic valve replacement.[10, 31] Significant nonfatal bleeding, usually cerebrovascular, averaged an additional four per cent per patient-year of treatment. Thus, according to these studies, acute heparinization followed by six months of oral anticoagulation exposes patients to a 1.8 per cent mortality from bleeding. In the Thrombolytic Trials, acute thrombolytic therapy was associated with fatal bleeding in approximately one per cent of patients and produced major bleeding in an additional 17 per cent.[11, 12] Despite alterations in hemostasis, recurrent pulmonary embolism has been reported in two to 23 per cent of patients,[9, 11, 12] with fatal recurrence in zero to three per cent.[9, 11, 26]

Table 7.   *Pulmonary Embolic Disease — Complications of Therapy*

TYPE OF THERAPY	MORTALITY (%)	SEVERE MORBIDITY (%)	RECURRENT EMBOLISM Fatal (%)	Total (%)
Alterations in Hemostasis				
Acute heparinization	1.2	13	0–3	2–23
Chronic anticoagulation°	1.2	4		
Thrombolytic therapy	1	17	1	8
Inferior Vena Caval Interruption				
External	15	10–50	0–2	0–50
Intracaval — umbrella	0.5	10	0.8	3
Intracaval — balloon	0	3	0	0
Pulmonary Embolectomy	40–100			

References: see text
° = per patient-year

INFERIOR VENA CAVAL INTERRUPTION

Contraindications to anticoagulation, bleeding complications, and recurrent embolization commonly precipitate venous interruption in patients diagnosed with pulmonary embolism. Utilizing extra-caval surgical techniques, operative mortality averages 15 per cent,[26, 28, 32-34] and significant morbidity from venous stasis occurs in 10 to 50 per cent of survivors.[28] Widely varying embolic recurrence rates have been reported, and one to two per cent of patients have fatal recurrence despite caval interruption.[26, 32] Mobin-Uddin's intra-caval umbrella occluder may be indicated in seriously ill patients for whom anticoagulants are contraindicated, although mortality, morbidity, and recurrence rates are appreciable.[35] If initial experience with the intra-caval balloon occluder is supported by further clinical application, this technique may well become the method of choice for inferior vena caval interruption.[36]

PULMONARY EMBOLECTOMY

This heroic and sometimes life-saving procedure has a mortality rate of approximately 75 per cent, and undoubtedly will be replaced by thrombolytic therapy in documented instances of massive pulmonary embolization with shock.[11, 13]

Decision Analysis in the Management of Suspected Pulmonary Embolism

Although some authors have criticized decision-analysis techniques in the management of individual patients,[4] suspected pulmonary embolism is an example par excellence of decision making in the face of uncertainty. Given the data base now available concerning the incidence of disease, the sensitivity, specificity, and risks of various diagnostic tests, and the hazards of various therapeutic alternatives, relatively simple calculations can be made to guide diagnostic management in the direction of optimal utility or overall patient benefit.

There is general agreement that pulmonary scintigraphy, including ventilation scanning, when possible, is the most effective screening technique in patients suspect for pulmonary embolism. The initial steps in diagnostic decision analysis based on lung scan results are depicted in Figure 5. Although the diagnostic accuracy of lung scanning can be assessed in terms of specific criteria sets, with their corresponding sensitivities, specificities, and degrees of true and false positivity and negativity (Table 2), scans are commonly interpreted in terms of probabilities for pulmonary embolism. The probability categories shown in Figure 5 have been proposed by McNeil[15] and are based on sufficient angiographic documentation to permit their utilization in an analysis of the relative value of routine pulmonary arteriography in patients with suspected pulmonary emboli.

Of the four commonly employed lung scan interpretations, two elicit

Pulmonary Embolic Disease

Decision Analysis Following Lung Scanning

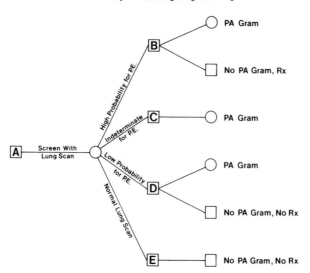

Figure 5. The initial steps in diagnostic decision analysis based on lung scan results. The probability categories shown have been suggested by McNeil.[15]

little or no controversy concerning the role of pulmonary arteriography. The finding of a normal perfusion lung scan virtually excludes the possibility of pulmonary embolism and the need for confirmatory arteriography (Fig. 5, Decision Node E). Lung scans having abnormalities associated with an 11 to 80 per cent true positivity for pulmonary embolism (or "predictive accuracy") are considered "indeterminate" for pulmonary embolism and require pulmonary arteriography for accurate diagnosis (Fig. 5, Decision Node C).

The remaining lung scan interpretations of high probability and low probability for pulmonary embolism form the basis for whatever controversy exists concerning the role of pulmonary arteriography in patients with suspected pulmonary embolism (Fig. 5, Decision Nodes B and D). McNeil and associates have considered "highly probable" those scanning abnormalities having an 81 to 100 per cent positivity for pulmonary embolism.[6, 15] When present on lung scanning, these abnormalities are considered sufficiently definitive to warrant initiation of therapy. Conversely, "low probability" is ascribed to those scanning abnormalities having one to 10 per cent true positivity for pulmonary embolism, and therapy is withheld.

THE RELATIVE VALUE OF PULMONARY ARTERIOGRAPHY VERSUS LUNG SCANNING ALONE IN HIGH- AND LOW-PROBABILITY SCANS

HIGH-PROBABILITY LUNG SCANS

Referring to Figure 6, the decision whether to perform pulmonary arteriography is indicated by square node B. If no arteriogram is performed, all patients with high-probability scans are candidates for anticoagulant thera-

Pulmonary Embolic Disease

Decision Analysis in High Probability Lung Scans

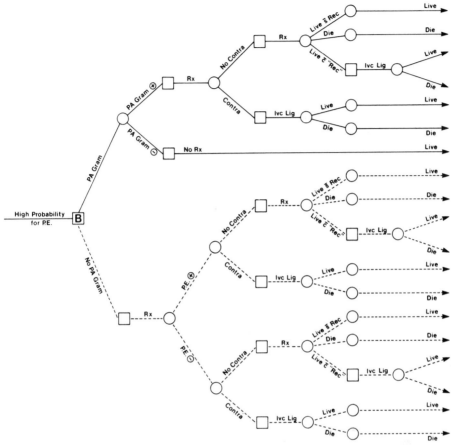

Figure 6. Decision analysis model in high-probability lung scans. (See text for discussion.)

py (Rx). Since high-probability scanning criteria include some patients without pulmonary embolism (false positivity), there is a chance (circular node) that a given patient either has the disease (PE+) or does not (PE−). In both situations, there is a chance that anticoagulant therapy is not contraindicated (No Contra) or is contraindicated (Contra). In the absence of contraindications, anticoagulant therapy is begun, resulting in the chances of living without recurrent pulmonary embolism (Live without Rec), dying of pulmonary embolism despite therapy or as a complication of treatment (Die), or living with true or spurious recurrent pulmonary embolism despite therapy (Live with Rec). In the latter circumstance, inferior vena caval interruption (Ivc Lig) is usually employed, resulting in the chances of living or operative mortality (Die).

If a pulmonary arteriogram is performed, there is a chance that it will be negative (PA Gram −) in patients with false positive lung scans. Therapy is withheld (No Rx) and the patient lives, unless mortality results from

Pulmonary Embolic Disease

Decision Analysis in Low Probability Lung Scans

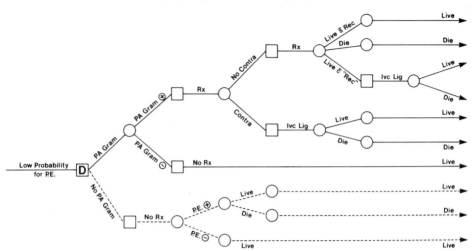

Figure 7. Decision analysis model in low-probability lung scans. (See text for discussion.)

the arteriographic study. If the arteriogram is positive (PA Gram +), therapy is appropriate, with the same sequence of decisions and chances of outcome described above, plus the mortality of arteriography.

LOW-PROBABILITY SCANS

Referring to Figure 7, the decision whether to perform pulmonary arteriography is indicated by square node D. If no arteriogram is performed, all patients with low-probability scans are considered not to have had pulmonary embolism, and treatment is withheld (No Rx). Since some patients with low-probability lung scans have pulmonary emboli (false negativity), there is a chance (circular node) that a given patient either has the disease (PE+) or does not (PE−). In either case, treatment is withheld, resulting in the chances of living or dying associated with no disease or untreated disease. If pulmonary arteriography is performed, there is a chance that it will be positive (PE+) in patients with false negative scans or negative (PE−). The decision concerning anticoagulant therapy, the chances of contraindications, caval ligation, recurrence, and ultimate outcome are identical to those described for high-probability scans followed by pulmonary arteriography.

Other possible outcomes, such as spurious embolic recurrence and significant morbidity, are not depicted in the decision models shown in Figures 6 and 7. Should pulmonary arteriography be performed in patients with high- and low-probability lung scans? Utilizing the data now available for solving the decision models, calculations of the relative values of pulmonary arteriography can be made as shown in Tables 8 and 9. The assumptions required for solving the decision models are as follows:

Table 8. *Distribution of High- and Low-Probability Lung Scans in 1000 Patients Studied for Possible Pulmonary Embolism*

	NUMBER OF PATIENTS*	LUNG SCAN PROBABILITY OF PULMONARY EMBOLISM			
		High		*Low*	
		n	%	n	%
With PE	400	304	76	8	2
Without PE	600	48	8	180	30
Total	1000	352		188	

*From population with incidence of 40 per cent.[6, 15, 16]
PE = pulmonary embolism.

Table 9. *Relative Values of Pulmonary Arteriography in Patients With High and Low Probabilities for Emboli by Lung Scanning*

	RESULTS OF SCANNING ONLY†				RESULTS OF ARTERI-OGRAPHY†	
	Probability					
	High		Low			
No. of patients	352		188		540	
Outcome	PE+	PE−	PE+	PE−	PE+	PE−
A. Presence of PE	304	48	8	180	312	228
B. Anticoag. Contra. (25%)[23]	76	12	−	−	78	−
C. Anticoag. Not Contra. (75%)	228	36	−	−	234	−
D. Survive s̄ Bleed						
(A − F)	−	−	5.6	180	−	228
[C − (E + F + G)]	176	30.4	−	−	181	−
E. Survive c̄ Bleed (0.13 × C)*	30	5	−	−	30	0
F. Die c̄ PE, s̄ Rx (30%)[3]	−	−	2.4	0	−	−
c̄ Rx (0.08 × C)[3]	18	0	−	−	19	0
G. Die c̄ Bleeding (0.018 × C)*	4	0.6	−	−	4	0
H. Rec. PE, s̄ Rx (50%)[7]	−	−	4	0	−	−
c̄ Rx (0.23 × D)[11]	40	0	−	−	42	0
I. Die c̄ Rec. PE, s̄ Rx (25%)[7]	−	−	2	0	−	−
c̄ Rx (0.03 × D)[11]	5	0	−	−	5	0
J. IVC Lig. (B + E + H)	146	17	−	−	150	0
K. Die c̄ IVC Lig. (0.15 × J)[28]	22	3	−	−	22	0
L. Die c̄ PA Gram (1.9%)*	−	−	−	−	0.6	0.4
M. Total Deaths (F + G + I + K + L)	49	3.6	4.4	0	50.6	0.4
	52.6		4.4			
	57				51	

*See text for references.
† Per 1000 patients with possible PE, 40 per cent incidence of disease.

1. Patients under consideration are drawn from the hospitalized population having a 40 per cent incidence of pulmonary embolism, as observed in McNeil's study.[6]

2. High- and low-probability lung scans are defined as demonstrating abnormalities having a predictive accuracy for pulmonary embolism of 81 to 100 per cent and one to 10 per cent, respectively.[15] The data provided by McNeil's arteriographic-lung scanning study indicate that high- and low-probability scans occur in approximately 76 per cent and two per cent, respectively, of patients with pulmonary emboli, and in eight per cent and 30 per cent, respectively, of patients without emboli (Table 8).

3. Pulmonary arteriography is considered the definitive indicator of the presence or absence of pulmonary embolism, since this assumption has been utilized in determining the diagnostic accuracy of lung-scanning criteria used in these decision analyses.[6]

Calculations of the type contained in Tables 8 and 9 are highly subject to error, and even minor changes in reported probabilities of various outcomes have significant impact on the cascading effects of compounded risks. Not included in these calculations are the benefits and costs of excluding spurious recurrent emboli by serial arteriography; nor are the inconvenience, discomfort, and minor morbidities of therapeutic alternatives adequately considered. Nonetheless, such decision analyses call attention to the complexity of optimal management in pulmonary embolic disease, Unfortunately, as Robin has stated, "Knowledge of the complexity of disease does not simplify management."[4] It also is clear that a much larger series of arteriographic-lung scanning correlations is needed.

Until more data are available, however, the decision models presented here strongly support the value of pulmonary arteriography in avoiding unnecessary mortality, bleeding, caval interruption, and costly therapy in patients suspected of having acute pulmonary embolic disease (Table 10). It

Table 10. *Major Benefits and Costs of Pulmonary Arteriography in Patients With High- and Low-Probability Lung Scans**

BENEFITS		ESTIMATED ECONOMIC VALUE
6	Deaths avoided	?
5	Major bleeds avoided @ $1000	$ 5000
13	IVC Ligations Avoided @ $2500	32,500
30	Courses of anticoagulation avoided @ $2000	60,000
630	Days of unnecessary hospitalization avoided @ $350/day	220,500
48	Erroneous diagnoses of "PE" avoided	?
		Total $318,000
COSTS		
540	Pulmonary arteriograms @ $600	$324,000
3	Non-fatal cardiac perforations	?
3	Non-fatal arrhythmias	?
		Total $324,000

*Per 1000 patients with possible PE, 40 per cent incidence of disease.

should be emphasized that as the incidence of disease increases in the population at risk, false negativity tends to increase, while the predictive accuracy of a positive lung scan also increases. The converse is true with decreasing disease incidence. Although false negativity contributes somewhat more to avoidable error than does false positivity, the value of pulmonary arteriography is retained throughout a wide range of disease incidence. In addition to reducing overall mortality, arteriography tends to confine complications to those patients with disease, while minimizing mortality in patients without disease.

Practical Implications of Performing Pulmonary Arteriography in Patients with Suspected Pulmonary Emboli

At the present time, adequate equipment and trained personnel for pulmonary arteriography are available in fewer than 20 per cent of hospitals in the United States. More serious, perhaps, is the inadequacy of resources for reliable pulmonary scintigraphy, including both ventilation and perfusion measurements. To place such facilities in all acute care institutions is clearly impractical and even undesirable. The development of logical and efficient educational, communication, referral, and transport networks has proven effective in many locales and must be implemented nationally if acute pulmonary embolism and a host of other complex problems are to receive optimal management.

Summary

Current knowledge has been presented concerning the incidence, pathophysiology, clinical presentations, diagnostic techniques, and therapy of suspected pulmonary embolism. By applying available data to relatively simple models of alternative forms of management, it is concluded that important benefits result from the performance of pulmonary arteriography in patients with suspected pulmonary embolism. If the data base applied to these analyses is reasonably accurate, routine pulmonary arteriography has the potential to reduce erroneous diagnosis, unnecessary bleeding complications, surgical intervention, and hospitalization. Most important, application of this relatively safe diagnostic technique can reduce unnecessary mortality in patients with suspected pulmonary embolism. Effective educational, referral, and transport networks must be developed, however, before these benefits can be achieved for substantial numbers of patients.

ACKNOWLEDGMENT

I wish to acknowledge the kindness of Dr. Barbara J. McNeil in providing data used in the preparation of this manuscript.

References

1. Modan B, Sharon E, and Jelin N: Factors contributing to the incorrect diagnosis of pulmonary embolic disease. Chest 62:388, 1972.
2. Hirsh J and Gallus AS: Diagnosis of venous thromboembolism: limitations and applications. In Madden JL, and Hume M (eds): *Venous Thromboembolism: Prevention and Treatment.* New York, Appleton-Century-Crofts, 1976.
3. Dalen JE, and Alpert JS: Natural history of pulmonary embolism. Prog Cardiovasc Dis 27:259–270, 1975.
4. Robin ED: Overdiagnosis and overtreatment of pulmonary embolism: the emperor may have no clothes. Ann Intern Med 87:775–781, 1977.
5. Bell WR, and Simon TL: A comparative analysis of pulmonary perfusion scans with pulmonary angiograms. Am Heart J 92:700–706, 1976.
6. McNeil BJ: A diagnostic strategy using ventilation-perfusion studies in patients suspect for pulmonary embolism. J Nucl Med 17:613–616, 1976.
7. Barritt DW, and Jordan SC: Anticoagulant drugs in the treatment of pulmonary embolism — a controlled trial. Lancet 1:1309, 1960.
8. Salzman EW, Deykin D, Shapiro RM, and Rosenberg R: Management of heparin therapy. Controlled prospective trial. N Engl J Med 292:1046–1050, 1975.
9. Glazier RL, and Crowell, EB: Randomized prospective trial of continuous vs intermittent heparin therapy. JAMA 236:1365–1367, 1976.
10. Isom OW, Dembrow JM, Glassman E, Pasternack BS, Sackler JP, and Spencer FC: Factors influencing long-term survival after isolated aortic valve replacement. Circulation 49(Suppl II):II–154, 1974.
11. The Urokinase Pulmonary Embolism Trial: A national cooperative study. Circulation 47 (Suppl II):II-1–II-108, 1973.
12. Urokinase-Streptokinase Pulmonary Embolism Trial, phase 2 results, A cooperative study. JAMA 229:1606–1613, 1974.
13. Sasahara AA: Therapy for pulmonary embolism. JAMA 229:1795–1798, 1974.
14. Dalen JE, Brooks HL, Johnson LW, Meister SG, Szucs MM, and Dexter L: Pulmonary angiography in acute pulmonary embolism: indications, techniques, and results in 367 patients. Am Heart J 81:175–185, 1971.
15. McNeil BJ: The value of diagnostic aids in patients with potential surgical problems. In Bunker JP, Barnes BA, and Mosteller F (eds): *Costs, Risks and Benefits of Surgery.* New York, Oxford University Press, 1977.
16. McNeil BJ: Personal communication.
17. Moser KM, Longo AM, Ashburn WL, and Guisan M: Spurious scintiphotographic recurrence of pulmonary emboli. Am J Med 55:434–443, 1973.
18. Fred HL, Bruderi JA, Gonzalez DA, et al: Arteriographic assessment of lung scanning in the diagnosis of pulmonary thromboembolism. N Engl J Med 275:1025, 1966.
19. Wilson JE 3rd, and Bynum LJ: An improved pulmonary angiographic technique using a balloon-tipped catheter. Ann Rev Resp Dis 114:1137, 1976.
20. Manual of Operations, Urokinase Pulmonary Embolism Trial, National Heart Institute, October, 1968.
21. Schwartz WB, Gorry GA, Kassirer JP, and Essig A: Decision analysis and clinical judgment. Am J Med 55:459–472, 1973.
22. Breckenridge RT, and Ratnoff OD: Pulmonary embolism and unexpected death in supposedly normal persons. N Engl J Med 270:298, 1964.
23. Gallus AS, and Hirsh J: Prevention of venous thromboembolism. Semin Thromb Hemostas 2:232–290, 1976.
24. Neu LT Jr, Waterfield JR, and Ash CJ: Prophylactic anticoagulant therapy in the orthopedic patient. Ann Intern Med 62:463, 1965.
25. Dalen JE, and Dexter L: Diagnosis and management of massive pulmonary embolism. Disease-a-Month, August, 1967.
26. Nabseth DC, and Moran JM: Reassessment of the role of inferior vena cava ligation in venous thromboembolism. N Engl J Med 273:1250, 1965.
27. Mant MJ, Thong KL, Birtwhistle RV, O'Brien BD, Hammond GW, and Grace MG: Haemorrhagic complications of heparin therapy. Lancet 1:1133–1135, May 28, 1977.
28. Silver D, and Sabiston DC Jr: The role of vena cava interruption in the management of pulmonary embolism. Surgery 77:1–10, 1975.
29. Jick H, Slone D, Borda IT, and Shapiro S: Efficacy and toxicity of heparin in relation to age and sex. N Engl J Med 279:284–286, 1968.

30. Emerson PA, Derek T, and Handley AJ: The application of decision theory to the prevention of deep vein thrombosis following myocardial infarction. Q J Med (new series) 43:389–398, 1974.
31. Solomon NW, Stinson EB, Griepp RB, and Shumway NE: Mitral valve replacement: long-term evaluation of prosthesis-related mortality and morbidity. Circulation 56(Suppl II):II-94, 1977.
32. McNamara MF, Creasy JK, Takaki HS, Conn J Jr, Yao JST, and Bergan JJ: Vena caval surgery to prevent recurrent pulmonary embolism. Proc Inst Med Chic 31:173–177, 1977.
33. Moran JM, Criscitiello MG, and Callow AD: Vena cava interruption for thromboembolism: Partial or complete? Influences of cardiac disease upon results. Circulation 39(Suppl 1):I-263, 1969.
34. Couch NP, Balduri SS, and Crane C: Mortality and morbidity rates after IVC clipping. Surgery 77:106, 1975.
35. Mobin-Uddin K, Utley JR, and Bryant LR: The inferior vena cava umbrella filter. Prog Cardiovasc Dis 17:391–399, 1975.
36. Hunter JA, Dye WS, Javid H, Najafi H, Goldin MD, and Serry C: Permanent transvenous balloon occlusion of the inferior vena cava. Experience with 60 Patients. Ann Surg 186:491–499, 1977.

Pulmonary Angiography Is Not Indicated in All Patients with Suspected Pulmonary Embolism

JAMES E. DALEN, M.D.

Department of Medicine, University of Massachusetts
Medical School, Worcester, Massachusetts

Pulmonary angiography is the most accurate diagnostic test currently available for the detection of pulmonary embolism. A technically ideal angiographic study interpreted accurately is rarely incorrect. However, not all pulmonary angiographic studies are of ideal technical quality. A variety of factors may cause an angiographic study to be of suboptimal quality, and the patient's condition may interdict further investigation. Not all angiographic studies are interpreted by experienced angiographers.

The angiographer often feels compelled to make a final, definite diagnosis of PE (pulmonary embolism) or no PE even though in some cases the angiographic findings are, in fact, equivocal.[1] These comments are not made to denigrate the value of pulmonary angiography. They only serve to remind that pulmonary angiography, though our best available diagnostic technique for the detection of pulmonary embolism, is not perfect.

It seems to me that before we decide that pulmonary angiography should be performed in all patients in whom pulmonary embolism is suspected, there are certain facts about pulmonary angiography that we must consider:

1. Pulmonary angiography is an invasive, uncomfortable procedure.
2. Pulmonary angiography requires hospitalization.
3. Pulmonary angiography is not available in all hospitals in the U.S.

1. PULMONARY ANGIOGRAPHY IS AN INVASIVE, UNCOMFORTABLE PROCEDURE

The mortality rate of pulmonary angiography when performed by experienced teams is very small, certainly less than one per cent.[1] The mortality

472

when it is performed by inexperienced teams is unknown. If an analogy with coronary arteriography is germane,[2] there is reason to believe that the mortality is higher when performed by inexperienced teams. The reported complications of pulmonary angiography are low, in the range of five per cent.[1] The incidence of complications when performed by inexperienced teams is unknown.

An additional fact about this procedure that needs to be considered is that the morbidity is essentially 100 per cent. After performing or helping to perform about 500 pulmonary angiograms, I have yet to encounter a patient who enjoyed the procedure or who was anxious to have another angiogram performed. The same might be said about all catheterization and angiographic procedures. However, the impact of the invasive nature of pulmonary angiography seems to be compounded by the circumstances under which it is performed. Unlike other cardiac diagnostic procedures, it is rarely elective. Most patients who undergo cardiac catheterization have had the opportunity to have their own physician explain the procedure and the reason it needs to be done. Most patients realize that elective cardiac catheterization needs to be performed to determine what therapy is needed to treat their often long-standing, symptomatic cardiac disease.

The circumstances of pulmonary angiography are, unfortunately, quite different. Pulmonary embolism occurs as a sudden, unwanted, unexpected complication of another condition. The necessity for pulmonary angiography is often seen by the patient as an additional sudden, unwanted, unexpected complication. It is my opinion that these circumstances increase the patient's anxiety and sense of discomfort during the procedure.

In essence, if someone were to tell me that I needed an emergency pulmonary angiogram, I would need to be convinced that the risks and potential complications and almost certain discomfort of pulmonary angiography would be outweighed *in my case* by the risks attendant to not performing pulmonary angiography.

2. PULMONARY ANGIOGRAPHY REQUIRES HOSPITALIZATION

Should all patients with suspected pulmonary embolism be hospitalized? Many patients with suspected pulmonary embolism do not have pulmonary embolism. How many patients would be admitted unnecessarily? Before we further increase the percentage of our gross national product devoted to medical care, we need to explore the basis upon which pulmonary embolism is suspected. Should the suspicion be based on clinical examination alone? Or should it be supplemented by the results of a chest x-ray, EKG, arterial blood gases, or lung scan?

3. PULMONARY ANGIOGRAPHY IS NOT AVAILABLE IN ALL HOSPITALS IN THE U.S.

Should it be? Do we have sufficient data to justify the need to install expensive angiographic suites and angiography teams in every hospital in the

U.S.? How many pulmonary angiograms would be done per year in a 100-bed hospital? (There are 3500 hospitals in the U.S. with less than 100 beds.)

As an alternative to establishing angiographic facilities in all hospitals, maybe we should transfer patients who are suspected to have pulmonary embolism to hospitals with active angiographic teams. Before we recommend this, we should wonder how often (and on what basis) pulmonary embolism is suspected in hospitals not currently performing pulmonary angiography.

Given the fact that pulmonary angiography is an invasive, uncomfortable procedure that requires hospitalization, we must ask: *What is the basis for suspecting pulmonary embolism?* None of the symptoms associated with pulmonary embolism are diagnostic.[4] Dyspnea, pleuritic pain, hemoptysis, and syncope all may be caused by a variety of other disorders. Similarly, the physical findings associated with pulmonary embolism are not unique to this disease. Thus, if we were to perform pulmonary angiography on all patients with dyspnea, pleuritic pain, or tachypnea, the yield of patients with documented pulmonary embolism would be very small. The cost-benefit ratio would be unacceptably high.

When clinical findings are supplemented by standard laboratory tests, such as chest x-rays, EKG, and arterial blood gases, the accuracy of clinical diagnosis increases somewhat.[5] Of all available diagnostic tests, the one that agrees best with pulmonary angiography is the lung scan. Since lung scanning is a non-invasive, outpatient procedure, we must at least consider its potential impact on deciding which patients need to have pulmonary angiography.

The Role of the Lung Scan in Patients Suspected of Pulmonary Embolism

The first question we might ask about lung scans is: How often are they normal in patients with suspected pulmonary embolism? In the Urokinase Pulmonary Embolism Trial, pulmonary embolism was suspected clinically in 2227 patients. When lung scans were performed, 492 (24 per cent) were entirely normal.[6] In a series of 97 patients under age 40 in whom pulmonary embolism was suspected because of acute pleuritic pain, 42 (43 per cent) had normal lung scans.[7] These two studies make it clear that it is not uncommon to find a normal lung scan in a patient suspected to have pulmonary embolism.

The next question we must ask is: What does it mean when a patient suspected to have pulmonary embolism has a normal lung scan? There are two possible explanations: Either the clinical diagnosis is wrong, or the scan is wrong — that is, it is a "false negative." Nearly all authorities in this field agree that false negative lung scans are exceedingly rare, if they exist at all.[8]

There are no large series of patients with normal perfusion lung scans who have then had pulmonary angiography or postmortem examination. However, listed below is a tabulation of reported angiographic results in patients with normal perfusion scans.

In reviewing the literature, I can find only one report of pulmonary embolism documented by pulmonary angiography within 24 hours of a normal lung scan. This patient, reported by Fred et al.[10] in 1966, had obstruction of a segmental artery in the right lower lobe. However, the lung scan consisted of a single, posterior view. At the present time lung scans are performed in four views. I know of no reports of pulmonary embolism documented by angiogram in a patient who has had a normal four-view lung scan. I would conclude that if a patient suspected to have pulmonary embolism has a normal (four-view) perfusion scan, there is no reason to perform pulmonary angiography.

What if the perfusion lung scan is abnormal; that is, there are one or more perfusion defects? In the more than 10 years since the introduction of lung scans for the diagnosis of pulmonary embolism, it has become abundantly clear that a "positive" lung scan, that is, a lung scan showing one or more perfusion defects, is not diagnostic of pulmonary embolism. Perfusion defects are not specific and can be caused by a wide variety of pulmonary disorders, even when the chest x-ray is normal.[4]

The specificity of lung scans has been enhanced by improvements in technique and in their interpretation. We now know that perfusion defects are far more likely to be due to pulmonary embolism when they are segmental; that is, when they correspond to specific anatomical segments of the lung.[11] Patchy, diffuse, nonsegmental defects are far less likely to be due to pulmonary embolism.[11]

A further increase in the specificity of lung scans occurred with the introduction of ventilation scans. Perfusion defects that do not ventilate are rarely due to pulmonary embolism, whereas segmental perfusion defects that ventilate normally are highly suggestive of pulmonary embolism.[12]

At the present time it is clear that we should not try to interpret lung scans as being either positive or negative for pulmonary embolism. Rather, lung scans should be read as:

1. Normal.
2. Low probability of pulmonary embolism.
3. High probability of pulmonary embolism.

When lung scans are interpreted in this manner, they have a very important role in determining which patients should have pulmonary angiography.

It is my belief that patients who are suspected to have pulmonary embolism should have a perfusion lung scan. If the (four-view) perfusion scan is normal, the diagnosis of pulmonary embolism should be dismissed, and pulmonary angiography is not indicated. If the perfusion lung scan shows defects, a ventilation scan should be performed.

	NEGATIVE SCANS	POSITIVE ANGIOS
Szucs et al.[5]	12	0
Wagner and Strauss[4]	21	0
Linton[9]	11	0
Total	44	0

In the decision to proceed to pulmonary angiography, the following should then be considered:

1. The results of the ventilation-perfusion scan.
2. The specifics of the individual case (as outlined below).

INDICATIONS FOR PULMONARY ANGIOGRAPHY WHEN THE LUNG SCAN IS INTERPRETED AS "LOW PROBABILITY OF PULMONARY EMBOLISM"

There are several circumstances when the ventilation-perfusion scan findings have a low probability of pulmonary embolism:[12]

1. When perfusion defects are not segmental.
2. When perfusion defects match radiographic abnormalities.
3. When some or all of the perfusion defects have diminished or absent ventilation.
4. When a single defect is present.

In the presence of a low-probability scan, the probability of pulmonary embolism by angiography is quite low, in the range of 10 to 20 per cent.[12] Under these circumstances I would not proceed to angiography until I had considered the following:

1. How strong is the clinical evidence of pulmonary embolism? Are there alternative explanations for the patient's signs and symptoms? Are there other explanations for the lung scan abnormalities? If there are no other explanations for the patient's findings, it may be appropriate to proceed to pulmonary angiography.

2. Is there evidence of deep venous thrombosis? When it is available, the impedance plethysmogram (IPG) is very useful in detecting deep venous thrombosis. This non-invasive test has an accuracy of about 90 per cent as judged by its correlation with venograms.[13] If the lung scan has a low probability of pulmonary embolism and the IPG shows no evidence of deep venous thrombosis, I would feel quite justified in dismissing the diagnosis of pulmonary embolism. If the IPG were positive or even equivocal, I would usually proceed to pulmonary angiography.

In summary, when the results of a ventilation and perfusion scan are of low probability for PE, I see no need to proceed to pulmonary angiography unless there is evidence of deep venous thrombosis by IPG or if the clinical evidence of pulmonary embolism is especially compelling.

INDICATIONS FOR PULMONARY ANGIOGRAPHY IN THE PRESENCE OF A HIGH-PROBABILITY LUNG SCAN

If there are multiple segmental perfusion defects that ventilate normally, the probability of pulmonary embolism approaches 90 per cent.[12] In this circumstance, I do not believe that pulmonary angiography is necessary unless one of the following problems is present:

1. Contraindication or relative contraindication to anticoagulant therapy. In this circumstance the risk of anticoagulants is increased, or the patient may require venous interruption. In either event, I would want to be certain that he does, in fact, have acute pulmonary embolism.

2. Recurrent pulmonary embolism or evidence of prolonged predisposition to venous thrombosis. In this setting, one has to think of long-term anticoagulation or venous interruption. Again, I would want to be certain of the diagnosis of pulmonary embolism.

3. There is potential indication for pulmonary embolectomy. In this circumstance pulmonary angiography is a necessity.

PULMONARY ANGIOGRAPHY WITHOUT LUNG SCAN

In the critically ill, hypotensive patient with suspected massive pulmonary embolism, I would usually proceed directly to pulmonary angiography without obtaining a lung scan. It also may be prudent to proceed directly to pulmonary angiography in patients with significant chronic lung disease as evidenced by chest x-ray.

In summary, although pulmonary angiography is the best test we have for the diagnosis of pulmonary embolism, I do not believe that it is indicated in all patients in whom pulmonary embolism has been suspected for any possible reason. One cannot ignore the fact that the procedure is invasive, uncomfortable, and requires hospitalization. Furthermore, one cannot ignore the fact that perfusion and ventilation lung scans very clearly enhance the accuracy of the clinical diagnosis of pulmonary embolism. If on the basis of the clinical findings and a lung scan one can reduce the probability of pulmonary embolism to the 10 per cent range, I would rarely proceed to pulmonary angiography. Similarly, when the probability of pulmonary embolism is in the range of 90 per cent, I would not perform pulmonary angiography unless there were specific problems in the individual case, as outlined above.

References

1. Dalen JE, Brooks HL, Johnson LW, et al: Pulmonary angiography in acute pulmonary embolism: Indications, techniques, and results in 367 patients. Am. Heart J 81:175–185, 1971.
2. Adams DF, Fraser DB, and Abrams HC: The complications of coronary arteriography. Circulation 48:609–618, 1973.
3. Glaser RJ: The teaching hospital and the medical school. In Knowles JH(ed): The Teaching Hospital. Cambridge, Harvard University Press, 1966.
4. Wagner HN Jr, and Strauss HW: Radioactive tracers in the differential diagnosis of pulmonary embolism. Prog Cardiovasc Dis 17:271–282, 1975.
5. Szucs MM Jr, Brooks HL, Grossman W, et al: Diagnostic sensitivity of laboratory findings in acute pulmonary embolism. Ann Intern Med 74:161–166, 1971.
6. The Urokinase Pulmonary Embolism Trial. Circulation 47(Suppl II):II-1-108, 1973.
7. McNeil BJ, Hessel SJ, Branch WT, et al: Measures of clinical efficacy. III. The value of the lung scan in the evaluation of young patients with pleuritic chest pain. J Nucl Med 17:163–168, 1976.

8. Greenspan RH: Does a normal isotope perfusion scan exclude pulmonary embolism? Invest Radiol 8:97, 98, 1973.
9. Linton DS Jr, Bellon EM, Bodie JF, et al: Comparison of results of pulmonary arteriography and radioisotope lung scanning in the diagnosis of pulmonary emboli. J Roentgenol Radium Ther Nucl Med 112:745–748, 1971.
10. Fred HL, Burdine JA Jr, Gonzalez DA, et al: Arteriographic assessment of lung scanning in the diagnosis of pulmonary thromboembolism. N Engl J Med 275:1025–1032, 1966.
11. Poulose KP, Reba RC, Gilday DL, et al: Diagnosis of pulmonary embolism. A correlative study of the clinical, scan, and angiographic findings. Br Med J 3:67–71, 1970.
12. McNeil BJ: A diagnostic strategy using ventilation-perfusion studies in patients suspect for pulmonary embolism. J Nucl Med 17:613–616, 1976.
13. Hull R, Hirsh J, Sackett DL, et al: Combined use of leg scanning and impedance plethysmography in suspected venous thrombosis. N Engl J Med 296:1497–1500, 1977.

Comment

Both Drs. Messer and Dalen agree that pulmonary arteriography is the most accurate diagnostic test that is currently available to establish the presence or absence of pulmonary embolism. Not all hospitals are equipped to perform this procedure, and it is accompanied by a distinct morbidity and, on rare occasions, mortality. Furthermore, at times, the pulmonary arteriogram may be technically unsatisfactory or incorrectly interpreted. Because of the above, the question arises as to whether pulmonary arteriography should be employed routinely when a patient is suspected of having a pulmonary embolism.

Dr. Messer has presented a very thorough and scholarly presentation to support his thesis that pulmonary arteriography should be performed routinely in patients with suspected acute pulmonary emboli. He emphasizes that routine pulmonary arteriography will reduce erroneous diagnosis, reduce unnecessary bleeding complications through elimination of the use of anticoagulants when they are not indicated, decrease unnecessary surgical intervention, and cut down the period of hospitalization. At the same time, he also emphasizes that it can establish a diagnosis and permit appropriate treatment when this may otherwise not be done.

Dr. Dalen, on the other hand, relies heavily on the use of pulmonary scintigraphy as a screening device. He points out (as does Dr. Messer) that a normal pulmonary scintigram virtually excludes the diagnosis of a recent acute pulmonary embolus. When such scintigrams are positive, he further evaluates the likelihood that the defect is secondary to acute pulmonary embolus by performing ventilation studies, since the probability that an unventilated area associated with a perfusion defect is due to an acute pulmonary embolism is remote.

My own approach is somewhat more selective than that of Dr. Messer in recommending pulmonary arteriography for patients suspected of acute pulmonary emboli. For example, I do not perform pulmonary arteriography in patients with acute tricuspid valve endocarditis when the chest film reveals multiple infiltrates from presumed septic pulmonary emboli and the clinical picture (including blood culture) has established a diagnosis of acute infective endocarditis. Similarly, I have not recommended pulmonary arteriography when the clinical picture has, in my judgment, been classic, such as in a patient with obvious peripheral evidences of thrombophlebitis or phlebothrombosis who has had a typical clinical episode associated with the usual laboratory abnormalities detailed by Drs. Dalen and Messer. Under these circumstances, I feel that our diagnostic accuracy outweighs the morbidity, expense, delay, and potential mortality of pulmonary arteriography, and I

479

begin anticoagulant therapy with intravenous heparin. Only if the patient continues to demonstrate evidence of repeated pulmonary emboli while fully anticoagulated, so as to suggest the need for a surgical form of intervention, will I go on to perform pulmonary arteriography.

There is, however, one area in which I feel that pulmonary arteriography is particularly desirable. That is in patients in whom recurrent or relatively silent pulmonary emboli are suspected. The potential danger of this problem leading to unrecognized severe pulmonary vascular disease with irreversible pulmonary hypertension makes it desirable to insure that these patients are not undergoing repeated episodes of relatively small, clinically silent, or minimally symptomatic emboli. One should not hesitate to perform pulmonary arteriography in this group of patients.

ELLIOT RAPAPORT, M.D.

Twenty

Does Low-Dose Heparin Significantly Reduce the Incidence of Postoperative Pulmonary Emboli and Should It Be Used Routinely in General Abdominal Surgery?

THE CASE AGAINST LOW-DOSE HEPARIN

D. E. Strandness, Jr., M.D.

LOW-DOSE HEPARIN SIGNIFICANTLY REDUCES THE INCIDENCE OF POSTOPERATIVE PULMONARY EMBOLI AND SHOULD BE USED ROUTINELY IN GENERAL ABDOMINAL AND THORACIC SURGERY

Stanford Wessler, M.D.

COMMENT

The Case Against Low-Dose Heparin

D. E. STRANDNESS, JR., M.D.

Professor of Surgery, University of Washington School of
Medicine, Seattle, Washington

There is no doubt that acute venous thrombosis is the most common vascular disease that develops in hospitalized patients. It produces problems in a variety of ways: (1) it may lead to fatal or non-fatal pulmonary embolism; (2) it prolongs the period of hospitalization, increasing the costs to the patient; (3) the requirement for anticoagulants to control extension of the thrombosis involves additional risks for the patient, which may, on occasion, be life-threatening; and (4) the destruction of the venous valves may lead to the development of the postphlebitic syndrome.

The introduction of the ^{125}I-labeled fibrinogen test permitted for the first time prospective studies of both the incidence of calf-vein thrombosis and the effects of the variety of prophylactic measures designed to minimize or eliminate the process entirely. While prevention of the postphlebitic syndrome alone would be a major accomplishment, the principal emphasis has been on the problem of pulmonary embolism. A discouraging feature of the clinical course in patients with fatal pulmonary embolism is that approximately 80 per cent will succumb suddenly without prior premonitory symptoms or signs. For this group of patients, prevention is probably the only answer, short of some reliable testing procedure that is sensitive enough to detect the disease at a stage that may be treatable.

The labeled fibrinogen method has shown clearly that calf-vein thrombosis does occur in a high percentage of patients 40 years of age or older who undergo major, elective abdominothoracic surgery.[1] It has also been demonstrated that low-dose heparin is effective in reducing the incidence of scan-detected calf-vein thrombosis. Proof of its efficacy in reducing the incidence of fatal pulmonary embolism awaited the results of the multicenter trial that were published in 1975.[2] This randomized trial from 28 centers included 4121 patients and demonstrated a significant reduction in fatal pulmonary embolism, 16 in the control group, two in the low-dose heparin group ($p < 0.005$). The treated patients received 5000 units of heparin subcutaneously two hours prior to operation and every eight hours thereafter until fully ambulant. The study population included a variety of elective major surgical procedures in patients over the age of 40 years.

483

A special report by the Council on Thrombosis of the American Heart Association has proposed that if 5000 units of heparin were given two hours prior to operation and continued twice daily until the patient is discharged, this could possibly save 4000 to 8000 lives annually in patients 40 years or older undergoing major elective abdominal and thoracic surgery.[3] To achieve this reduction in mortality, it is estimated that at least five million patients annually in the United States would constitute the target population for this method of prophylaxis.

This recommendation appears to be based upon two observations: the reduction in calf-vein thrombosis achieved by low-dose heparin and the results reported in the report of the multicenter trial.[2] At this point, it must be emphasized that the multicenter study did not demonstrate a reduction in overall mortality rate between the heparin and control groups. Although the study was a randomized trial, it was not double blind, which in and of itself raises some question; but in general, the conclusions have been accepted as valid.

However, a report by one of the participating centers recently appeared that pointed out some difficulties in the study that cannot be overlooked.[4] Furthermore, a subsequent publication prepared in response to this paper by the director of the multicenter trial, Mr. V. V. Kakkar,[5] appears, to this author at least, to confuse the issue even further rather than to clarify the discrepancies that are apparent in reviewing the two articles. It will, of course, be up to the individual reader to evaluate these two reports, but in light of the recommendation of the American Heart Association, the details and controversy raised by these publications should be reviewed carefully and placed in perspective, if that is possible.

In the report by Gruber et al.,[4] the patients from this contributing group were analyzed in detail: (1) There were 194 patients (100 control, 94 in the heparin group) who *apparently* satisfied the original protocol, at least as interpreted by this group. (2) There were four fatal pulmonary emboli in the control group and six in the heparin group. The number of fatalities in the heparin group was four more than reported from the other 27 centers, and they were not included in the final report of the multicenter trial. (3) All of the fatalities in the heparin group and one of the four patients in the control group had negative leg scans in the first postoperative week. (4) The time of death was after day seven in all four patients in the control group and in three of the six patients in the heparin group. These were apparently in patients considered ambulant and thus not on heparin. Furthermore, Gruber et al. maintain that the protocol did not define either what ambulant meant or when the postoperative period was considered over. (5) Apparently the complete data from all the centers were not made available to the participants, since Gruber et al. were not aware of the time of death in the control patients other than the average figures that appeared in the final report of the trial.

The response by Kakkar[5] to this report was surprising. Rather than trying to reconcile the obvious discrepancies, the data were reanalyzed totally, excluding the material provided by Gruber's group. This, of course, tended to further support the conclusions of the trial, since by removing these data entirely, there were no deaths from pulmonary embolism in the heparin group. The reasons for taking this approach were given, but tend to confuse the issue even further: (1) Of the 223 proformas submitted by Gruber et al.[4] to the multicenter trial, 123 (59.6 per cent) were excluded because the randomized procedure had not been followed during the latter part of the trial. On the other hand, according to Gruber et al., there were 232 patients initially entering the trial, with only 38 being excluded because their protocols were incomplete (16.3 per cent). (2) Kakkar[5] states that the data sent to the multicenter trial indicated there were three fatal emboli and one contributory embolus in the 110 patients given heparin. In the subsequent report by Gruber et al., this number was reported to be six out of the 94 patients who received heparin. (3) Kakkar reports as a disturbing feature the high incidence of pulmonary embolism in the group of Gruber et al. (3.1 per cent) as compared to only 0.4 per cent from the other 27 participating centers. It appears that in the final analysis of the trial, only 89 patients from Gruber et al.'s entire contribution were allowed to be included, and in this group, there were three fatal pulmonary emboli, two in the heparin and one in the control group. Kakkar states that these patients were included to ensure that the analysis of the center results could not be criticized as being biased.

It is clear that the figures in Kakkar's report with regard to the contribution by Gruber et al. to the trial are not consistent. For example, Kakkar states that of the 223 patients submitted, 123 were excluded, leaving 100 patients. However, later in the same report, it is stated that only 89 patients had complete protocols. What happened to the other 11 patients?

Finally, with regard to the problem of the patients excluded in the report of the multicenter trial, this issue was raised in the discussion of this study sponsored by the NHLI in a workshop convened in April, 1975. Shaw[6] raised the point that one technique often used is to put the excluded patients back into the study to see how it affects the findings. Kakkar[6] indicated that this had been done and the differences were still highly significant. Yet in the latest published report by Kakkar,[5] the opposite was done, suggesting that the results and the conclusions might have been different.

Clearly, it is impossible for this author to reconcile the differences, but the discrepancies in the two reports are obvious and must be considered pertinent to the entire question. Furthermore, since this is the only study that gives credence to the recommendations of the American Heart Association, serious questions will remain until the issues are clarified further.

Even disregarding for a moment the concerns expressed with the multicenter trial, there are other compelling reasons for questioning the widespread application of low-dose heparin prophylaxis. Most experts agree that the thrombi of greatest significance are those that have either propagated into the major deep veins or form *de novo* in large veins at sites removed from the calf.

The report by Gallus et al.[7] in which 820 surgical patients were randomized produced some interesting results. These authors reported the incidence of femoropopliteal thrombosis to be 2.9 per cent in the control group and 1.0 per cent in the heparin group (p < 0.04). There was not a single case of ileofemoral venous thrombosis reported in the entire series. The heparin in this study was 5000 units given two hours prior to operation and every eight hours thereafter for at least seven days unless the patients were discharged earlier.

Most important, the study by Gallus et al. analyzed in detail the problems associated with the use of low-dose heparin even in an institution that is known for its careful clinical studies. Their findings are of particular importance when the implications for widespread usage are considered: (1) dispensing errors on the part of the nursing staff occurred in 46 patients (11.2 per cent); (2) the prophylaxis was withdrawn because of possible complications in 31 of the 362 patients who received the heparin as ordered (8.6 per cent); (3) wound hematomas developed in 10 (2.8 per cent) patients in the heparin group as compared to two (0.5 per cent) of the control patients (p <0.01); and (4) the blood loss in the heparin group and the hematocrit fall in the treated group were significantly greater (p <0.05).

Clearly, based on the above figures, low-dose heparin is not the ideal prophylactic agent. One in five of the patients did not get the drug as prescribed or had it stopped because of complications. Furthermore, the increased incidence of wound hematomas and greater blood loss are of serious concern. Also, wound hematomas require drainage, which will prolong hospitalization and possibly lead to a higher incidence of wound complications, including infection.

The recommendations of the American Heart Association have tried to minimize the potential complications above by recommending that the heparin be given every 12 hours rather than three times daily, as administered in the multicenter trial[2] and in that reported by Gallus et al.[7] However, as Gallus et al. concluded, "The relative advantages and risks of prophylaxis with twice-daily or three-times-daily heparin injections can only be assessed by careful prospective comparative studies." It is a fact that such studies have not been done, and thus the issue remains unsettled.

Finally, it must be emphasized that nearly all of the studies upon which the Heart Association based its recommendations were done outside this country. It is not sufficient to assume that the incidence, indeed the magnitude, of the problem is the same in the United States. For example, Covey et al.[8] studied 105 patients over 40 years of age undergoing major surgery and found an incidence of calf-vein thrombosis of 9.6 per cent in the control group and 7.5 per cent in patients receiving heparin twice daily.

What, then, is the answer? Clearly, to this author at least, the whole issue remains unsettled. The recommendations of the Heart Association cannot be accepted until carefully controlled studies are done in this country. The problems that have surfaced with the multicenter trial raise serious questions that require answers. This can only be accomplished by a reexamination of the entire issue, which must include a look at other methods of prophylaxis and, finally, a better definition of what in fact constitutes a "high-risk" patient.

References

1. Nicolaides AN, and Irving D: Clinical factors in the risk of deep venous thrombosis. *In* Nicolaides AN (ed): *Thromboembolism: Etiology, Advances in Prevention and Management*. Baltimore, University Park Press, 1975, Chapter 13.
2. Prevention of fatal postoperative pulmonary embolism by low doses of heparin: an international multicentre trial. Lancet 2:45, 1975.
3. Prevention of venous thromboembolism in surgical patients by low-dose heparin: prepared by the Council on Thrombosis of the American Heart Association. A special report issued by the American Heart Association, 1977.
4. Gruber, UF, Duckert F, Fridrich R, Torhorst J, and Rem J: Prevention of postoperative thromboembolism by Dextran 40, low doses of Heparin or Xantinol Nicotinate. Lancet 1:207, 1977.
5. Shaw L: In discussion of efficacy of low-dose heparin in preventing postoperative fatal pulmonary embolism: results of an international multicenter trial. *In* Prophylactic Therapy of Deep Vein Thrombosis and Pulmonary Embolism. DHEW Publ #(NIH) 76-866, 1975, p 225.
6. Prevention of fatal pulmonary embolism by low doses of heparin: international multicentre trial. Lancet 1:567, 1977.
7. Gallus AS, Hirsh J, O'Brien SE, McBride JA, Tuttle RJ, and Gent M: Prevention of venous thrombosis with small subcutaneous doses of heparin. JAMA 235:1980, 1976.
8. Covey TH, Sherman L, and Baue AE: Low-dose heparin in postoperative patients. Arch Surg 110:1021, 1975.

Low-Dose Heparin Significantly Reduces the Incidence of Postoperative Pulmonary Emboli and Should Be Used Routinely in General Abdominal and Thoracic Surgery*

STANFORD WESSLER, M.D.

Professor, Department of Medicine, New York University
School of Medicine, New York, New York

Venous thromboembolism is a ubiquitous and frequently lethal complication of a broad spectrum of medical and surgical diseases and of sedentary living. Its hazard to a productive life has been masked by a lack of awareness of its true incidence and by the fact that it is not itself a disease, but rather a complication of a host of major disease states. Recent data have documented not only its remarkable scope, its increasing prevalence in our society, its mechanism of action at the molecular level, but most importantly, have provided new methods of primary prophylaxis that are now available for general use by physicians and surgeons. In short, it can be suggested that venous thromboembolism may become in large measure a preventable complication of disease.

*Supported by National Heart, Lung, and Blood Institute Grant #2 R01 HL18333, National Institutes of Health, Department of Health, Education, and Welfare.

488

It has been conservatively estimated that venous thromboembolism causes 50,000 deaths annually in the United States. The cost of the hospitalization of another 250,000 who survive has been calculated to exceed 750 million dollars per year. These figures do not include the disability, cost of treatment, or absenteeism from work among patients who recover from pulmonary embolism or who suffer from venous thrombosis and its limb sequelae alone.

Aside from its occurrence in the apparently healthy population at large, venous thromboembolism is prone to occur among the elderly, among subjects immobilized for any cause, and in individuals with a previous history of venous thrombosis. Similarly, venous thromboembolism tends to complicate traumatic, postoperative, and postpartum states, acute myocardial infarction, congestive heart failure, shock, estrogen therapy (including its use to prevent conception, lactation, postmenopausal symptoms, and the spread of certain malignancies), gram-negative sepsis, polycythemia vera, certain dysproteinemias, and several malignant tumors. In cancer, pulmonary embolism may, in fact, be the premature cause of death. There are, moreover, patients with genetic abnormalities, such as antithrombin III deficiency, who are prone to thrombosis.

Embolism to the lung is reported to be one of the most frequent acute pulmonary illnesses encountered in a general hospital and one of the most lethal processes seen at autopsy. Indeed, in hospitalized patients who die and come to necropsy, thorough autopsy examinations disclose evidence of grossly visible old and fresh pulmonary emboli in more than 50 per cent. Venous thromboembolism is a significant cause of death in patients hospitalized for major orthopedic procedures, the most frequent nonobstetrical cause of postpartum death, and a primary or contributory cause of mortality in our large population of patients with chronic cardiac and pulmonary disease.

Of further concern are the data showing that annual death rates from pulmonary embolism have been sharply increasing since World War II. This increase is not explained by the rise in total population and total deaths, the increase in the number of older people in the population, the increasing use of estrogens, selective data recording, or improved physician awareness.

Although many of the deaths from pulmonary embolism occur in patients suffering from terminal diseases for which prophylactic therapy cannot produce much enthusiasm, an appreciable number of patients do succumb to pulmonary emboli who, without this complication, would recover from their underlying illness. The present use of heparin in regular dosage, although documented to reduce the fatality rate from pulmonary embolism, does not presently have any measurable impact nationally in diminishing overall mortality from pulmonary embolism.

More specifically, there is one condition in which large numbers of otherwise salvageable patients are at risk of death from pulmonary embolism. Five million individuals over the age of 40 are subjected annually to major abdominal or thoracic surgery, 0.2 per cent of whom will die from pulmonary embolism. If antithrombotic therapy were 80 per cent effective in the primary prevention of venous thromboembolism following major general surgical procedures performed in patients over age 40, 8000 individuals per year would be saved from premature death. Such results would compare favorably with the benefits achieved in this country from the prevention of poliomyelitis by vaccination.

Finally, it should be emphasized that prevention of morbidity from venous thrombosis has almost as much to recommend it as a reduction in deaths and certainly applies to a population many times that mentioned in terms of life survival.

Despite the fact that heparin is an effective drug in the prevention of venous thromboembolism and has been in use for more than a quarter of this century, there has been no recognized decrease in overall deaths attributable to this agent. Several factors have contributed to this paradox: (1) the disparity between the high prevalence of thromboembolic events and the low incidence of associated mortality or disability which has rendered the required size of trial populations exceedingly large, cumbersome, and costly; (2) the major use of heparin has occurred after a thromboembolic event rather than as a means of primary prophylaxis; (3) the difficulties in regulating drug dosage persist, and serious hemorrhage remains an infrequent but real complication of therapy; and (4) the physician is invariably apprised of clinical failure (further thrombosis or hemorrhage) but rarely of success (no thrombosis). However, recent advances in our understanding of the mechanism of intravascular coagulation, of the pathophysiology of thromboembolism, and of the molecular basis of the anticoagulant action of heparin have begun to permit more effective use of this antithrombotic agent by employing low doses of heparin prior to the thrombotic event.

Low-Dose Heparin

As a relatively new concept in antithrombotic therapy, low-dose heparin holds promise of eliminating the risk of substantial hemorrhage as well as the need to monitor drug therapy. Moreover, the recent low-dose regimens have been the most rigorously evaluated for efficacy by clinical trial.[1]

In retrospect, hints about the possible prophylactic efficacy of low doses of heparin can be found among the earliest reports on the use of this compound to prevent thrombosis in animals and man. However, it was not until 1966 that the prophylactic use of small doses of heparin for the prevention of postoperative thrombosis was actually undertaken and reported.

STIMULUS TO CURRENT USE

There were at least three factors that, by 1970, led to renewed interest in low-dose heparin for the prophylaxis of postoperative thromboembolism.

First, there was the recognition that thrombi are of two predominant types: (1) the red or fibrin-erythrocyte thrombus that represents the major component of the venous lesion; and (2) the white or platelet thrombus that represents the primary arterial lesion. It is the red thrombus that can be prevented by prophylactic heparin therapy.

Second, improved techniques of phlebography revived interest in this method as an accurate measure of venous obstruction. Perhaps more important was validation of the ^{125}I-labeled fibrinogen scan as a practical laboratory tool for recognition of deep venous thrombosis in the lower limbs. At the same time, parallel improvements in pulmonary angiography and lung scanning became available. These technical developments, because of their precision and sensitivity, made it feasible to conduct clinical trials with smaller numbers of patients than would be practical if diagnostic reliance were placed solely on clinical evidence of venous thromboembolism.

The third factor was the emerging data and concepts surrounding the biochemistry of the anticoagulant action of heparin.

MOLECULAR BASIS FOR ANTITHROMBOTIC ACTION

Heparin cannot function as an anticoagulant without the presence of antithrombin III, a naturally occurring plasma protease inhibitor (molecular weight 63,000) that is identical to the inhibitor to activated Factor X(Xa) and heparin co-factor, has broad specificity, and plays an important role in maintaining the fluidity of circulating blood.[1] Antithrombin III is particularly effective against Xa and thrombin.

Biochemical data strongly suggest that the primary physiological target of antithrombin III, in terms of preventing thrombus formation, is Xa rather than thrombin. These observations are also consistent with the view that the enzymatic coagulation sequence functions as a biological amplification system. That is, it takes less energy to stop intravascular coagulation at the Xa step than at the subsequent thrombin stage. Heparin does not increase the amount of circulating antithrombin III, but small quantities of the drug increase the rate at which antithrombin III combines with Xa as well as with thrombin and other clotting proteases.[1]

Figure 1 shows these concepts schematically. There are two pathways

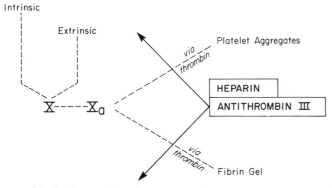

Figure 1.   Simplified schema of the clotting cascade. Prior to the initiation of intravascular coagulation, antithrombin III is particularly effective in inhibiting the action of Xa on prothrombin. Heparin acts as a catalyst to this antithrombin III–Xa reaction.

from the initiation of coagulation to the formation of the fibrin gel, the intrinsic cascade beginning with Hageman Factor and the extrinsic system initiated by tissue thromboplastin. These pathways lead via thrombin to fibrin formation and irreversible platelet aggregation. The protease inhibitor antithrombin III has the capacity, by itself, of inhibiting Xa. Antithrombin III also inhibits thrombin downstream in the final path, but requires more molecules for this latter step because of the biochemical amplification that occurs throughout the sequence.

Accordingly, it seemed reasonable to suggest that if a tendency to thrombosis were treated before intravascular coagulation were initiated, less heparin might be required than if therapy were begun after thrombin formation had occurred. One excellent clinical situation in which to test this thesis is the postoperative state, since the blood in most patients is not actively clotting prior to elective surgery and since the majority of thrombi begin to form at the time of operation. It would be, in essence, the presence of small amounts of exogenous plasma heparin augmenting the activity of antithrombin III to prevent the development of hypercoagulability that might diminish venous thrombosis in patients undergoing operation — and accomplish this task without risk of the hemorrhage associated with the more classical doses of this anticoagulant.

It was with this background that clinical trials of low-dose heparin were initiated in 1971 and continue to the present time, first in surgical cases, and then in other conditions associated with pulmonary embolism.

CLINICAL TRIALS

Venous thromboembolism is a common phenomenon accompanying surgical procedures. This knowledge has clearly been dramatized by the advances in non-invasive techniques presently available for the recognition of various forms of intravascular coagulation. However, in contrast to the high incidence of thromboembolic events, there stands the infrequency with which these forms of intravascular coagulation cause death or major disability. It is this disparity between the high prevalence of lesions on the one hand and the low incidence of associated mortality or disability on the other that has rendered the design of trials difficult. Pathologists, moreover, can define fatal acute pulmonary embolism at necropsy over only a narrow range, leaving a large number of deaths with embolism in which, in each case, the relative importance of embolism must be weighed against other coexisting factors that can augment the effects of emboli. Regardless of uncertainty or controversy over the lethality of certain forms of embolism, death is not the only outcome of thromboembolism. Clearly, morbidity must also be considered a major consequence of thromboembolic disease. Thus, the question of lethality can be legitimately bypassed, and instead, the total number of defined massive fresh pulmonary emboli can be compared in treated and control groups.

In the four-year period, 1971 to 1975, more than 20 trials of low-dose heparin in over 2000 surgical patients monitored by ^{125}I-labeled fibrinogen limb scanning and/or venography demonstrated, with only one exception, that there was a significant decrease in deep vein thrombosis in the treated compared to the control groups.[1] Because of the small number of patients in each of these trials, however, no conclusions could be reached concerning the prevention of postoperative pulmonary emboli.

To determine whether low-dose heparin in surgical patients prevented postoperative pulmonary emboli, two large clinical trials were initiated. In the first of these trials 4121 patients were involved,[2] and in the second there were 500 patients.[3] Although neither trial contained enough patients to demonstrate a difference in mortality between treated and control groups, the autopsy findings revealed significant differences in the incidence of large pulmonary emboli (those that could have caused or contributed to death). Among the 4621 patients in the two trials, the ratio of large pulmonary emboli in the control versus the treated group was 5:1. The p value was less than 0.0005. Thus, despite the failure to demonstrate an overall mortality difference, it can reasonably be inferred that the survival benefit attributable to anticoagulants is real. It is on this inferential argument that the value of low-dose heparin in surgical patients is based — supported by the substantial number of trials in various countries demonstrating the decrease in postoperative deep venous thrombosis. Most trials, however, have also documented that low-dose heparin causes a definite but minor increase in bleeding.

RECOMMENDATIONS

These findings have led to the recommendation that a low-dose heparin regimen be used for all patients over the age of 40 subjected to elective abdominal and thoracic surgery with the following important caveats, limitations, and exceptions. Prior to a low-dose heparin regimen, all patients should receive a laboratory screening, including hematocrit, prothrombin time, partial thromboplastin time, and platelet count. It should be determined prior to operation that the patient is not receiving oral anticoagulants and did not receive platelet anti-aggregating agents, such as aspirin, within five days before surgery, since these drugs together with heparin can augment operative or postoperative bleeding. Low-dose heparin regimens are presently of limited value in open prostatectomy and major orthopedic procedures, especially repair of femoral fractures and reconstructive operations on the hip and knee. No data are available on low-dose heparin prophylaxis for emergency operations or trauma. Nor are substantive data currently available to justify prophylaxis in patients undergoing spinal or epidural anesthesia, or operations on the brain or eye; with further experience, the anesthesia restrictions may be removed. Low-dose heparin prophylaxis is also considered inadequate for patients undergoing operation during an active thrombotic process. Whether to continue anticoagulant therapy in selected patients after discharge should be decided on an individual basis.[4]

Most trials have used doses of heparin ranging between 10,000 and

15,000 units per day subcutaneously in divided doses. In surgical patients, the most common regimens have been 5000 units starting two hours before operation and repeated every eight or 12 hours until the patient is ambulatory or discharged.

Available evidence on general abdominothoracic surgery suggests that 5000 units twice daily is as effective as and is associated with less bleeding than the same quantity administered every eight hours. This issue is complicated by claims that the USP heparin unit is 10 to 15 per cent more potent than the International unit that has been used in all Canadian and European studies. Thus, 15,000 USP units may be equivalent to 16,500 to 17,250 International units; whereas 10,000 USP units may be equivalent to 11,000 to 11,500 International units. These are the reasons why, in the United States, the dosage for the present should be restricted to 10,000 units per day in surgical patients.

When using heparin on a low-dosage schedule, there is no need to monitor the effect of the drug by laboratory test. Before low-dose heparin regimens are used widely throughout the country, however, it is anticipated that the pharmaceutical industry will make available a heparin vial packaged with an attached syringe that allows accurate delivery of 5000 units to reduce the inadvertent human error of administering an excess of the drug.

Although this formulation can be helpful to physicians, it must be recognized that all possible complications of the recommended prophylaxis cannot be foreseen. Accordingly, there will be instances in which the individual physician will correctly decide in special situations, or in patients at extremely low risk of venous thromboembolism, not to employ low-dose heparin prophylaxis. Conversely, in patients under the age of 40 who are at increased risk (e.g., those with previous phlebitis or pulmonary embolism, cancer, congestive heart failure, or on estrogen therapy), the physician may wish to use the low-dose heparin regimen.

IMPLICATIONS OF LOW-DOSE HEPARIN IN GENERAL SURGERY

The option presented to surgeons is an unusual one in that for the first time a plausible therapy is available for the primary prevention of postoperative pulmonary embolism. Yet, the individual surgeon will rarely, if ever, see the success of and will occasionally be confronted with the failures of this prophylactic regimen.

If a general surgeon annually performs 300 elective major abdominal procedures exclusive of trauma without anticoagulant or other prophylaxis among patients over the age of 40, he can anticipate one to two deaths from pulmonary emboli every three years; if his annual work load of such cases is 200, he can expect only one to two deaths from pulmonary emboli every five years. Since the pulmonary embolic deaths will tend to occur in the older patients who have other major diseases, it will be difficult, in any individual patient, to determine wheter the emboli were causal, contributory, or incidental to the postoperative death. He will also be concerned whether any excessive bleeding stemmed from the use of heparin, for it must be clearly recognized that a low-dose heparin regimen may increase the likelihood of hemorrhage, even though the increase will be minimal.

Another implication of low-dose heparin, not previously stressed, also warrants consideration. There is in the United States a large group of individuals incapacitated by chronic venous insufficiency. This is a disabling syndrome with high in-hospital and out-patient costs. Most of these syndromes begin as a result of deep venous thrombosis. It is also known that deep venous thrombosis has a high recurrence rate. The data on the prevention of postoperative deep venous thrombosis by low-dose heparin strongly suggest that in addition to preventing massive pulmonary embolism, this therapeutic regimen may also prevent the onset of chronic venous insufficiency.

REMAINING OBSTACLES TO THE WIDESPREAD USE OF LOW-DOSE HEPARIN IN SURGICAL PATIENTS

Even if the validity of primary prophylaxis is accepted on a statistical basis, there remain two additional hurdles to overcome beyond that of the physician's ability to recognize benefit in this individual practice.

The first hurdle is one of the visibility of benefit in the total population. This can be illustrated by contrasting two pathologic processes with numerically comparable sequelae of differing visibility. Poliomyelitis prophylaxis protects 10,000 individuals per year from severe neurologic defects, and nationally this benefit is readily apparent to physician and layman alike. But a diminution in lethal postoperative pulmonary embolism comparable in numbers to the poliomyelitis cases will not be clearly appreciated, for it will be submerged in autopsy statistics that will never see the light of day — and it is doubtful that this handicap can ever be overcome.

The second and more important hurdle is the demonstrable risk of heparin-induced hemorrhage, even though the bleeding is minor. A partial resolution of this dilemma is provided by two pieces of information. First, in the large trial referred to earlier, there was excessive blood loss during surgery and a substantive number of wound hematoma in the control patients who received no anticoagulant in relation to their surgery.[2] Second, in all published trials of low-dose heparin, no effort was made to eliminate aspirin for five days preceding the operative procedure. Aspirin itself can cause bleeding in surgical patients, and the combination of aspirin and low doses of heparin induces a double hemostatic defect with a likelihood of hemorrhage greater than with either drug alone. Aspirin may, in fact, account for some of the bleeding observed among control patients in many of the trials. Thus, if the caveat is honored that patients given low-dose heparin should not receive aspirin for five days prior to operation, it can be anticipated that there will be even less bleeding from heparin than has been recorded in past trials.

Because of the problem of hemorrhage, some investigators are recommending that the dose of heparin be varied from patient to patient, whereas others are suggesting that prophylaxis be limited to patients at increased risk of venous thromboembolism. While these views are understandable, they will, if followed, never permit low-dose heparin regimens to exert a favorable impact on national mortality from pulmonary embolism. The eventual arbiters of this dilemma will be the medical community.

References

1. Fratantoni J, and Wessler S (eds): Prophylactic Therapy of Deep Vein Thrombosis and Pulmonary Embolism. Washington, DC, United States Government Printing Office. DHEW Publication No (NIH) 76-866, 1975.
2. Prevention of fatal postoperative pulmonary embolism by low doses of heparin. An international multicentre trial. Lancet 2:45, 1975.
3. Sagar S, Massey J, and Sanderson JM: Low-dose heparin prophylaxis against fatal pulmonary embolism. Br Med J 4:257, 1975.
4. Prevention of venous thromboembolism in surgical patients by low-dose heparin: prepared by the Council on Thrombosis of the American Heart Association. Circulation 55:423A, 1977.

Comment

Dr. Wessler was one of the chief architects of the American Heart Association Council on Thrombosis recommendation advocating the use of low-dose heparin in older patients undergoing general abdominal and thoracic surgery. His essay presents the general justification for these recommendations. He does point out certain important limitations and exceptions, however, and adds to this the suggestion that aspirin, if used, should be discontinued five days or so before such patients go to surgery and before low-dose heparin is used. The major rationale for the use of low-dose heparin is its demonstrable ability to reduce the incidence of deep vein thrombosis, despite the fact that the death rate from pulmonary emboli was not significantly lowered among those receiving low-dose heparin compared to control groups in the multi-center trial.

Dr. Strandness emphasizes some of the problems that arose in the multi-center trial report. He questions, specifically, the exclusion of one of the participating centers whose results appear to have been different from the other 27 centers and, therefore, were not included in the final report. If these controversial data had been included, Dr. Strandness suggests that the conclusions of this report would have been less clear-cut. Dr. Strandness questions whether the complications of low-dose heparin, including such problems as dispensing errors by the nursing staff, wound hematomas, and significant blood loss, justify the apparent slight reduction that occurs in the incidence of deep vein thromboses.

I suspect that if one strictly observes the indications, exceptions, and caveats detailed by Dr. Wessler, the use of low-dose heparin can be implemented with very little risk to the patient, while providing some distinct benefits. Unfortunately, medical practice often results in others ignoring the restrictions and limitations suggested by advocates of a particular regimen, producing results less rewarding than those of the original proponents. Thus, I favor the use of low-dose heparin in older patients undergoing extensive abdominal and thoracic surgical procedures, since I believe that a reduction in the incidence of deep vein thrombosis ultimately will save some unnecessary deaths due to fatal pulmonary emboli (even if this is not demonstrated statistically in multicenter trials). Since low-dose heparin programs offer very little risk to the patient, this seems to be a rational approach within the limitations proposed. I think it should be recognized, however, that there is a significant body of general surgeons who do not share this view and who, therefore, do not carry out this recommendation of the American Heart Association Council on Thrombosis.

ELLIOT RAPAPORT, M.D.

Twenty-one

Is Extensive Work-Up for the Newly Discovered Hypertensive Unnecessary?

EXTENSIVE WORK-UP FOR THE NEWLY DISCOVERED
HYPERTENSIVE IS UNNECESSARY
   Frank A. Finnerty, Jr., M.D.

COMPREHENSIVE HYPERTENSIVE EVALUATION: PRO
   James C. Melby, M.D.

COMMENT

Extensive Work-Up for the Newly Discovered Hypertensive Is Unnecessary

FRANK A. FINNERTY, JR., M.D.

Clinical Professor of Medicine, George Washington
University Medical Center, Washington, D.C.; Director,
Hypertension Center of Washington, D.C.

The diagnostic aspects and complications of hypertension have unfortunately received more emphasis than its therapeutic aspects in medical schools, house-officer training, and postgraduate educational programs. Usually, the only contact that the student or house staff has with hypertensive patients is when such patients are hospitalized for stroke, congestive heart failure, or renal failure. Often, it is not appreciated or emphasized that each of these is a direct and preventable complication of hypertension and that the patient is actually in the hospital because of inadequate or no treatment.

Similarly, most hypertension clinics in university hospitals place major emphasis on diagnosis or on following up cases of severe or unusual disease. They are not interested in asymptomatic patients with mild or moderately severe hypertension. A quick review of the contents of the average postgraduate seminar on hypertension readily discloses the overwhelming emphasis on the rare forms of hypertension and on the importance of chemical and endocrinological profiles. No one tells the practicing physician that controlling blood pressure in patients with mild and moderately severe disease prevents complications; no one teaches him how to treat these patients, who must be motivated if they are going to remain under medical care for the rest of their lives.

The cause of essential hypertension remains unknown. There is no doubt, therefore, that continued basic research into the mechanisms of disease processes must be encouraged and supported. Indeed, 50 per cent of federal funding for hypertension is being spent on just this type of basic research. It must be emphasized, however, that this type of research must be carried on in university centers by trained personnel on selected pa-

501

tients and should not become part of the routine office investigation for the average asymptomatic hypertensive patient.

Gifford[1] has found that less than six per cent of 5000 consecutive hypertensive patients first seen at the Cleveland Clinic (where emphasis is on diagnosis of secondary types of hypertension) have secondary hypertension. I thoroughly agree with his conclusions that these observations would hardly warrant an exhaustive search for secondary hypertension in every patient. Indeed, one of the major drawbacks for the practicing physician who accepts the responsibility of caring for any hypertensive patient is the fear of criticism from his peers that he did not "work up" the patient completely or promptly. He is also reluctant to spend the patient's money for sophisticated, expensive, "routine" laboratory procedures.

Since 85 to 90 per cent of the hypertensive population have essential hypertension, with a 75 per cent chance of having a mild, readily treatable form of the disease, and since 70 per cent of hypertensive patients are over 40 years of age, we recommend the following work-up for the asymptomatic patient in this age group:

1. Recording of a diastolic pressure over 95 mm Hg on at least three independent visits.
2. A careful history, with emphasis on the cardiovascular and renal systems, and a complete physical examination.
3. Laboratory evaluation of serum levels of glucose (preferably two hours postprandial), creatinine, potassium, and cholesterol. (Although not directly related to hypertension, an elevated cholesterol value represents an important risk factor for coronary disease.)
4. Urinalysis.
5. Electrocardiogram.

These examinations are readily available, easy to perform, relatively inexpensive, and conform in general to the recommendations of the Hypertension Study Group of the Inter-Society Commission for Heart Disease Resources.[2] The history and physical examination are most important. They not only establish the degree of vascular disease and the presence or absence of target-organ involvement, but also frequently provide telltale clues of the presence of secondary types of hypertension. Most types of secondary hypertension can at least be suspected from a careful history, physical examination, and simple laboratory data.

It should be emphasized that at any age, patients with accelerated hypertension, patients who do not respond satisfactorily to treatment, or patients who cannot or will not tolerate effective doses of antihypertensive drugs need an exhaustive work-up for secondary hypertension. Secondary hypertension should also be ruled out in whites under the age of 30 years and in blacks under the age of 20 years when there is evidence of target-organ disease; the younger the patient, the more extensive the work-up.

Asymptomatic patients over 40 years of age whose hypertension has been verified on at least three visits and who demonstrate no evidence of secondary hypertension from history, physical examination, or simple laboratory data should be treated without further investigation.

A few comments seem in order regarding the exclusion of the chest x-rays, intravenous pyelogram, and renin determinations from the recommended *routine* work-up. It is felt that one can learn as much about heart size and more about strain and coronary artery involvement from the electrocardiogram than from the x-ray. Surely, there is no argument that if the physician treating the patient is the primary physician, a chest x-ray once a year is sound medical practice. The government-supported Hypertension Detection and Follow-Up Program does include a chest x-ray in the routine work-up, but this is used more to detect pulmonary tuberculosis in the many black populations than to document cardiac involvement.

Many physicians still feel that a pyelogram should be performed routinely and that if it is not done, second-class medicine is being practiced. In my experience, both in the clinic and in private practice, a careful history, physical examination, and an accurate urinalysis, with the microscopic examination performed on freshly voided urine, is sufficient to rule out intrinsic renal disease. The National High Blood Pressure Information Program agrees with this recommendation.[3]

A final point that truly needs emphasis is the uselessness of measuring renin *routinely* from the diagnostic, prognostic, or therapeutic standpoint. There is only one indication for a determination of peripheral renin activity and that is in the patient with a history suggesting primary aldosteronism whose serum reveals a low potassium. The only indication for a renal-vein renin determination is when one suspects renovascular disease as the cause of hypertension. In this situation, in order to keep procedures and cost to a minimum, the renal-vein renin determinations should be performed at the time of renal angiography following furosemide. A difference greater than 2.5 times in the two samples strongly suggests that the involved kidney is the cause of the hypertension.

Data from a variety of centers, including our own, demonstrate that patients with low renin have the same incidence of cardiovascular complications as those with high renin. Finally, selecting an antihypertensive agent because of its renin-lowering activity does not seem to be clinically sound for several reasons:

1. Most investigators feel that propranolol — highly publicized as a renin-lowering agent — exerts its major antihypertensive effect through some central mechanism rather than by lowering renin.
2. Many other beta blockers more antihypertensive than propranolol actually do not lower renin.
3. Most investigators would agree that diuretics should be the cornerstone of all antihypertensive therapy, and diuretics consistently elevate renin.
4. Finally, one of the drugs of choice for the therapy of hypertensive encephalopathy or malignant hypertension is diazoxide, which is the greatest stimulus to renin.

We should look upon renin as one part of the huge renin-angiotensin system, in the same way that CO_2 is part of the Krebs cycle. Basic research should certainly continue, since it may lead to a better understanding of hypertension. Such research, however, should not be done routinely in the doctor's office on the average patient; it should be done on selected patients in university centers for a particular purpose. If the incidence of strokes, congestive heart failure, and end-stage renal disease is to be reduced, physicians should give more attention to treating their patients rather than investigating them.

References

1. Gifford RW Jr: Evaluation of the hypertensive patient with emphasis on detecting curable causes. Milbank Mem Fund Q 47:170, 1969.
2. Report of the Inter-Society Commission for Heart Disease Resources: Guidelines for the detection, diagnosis, and management of hypertensive populations. Circulation 44:A263, 1971. (Revised August 1972.)
3. Report of the Joint National Committee on Detection, Evaluation, and Treatment of High Blood Pressure: A cooperative study. JAMA 237:255, 1977.

Comprehensive Hypertensive Evaluation: Pro

JAMES C. MELBY, M.D.

Professor of Medicine; Head, Section of Endocrinology
and Metabolism, Boston University School of Medicine,
Boston, Massachusetts

The Problem

Approximately one in five adult Americans has systemic arterial hypertension (blood pressures of 160/95 mm Hg or above). It is generally held that prompt, continuous, effective treatment will protect against the excess cardiovascular-cerebrovascular-renal morbidity and mortality of hypertension. Although the efficacy of antihypertensive drug therapy for mild hypertension (diastolic blood pressures consistently below 105 mm Hg) in terms of eliminating or reducing excess cardiovascular-cerebrovascular-renal morbidity and mortality has yet to be established conclusively, it is generally conceded that it is probably desirable to detect and to treat all hypertensive patients.

The Nature of Comprehensive Hypertensive Evaluation

Because of the epidemic proportions of the hypertension problem, conscientious and thoughtful physicians, as well as public health officials, health insurance carriers, and not least, the patients, would like to reduce diagnostic procedures, cost of work-up, and inconvenience to an essential minimum. Once the remediable causes of hypertension have been excluded, it is to the patient's best interest to commence immediately on one of the several sequential treatment programs now being recommended. It is the thesis of this essay that we should attempt to characterize the pathophysiology of hypertension as accurately as possible in every patient, so as to allow the most reasonable therapeutic program. Hard data on the cost:benefit ratio or risk:benefit ratio are lacking. Furthermore, there exists no general agreement as to what comprises a comprehensive hypertensive evaluation. There are only a hand-

505

ful of studies that relate hypertensive evaluation to the outcome of treatment. Nearly all studies involving extensive hypertensive evaluation include some form of renal angiography, renin profiling, aldosterone profiling, and urinary metanephrine excretion. It should be emphasized that it is illogical to quantify the prevalence of secondary hypertension in the general hypertensive population or to quantify disordered renin and aldosterone secretion in this population if one does not use procedures that will identify abnormalities of the renal vasculature, epinephrine or norephinephrine excretory products, and the behavior or renin and aldosterone before and after provocation with acute volume-induced plasma volume change. It is distressing that the prevalence of a disease such as primary aldosteronism is generally derived from studies in which measurement of aldosterone was not made.

A Rationale of Comprehensive Hypertensive Evaluation

There is considerable tactical advantage in subjecting a patient to a comprehensive hypertensive evaluation prior to the institution of therapy, because nearly all therapeutic agents used in the treatment of hypertension affect renin and aldosterone profiling at least, and in some instances, urinary metanephrines. In this clinic, it is our habit to discontinue antihypertensive medications, including diuretics, for at least four to six weeks prior to comprehensive evaluation, during which time the patient will ingest a normal amount of sodium and chloride in his diet. The comprehensive approach espoused in this clinic is extremely well accepted by the hypertensive population and has resulted in the recognition of curable hypertension and altered renin and aldosterone metabolism to a much greater extent than would have been anticipated from the existing literature. Routine hypertensive work-up, including electrocardiogram and determination of plasma and serum electrolytes and creatinine levels and augmented by rapid-sequence excretory urography, urinary metanephrine excretion, and appropriate aldosterone and renin profiling, permits the recognition of curable secondary hypertension with few false-negative results. Where is this more evident? Description of the behavior of the renin-angiotensin-aldosterone system permits greater therapeutic specificity or tailoring of therapy for the patient. This view is controversial.[1-4] Our own views have been stated previously, supporting the extensive work-up.[5] Certainly, the lack of patient compliance in the self-administration of antihypertensive drugs is so great (in some studies between 60 and 80 per cent) because of the lack of symptoms of arterial hypertension, the distressing side effects of certain of the antihypertensive preparations, and the inconvenience of dose schedule; patient compliance can be improved with a more reasoned tailoring of therapy to the individual patient and identification of curable hypertension by an appropriate diagnostic evaluation. In our own clinic, the frequency of altered regulation of renin-angiotensin-aldosterone secretion and presence of secondary hypertension approaches 40 to 50 per cent.

Identifying Curable Secondary Hypertension

For many years, it was believed that curable secondary hypertension accounted for five to 10 per cent of the entire hypertensive population. Since there are approximately 24 million Americans with blood pressures of 160/95 or higher, the possibility exists that there are some 2.4 million Americans with surgically remediable hypertension. Of the more conservative estimates of the prevalence of curable hypertension, a large clinical population that was well studied is that of Gifford,[6] who found that slightly less than six per cent of some 5000 hypertensive patients seen at the Cleveland Clinic had curable forms of hypertension. The distribution of the potentially curable forms of secondary hypertension identified by Gifford is found in Table 1. The Gifford study, which has been the classic reference for any discussion of prevalence of various forms of curable secondary hypertension, was first published in 1969, at a time when the application of renin profiling, as well as analysis of the behavior of aldosterone, had just begun. It is highly likely that these measurements were not made in the majority of the patients unless they had hypokalemia. A more modern study from the Mayo Clinic, performed from 1973 through 1975, suggests that the prevalence of curable secondary hypertension is much lower than even the previous Gifford study had demonstrated.[7] Tucker and LaBarthe examined the frequency of surgical treatment of hypertension in adults at the Mayo Clinic and related this to the number of patients whose diastolic blood pressures were consistently above 95 mm Hg. Their astonishing findings are shown in Table 1. The number of patients studied by comprehensive evaluation of hypertension in the Tucker and LaBarthe series is probably very low. However, the results expressed by Tucker and LaBarthe cannot be validly compared with those given by Gifford. Nevertheless, the study of Tucker and LaBarthe can be challenged because sufficient data on diagnostic cues suggesting the presence of curable secondary hypertension are not given. Of great interest is that Tucker and LaBarthe show a high percentage of positive renal arteriograms in patients who had undergone this procedure. It cannot be considered valid to dismiss the possibility of evolving primary aldosteronism or evolving fibromuscular dysplastic lesions of the renal arteries if the appropriate maneuvers were not made. Grim and colleagues[8] observed an astonishingly high incidence of curable secondary hypertension in 236 hypertensive patients referred to the University of

Table 1. *Prevalence of Curable Hypertension in the United States*

| | NO. (%) OF ALL HYPERTENSIVE CASES | | | |
INVESTIGATORS	Renovascular Disease	Coarctation of the Aorta	Primary Aldosteronism	Pheochromocytoma
Gifford[6]	960,000 (4)	240,000 (1.0)	120,000 (0.5)	48,000 (0.2)
Tucker and LaBarthe[7]	43,200 (0.18)	not reported	2400 (0.01)	9600 (0.04)
Grim et al.[8]	3,840,000 (16)	not reported	2,832,000 (11.8)	not reported

Indiana Specialized Center of Research in Hypertension by primary care physicians from January 1, 1974, through December 31, 1976. In this study, Grim and his colleagues performed renal arteriograms on most of the patients whether or not the rapid-sequence excretory urogram was positive. It resulted in an enormous yield of patients who had functional arterial stenosis, with agreement that the lesions were functional by the differential renin levels from the renal veins. Sixteen per cent of the patients in this study had renovascular disease, and 11.8 per cent were shown to have primary aldosteronism confirmed by surgical intervention. These investigators also demonstrated marked alterations in the behavior of the renin-angiotensin-aldosterone system in a high percentage of patients. Grim and his colleagues do not suggest that their experience is representative of the hypertensive population at large. It can be inferred, however, that comprehensive evaluation will markedly increase the recognition of curable secondary hypertension. The Tucker and LaBarthe study, based on the results of accomplished surgery and with relationship to computerized information on the percentage of patients with diastolic pressures above 95 mm Hg, is hardly more valid than the study of Grim and his colleagues.

RENOVASCULAR DISEASE

The most common form of curable secondary hypertension is renovascular disease, and frequently it can be recognized by utilizing rapid-sequence excretory urography. It is estimated that 15 to 25 per cent of the rapid-sequence excretory urography gives false-negative results in the presence of functional renal arterial stenosis. About 50 per cent of patients who have renovascular hypertension have elevated resting levels of plasma renin activity, and nearly all patients who have renovascular disease respond to the administration of converting enzyme inhibitor (inhibiting the conversion of angiotensin I to angiotensin II) with a reduction of blood pressure, often into the normal range.[1] Since renovascular disease is the most common form of secondary hypertension in man and since rapid-sequence excretory urography is the most convenient diagnostic aid, except for perhaps the injection of the converting enzyme inhibitor, it is our view that rapid-sequence urography should be used because of its high yield of information. A routine hypertensive intravenous pyelogram is not recommended by the American Heart Association or by those who prefer a more abbreviated work-up, because they feel that the false-negative percentage is excessive. If the patient is young and has an elevated renin level or an aberration of electrolyte metabolism, it may be well to go on with a renal arteriogram and bilateral renal-vein renin testing after stimulation with a diuretic. A rapid-sequence excretory urogram should be performed on all patients with hypertension of recent onset, particularly rapid onset after age 50 and in patients during the first three decades of life, regardless of the duration of the hypertension in the latter.

PRIMARY ALDOSTERONISM

The prevalence of primary aldosteronism is controversial and will remain so until all members of an unselected hypertensive population are studied by appropriate maneuvers that will demonstrate autonomous hypersecretion of aldosterone and concomitant suppression of renin secretion. It is reasonably clear that neither the Mayo Clinic or Cleveland Clinic populations were studied by maneuvers that would alter aldosterone secretion, such as suppression and stimulation of plasma aldosterone and plasma renin activity, in any systematic way, and it is our view that these studies do not reflect the prevalence of primary aldosteronism. One need only look at the statistics offered by Tucker and LaBarthe[7] from the Mayo Clinic, which state that approximately 2.7 patients per year undergo adrenalectomy for primary aldosteronism. Approximately six to 10 patients are operated yearly at our clinic for primary aldosteronism in a hospital with only 350 beds, whereas the Mayo Clinic has at its disposal several thousand beds. Our own experience more exactly mirrors the experience of Grim et al.[8] from the University of Indiana. It is generally accepted that patients with hypertension who exhibit spontaneous hypokalemia have a 50 per cent chance of having an aldosterone-producing adenoma as a cause of their hypertension and spontaneous hypokalemia. The occurrence of spontaneous hypokalemia and hypertension is greater than that observed in the general population and is more apt to occur when plasma renin activity is suppressed, as has been shown by Padfield et al.[9] There is no feature of the hypertension of primary aldosteronism that is distinctive. It occurs most frequently between the third and fifth decades, and more often in women. Spontaneous hypokalemia is observed in almost 80 per cent of patients, but 20 per cent or more have a perfectly normal serum potassium level.[10] It is highly likely that potassium depletion follows the rise in blood pressure that is observed in primary aldosteronism in the young, because approximately 12 per cent of patients labeled as having low-renin hypertension have normal aldosterone levels, which are really quite inappropriate for the very suppressed levels of plasma renin activity. Patients who have intermittent spontaneous hypokalemia may never exhibit hypokalemia during the time they are under a physician's observation. The only sign of any mild potassium deficiency may be the presence of nocturnal polyuria. These patients often show a marked sensitivity to the thiazides in terms of production of hypokalemia, which may be associated with appearance of a cardiac irregularity, paralysis, and tetany. Acute precipitation of potassium depletion by thiazide diuretics in the routine treatment of the hypertensive patient should immediately suggest the possibility of primary aldosteronism. The diagnosis of primary aldosteronism should be suspected in any hypertensive patient who has episodic or persistent spontaneous hypokalemia or who has become hypokalemic shortly after the initiation of thiazide or loop diuretic therapy or after ingestion of large amounts of sodium chloride. It has long been known that in primary aldosteronism, sodium loading intensifies potassium depletion and that sodium deprivation permits potassium repletion. When aldosterone secretion is suppressed by salt ingestion in healthy subjects, the distal tubular

stimulus to sodium reabsorption is quickly dissipated; patients with autonomous aldosterone secretion exhibit continued distal tubular sodium reab-
sorptive activity in response to a marked increase in the filtered load of
sodium. If one ingests more than 200 mEq of sodium per day (nine one-
gram sodium chloride tablets per day) for four days and this does not influence serum potassium, one can exclude for all practical purposes the
diagnosis of primary aldosteronism. Hypokalemia induced by a sodium load is
strong indirect evidence for sustained excessive secretion of aldosterone. The
diagnosis of primary aldosteronism rests on the demonstration of increased
aldosterone secretion or plasma concentrations in the presence of very low or
suppressed plasma renin activity. The most simple and rewarding method for
diagnosis is to obtain blood specimens simultaneously for plasma aldosterone
concentration and plasma renin activity before and after maximal stimulation
by acute volume depletion. One must be certain that these tests are carried
out in the early morning hours, since aldosterone levels in plasma in patients
with primary aldosteronism fall during the day because they are exclusively
under the control of ACTH (adrenocorticotropic hormone) secretion. In Figure 1, the measurement of plasma aldosterone is useful in determining the
nature of the adrenal lesion involved. Specimens of blood for aldosterone
measurement should be obtained at 8 AM and again at noon to determine the
cause of primary aldosteronism. The patient should also be encouraged to be
up and about. Plasma aldosterone levels in patients with Conn's syndrome
due to an aldosterone-producing adenoma have a lower plasma aldosterone
level at noon than they do at 8 AM; in fact, it may be in the normal range. This
is one of the reasons that tests for aldosterone in the plasma must be carried
out before 9 AM. In idiopathic aldosteronism due to bilateral macronodular

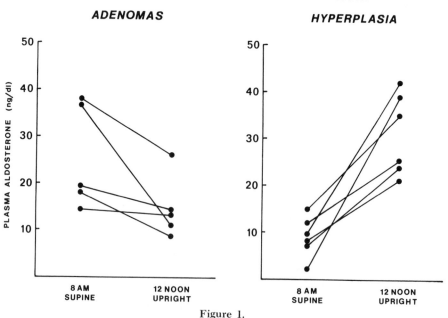

Figure 1.

and micronodular hyperplasia of the adrenals, the noon aldosterone level is usually above the 8 AM level, with a slight increment in renin activity. This biochemical determination of the etiology of the disease has been repeatedly confirmed and is extremely useful.

CUSHING'S SYNDROME

This rare cause of secondary hypertension is sufficiently obvious under most circumstances to preclude initial special laboratory examination for its presence. The best single screening test for the presence of Cushing's syndrome is a 24-hour urinary excretion of "free" cortisol. Urinary "free" cortisol is generally below 80 μg/24 hours.

PHEOCHROMOCYTOMA

Elevation of urinary metanephrine excretion in the persistently hypertensive patient and in the patient with paroxysmal bouts of hypertension, especially during a hypertensive episode, is diagnostic for pheochromocytoma. This test should not be a part of the usual hypertensive work-up unless there is some clinical indication for the application of this test. The urinary metanephrines are least affected by a variety of antihypertensive drugs, but nevertheless, they should be collected in acid 48 hours after the last dose of the antihypertensive drug. Urinary metanephrines have approximately a 20 per cent edge on urinary catecholamines and VMA excretion for accuracy in diagnosis.

In summary, curable secondary hypertension can be recognized in most patients if a rapid-sequence excretory urogram is undertaken and if measurements of basal and stimulated plasma renin activity and aldosterone concentrations are obtained.

Determining Appropriate Treatment

HYPERRENINEMIC HYPERTENSION

Laragh has introduced a new taxonomy of hypertension utilizing renin profiling with so-called basal vasoconstriction-volume analysis.[2] A modification of this classification of hypertension based on renin profiling and sodium dependence of blood pressure is presented in Table 2. The Laragh group contends that intensive treatment to reduce renin activity in patients with hyperreninemic hypertension is effective of itself in reducing blood pressure. The Laragh laboratory has provided a great deal of evidence to support their concept that the primary antihypertensive effect of the β-adrenoceptors is to reduce renin activity and that perhaps this is also true of clonidine, which is a sympathetic outflow inhibitor acting in the central nervous system. The treatment of hypertension based on the behavior of the

Table 2. *Classification of Systemic Arterial Hypertension Based on Renin Profiling*

I. ANGIOTENSIN DEPENDENCE PREDOMINANT (15%)

Hyperreninemia, increased peripheral resistance (vasoconstructive) ++++, unresponsive to diuretics:
 1° — *Juxtaglomerular cell and Wilms' tumors*
 2° — *Accelerated, renovascular, OC hypertension*

II. SODIUM DEPENDENCE PREDOMINANT (15–25%)

Hyporeninemia, blood and ECF volumes increased 0–++++, responsive to diuretics:
 Low-renin hypertension
 Mineralocorticoid-hypertensive syndrome

renin-angiotensin-aldosterone system is shown in Table 3. The majority of patients exhibit both partial angiotensin II dependence and partial sodium dependence in terms of blood pressure response. The Laragh group has demonstrated clearly by the appropriate application of the converting enzyme inhibitor that angiotensin II has a central role in the perpetuation and intensification of hypertension when its levels are elevated in patients with hypertension; that sodium has this reciprocal role in patients with suppressed renin activity; and that the inhibition of converting enzyme in patients with low-renin hypertension or sodium-dependent hypertension has very little effect on blood pressure. Renin profiling for the classification of hypertension based on renin-volume relationships is not thought to be essential by a large segment of investigators in hypertension. It is more often suggested that response to specific inhibitors and diuretics be the determinants of the final treatment program. Unfortunately, the theory of sodium predominance is harder to prove than that of angiotensin II. In order to identify the high-renin group, it is necessary to collect the blood sample for determination of plasma renin activity when the patient has been recumbent overnight and on a normal salt intake. Patients with accelerated or malignant hypertension often exhibit increased plasma renin activity, and these patients deserve intensive comprehensive therapy with multiple doses of renin inhibitors, such as the converting enzyme inhibitor, the β-adrenoceptor inhibitors, or the central active outflow

Table 3. *Appropriate Treatment Based on Renin Profiling*

1. TREATMENT OF ANGIOTENSIN II–DEPENDENT HYPERTENSION

Converting enzyme inhibitor
Saralasin (angiotensin II inhibitor)
β-adrenoceptor inhibitor (propranolol, and so on)
Centrally active sympathetic inhibitor
 α-methyldopa
 clonidine

2. SODIUM-DEPENDENT HYPERTENSION

Diuretic agents

inhibitors such as clonidine, in addition to diuretic therapy and perhaps direct vasodilator therapy. It should be emphasized that diuretic therapy alone in a patient with elevated renin activity may cause even a further increment in peripheral resistance and a rise in blood pressure. Diuretics usually have to be given to patients who are receiving sympathetic inhibitors acting at a variety of levels, because with nearly all sympathetic inhibition, there is marked sodium retention, a tendency toward volume expansion, and ultimately, a rise in blood pressure. In young, labile hypertensives with only modest elevations of plasma renin activity, it has been recommended by the Laragh group that β-adrenoceptor inhibition be tried alone, without superimposing diuretic therapy. Evidence that angiotensin II is the sole determinant of hypertension in patients with essential hypertension is lacking. Evidence that angiotensin II is the central cause of hypertension in patients with renovascular disease is very substantial. Primary hyperreninism due to a juxtaglomerular cell tumor or to a Wilms' tumor in children is a rare event and is often hard to recognize; it has been most often recognized post mortem. Bilateral venous catheterization of the kidneys would be in order if one suspected the presence of a renin-producing tumor of the kidney because of subtle distortions of the rapid-sequence excretory urogram.

It would appear that the converting enzyme inhibitor is active orally, and this compound will probably emerge as an important therapeutic agent in the treatment of high-renin hypertension. Since we have such highly specific inhibitors that could neutralize the renin-angiotensin system with virtually no other vascular disturbance, it is likely that there would be a continued need to undertake renin profiling in patients with severe hypertension, particularly those who were not responsive to the usual sympathetic inhibitor therapy combined with diuretics.

NORMAL RENINEMIC HYPERTENSION

The presence of normal reninemic hypertension is determined by stimulation of plasma renin activity using an acute loop diuretic to reduce plasma volume. The patient is asked to discontinue diuretic therapy for at least three weeks and inhibitors of renin secretion for at least one week before the tests are performed. The patient is asked to eat a diet containing at least 100 mEq of sodium per day. On the morning of the test, 80 mg of furosemide is ingested, and a blood specimen for the determination of renin activity is obtained within two hours. It is useful to also obtain blood for aldosterone analysis if required. It is important that this study be carried out as early as possible in the day, so as not to introduce ambiguity if primary aldosteronism is present.

Normal reninemic patients include those with labile hypertension who are often responsive to β-adrenoceptor inhibitors such as propranolol. Varying degrees of increments in resistance of the peripheral circulation are seen in this group of patients, but the increased peripheral resistance is of a lower order of magnitude than is observed in patients with high-renin hypertension and patients with more severe hypertension. Generally, these normal reninemic patients respond well to the combination of a β-adrenoceptor inhibitor or a centrally active sympathetic outflow inhibitor, such as clonidine, associated with a long-acting diuretic.

HYPORENINEMIC HYPERTENSION

A subgroup of patients have been identified who seemingly have essential hypertension, but who also exhibit suppressed or hyporesponsive plasma renin activity when challenged by any maneuver that will acutely produce substantially negative sodium balance. This subgroup of patients represents approximately 20 to 25 per cent of the hypertensive population. Interestingly, the only other situation in which untreated patients with hypertension have suppressed plasma renin activity is in the mineralocorticoid-hypertensive syndrome.[11] Increased exchangeable sodium, extracellular fluid volume, and plasma volume have all been demonstrated in low-renin hypertension, but not consistently, as they have been demonstrated in patients with mineralocorticoid excess. Both patients with mineralocorticoid excess and those with so-called low-renin hypertension have a reduction in blood pressure when sodium is deprived or when diuretics are used intensively. The response to diuretics and particularly to anti-mineralocorticoids in patients with low-renin hypertension is identical to that of patients with primary aldosteronism in terms of reduction in blood pressure. It is therefore suggested that sodium and water retention is an immediate cause of a volume-dependent hypertension in both disorders — that is, low-renin hypertension and acknowledged mineralocorticoid excess. There is compelling evidence from a variety of investigators to support the idea that adrenal mineralocorticoid excess has a primary role in the genesis of low-renin hypertension.[11] To date, some five separate adrenocortical hormonal steroids have been implicated as causal agents for the development of low-renin hypertension.[12] It is tempting to conclude that this subgroup of patients with low plasma renin activity is afflicted with mineralocorticoid hypertensive syndrome and that any mineralocorticoids involved have yet to be characterized because of the recently rapidly accumulating demonstrations of altered adrenal steroidogenesis in the low-renin hypertensive population.

Low-renin hypertension is identified by a stimulated plasma renin activity measurement in conjunction with plasma aldosterone determination, which is preceded by 80 mg of furosemide given when the patient has been off diuretic therapy for several weeks and off inhibitors of renin secretion for at least one week. It is important that these studies be begun at 7 AM and end at or about 9 AM so as not to receive ambiguous results in patients with evolving primary aldosteronism whose plasma aldosterone responds mainly to secreted ACTH. Increments in plasma renin activity after stimulation with furosemide are often imperceptible and generally well below 2 ng/ml/hr. If the aldosterone level is inappropriately elevated for the level of plasma renin activity, even if it is as low as 10 ng per cent, the diagnosis of primary aldosteronism is nearly assured. If it is low, it suggests the possible presence of another hypertensinogenic mineralocorticoid.

Treatment of low-renin hypertension consists of diuretic therapy alone. This treatment is remarkably successful in most patients over a relatively brief period of time. Long-term thiazide therapy is often associated with hypo-kalemia, as is the tendency toward development of spontaneous hypokalemia in these patients. Spironolactone therapy should be substituted if the hypo-kalemia supervenes. Hypokalemia may be much more dangerous than has been previously reckoned in patients who have risk factors for coronary atherosclerosis, such as hypertension.[13]

Conclusion

History, physical examination, routine laboratory work-up with electro-lytes, stimulated and unstimulated plasma renin activity determinations, and determination of plasma aldosterone concentrations should be performed. A rapid-sequence excretory urogram should be carried out. These maneuvers will identify almost all patients with curable secondary hypertension. Deter-mination of plasma aldosterone in those with stimulated plasma renin activity will permit development of therapeutic regimens that are more likely to be effective using the least amount of drugs in patients with elevated, normal, and suppressed plasma renin activity. The additional expense, inconven-ience, and discomfort to the patient are less important considerations com-pared with the significant benefits of detecting curable secondary hyper-tension.

It is not possible to include or exclude patients for comprehensive evalua-tion of their hypertension on the basis of their age. We now recognize that most juvenile and adolescent hypertension is in family arrogation and may have no more tendency toward secondary hypertension than seen in the young adult. It is true that glomerulonephritis is a significant cause of hyper-tension in children under 10 years of age.

A comment should be made about the cost and yield of the comprehen-sive hypertensive evaluation. In 1975, Ferguson estimated the cost of an extensive evaluation to be $2083. In his own investigations, he found that 26 cases of secondary hypertension were discovered and that of these, 21 could be recognized by history and physical examination alone. Are we to be led to believe that the diagnostic studies would end there if the history and physical examination were very positive? This is not our experience.[14] It is possible to evaluate patients as extensively as I have recommended for as little as $300 when studied in the outpatient department. Isn't it possible that the public health approach to the diagnosis and treatment of hypertension has over-looked the enormously rapid development of relatively inexpensive laborato-ry procedures? Is it possible that this type of approach (epidemiologic and so on) may reinforce an attitude that will promote non-compliance of therapy when side effects from unnecessary drugs appear?

The sheer number of patients with hypertension tempers our insistence on comprehensive evaluation of each patient, especially when there are regional differences in the nature and extent of hypertension in the United

States. However, when the causes of curable secondary hypertension have been sought, an unexpected number of causes appear.

References

1. Case DB, Wallace JM, Keim HJ, Weber MA, Sealey JE, and Laragh JH: Possible role of renin in hypertension as suggested by renin-sodium profiling and inhibition of converting enzyme. N Engl J Med 296:641–646, 1977.
2. Laragh JH: Modern system for treating high blood pressure based on renin profiling and vasoconstriction-volume analysis: a primary role for beta blocking drugs such as propranolol. Am J Med 61:797–810, 1976.
3. Kaplan NM: Renin profiles: the unfulfilled promises. JAMA 238:611–613, 1977.
4. Guthrie GP Jr, Genest J, and Kuchel O: Renin and the therapy of hypertension. Annu Rev Pharmacol Toxicol 16:287–309, 1976.
5. Melby JC: Extensive hypertensive work-up: pro. JAMA 231:399–401, 1975.
6. Gifford RW Jr: Evaluation of the hypertensive patient with emphasis on detecting curable causes. Milbank Mem Fund Q 47:170–186, 1969.
7. Tucker RM, and LaBarthe DR: Frequency of surgical treatment for hypertension in adults at the Mayo Clinic from 1973 through 1975. Mayo Clin Proc 52:549–555, 1977.
8. Grim CE, Weinberger MH, Higgins JT, and Kramer NJ: Diagnosis of secondary forms of hypertension — a comprehensive protocol. JAMA 237:1331–1335, 1977.
9. Padfield PL, Brown JJ, Lever AF, et al: Is low-renin hypertension a stage in the development of essential hypertension or a diagnostic entity? Lancet 2:548–550, 1975.
10. Conn JW, Rovner DR, Cohen EL, and Nesbit RM: Normokalemic primary aldosteronism. Its masquerade as "essential" hypertension. JAMA 195:21–26, 1966.
11. Melby JC, and Dale SL: New mineralocorticoids and adrenocorticosteroids in hypertension. Am J Cardiol 38:805–813, 1976.
12. Melby JC, and Dale SL: Role of 18-hydroxy-11-deoxycorticosterone and 16α, 18-dihydroxy-11-deoxycorticosterone in hypertension. Mayo Clin Proc 52:317–322, 1977.
13. Duke M: Thiazide-induced hypokalemia: association with acute myocardial infarction and ventricular fibrillation. JAMA 239:43–45, 1978.
14. Ferguson RK: Cost and yield of the hypertensive evaluation: experience of a community-based referral clinic. Ann Intern Med 82:761–765, 1975.

Comment

Hypertension is a major public-health problem in the United States. Recently, the National High Blood Pressure Education Program of the National Institutes of Health suggested that the prevalence of high blood pressure is higher than the figure of 24 million people so frequently quoted. Present estimates suggest that close to 35 million people in the United States suffer from hypertension. The extent of the problem and its neglect in the past have led to an intensive educational program directed both to the public and the profession that is designed to improve the detection, evaluation, and treatment of hypertension. To encourage greater patient compliance and to keep health-care costs down, it has been proposed that a minimum work-up be carried out, one similar to that described by Dr. Finnerty, and that treatment be approached in a so-called stepped-care fashion; that is, therapy is begun initially with a thiazide type of diuretic, and if this is unsuccessful, one adds several alternative Step 2 drugs, including propranolol. If the Step 2 addition is unsuccessful and a third step is needed, hydralazine or a comparable vasodilator is added to the regimen. If treatment is still ineffective, it is then urged that specific causes of unresponsiveness be investigated. If no clear-cut reason for lack of responsiveness is uncovered, guanethidine is then recommended as a Step 4 drug.

The basic rationale of this approach is that approximately 85 to 90 per cent of patients with hypertension have essential hypertension, for which detailed laboratory studies will not alter basic management. It is suggested by the proponents of this approach that more detailed laboratory investigations, such as proposed by Dr. Melby, be reserved for situations in which the patient has failed to respond to the usual program or in which history or physical examination has uncovered suggestive evidence of a specific curable type of secondary hypertension.

I have no argument with the logic presented by Dr. Melby or the academic desirability of carrying out the program he proposes. The question revolves around the cost-benefit ratio as applied to large-scale detection and referral programs and compliance of both physicians and patients with this type of program. Working in an academic center, I tend to carry out more extensive diagnostic studies than might be carried out by the general practitioner who frequently is the one who must manage the problem. I do believe that a chest x-ray is always desirable, in contrast to the position taken by Dr. Finnerty. However, renin assays or, for that matter, intravenous pyelograms may not be necessary routinely and could be reserved for patients who are either very young, have no family history of hypertensive disease, have an unusual history or finding on physical examination, have an abnormality on urinalysis, or fail to respond to usual therapy.

Whether one undertakes a comprehensive physical and laboratory examination in an attempt to uncover all of the potential secondary curable causes of hypertension or not, one must not lose sight of the importance of adequate drug management of hypertension. Essentially all patients with hypertensive disease must be treated adequately. Whatever is necessary to accomplish this, whether it includes more extensive investigations or not, must be done to insure that the blood pressure of hypertensive patients is brought back into the normal range.

ELLIOT RAPAPORT, M.D.

Twenty-two

Is the Determination of Plasma Renin Levels Helpful in the Management of Patients with Hypertensive Disease?

RENIN-SODIUM PROFILING IS HELPFUL FOR MODERN MANAGEMENT OF HYPERTENSIVE PATIENTS
John H. Laragh, M.D.

ROUTINE MEASUREMENT OF PLASMA RENIN ACTIVITY
Harriet P. Dustan, M.D.

COMMENT

Renin-Sodium Profiling Is Helpful for Modern Management of Hypertensive Patients

JOHN H. LARAGH, M.D.

Director, Hypertension and Cardiovascular Center; Chief,
Division of Cardiology, The New York Hospital-Cornell
Medical Center, New York, New York

In the last 18 years or so, we and others associated with us have developed a diagnostic and therapeutic approach to hypertension based on our concurrently acquired knowledge of how the renin system participates in hypertensive states. Our basic tool for applying this approach is the renin-sodium profile. With this tool we have demonstrated the pathophysiologic heterogeneity of so-called essential hypertension.

We have proposed four major clinical applications for renin profiles: (1) definitive diagnosis of surgically curable renovascular hypertension; (2) definitive diagnosis of adrenocortical hypertensions; (3) acquisition of baseline information about hypertensive mechanisms of essential hypertension in order to plan simpler, more specific, and more predictable therapy; and (4) evaluation of the pace, severity, and prognosis of the native disorder.

Many aspects of our new analysis have already found their way into conventional medical practice, but some elements continue to be touched by controversy, particularly the utility of our method for diagnosing and managing essential hypertension.

This article, in reviewing the basis for our reliance on renin-sodium profiling in all hypertension, touches on some of the more critical points of debate and attempts to clarify areas of misunderstanding or misinterpretation.

At the outset, it is important to make clear that the concept we describe does not in any way presuppose that the renin system is causing any particular hypertensive state. Rather, it contends that measurement of the components of the system will always have value because the system, being inextricably involved in the regulation of blood pressure events, must either cause, support, or react to high blood pressure in one of the following ways: (1) by producing primary excesses of a hormone that causes the hy-

521

pertension; (2) by failing to react to other pressor factors with appropriate shutoff, thus contributing to maintenance of the hypertension; or (3) by appropriately suppressing its hormonal activity, and thus its basic vasoconstrictive and volume effects in reaction to other pressor or volume factors.

It scarcely needs to be restated that the ultimate causes of hypertension remain to be fully exposed. The renin approach neither excludes nor ignores the possibility that other factors may have etiologic importance, including the participation of such pressor or depressor hormones as the catecholamines, vasopressin, bradykinin, and the prostaglandins. However, with present knowledge, the precise role of these other factors is much less certain, and reliable methods of measurement are not often generally available. It is our position that whatever the influences of other factors, major or minor, they will in all likelihood also be reflected in changes in the renin system, which at the present time offers the only clear peephole we have into the complex biochemistry of human hypertension. The operational validity of the renin control system approach should not be impugned because we do not yet understand the role of other factors.

In the same context, the validity of this hypothesis should not suffer because we do not yet understand all aspects of the renin system itself. It may be advisable to emphasize, parenthetically, what should be taken for granted but, for some puzzling reason, is not: The renin approach, like most diagnostic and therapeutic strategies, is not 100 per cent reliable or effective. In this, as in most medical areas, nature still withholds certain secrets, a fact that should surprise no one, in view of the relatively recent state of our understanding of the renin system and its role in hypertension. That the approach we shall describe is effective and predictive *most* of the time seems sufficient evidence that it is useful and truthful and that it represents an important closure of gaps in our understanding and therapy of hypertension. The claim that it should be discarded because it does not *always* work bewilders me; if this notion were to gain currency, virtually every theory and therapeutic modality in medicine would have to be abandoned. Actually, exceptions to the rule are exposed by our approach, so that they themselves become the focus for new research.

Exposure of the Renin-Angiotensin-Aldosterone Axis

The renin "axis" was first revealed in 1960 by studies of a disease state in which its most flagrant abnormalities are expressed: malignant hypertension. We found that patients with malignant hypertension, quite unlike those with benign essential hypertension, had massive oversecretion of the adrenal cortical sodium-retaining hormone aldosterone.[1] This oversecretion proved to be a consequence of kidney damage that was causing inappropriate secretion of the enzyme renin into the bloodstream, with resultant generation in plasma of marked excesses of the vasoconstrictor hormone angiotensin II. The key to establishing this link was the demonstration that angiotensin II, unlike other pressor agents, selectively stimulates the adrenocortical secretion of aldosterone in normal persons.[2, 3] Angiotensin II thus emerged as a major physiologic stimulus for aldosterone, and the excesses of this hormone therefore explained the aldosterone oversecretion in malignant hypertension.

This research placed a new perspective on an important, but long overlooked, study by Kahn, Skeggs, Shumway, and Wisenbaugh,[4] who had shown marked hyperangiotensinemia in patients with malignant, but not with benign, hypertension. We proposed that the strikingly excessive levels of angiotensin II and aldosterone in malignant hypertension caused not only the severe hypertensive condition, but also the attendant diffuse vascular damage.[2, 3] This suggestion has been borne out by subsequent animal studies in which malignant vasculitis and death have been produced by the combined administration of renin, aldosterone, and salt[5] and by a number of subsequent clinical studies in which malignant hypertension has been dramatically arrested or cured by three means of renin deletion: beta-adrenergic blockade,[6, 7] angiotensin II blockade,[8, 9] or total nephrectomy.[5]

Following this research, the renin-angiotensin-aldosterone system became recognized as a cascading, sequential hormonal "axis" involving renin secretion by the kidney, angiotensin generation in plasma, and increased adrenal aldosterone secretion (Fig. 1). It has been our view that this system is designed to respond to changes in renal perfusion in order to

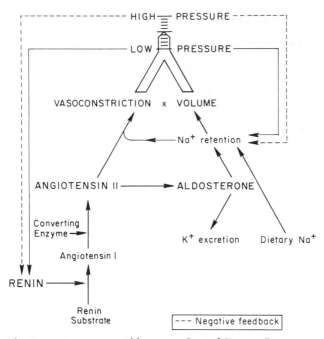

Figure 1. The Renin-Angiotensin-Aldosterone Control System. Renin, an enzyme secreted in response to reduced arterial pressure or renal tubular sodium supply, acts on a plasma protein to release inactive angiotensin I. This is hydrolyzed by converting enzymes to angiotensin II, the most powerful natural pressor known, and it quickly constricts arterioles and raises blood pressure. Angiotensin II also stimulates the secretion of aldosterone, which acts more slowly to retain sodium at potassium's expense, expanding fluid volume and restoring tissue perfusion. In normal persons, combined vasoconstriction and volume effects shut off the initial signal for renin secretion.

simultaneously maintain arterial blood pressure and sodium balance.[5] Renin is secreted in response to factors that reduce arterial pressure and cause poor renal perfusion, such as shock, hemorrhage, heart failure, or reduced flow in the distal tubule found during sodium depletion.

Renin has no physiologic action of its own but acts enzymatically on a plasma globulin to release the inactive decapeptide angiotensin I, which is then rapidly hydrolyzed to the octapeptide angiotensin II by pulmonary, plasma, and tissue converting enzymes. Angiotensin II, the most potent natural pressor substance known, restores blood pressure quickly by its direct vasoconstrictor action. At the same time, angiotensin II stimulates aldosterone secretion, and aldosterone acts over the next several hours to increase renal sodium retention and potassium excretion. The induced positive sodium balance leads secondarily to retention of water, expansion of extracellular fluids, and further indirect support of blood pressure. The immediate action of angiotensin restores pressure, while the action of aldosterone restores effective volume and flow. Together, the two hormones restore systemic flow and renal perfusion and compensate the system. Since the stimulus for renin secretion is reduced renal perfusion, the subsequent increases in pressure and flow that it induces provide the negative feedback signals that shut off renin release. Most likely, baroreceptor mechanisms in the afferent arterioles, as well as a sodium-load sensitive receptor in the macula densa of the renal tubules, are both involved, and it is a reasonable surmise that beta-adrenergic processes negotiate part of the former communication.[6, 7]

Evaluating the Renin System: The Assay

The diagnostic and therapeutic concepts presented here concerning involvement of the renin system were laboriously constructed on the measurement of the renin system in normal subjects, in the various hypertensive states, and in a variety of therapeutic protocols. A key aspect of this exploration was the development of a method that would be accurate, sensitive, responsive to variables, and free of artifactual distortions. Consistency and refinement in method are of particular importance in this area because of the extremely small concentrations of measurable hormones involved, the need to discriminate subnormal values, the significance of even the tiniest variation in concentration, and the many distortions that can be introduced by chemical and physical artifact. In addition, it must be recognized that one is evaluating a relative, not an absolute, value; the activity level of a control system cannot be considered normal or abnormal unless it is related to the conditions it is intended to control.

Scientific protocol is rather insistent on the axiom that to duplicate results one must duplicate the method. This prescription is especially relevant in view of the disparate results obtained by certain investigators, a circumstance that is usual when critical methodologic and physiologic conditions are overlooked. Therefore, before summarizing our findings and their implications, it may be useful to describe our methods briefly and to review their rationale.

A key requirement for full diagnostic exploitation of renin profiling is the use of a renin assay method sufficiently reliable and sensitive to explore and discriminate renin activity values below the normal range. This is especially important in identifying low-renin states and for characterizing the effects of renin-lowering agents. In this context, the clinician should be especially wary of methods in which the normal range includes or reports many values of zero or near zero at sodium excretion rates under 120 mEq/day. The sensitivity of such methods is inadequate.

To achieve adequate sensitivity requires a laboratory method that both controls pH and employs the pH optimum for renin (5.5 to 6.0) during incubation of the plasma sample and that also provides for complete inhibition of plasma angiotensinases for prolonged periods of time, so that low activity samples can be incubated up to 18 hours.[10-12] The prolonged incubation obviates the need for blank subtraction, and thus greatly increases accuracy as well as sensitivity and simplicity of the measurements. To date, such complete angiotensinase inhibition can be achieved only with the use of EDTA (edetate), a bacteriostatic agent, and either DFP (diisopropyl fluorophosphate)[13] or PMSF (phenylmethylsulfonyl fluoride)[14] at the acid pH optimum for renin.[10-12] Confusion in the field has resulted from the fairly common use of a method[15] that provides no pH control, does not employ the pH optimum, and recommends the agents BAL (dimercaprol) and 8-OH quinoline, agents that do not adequately inhibit angiotensinases.[16]

In addition, artificially high renin values have been produced by certain methods[17, 18] that acidify plasma to below pH 4 in order to destroy substrate and angiotensinases. The high values are a result of this acidification, which activates an inactive form of renin.[19] Our studies establish that chilling should be avoided in the blood collection process because of cryoactivation of "prorenin,"[20] a phenomenon that can increase the renin activity measurement.

Failure to take these considerations into account undoubtedly explains discrepant findings in some clinical reports; in fact, two groups have now explained their earlier failures to demonstrate renin suppression with beta-adrenergic blocking drugs as due to inadvertent acid-activation of renin.[21, 22] All of these problems can be avoided by the use of methods and procedures that we have described.[10-12] A simple and reliable renin assay procedure has been updated,[12] and kits using similar principles and procedures have recently become commercially available.

Evaluating Behavior of the System: The Renin-Sodium Profile

Even the most accurate and sensitive assay of plasma renin activity would have little physiologic meaning unless referenced against a dependable measurement of factors known to participate in the stimulus/response ambiance in which the renin system plays either an appropriate or inappropriate role.

The major countervailing force of the renin system is the state of sodium balance; indeed, one limb of the system's action is concerned with corrective adjustment of sodium balance (Fig. 1). In normal individuals, a rise in sodium balance depresses renin production, while a fall in sodium balance increases it. To express this normal, appropriate relationship, we have developed a procedure that we call renin-sodium profiling,[5, 23, 24] or renin profiling for short, in which the measured plasma renin activity (PRA) is referenced against the state of salt balance as determined from the sodium assay of a 24-hour urine collection.

Figure 2 is the nomogram charting this relationship in normal subjects. Several points must be made about this. First, the nomogram demonstrates most graphically the inverse curvilinear relationship between renin and sodium levels and emphasizes the necessity for this kind of indexing. Second, the nomogram allows evaluation of normal values on a more continuous index from low to high and within a narrower profile than does the use of bracketed ranges, which tends to obscure the meaning of values lying in the overlap of brackets. It should be further stated that while we commend the method to all, it would be wrong to employ our plotting of normal in the study of particular populations with possible different characteristics. Unfortunately, this has been done, and accounts for some confusing results.

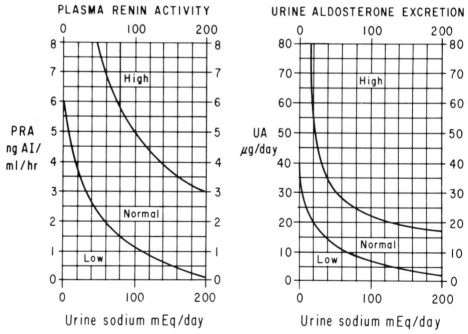

Figure 2.   Correlation of plasma renin activity and urine aldosterone excretion with sodium excretion. Renin activity was measured in plasma samples obtained at noon and aldosterone in 24-hour urines of normal subjects. A similar dynamic hyperbolic relationship is evident between the secretion of each hormone and the daily rate of sodium excretion. Subjects studied on random diets outside the hospital exhibited similar relationships, a finding that validates the use of this graph for studying outpatients and subjects not on constant hospital diets. AI = angiotensin I.

Normal control values of renin, like those for any assayable substance, should be obtained locally.

To be sure, the state of salt balance can be obtained in the traditional manner in the salt balance ward, and we did so before adopting the 24-hour salt excretion. In comparing the two methods,[5] we found the 24-hour urine collection to be as accurate a reflection of salt intake as the balance ward study and, frequently, an even more sensitive indicator of salt balance. True, it relies on patient compliance, but in actuality, no more than in the balance ward. Calculations are simpler, fewer personnel are involved, and outpatient procedures can be used, allowing the study of large numbers of subjects and patients. What is more, the method reduces the importance and the labor of the dietary history; the 24-hour salt excretion provides an irrefutable summary, automatically averaged, of the subject's salt life as it really is. Actually, because of the basic relationship between arterial blood pressure and renal sodium excretion, this measurement is a close function of the degree of arterial filling, and so provides an insight into the fundamental arterial pressure/volume relationship (also called the renal function curve by Guyton and his associates[25]) that we consider highly relevant to the analysis of hypertensive mechanisms.

In the same way, an aldosterone-sodium profile provides a pre-processed, pre-averaged indication of aldosterone production.[23, 26] This can be measured by assaying the acid-labile conjugate, the result being "profiled" as the daily aldosterone excretion related to the daily urinary sodium excretion, all from the same urine collection. This means of evaluating aldosterone production is particularly useful, because plasma aldosterone measurements vary widely during the day in response to transient phenomena.

Because renin levels normally fall toward zero at high levels of salt intake (Fig. 2), patients are best evaluated while on a moderately restricted sodium diet, one that will provide a urinary excretion rate from 40 to 100 mEq per day.[24] This mild stimulation of renin secretion enables more efficient separation of patients into low-, medium- or high-renin subgroups. Too drastic a salt restriction, however, would make accurate discrimination of high-renin patients difficult, because even normal subjects respond to such conditions with very high renin levels.

The 24-hour urine collection, then, is an extremely valuable diagnostic tool when used in properly prepared patients. We give each patient written instructions on how to perform a 24-hour urine collection, and we provide a suitable container — in the case of women, a wide-mouth vessel. We also provide written instructions for a moderate low-sodium diet containing somewhat less than 100 mEq of sodium per day, with a detailed list of foods that can or cannot be eaten.[24] The diet is instituted five to seven days before the blood and urine collections.

To standardize a second major factor that normally influences renin secretion, i.e., posture, the blood sample for renin determination is collected before noon while the patient is quietly seated, but after he or she has been up and about for at least an hour. Thus, the normal neurogenic drive to renin secretion is included in the evaluation.

Inasmuch as the purpose of the test in patients is to obtain a baseline estimate of the native renin contribution to hypertension (and by association, of sodium/volume status as well), the patient should be studied in the untreated state. Since renin is central to a control system that regulates blood pressure and sodium balance, practically all antihypertensive drugs and diuretics can be expected to affect renin secretion. If patients have been receiving treatment, the drugs should be withheld under supervision of a physician for at least three weeks prior to testing.

Having reviewed the method of renin evaluation that underlies our approach, let us go on to review what we have learned about renin and the hypertensions.

The Renin System in the Hypertensions

By now, the causal involvement of the renin system is well established in malignant hypertension[1, 2] and in primary aldosteronism.[5] These disorders express the polar extremes of oversecretion of the two hormonal limbs of the system: primary renin excess (i.e., angiotensin II) in the former and primary aldosterone excess in the latter. It is noteworthy, in view of a discussion to follow concerning the physiologic effects of hyperreninemia, that primary aldosteronism, in which PRA is suppressed and the hypertension is volume-dependent, is a benign disease, while malignant hypertension, in which PRA and aldosterone are both in excess, is a virulent disorder associated with diffuse necrotizing arteriolitis, uremia, and often, early death.

Renin-sodium profiling is helpful in characterizing both of these disorders. In *malignant hypertension*, the profile establishes the presence and extent of the renin involvement. It also affords a guide to appropriate antirenin treatment in various other renin-induced hypertensive emergencies discussed later. In *primary aldosteronism*, the demonstrations of low PRA, elevated urinary aldosterone, and hypokalemia establish the diagnosis of adrenocortical hypertension and distinguish it from low-renin essential hypertension, in which the latter two findings are absent. One can then go on to distinguish primary from pseudoprimary aldosteronism by testing the rise or fall in plasma aldosterone in response to upright posture.[24]

For some time, it has not been clear whether or not abnormal renin levels contribute to *renovascular hypertension*. Thus, in the recent series of studies of the National Cooperative Study Group, renin measurements were not included in the evaluation. However, recent research makes it evident that here, too, renin involvement is diagnostic. This has resulted from the appreciation of the renin relationship to sodium balance, from improved assay methods, and from a new understanding that patients with unilateral disease have high peripheral renin profiles, whereas those with bilateral renal involvement usually have low or normal circulating renin values.[27-29] These new correlations and concepts have been verified in humans using angiotensin blocking drugs.[9, 30]

If one accepts, as most do, a causal role for renin system derangements in malignant and renovascular hypertension and in primary aldosteronism, and therefore, the basic value of renin profiling for diagnosis and treatment of these disorders,[24] the next step is to consider the involvement of renin in essential hypertension, its etiologic significance, the utility of renin measurements in diagnosis, and the place of anti-renin therapy in management. I shall summarize the evidence for our thesis that the renin system also plays an important role in this group of hypertensive disorders, that the degree of its involvement can be diagnosed by renin-sodium profiling, and that this also provides a strong (but not infallible) prediction of the effect of specific anti-renin or anti-volume therapy. The corollary will also emerge that anti-renin therapy or anti-volume therapy, when indicated, is lesion-specific and to be preferred over the blanket application of volume depletion or vasodilation. The reasons for these preferences will be given.

Differentiation of Essential Hypertension

The first line of evidence for our thesis stems from our definition of a physiologically-related biochemical multiformity in essential hypertension, a description that was made possible by applying renin-sodium profiling to this group of patients according to the methods described above. Thus, Brunner et al., when studying 219 patients in the untreated state, found that about 15 per cent had high, 55 per cent had "normal," and 30 per cent had low plasma renin activity.[31] Many studies the world over have described similar patterns of distribution. The "normal" value, of course, refers to the concentrations shown by normal volunteers and charted on the nomogram previously described. More will be said later concerning the meaning of a "normal" renin value in a hypertensive patient.

We also found in this study that the three renin subgroups differed epidemiologically. As groups, those with high or normal plasma renins exhibited significantly higher incidences of heart attack and stroke than did the low-renin patients.[31] The low-renin patients' relative protection from cardiovascular sequelae seemed even more significant in view of the attendant findings that as a group, they were nine years older, with at least as long a duration of disease, and with an even *higher* average level of blood pressure than the normal-renin patients—all factors that could be presumed to increase their risk of such sequelae.

Based on these findings, we suggested that a relative or absolute renin excess such as that found in the normal-renin and high-renin patients might be vasculotoxic and so predispose these hypertensive patients to cardiovascular injury by virtue of its vasoconstrictor effect or other effects not yet known. Conversely, low-renin hypertensive patients with little or no angiotensin-vasoconstriction appear to have a better prognosis, with a relative protection from stroke or heart attack.

This suggestion has caused some dispute. However, as pointed out in a recent review by Kirkendall et al.,[32] most of those who disagree have not bothered to use the renin-sodium profile, or even an adequately sensitive renin assay, to test the hypothesis. Indeed, only two such studies have even measured urinary sodium excretion, and in these studies, the preponderance of very low values provides almost certain evidence for inadequate urine collections.[33] One such study, in solo counterdiscordance, actually produced the result that low-renin patients are at significantly *greater* risk of heart attack or stroke than normal-renin patients.[34] This study used the only renin assay that employs no angiotensin inhibitor, not even EDTA, a renin method that has since been generally abandoned.

The logic of one objection to our research is worth considering. It is argued that our renin profiles were obtained from untreated patients, while morbidity data were compiled from the experience of treated, and ostensibly controlled, patients, and that, therefore, the baseline renin profile could hardly predict the "natural" history of the disorder in these patients. Actually, this is not correct. These studies were carried out in an era when most patients were likely to have had their hypertension for a longer time before detection. Furthermore, in this era most patients in our clinic at the Presbyterian Hospital were not treated, and in the others, compliance and control were usually not adequate. Moreover, the only therapies generally used at that time were diuretics and reserpine.

A further criticism suggests that the possible epidemiologic differences of blacks have not been taken into account. Although there may be theoretical validity to the charge that our normal values did not include black controls, actually, it is highly doubtful that such an inclusion would have changed the picture; there is little evidence that normotensive blacks have different renin profiles from whites except perhaps in males over age 50. In the same context, it is pointed out that black hypertensive patients have more cardiovascular complications than white patients. This is a true overall statement, but when properly qualified, it supports the prognostic application of renin profiling.[33] The high rate of cardiovascular complications among blacks is known to be concentrated among those under 50 years of age, in whom normal-renin or high-renin hypertension prevails, while the older blacks, who tend to have a more benign and long-standing type of hypertension, are usually characterized by a low renin level.[35] One may also speculate, of course, that the renin profile might change in time, but no one has yet documented crossovers from high-renin to low-renin hypertension. Available evidence suggests that the observed patterns usually tend to persist.

On the other hand, four lines of evidence now appear to be converging in support of the suggestion that low-renin patients are relatively protected from cardiovascular injury.[24, 33] First is the broadly verified observation that low-renin patients are, on the average, actually *more* hypertensive than the normal-renin patients and are also significantly older, by some nine years.[31] Since both greater age and more hypertension both *per se* increase the likelihood of heart attack or stroke, the most likely explanation for the less frequent occurrence of these cardiovascular injuries in low-renin hypertensive patients is that they are relatively protected from cardiovascular damage. The second line of evidence derives from animal studies showing that injections of renin with sodium produce vascular damage in the brain, heart, and kidneys.[5, 24, 36] Third is the recent evidence to be discussed,[8, 9, 30, 43-46] which shows that renin measurements are really a direct measure of its active vasoconstriction. It is such vasoconstriction, with attendant poor tissue perfusion, that we suggest might be critically involved in predisposing to heart attack or stroke. Fourth, a new clinical study has shown that rebound hypertension after withdrawal of angiotensin blockade is associated with marked rebound hyperreninemia and with encephalopathy and coma, even though blood pressure levels do not exceed baseline values.[37] This latter study complements certain phenomena already well known to clinicians. Thus, malignant hypertension with very high renin levels is associated with encephalopathy and with strokes. The same can also occur following acute renal injury, upon the closure of a renal artery graft, or with a renin-secreting tumor.[38] In all, hyperreninemia looms as the likely factor inducing the vascular injury.

Altogether, these findings buttress the proposal[31, 35] that inappropriate renin-induced vasoconstriction exerts an added adverse influence in hypertensive patients.[24] It seems reasonable that this vasoconstriction, directly or indirectly, perhaps by impairing microcirculatory flow and capillary exchange, by inducing hemoconcentration and increased viscosity, or by other unknown effects, renders the hypertensive patient less resistant to cardiovascular damage in the brain, heart, and kidneys. Surely the fact that low-renin patients live longer despite greater hypertension raises the possibility that renin excess is vasculotoxic in some way other than by virtue of the high blood pressure level.[39] Thus, given an equal level of high blood pressure, there is reason to believe that the patient with a high renin level is at greater risk than the one with a low renin level.

The final answer to this important question must come from prospective research in which renin-sodium profiling is properly applied. Whatever the outcome, this biochemical and clinical heterogeneity indicates that essential hypertension is not all alike, and that it possibly can no longer be considered as a single entity either genetically, pathophysiologically, or epidemiologically.

Renin Participation in Essential Hypertension: The Physiologic Evidence

With only the above evidence to go on, the involvement of renin in essential hypertension could perhaps be considered a speculation of academic interest, and renin-sodium profiling a laboratory exercise. Thus, even if malignant hypertension is renin-dependent, the various renin patterns observed among patients with benign essential hypertension might not lead one to question the traditional view that renin has nothing to do with their high blood pressure. This is especially true when one considers that for this group, *lumped together* as one, renin levels bear no relation to the blood pressure levels. Actually, taken absolutely rather than relative to their hypertensive situation, many of these patients exhibit ostensibly "normal" plasma renin values.

However, in view of the powerful pressor actions of angiotensin[40] and of aldosterone, our research group has long believed that this control system must participate in some way in all hypertension. A key question was whether "normal" circulating levels of these hormones are sufficient to contribute to the hypertension. Our own research on this question suggested an affirmative answer, since we were able to demonstrate that the prolonged infusion of angiotensin for up to 11 days, in diminishing amounts that approached "normal" levels, could produce sustained increases in blood pressure in normal people.[40] This hypertension was uniquely dependent on concurrent angiotensin-induced sodium retention and could not be reproduced with norepinephrine.

An important series of clinical investigations has changed traditional thinking on the role of renin in essential hypertension. A giant stride forward was taken in 1972 when Bühler and associates[6] reported the first evidence that plasma renin activity really does contribute to the elevated blood pressure of most patients with essential hypertension. In this study, the degree to which the beta-blocking drug propranolol lowered blood pressure was directly related to the height of the pretreatment plasma renin level and to the degree that the drug reduced that level. Dramatically, this drug alone was often completely effective in lowering blood pressure in patients with malignant hypertension. Beyond this, propranolol alone was partially or completely effective in more than half of an unselected group of 74 patients with essential hypertension, including all high-renin and many "normal"-renin patients. Thus, in the latter group, what had been considered "normal" renin may not really be normal,[1] since their renin secretion should be suppressed by their hypertension (Fig. 1).

Our interpretation has been that the antihypertensive effect of beta-adrenergic blockade is largely a consequence of its suppression of renin, probably by blockade of specific renin-associated adrenergic receptors. This is not a completely accepted idea. Some observers suggest that it may reduce hypertension because it initially reduces cardiac output, which somehow induces a long-term adaptation in the total peripheral resistance. This suggestion does not stand up to the demonstration that the drug reduces cardiac output but not blood pressure in low-renin patients and normotensive subjects. Also, in studying the hemodynamics of various analogs, Frohlich and his co-workers conclude that changes in cardiac output are not essentially involved.[41]

It has been claimed by others that certain beta blockers can reduce hypertension without reducing renin, but more recent studies show that probably all beta blockers do, in fact, rather sharply reduce renin secretion.[42] Two analogs with intrinsic beta-agonist activity, bufuronal and pindolol, may show no renin-lowering effect except under very special circumstances.[42, 51] The literature is still not entirely consistent on this issue, but two of the groups who had failed to show renin suppression during beta blockade have now attributed their early failures to the use of renin assay methods that acid-activate prorenin.[21, 22]

At the same time, the proposition that renin really does participate in maintaining the blood pressure in major fractions of essential hypertension has been confirmed and extended using other drugs that specifically block either the action of angiotensin II (saralasin)[8, 9, 30] or its formation (converting enzyme inhibitor).[43-46] Our experience with the latter agent, which, unlike saralasin, has no intrinsic pressor action, completely parallels and extends the earlier observations with propranolol; the response to both these drugs indicates that a renin factor actively contributes to the hypertension in from 50 to 70 per cent of all patients with essential hypertension.[6, 7, 46]

The parallelism of antihypertensive effectiveness among propranolol, saralasin, and converting enzyme inhibitor strongly suggests that all three block the same mechanism — namely, renin-induced vasoconstriction. The differences in effectiveness reflect differences in the degree of blockade. Saralasin, because of its intrinsic agonism,[44] is effective in the smallest fraction of the essential hypertension population, that 12 to 15 per cent with high renin levels. Propranolol lowers blood pressure in about 50 per cent of patients[6] — all the high-renin and many normal-renin patients, but it does not completely block renin secretion, since it fails to block that secretory component affected by sodium depletion. The converting enzyme inhibitor SQ20881 is the most complete blocker, lowering blood pressure in up to 70 per cent of patients with essential hypertension.

Altogether, these studies with three different types of renin-system blockers establish that with a proper baseline plasma renin measurement, the extent of each of their blood pressure–lowering responses can be predicted. Accordingly, the renin level *per se* is a valid indicator of the extent of active renin vasoconstriction, while the 24-hour urinary sodium measurement defines the appropriateness of the vasoconstriction for fluid volume status of the patient.

Perhaps of equal interest conceptually is that other 30 per cent of patients with essential hypertension who have subnormal renin values and in whom all three anti-renin system drugs are ineffective. In this low-renin subgroup, diuretic treatment by itself is uniquely effective, suggesting that their high blood pressure is instead predominantly volume-dependent.[47]

Confirmations

An impressive body of research has been accumulated that confirms and further characterizes the differing response patterns of hypertensive patients within the renin subgroups to beta blockade as opposed to diuretic therapy. These studies to date are listed in Table 1.

That propranolol and other beta blockers sharply reduce renin secretion, that this is a likely major factor in lowering the blood pressure, and that baseline renin profiles are in turn highly predictive of the antihypertensive response have been widely confirmed (Table 1). The predictive value of the baseline renin profile and the unresponsiveness of low-renin patients to propranolol have been reaffirmed and extended in studies using propranolol,[48–51] acebutolol,[52] atenolol,[53, 54] and either intravenous propranolol or pindolol.[55] This pattern has also been shown in pediatric patients,[56] and MacGregor and Dawes have shown that control plasma angiotensin II levels also predict response to propranolol or spironolactone.[57] An important study by Pettinger and Mitchell[58] has demonstrated overlap effectiveness be-

Table 1.   *The Selective Effectiveness of Antihypertensive Drugs*

BETA BLOCKERS ARE PREFERENTIALLY EFFECTIVE IN HIGH- AND NORMAL-RENIN PATIENTS	DIURETICS ARE PREFERENTIALLY EFFECTIVE IN LOW-RENIN PATIENTS
Bühler et al, N Engl J Med 287:1209, 1972	Crane et al, Am J Med Sci 260:311, 1970
Bühler et al, Am J Cardiol 32:511, 1973	Spark et al, Ann Intern Med 75:831, 1971
Bühler et al, Am J Cardiol 36:652, 1975	Crane et al, Am J Med 52:457, 1972
Castenfors et al, Acta Med Scand 193:189, 1973	Carey et al, Arch Intern Med 130:849, 1972
Pettinger et al, N Engl J Med 292:1214, 1975	Adlin et al, Arch Intern Med 130:855, 1972
Karlberg et al, Am J Cardiol 27:642, 1976	Vaughan et al, Am J Cardiol 32:523, 1973
Hollifield et al, N Engl J Med 295:68, 1976	Castenfors et al, Acta Med Scand 193:189, 1973
Weidmann et al, Klin Wochenschr 54:765, 1976	Distler et al, Dtsch Med Wochenschr 99:864, 1974
Menard et al, Am J Med 60:886, 1976	Douglas et al, JAMA 227:518, 1974
Stumpe et al, Am J Med 60:853, 1976	Karlberg et al, Am J Cardiol 37:642, 1976
MacGregor et al, Clin Sci Mol Med 50:18p, 1976	MacGregor et al, Clin Sci Mol Med 50:18p, 1976
Boerth, Pediatr Res 10:328, 1976	
Moore et al, Lancet 2:67, 1976	
Bahr et al, Clin Pharm Ther 20:130, 1976	
Zech et al, Postgrad Med J 53(Suppl III):134, 1977	
Philipp et al, Dtsch Med Wochenschr 102:569, 1977	

BETA BLOCKERS CAN ACTUALLY RAISE PRESSURE IN LOW-RENIN PATIENTS	DIURETICS CAN ACTUALLY RAISE PRESSURE IN HIGH-RENIN PATIENTS
Drayer et al, Am J Med 60:897, 1976	Baer et al, Ann Intern Med 86:257, 1977

tween propranolol and saralasin in the same patients, while still other studies[59] have even related the degree of benefit of adding propranolol to a diuretic regimen to its renin-lowering action. (This latter relationship is more difficult to demonstrate since, as discussed, beta blockade does not block that component of renin secretion activated by sodium depletion.)

On the opposite side of the coin too (Table 1), the worldwide experience to date[47, 60-66] clearly indicates that diuretic therapy works on the end of the spectrum opposite from that influenced by beta blockade (volume rather than vasoconstriction). Low-renin patients respond best, normal-renin patients exhibit an intermediate response, and high-renin patients exhibit the poorest antihypertensive response to diruresis. Indeed, in the latter group, often already vasoconstricted to the point of dehydration and azotemia, diuretic therapy can actually be contraindicated,[67] since it could further impair central blood volume microcirculatory flow and organ perfusion.

An additional support to this scheme is the reciprocal effects, also shown in Table 1, which reinforce these basic pharmacologic relationships; not only is propranolol usually ineffective in low-renin patients, but, like saralasin, it can be overtly *pressor* in them.[66] Furthermore, diuretics, uniquely effective in low-renin patients, can actually be *pressor* in the high-renin patients.[69] Presumably, these already vasoconstricted and hypovolemic patients react to more dehydration with an overshoot renin response. The renin-volume interplay appears as a seesaw. Some patients given diuretics respond with vigorous hyperreninemia, explaining the failure of their blood pressure to fall.[43] Conversely, patients given anti-renin agents may not respond because of reactive sodium retention. Altogether, these results are the scientific underpinning opening the door to a new era of predictable and selective drug therapy for essential hypertension.

The Role of the Renin System in Renovascular and Renal Hypertensions

A parallel series of investigations, in which we used angiotensin blockade in both animal and human forms of renovascular hypertension, has revealed that the same two pressor mechanisms are operative (renin excess and sodium-volume excess).[27] Patients with bilateral renal disease[27-29] and their animal counterparts[70-72] have normal or low renin profiles and do not respond to angiotensin blockade, while those with unilateral renovascular disease have high renin profiles and respond to angiotensin blockade. Accordingly, the peripheral renin profile becomes the basic screening test for surgically curable renovascular hypertension with unilateral hypersecretion of renin (1) because it is a direct measure of renin secretion;[28] (2) because most cured patients have high renin profiles, and none are low;[29] and (3) because the circulating plasma renin level predicts the response to angiotensin blockade.[8, 9, 30, 43-46] The diagnosis is then established by a renal-vein renin study, using a mathematical analysis[29] in order to show that renin hypersecretion is (1) unilateral and (2) accompanied by ipsilateral ischemia and (3) by the absence of contralateral renin secretion; all three criteria are valuable for predicting surgical cure.[27, 29] In this new clinical approach, only after the peripheral-vein and then renal-vein renin studies are done, and when surgery seems a likely possibility on clinical grounds, do the more invasive, more costly, and less specific tests of intravenous pyelography and renal arteriography become necessary.

The Vasoconstriction-Volume Hypothesis

Based on these clinical and animal studies, we have constructed a hypothesis to analyze, understand, and treat all types of hypertension.[67] In this hypothesis, hypertension is viewed as a spectrum ranging between a predominant excess of either vasoconstriction or "effective" volume (the volume between the aortic valve and the capillaries), with intermediate forms exhibiting inappropriate excess of one relative to the other (Fig. 3). Malignant hypertension and primary aldosteronism are the polar extremes of the spectrum. They are due *largely* to excess renin-vasoconstriction or to excess volume, respectively, and are totally correctable by elimination of the excess. Other common clinical entities fall at intermediate points within the spectrum (Fig. 3), as identified by the renin profile.[24]

Our analytic model has been contested; but the fact is that one of the

THE VASOCONSTRICTION-VOLUME SPECTRUM IN HYPERTENSION

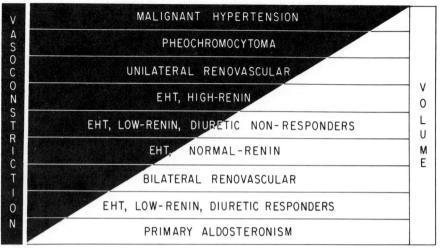

Figure 3. The vasoconstriction-volume spectrum that is hypertension. EHT = essential hypertension. (From: Laragh JH, Letcher RL, Pickering TG: Renin profiling for modern diagnosis and treatment of hypertension. JAMA *241*:151–156, 1979.)

patterns can be demonstrated in all hypertensive patients by renin profiling and can be verified and quantified by administration of anti-renin or volume-reducing agents.[73] Moreover, those unusual patients whose hypertension does not respond as expected are picked out by the vasoconstriction-volume analytical model as likely to have another type of vasoconstrictor hypertension, such as that due to a pheochromocytoma.[24] The practical advantage of this bipolar model is that by exposing mechanisms, it suggests more precise and predictably effective drug therapies for a majority of patients.

The exceptions exposed by the model are worth an illustration. For some time, we have pointed out that low-renin patients are heterogeneous[74] and that the renin profile does not predict successful therapy in a third or so of the low-renin patients.[47] The analytic model actually exposes a subgroup of the low-renin group in whom, after volume and renin are excluded, the presence of another pressor agent (that suppresses renin) is a likely possibility.

The vasoconstriction-volume analytic model predicts that low-renin hypertension is due to a relative volume excess causing the suppression of renin secretion, whereas high-renin patients demonstrate instead a predominance of renin-vasoconstriction and relative hypovolemia.[67] Accordingly, *for an equal degree of hypertension,* high-renin patients would be expected to exhibit a higher peripheral resistance and a lower blood volume than low-renin patients, and for an equal degree of total peripheral resistance, low-renin patients will have a greater effective blood volume than high-renin patients. Thus, low-renin patients are less vasoconstricted (or comparatively vasodilated) and presumably have a greater microcirculatory flow. Since cardiac output may be closely related to the critical volume, the model also suggests that for an equal cardiac output, high-renin patients will have more hypertension.

We need more hard data to characterize the hemodynamic and extracellular fluid volume status of patients within different renin subgroups. It is known that plasma volume, for example, is usually lower in hypertensive people than in normotensive people.[75-81] Therefore, it is important to compare patients with similar hypertension but different renin profiles. Meanwhile, it is of interest to note that all available published results of space measurements (Table 2) are in keeping with what the vasoconstriction volume model suggests[67] — namely that low-renin patients are relatively hemodiluted and have expanded blood volumes. They have lower blood urea,[35] hematocrit, and hemoglobin values, and their total and central blood volumes, cardiac output values,[82] and extracellular fluid volumes are, almost without exception, at least as high as or higher than those of normal-renin patients (Table 2).[77, 79, 83] The converse is also true. Whenever hypervolemia is present, renin values are considerably reduced.[75] Thus, all the published data support the concept that low-renin patients tend to be hypervolemic and are never hypovolemic.

Moreover, these consistent trends have emerged even though many of the tabulated studies (Table 2) were performed with more primitive renin methods and the blood volume measurements, too, often were not done with the most precise method. More research is needed that compares high-renin patients with low-renin patients at similar sodium intakes, especially in light of errors inherent in space measurements and since the critical arterial volume is an unmeasurable fraction of total blood volume. Actually, to date, only the study by Weidmann et al.[81] (Table 2) has done this and also used a renin method that reliably separates low from high renin values.

Criticism of the Hypothesis

The validity of our observations and the effectiveness of our approach have been questioned, at times sharply, by a few investigators or reviewers, particularly in its application to essential hypertension. Such critics cling to the dated view that renin usually has little or nothing to do with high blood pressure and prefer the trial-and-error treatment methods of the past.

This criticism ignores the mass of published evidence that describes the renin dependency of high-renin and normal-renin patients and the volume dependency of low-renin patients (Table 1), and it also ignores the existence of numerous confirmatory studies using specific angiotensin-blocking drugs.[8, 9, 30, 43-46]

Part of the disagreement or confusion about the role of renin arises from conflicting results flawed by procedural or methodologic problems.[24] The nature of the renin-sodium interaction being what it is, as indicated already, studies must be discounted that do not relate renin levels to an index of sodium balance or that do not evaluate the postural stimulus in ambulatory patients, as must studies that use renin assay methods that yield inaccurate results because they fail to control pH between 5.5 and 6.0 or fail to use DFP or PMSF to inhibit angiotensinases during incubation.

Another basis for disagreement or confusion about the role of renin is those conflicting results based purely on procedural problems. An example is the study by Woods et al.,[84] which, contradicting an almost unanimous experience, found that propranolol was virtually ineffective as an antihypertensive

Table 2.   *Body Fluid Volumes in Essential Hypertension*

	N	LOW-RENIN GROUP	N	NORMAL-RENIN GROUP	p
A. PLASMA VOLUME					
1. Helmer et al, Circulation 38:965, 1968	8	117%*	12	104%*	NS
2. Jose et al, Ann Intern Med 72:9, 1970	5	1.53 L/M²	7	1.28 L/M²	>0.05
3. Woods et al, Arch Intern Med 123:366, 1969	9	31 ml/kg	5	30 ml/kg	NS
4. Schalekamp et al, Lancet 2:308, 1974	17	2.7 L/1.73 M²	38	2.65 L/1.73 M²	NS
5. Distler et al, Research on Steroids, North Holland-Elsevier, 1975	17	1.71 L/M²	17	1.57 L/M²	<0.025
6. Tarazi, Circ Res 38(Suppl II):II-73, 1976	13	33.4 ml/cm⁺	26	26.2 ml/cm⁺	<0.001
7. Weidmann et al, Am J Med 62:209, 1977	15	110%*	48 (8) (high-renin patients)	102%* (92%)	<0.05 (<0.02)
B. EXTRACELLULAR FLUID VOLUME					
1. Jose et al, Arch Intern Med 123:141, 1969	11	9.6 L/M²	36	9.5 L/M²	NS
2. Jose et al, Ann Intern Med 72:9, 1970	6	9.6 L/M²	7	7.7 L/M²	<0.01
3. Schalekamp et al, Lancet 2:310, 1974	12	11.2 L/1.73 M²	29	11.1 L/1.73 M²	NS
C. EXCHANGEABLE SODIUM					
1. Woods et al, Arch Intern Med 123:366, 1969	9	37.9 mEq/kg	5	32.3 mEq/kg	<0.05
2. Lebel et al, Lancet 2:308, 1974	12	95%*	33	98%*	NS
3. Distler et al, Research on Steroids, North Holland-Elsevier, 1975	18	1609 mEq/M²	15	1549 mEq/M²	NS
4. Padfield et al, Lancet 1:548, 1975	23	101%*	42	98%*	NS

*Figures given expressed as % normal control.
⁺Figure given is total blood volume calculated from plasma volume.

agent and, just as discordantly, that a diuretic was equally effective in both low-renin and normal-renin patients. Undoubtedly, most of these patients really had low-renin hypertension and were misclassified by the renin assay and data-analysis procedures.[84] Actually, anomalous reports like this allow one to appreciate how the great value of propranolol in high-renin and normal-renin patients might be obscured or missed if most patients have low renin levels or if positive results are averaged together with its lack of effect in the low-renin group.

The New, Integrated Plan for Diagnosis and Treatment

Based on these research findings, we believe that the renin profile has four clinical applications: (1) definitive diagnosis of surgically curable renovascular hypertension: (2) definitive diagnosis of adrenocortical hypertension; (3) acquisition of baseline information for planning simpler, more specific, and predictable therapy; and (4) evaluation of the pace, severity, and prognosis of the underlying disorder. These four applications become mutually reinforcing when used as the matrix of a complete system for diagnosis and treatment. If renin profiling is not available, the new system can be applied empirically,[24, 73] but having the renin profile in hand allows much greater speed and precision. The plan itself illustrates the coherence of the analytic model and demonstrates a well-directed passage through the complicated maze of hypertensive phenomena.

The new method, which is outlined in Figure 4, is for patients who have significant, sustained hypertension and are clearly in need of therapy. A simple, but extremely important, primary screening step is the establishment of normokalemia or hypokalemia (<3.5 mEq/L), because it is unnecessary to pursue adrenocortical causes in patients who are normokalemic. For normokalemic patients over age 60, a trial of diuretic therapy alone may be undertaken without any further tests, since with increasing age, diuretic-responsive low-renin hypertension becomes more common, while the surgical curability of renovascular hypertension diminishes. If a diuretic trial fails, the drug is stopped, and the patient is returned to the basic plan.

For the majority of patients, the baseline renin profile guides further diagnostic work-up. Patients with high renin profiles are prime candidates for procedures to exclude surgically curable renovascular hypertension. This route is especially recommended if the hypertension is severe, of recent onset, occurs in a younger person, or is accompanied by a bruit or hypokalemia. A positive response to either propranolol or to an angiotensin-blocking drug points to a renin excess but provides no information about its lateralization. In these circumstances, the definitive test is a renal-vein renin study, using three renin samples and a mathematical analysis to demonstrate whether or not *all* of the renin is being secreted from the suspect side and *none* from the contralateral kidney and to evaluate renal ischemia.[24, 27-29] The more invasive, expensive tests — intravenous pyelography and renal arteriography — are thus reserved for patients likely to require surgery.

Patients with low renin profiles and hypokalemia are evaluated for the

A FLOW SHEET FOR DIAGNOSIS AND TREATMENT OF HYPERTENSION

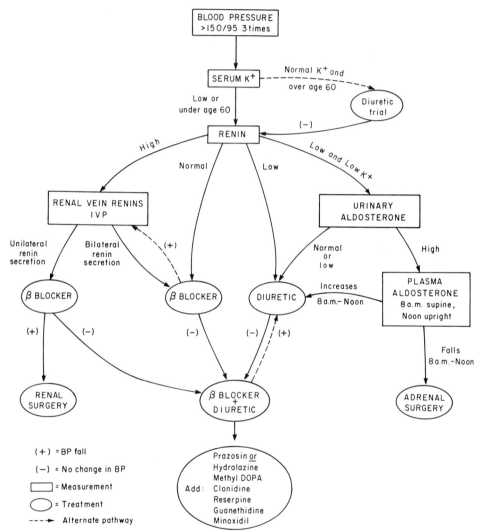

Figure 4. Normokalemic patients over 60 may be first tried on diuretics because of the higher prevalence of low-renin hypertension in this group. Low-renin patients with hypokalemia (serum K+ <3.5) are evaluated for adrenocortical disease and high-renin patients for renovascular disease. A mathematical analysis of the renal vein renins indicates ipsilateral hypersecretion with ischemia and no secretion contralaterally.[4, 18, 23] Surgically noncurable patients return to the basic treatment program. Normal- and high-renin patients are started on beta-blocker and low-renin patients on a diuretic. If either course is only partly corrective, the two are combined. Altogether, this normalizes about 85 per cent of patients. Unlike "stepped care," drug subtraction and dose reduction are performed whenever pressure is normalized, to achieve fewest drugs in smallest doses. Only for the small residual resistant group are other, less palatable drugs superimposed in traditional trial-and-error fashion.

surgically curable adrenocortical causes, primary and pseudoprimary aldosteronism. Details of this diagnostic process have been published[24] (Table 1). If this work-up is negative, the patients are treated with the normokalemic low-renin group.

For the remainder of patients, the treatment plan is determined by the baseline renin profile. The first step in treatment for both high-renin and "normal"-renin patients is the administration of a beta-blocking drug to reduce renin secretion. Low-renin patients are treated first with a diuretic. For many patients in each subgroup, such single-drug therapy is the only treatment needed.

A positive response to propranolol alone becomes another indication for renal vein studies in those who had bypassed this test. Conversely, the lack of a full response to either a beta blocker or to a diuretic alone is followed by a trial of the two agents together. In our experience, either single-drug therapy or the combination of the two types fully controls some 85 per cent of patients.[24, 73] Those on combined treatment are subjected to a trial subtraction of the first drug and a dose reduction trial. Contrary to the "stepped care" approach, the aim is to maintain the patient on the fewest number of drugs in the smallest effective dose.

The average effective dosage for propranolol, the first beta blocker available in the United States, seems to be 40 mg q.i.d. or 80 mg b.i.d. For metoprolol, 50 mg b.i.d. is about as effective as 40 mg b.i.d. of propranolol. For diuretic therapy, we employ either hydrochlorothiazide, 25 mg b.i.d., or chlorthalidone, 50 mg once daily, to start and then double the dose if necessary. Other sulfonamides, spironolactone, or triamterene are reasonable alternatives, the latter two when hypokalemia becomes a problem. Details of these alternatives have been discussed.[73]

The clinician should be alert to those uncommon circumstances in which propranolol may be contraindicated, especially if renin profiling is not available. These include some patients over age 60, in whom low-renin hypertension is more common, and patients with a history of asthma, congestive heart failure, undue bradycardia, or peripheral vascular disease. In these cases, treatment should begin with a diuretic.

In about 10 to 15 per cent of patients, hypertension cannot be controlled fully by specific anti-renin or volume-reducing therapy or by a combination of the two. For this more refractory group, the clinician must revert to the classic trial-and-error approach and add serially such drugs as hydralazine, prazosin, clonidine, methyldopa, reserpine, or guanethidine until full control is achieved. Here, too, we recommend that after control is secured, serial subtraction and dose reduction be tried to establish a regimen for the long term, based on the minimum number of drugs in their lowest effective dosage.[24, 73]

Clinical Illuminations and Rewards

The new system enables both the clinician and the patient to reap advantages and satisfactions. Especially rewarding is the frequent total long-term control of high-renin and many normal-renin patients with nothing but a beta blocker, and sometimes in surprisingly small doses. In the traditional "stepped care" treatment, this sizable fraction of the essential hypertension population would be started on a diuretic and would likely exhibit a poor or no blood pressure response, compounded by a now much higher renin. We suspect that acceleration of this type of hypertension can actually be induced by such therapy. Then drugs such as methyldopa, reserpine, vasodilators, or guanethidine would be added. The patient could wind up with only partial blood pressure correction, dehydrated and weak, and possibly with impaired mentation, hypokalemia, and impotence.

In our system, such a patient would have perhaps a 75 per cent chance of responding to a beta blocker alone, without side effects, and with the possible bonus of cardioprotection.[73] Addition of a diuretic would then correct most of the rest. At the low-renin end of the spectrum, too, our method leads to the direct control of patients on a diuretic alone, again sometimes in surprisingly low doses.

The system permits more precise diagnosis over the entire range of hypertension. Consider the not uncommon younger patient with severe hypertension of recent onset who exhibits a greater than 2:1 renin ratio on renal vein study and has a positive arteriogram. If a preliminary renin profile is not obtained to establish peripheral hypersecretion[27] or if an inferior vena caval sample is not collected with the renal vein samples,[28] the lack of complete suppression of renin secretion in the contralateral kidney can be missed, and needless surgery might be performed.[29]

For another example, consider two clinically similar patients, each with a blood pressure of 220/120 mm Hg, one with a low renin-sodium profile and the other with a very high renin-sodium profile. Without reason to think otherwise, the clinician should certainly feel differently about these two patients in terms of the pace and severity of their disorder and, therefore, about the urgency and direction of their work-up and treatment.[9, 24, 25, 32, 33]

The new framework also prepares clinicians to understand and treat promptly more urgent hypertensive phenomena. A recent study described saralasin withdrawal that triggered marked rebound hyperreninemia and hypertension accompanied by encephalopathy and coma.[37] This description retraces the fulminant vascular events observed with high renin levels in acute or malignant hypertension, in instances of renal injury, following closure of a renal artery graft, or with renin-secreting tumors.[38] In all these, acute hyperreninemia looms as the culprit. Its early identification or exclusion allows better care of the acutely ill patient, especially if one considers that here, too, often when anti-renin therapy is appropriate, diuretic therapy is contraindicated, and vice versa.

Altogether then, this rational new system assures complete diagnosis and more precisely targeted treatment. It entails fewer drugs, lower costs, and fewer disturbances of physical or mental function. This means greater patient compliance and better results.

Conclusion

If one accepts the evidence that all essential hypertension is not alike biochemically, physiologically, or epidemiologically, it is only reasonable that the condition not be strait-jacketed into unimodular treatment systems.

The evolution of renin-sodium profiling, which demonstrates that essential hypertension is, in fact, a heterogenous disorder with pathophysiologic correlates, led us to construct the all-encompassing vasoconstriction-volume hypothesis to analyze and treat hypertension. In this model, all hypertension is viewed as a spectrum in which degrees of excess vasoconstriction or volume are involved in pathogenesis. Renin profiling exposes the degree of these involvements, and so leads to a more logical course of therapy. The evidence developed from profiling and from the use of renin system blocking drugs for the active participation of a renin factor in major fractions of the essential hypertension population and for the reciprocal participation of a sodium-volume excess in a lesser but large fraction is now beyond reasonable doubt.

Any clinician who has used this analytic model for understanding and treating blood pressure cannot help but be impressed by its workability, its simplicity, its coherence, and its receptivity to new information. The model is successful most of the time, and the clinical payoffs are impressive. Undoubtedly, it will be improved and more richly informed as other vasoconstrictor mechanisms are identified and fitted into the framework.

No matter what the criticism of the hypothesis, one also has to be impressed by the high success rate in treating that 70 per cent of essential hypertensive patients with high renin or normal renin profiles, sometimes with as little as 20 mg propranolol twice a day, and often without the need for a second drug. The specificity and freedom from side effects can be remarkable. There is no volume depletion with its untoward effects on plasma viscosity and uric acid, cholesterol,[85] and renin levels; the myocardium is protected, and hypokalemia and diabetes are avoided. At the same time, similar single-drug therapy with a diuretic, selected for low-renin patients, produces an equally satisfied and physiologically corrected patient, since in this group, diuresis corrects a postulated volume excess. Accordingly, the new system offers, for major fractions of all hypertensive patients, for the long-term or lifetime commitment, therapy with one drug instead of two, or two instead of three or more, with the attraction that the right drug is given to contain the physiologic lesion, i.e., anti-renin therapy or anti-volume therapy as revealed by the renin profile.

The physician armed with this analytic approach will find that he achieves a complete diagnosis while also reaching effective therapy more quickly, not only with the use of fewer drugs and with more compliant patients who experience fewer reactive aberrations and side effects, but also with a sense of order and control not afforded by the traditional trial-and-error methods. Accordingly, until better approaches are developed, it seems unlikely that informed physicians will continue to prefer empiricism to the order that can be gained by the application of a simple, now reliable, and non-invasive blood and urine test, especially when this approach, at the same time, reduces the need for and aids in selection of patients for the invasive tests of pyelography and arteriography.

One or two pieces of circumstantial evidence can serve only to alert the investigator; but when the evidence mounts from all directions, fitting together the entire picture, in jigsaw fashion, it is time to act. Such evidence comes from classification by renin-sodium profiling, the experiences with malignant hypertension and renovascular and adrenocortical hypertensions, the correlations provided by pharmacologic probes in essential hypertension, and — importantly — the clinical experience in *all* the hypertensions. The system hangs together; it is coherent. The diagnosis and treatment of hypertension can never be the same as it was.

The recent development and clinical trials of an orally active converting enzyme inhibitor (Captopril) verify[86, 87] over the long term what was previously demonstrated with propranolol, saralasin, and the intravenous converting enzyme inhibitor. The broad effectiveness of this drug is closely related to the control renin levels. This new pharmacologic approach adds a practical dimension for diagnosis and specific treatment of the renin factor in human hypertension.

Summary

Recent research has revealed and delineated the role of the renin-angiotensin-aldosterone axis for maintaining or causing high blood pressure in the majority of patients and has demonstrated anew that renin-sodium profiling defines this involvement. Performed along with a serum potassium measurement, this now simple and reliable test is useful for primary screening and then, in conjunction with renal-vein renin studies or an aldosterone profile, for the definitive diagnosis or exclusion of surgically curable forms of renovascular or adrenocortical hypertension. For the remaining majority of hypertensive patients, renin profiling helps define the relative participation of vasoconstriction and volume factors, and thus guides simpler, more specific, and more predictable anti-renin or anti-volume treatments. In particular, renin profiling picks out those hypertensive patients who should be started with a beta blocker or a newer anti-renin drug (e.g., Captopril), as opposed to a diuretic, and it also provides baseline information about the pace, severity, and prognosis of the disease in individual patients.

References

1. Laragh JH, Ulick S, Januszewics V, Deming QB, Kelly WG, and Lieberman S: Aldosterone secretion and primary and malignant hypertension. J Clin Invest 39:1091–1106, 1960.
2. Laragh JH, Angers M, Kelly WG, and Lieberman S: Hypotensive agents and pressor substances: the effect of epinephrine, norepinephrine, angiotensin II and others on the secretory rate of aldosterone in man. JAMA 174:234–240, 1960.
3. Laragh JH: The role of aldosterone in man: evidence for regulation of electrolyte balance and arterial pressure by renal-adrenal system which may be involved in malignant hypertension. JAMA 174:293–295, 1960.
4. Kahn JR, Skeggs LT Jr, Shumway NP, and Wisenbaugh PE: Assay of hypertension from arterial blood of normotensive and hypertensive human beings. J Exp Med 95:523–529, 1952.
5. Laragh JH, Baer L, Brunner HR, Bühler FR, Sealey JE, and Vaughan ED Jr: Renin, angiotensin and aldosterone system in pathogenesis and management of hypertensive vascular disease. Am J Med 52:633–652, 1972.
6. Bühler FR, Laragh JH, Baer L, Vaughan ED Jr, and Brunner HR: Propranolol inhibition of renin secretion: a specific approach to diagnosis and treatment of renin-dependent hypertensive diseases. N Engl J Med 287:1209–1214, 1972.

7. Bühler FR, Laragh JH, Vaughan ED Jr, Brunner HR, Gavras H, and Baer L: Antihypertensive action of propranolol: specific anti-renin responses in high and normal renin forms of essential, renal, renovascular and malignant hypertension. Am J Cardiol 32:511–522, 1973.
8. Brunner HR, Gavras H, and Laragh JH: Angiotensin II blockade in man by Sar¹-ala⁸-angiotensin II for understanding and treatment of high blood pressure. Lancet 2:1045–1048, 1973.
9. Brunner HR, Gavras H, Laragh JH, and Keenan R: Hypertension in man: exposure of the renin and sodium components using angiotension II blockade. Circ Res 34(Suppl I): I-35–I-45, 1974.
10. Sealey JE, Gerten-Banes J, and Laragh JH: The renin system: variations in man measured by radioimmunoassay or bioassay. Kidney Int 1:240–253, 1972.
11. Sealey JE, and Laragh JH: Radioimmunoassay of plasma renin activity. Semin Nucl Med 5:189–202, 1975.
12. Sealey JE, and Laragh JH: How to do a plasma renin assay. Cardiovasc Med 2:1079–1092, 1977.
13. Pickens PT, Bumpus F, Merlin F, Lloyd AM, Smeby RR, and Page IH: Measurement of renin activity in human plasma. Circ Res 17:438–448, 1965.
14. Goodfriend TL: Radioimmunoassay of angiotensins and renin activity. In Berson SA, and Yalow RS (eds): Methods in Investigative and Diagnostic Endocrinology. Amsterdam, Elsevier, 1973, Vol 2B, pp 1158–1168.
15. Haber E, Koerner T, Page LB, and Kliman B: Application of a radioimmunoassay for angiotensin I to the physiologic measurements of plasma renin activity in normal human subjects. J Clin Endocrinol Metab 29:1349–1355, 1969.
16. Sealey JE, and Laragh JH: Searching out low renin patients. Limitations of some commonly used methods. Am J Med 55:303–314, 1973.
17. Brown JJ, Davies DL, Lever AF, Robertson JIS, and Tree M: The estimation of renin in human plasma. Biochem J 93:594–600, 1964.
18. Skinner SL: Improved assay methods for renin concentration and activity in human plasma: methods using selective denaturation of renin substrate. Circ Res 20:391–402, 1967.
19. Lumbers ER: Activation of renin in human amniotic fluid by low pH. Enzymologia 40:329–336, 1971.
20. Sealey JE, Moon C, Laragh JH, and Atlas SA: Plasma prorenin measurements in normal, hypertensive, and anephric subjects and its effect on renin measurements. Circ Res 40(Suppl I):I-41–I-45, 1977.
21. Amery A, Lijnen P, Fagard R, and Reybrouck T: Inactive renin in human plasma. Lancet 2:849, 1976.
22. Derkx FHM, v Gool JMG, Wenting GJ, et al: Inactive renin in human plasma. Lancet 2:496–499, 1976.
23. Laragh JH, Sealey JE, and Sommers SC: Patterns of adrenal secretion and urinary excretion of aldosterone and plasma renin activity in normal and hypertensive subjects. Circ Res 18(Suppl I):I-158–I-174, 1966.
24. Laragh JH, and Sealey JE: Renin-sodium profiling: How, when and why in clinical practice. Cardiovasc Med 2:1053–1075, 1977.
25. Guyton AC, Coleman TG, Cowley AW Jr, Scheel KW, Manning RD Jr, and Norman RA Jr: Arterial pressure regulation. Overriding dominance of the kidneys in long-term regulation and in hypertension. In Laragh JH (ed): Hypertension Manual. New York, Dun-Donnelley, 1974, pp 111–134.
26. Sealey JE, Bühler FR, Laragh JH, Manning EL, and Brunner HR: Aldosterone excretion: physiologic variations in man measured by radioimmunoassay or double isotope dilution. Circ Res 31:367–378, 1972.
27. Laragh JH, Sealey JE, Bühler FR, Vaughan ED Jr, Brunner HR, Gavras H, and Baer L: The renin axis and vasoconstriction volume analysis for understanding and treating renovascular and renal hypertension. Am J Med 58:4–13, 1975.
28. Sealey JE, Bühler FR, Laragh JH, and Vaughan ED Jr: The physiology of renin secretion in essential hypertension: estimation of renin secretion rate and renal plasma flow from peripheral and renal vein renin levels. Am J Med 55:391–401, 1973.
29. Vaughan ED Jr, Bühler FR, Laragh JH, Sealey JE, Baer L, and Bard RH: Renovascular hypertension: renin measurements to indicate hypersecretion, and contralateral suppression, estimate renal plasma flow and score for surgical curability. Am J Med 55:402–414, 1973.
30. Streeten DHP, Anderson GH, Freiburg JM, et al: Use of an angiotensin II antagonist (saralasin) in the recognition of "angiotensinogenic" hypertension. N Engl J Med 292:657–662, 1975.

31. Brunner HR, Laragh JH, Baer L, Newton MA, Goodwin FT, Krakoff LR, Bard RH, and Bühler FR: Essential hypertension: renin and aldosterone, heart attack and stroke. N Engl J Med 286:441–449, 1972.
32. Kirkendall WN, Hammond JJ, and Overturf ML: Renin as a predictor of hypertensive complications. Ann NY Acad Sci 304:147–160, 1978.
33. Laragh JH: Renin as a predictor of hypertensive complications: discussion. Ann NY Acad Sci 304:165–177, 1978.
34. Gulati SC, Adlin EV, Biddle CM, et al: The occurrences of vascular complications in low renin hypertension (abstr). Ann Intern Med 78:828, 1973.
35. Brunner HR, Sealey JE, and Laragh JH: Renin as a risk factor in essential hypertension: more evidence. Am J Med 55:295–302, 1973.
36. Gavras H, Brunner HR, and Laragh JH: Renin and aldosterone and the pathogenesis of hypertensive vascular damage. Prog Cardiovasc Dis 17:39–49, 1974.
37. Keim HJ, Drayer JI, Case DB, Lopez-Ovejero JA, Wallace JM, and Laragh JH: A role for renin in rebound hypertension and encephalopathy after infusion of Sar^1-ala^8-angiotensin II. N Engl J Med 295:1175–1177, 1976.
38. Orjavik OS, Aas M, Fauchold P, et al: Renin secreting tumors with severe hypertension. Acta Med Scand 197:329–336, 1975.
39. Möhring J: Editorial: Controversy in clinical science. The case for humoral factors as well as pressure, and high arterial pressure versus humoral factors in the pathogenesis of the vascular lesions of malignant hypertension. Clin Sci Mol Med 52:111–117, 1977.
40. Ames RP, Borkowski AJ, Sicinski AM, and Laragh JH: Prolonged infusions of angiotensin II and norepinephrine and blood pressure, electrolyte balance, aldosterone and cortisol secretion in normal man and in cirrhosis with ascites. J Clin Invest 44:1171–1186, 1965.
41. Frohlich ED, Dunn FG, and Chrysant SG: Beta blocking agents: Nonessentiality of cardiac output (CO) in antihypertensive action (abstr.). Circulation 52(Suppl II):II-184, 1975.
42. Bühler FR, Burkhart F, and Lütold BE: Antihypertensive beta blocking action as related to renin and age. A pharmacologic tool to identify pathogenic mechanisms in essential hypertension. Am J Cardiol 38:653–669, 1975.
43. Gavras H, Brunner HR, Laragh JH, Sealey JE, Gavras I, and Vukovitch RA: An angiotensin converting enzyme inhibitor to identify and treat vasoconstrictor and volume factors in hypertensive patients. N Engl J Med 291:817–821, 1974.
44. Case DB, Wallace JM, Keim JH, Sealey JE, and Laragh JH: Usefulness and limitations of saralasin, a partial competitive agonist of angiotensin II, for evaluating the renin and sodium factors in hypertensive patients. Am J Med 60:825–836, 1976.
45. Case DB, Wallace JM, Keim JH, Weber MA, Drayer JI, White RP, Sealey JE, and Laragh JH: Estimating renin participation in hypertension: superiority of converting enzyme inhibitor over saralasin. Am J Med 61:790–796, 1976.
46. Case DB, Wallace JM, Keim JH, Weber MA, Sealey JE, and Laragh JH: Possible role of renin in hypertension as suggested by renin-sodium profiling and inhibition of converting enzyme. N Engl J Med 296:641–656, 1977.
47. Vaughan ED Jr, Laragh JH, Gavras I, et al: The volume factor in low and normal renin essential hypertension: its treatment with either spironolactone or chlorthalidone. Am J Cardiol 32:523–532, 1973.
48. Bühler FR, Burkhart F, and Lütold BE: Antihypertensive beta blocking action as related to renin and age: A pharmacologic tool to identify pathogenic mechanisms in essential hypertension. Am J Cardiol 38:653–669, 1975.
49. Karlberg BE, Kagedal B, and Tegler L: Controlled treatment of primary hypertension with propranolol and spironolactone. A crossover study with special reference to initial plasma renin activity. Am J Cardiol 37:642–649, 1976.
50. Hollifield JW, Sherman K, Zwagg RV, et al: Proposed mechanisms of propranolol's antihypertensive effect in essential hypertension. N Engl J Med 295:68–73, 1976.
51. Weidmann P, Beretta-Piccoli C, Ziegler W, et al: Interrelations among blood pressure, blood volume plasma renin and urinary catecholamines during beta blockade in essential hypertension. Klin Wochenschr 54:765–773, 1976.
52. Menard J, Bergagna X, N'Guyen PT, et al: Rapid identification of patients with essential hypertension sensitive to acebutolol (a new cardioselective beta-blocker). Am J Med 60:886–890, 1976.
53. Zech PY, Labeeuw M, Pozet N, et al: Response to atenolol in arterial hypertension in relation to renal function, pharmokinetics and renin activity. Postgrad Med J 53:(Suppl III):134–141, 1977.
54. Philipp T, Cordes U, and Distler A: Sympathetic responsiveness and antihypertensive effect

of beta-receptor blockade in essential hypertension: the effect of atenolol. Dtsch Med Wochenschr *102*:569–574, 1977.

55. Stumpe KO, Kollach R, Better H, et al: Acute and long-term studies of the mechanisms of action of beta-blocking drugs in lowering blood pressure. Am J Med *60*:853–865, 1976.

56. Boerth RC: The effect of propranolol in the treatment of hypertension in children (abstr). Pediatr Res *10*:328, 1976.

57. MacGregor GA, and Dawes P: Antihypertensive effect of propranolol and spironolactone in relation to plasma angiotensin II. Clin Sci Mol Med *50*:18p, 1976.

58. Pettinger WA, and Mitchell HC: Renin release, saralasin and the vasodilator-beta-blocker drug interaction in man. N Engl J Med *292*:1214–1217, 1975.

59. Castenfors J, Johnsson H, and Orö L: Effect of alprenolol on blood pressure and plasma renin activity in hypertensive patients. Acta Med Scand *193*:189–195, 1973.

60. Crane MG, and Harris JJ: Effect of spironolactone in hypertensive patients. Am J Med Sci *260*:311–330, 1970.

61. Spark RF, and Melby JC: Hypertension and low plasma renin activity: Presumptive evidence for mineralocorticoid excess. Ann Intern Med *75*:831–836, 1971.

62. Crane MG, Harris JJ, and Johns UJ: Hyporeninemic hypertension. Am J Med Sci *260*:311–330, 1970.

63. Carey RM, Douglas JG, Schweikert JR, et al: The syndrome of essential hypertension and suppressed plasma renin activity. Normalization of blood pressure with spironolactone. Arch Intern Med *130*:849–854, 1972.

64. Dustan HP, Bravo EL, and Tarazi RC: Volume-dependent essential and steroid hypertension. Am J Cardiol *31*:606–615, 1973.

65. Adlin EV, Marks AD, and Channick BJ: Spironolactone and hydrochlorothiazide in essential hypertension: Blood pressure response and plasma renin activity. Arch Intern Med *130*:855–858, 1972.

66. Douglas JG, Hollifield JW, and Liddle GW: Treatment of low-renin essential hypertension. JAMA *227*:518–521, 1974.

67. Laragh JH: Vasoconstriction volume analysis for understanding and treating hypertension: the use of renin and aldosterone profiles. Am J Med *55*:261–274, 1973.

68. Drayer JI, Keim JH, Weber MA, et al: Unexpected pressor responses to propranolol in essential hypertension: An interaction between renin, aldosterone and sympathetic activity. Am J Med *60*:897–904, 1976.

69. Baer L, Parra-Carrillo JZ, Radichevich I, and Williams GS: Detection of renovascular hypertension with angiotensin II blockade. Ann Intern Med *86*:257–260, 1977.

70. Brunner HR, Kirshman JD, Sealey JE, et al: Hypertension of renal origin: Evidence for two different mechanisms. Science *174*:1344–1346, 1971.

71. Gavras H, Brunner HR, Vaughan ED Jr, et al: Angiotensin-sodium interaction in blood pressure maintenance of renal hypertensive and normotensive rats. Science *180*:1369–1371, 1973.

72. Gavras H, Brunner HR, Thurston H, and Laragh JH: Reciprocation of renin dependency with sodium volume dependency in renal hypertension. Science *188*:1316–1317, 1975.

73. Laragh JH: Modern system for treating high blood pressure based on renin profiling and vasoconstriction-volume analysis: a primary role for beta blocking drugs such as propranolol. Am J Med *61*:797–810, 1976.

74. Laragh JH, Sealey JE, and Brunner HR: The control of aldosterone secretion in normal and hypertensive man: Abnormal renin-aldosterone patterns in low renin hypertension. Am J Med *53*:649–662, 1972.

75. Tarazi RC: Hemodynamic role of extracellular fluid in hypertension. Circ Res 38(Suppl II):II-73–II-83, 1976.

76. Helmer OM, and Judson WE: Metabolic studies on hypertensive patients with suppressed plasma renin activity not due to hyperaldosteronism. Circulation *38*:965–976, 1968.

77. Jose A, Crout JR, and Kaplan NM: Suppressed plasma renin activity in essential hypertension: roles of plasma volume, blood pressure, and sympathetic nervous system. Ann Intern Med *72*:9–16, 1970.

78. Woods, JW, Liddle GW, and Stant BC Jr: Effect of an adrenal inhibitor in hypertensive patients with suppressed renin. Arch Intern Med *123*:366–370, 1969.

79. Schalekamp MA, Beevers DG, Kosters G, Lebel M, Fraser R, and Birkenhager WH: Body fluid volume in low-renin hypertension. Lancet *2*:310–311, 1974.

80. Distler A, Kim HJ, Philipp TH, Philippi A, Werner E, and Wolff HP: Exchangeable sodium, plasma volume and the effects of various diuretics in patients with low renin hypertension. *In* Brener H, Nuglis A, Klopper A, et al (eds): *Research on Steroids*, Vol 1. New York, North Holland-Elsevier, 1975.

81. Weidmann P, Hirsch D, Beretta-Piccoli C, and Reubi FC: Interrelations among blood pressure, blood volume, plasma renin activity and urinary catecholamines in benign essential hypertension. Am J Med 62:209–218, 1977.
82. Esler M, Randall O, Bennett J, et al: Suppression of sympathetic nervous function in low-renin essential hypertension. Lancet 1:115–118, 1976.
83. Jose A, and Kaplan NM: Plasma renin activity in the diagnosis of primary aldosteronism. Arch Intern Med 123:141–146, 1969.
84. Woods JW, Pittman AW, Pulliam CC, et al: Renin profiling in the treatment of hypertension. N Engl J Med 294:1137–1142, 1976.
85. Ames RP, and Hill P: Elevation of serum lipid levels during diuretic therapy of hypertension. Am J Med 61:748–757, 1976.
86. Case DB, Atlas SA, Laragh JH, Sealey JE, Sullivan PA, and McKinstry DN: Clinical experience with blockade of the renin-angiotensin-aldosterone system by an oral converting-enzyme inhibitor (SQ 14,225, Captopril) in hypertensive patients. Prog Cardiovasc Dis 21:195–206, 1978.
87. Laragh JH: The renin system in high blood pressure, from disbelief to reality: converting-enzyme blockade for analysis and treatment. Prog Cardiovasc Dis 21:159–166, 1978.

Routine Measurement of Plasma Renin Activity

HARRIET P. DUSTAN, M.D.

Professor of Medicine and Director, Cardiovascular Research and
Training Center, University of Alabama Medical Center,
Birmingham, Alabama

There is no doubt that measurements of plasma renin activity (PRA) have added much to our knowledge of renal and adrenal hypertensions. Measurement of PRA in renal venous blood has provided a useful method for helping to assess the contribution of the renal pressor system (RPS) to renovascular hypertension in unilateral renal arterial disease, although it is not so helpful when lesions are bilateral. Also, measurement of peripheral venous PRA has proved important in evaluating whether hypokalemia reflects primary or secondary hyperaldosteronism. In essential hypertension, knowing PRA adds an important dimension to understanding the mechanisms for elevated arterial pressure in any patient. However, since there are many factors that participate in blood pressure control, knowledge of plasma catecholamine levels, extracellular fluid volumes, total exchangeable sodium, systemic hemodynamic functions, and plasma aldosterone levels seems of equal importance.

Another point that bears emphasis here is that the RPS is one of the important systems that determine arterial pressure. For years, investigators have looked for positive correlations between PRA and pressure, but few have been found. This failure to find direct relationships between these two variables need not be looked upon as indicating that the RPS is unimportant in hypertension, but rather, that since many systems participate in determining pressure, measurement of only one cannot be expected to always produce high levels of correlation with arterial pressure.

These considerations, although important, are not at issue here; what is at issue is the value of routine measurement of peripheral PRA for indicating the prognosis of essential hypertension with regard to its atherosclerotic complications and for determining "specific" antihypertensive drug therapy.

PRA as Indicative of Prognosis

It all began in 1972, when Brunner and his colleagues[1] reported on the clinical courses of hypertensive patients in relation to their PRA levels off therapy. Of these patients, 59 had low PRA and 124 had normal PRA in

549

relation to sodium excretion. The 59 patients with low PRA suffered no vascular complications, while 11 per cent of the 124 patients with normal PRA did. These findings formed the basis for their hypothesis that renin is vasculo-toxic and results in atherosclerotic complications.

Now, seven years since that report, there seems to be ample evidence that low renin does not protect patients with hypertension from developing atherosclerotic complications. This evidence has been reviewed by Kaplan.[2] He collated the findings from eight studies (including that of Brunner et al.).[1, 3-9] These studies involved a total of 456 patients with low PRA and 728 patients with normal PRA. Vascular complications — heart attack, stroke, and dissecting aneurysm — occurred in 14.0 per cent of the former and in 13.5 per cent of the latter.

Some important aspects are addressed in these reports that were not assessed in the original publication of Brunner et al.[1] Kaplan[2] points out that none of the normotensive control subjects in Brunner's study were black, yet data from the all-white control group were used to classify the hypertensives into renin subgroups, although it was well known by 1972 that low-renin hypertension occurs more frequently in blacks than in whites. This raises the question of whether it is valid to group blacks and whites together according to a biochemical characteristic that shows marked racial differences.

Gulati et al.[9] examined PRA data in relation to age and found that the 85 patients with low PRA were significantly older than the 116 with normal PRA (50 versus 43 years, p < 0.01). In the entire group, the occurrence of "low-renin hypertension" increased progressively with age, being 21 per cent for those 30 years of age or younger, 40 per cent for those between 31 and 50 years of age, and 58 per cent among those older than 50. In this study, strokes or heart attacks occurred in 15 per cent of the patients with low PRA and in five per cent of those with normal PRA.

Christlieb et al.[7] found that the 16 "low-renin hypertensive" patients they followed for five years had no vascular complications, in contrast to 23 per cent of 45 patients with normal PRA and 33 per cent of six patients with high PRA who did have complications. However, they pointed out that patients who suffered complications had higher mean arterial pressures and more electrocardiographic abnormalities than those who did not. Furthermore, they found that the known risk factors for atherosclerotic complications — mean arterial pressure greater than 130 mm Hg, hypercholesterolemia, and ECG evidences of left ventricular hypertrophy or previous myocardial infarction — were independent of PRA levels.

Throughout these seven years of controversy over the importance of PRA in the prognosis of hypertension, there have been two other puzzling features. One is that although low PRA occurs more frequently in black hypertensives than in white hypertensives, hypertension is well known to cause more complications (at least strokes) in blacks than in whites. Also, "renin profiling"[10] (i.e., classifying patients according to whether PRA is high, normal, or low) is done only when patients are untreated or have discontinued treatment for at least two weeks; yet whatever the PRA level is at that time, it is unlikely to remain there, because drug therapy will usually modify it. It is well recognized that low PRA does not remain low during long-term diuretic therapy, that vasodilators also raise PRA, and that sympatholytic drugs do not predictably reduce PRA, although they may suppress the increased renin release that occurs with standing. Thus, it seems unlikely that pretreatment measurement of PRA would bear any relationship to complication rate during treatment even if renin has any important influence on the course of atherosclerosis.

Renin as a Vasculotoxic Agent

Much stress has been given to renin as being a vasculotoxic agent. For the purpose of this presentation, it seems worthwhile to review the evidence for this and to assess what bearing it has on the atherothrombotic complications of hypertension.

It was the early study of Winternitz[11] that suggested that the kidney contains a substance that damages arterioles. Somewhat later, in a series of experiments, Masson and his colleagues[12-16] clearly showed the substance to be renin, and from these studies came the phrase "the vasculotoxic effect of renin." Giese's review[17] is a masterful presentation of the evidence, relating the renal pressor system to acute arteriolar lesions. He points out that although, experimentally, hyperreninemia or hyperangiotensinemia (either endogenous or exogenous) is associated with vascular lesions, these can also occur in nephrectomized animals that are salt-loaded. These lesions are arteriolar in location; they are caused by escape of plasma into the vessel wall, and this escape is the result of high intra-arterial pressure.

The relevance that these arteriolar lesions have to the accelerated atherosclerosis that characterizes hypertension is difficult to determine. There is some evidence that angiotensin II can cause endothelial cells to contract, widening intercellular junctions, and thus allowing the escape of plasmatic components into arterial walls.[18, 19] If this occurs in man, it could be one of the many causes of atherosclerosis, but the evidence for this possibility has not been produced.

If the RPS is shown to play a role in development of atherosclerotic plaques, then renin can be said to be vasculotoxic. At the present time, however, the vasculotoxicity of renin refers to the damaging effect of high blood pressure in animals with experimental hyperreninemia. Again it should be stressed that this vascular damage results from high blood pressure, and not the hyperreninemia *per se*.

Renin Levels as Guides to Pathophysiology and Therapy

The matter at issue here is whether PRA levels reliably indicate the predominant mechanisms of essential hypertension and can therefore be used as a guide to specific antihypertensive drug therapy. This proposal is based on Laragh's hypothesis that an elevated PRA indicates that vasoconstriction is maintaining the hypertension, while a low PRA indicates an expanded extracellular fluid volume as the cause of hypertension.[20] This, then, means that suppression of renin release, as with propranolol treatment,[21] will reduce arterial pressure in the former condition, while in the latter, the drug of choice is some form of diuretic therapy.[22]

This proposition has been extended to include a number of physiologic functions that can be predicted from the PRA level. Thus, Laragh[20] suggests that when PRA is high, the following abnormalities should be found: an elevated total peripheral resistance and aldosterone secretion; low plasma volume and cardiac output; elevated hematocrit, blood viscosity, and blood urea; low tissue perfusion; and finally, orthostatic hypotension. Low-renin hypertension, which he calls the vasodilated form of hypertension, is also considered to be associated with elevated total peripheral resistance. (He does not explain how vasodilation and elevated vascular resistance can co-exist.) In addition, aldosterone would be low or high (as in primary aldosteronism); plasma volume and cardiac output elevated; hematocrit, blood viscosity, and blood urea low; tissue perfusion elevated; and finally, no orthostatic hypotension.

It is an attractive proposal, because what physicians need in treating any disease is a simple method that indicates the basic abnormality and a treatment that will correct that abnormality. What follows are assessments of certain aspects of the vasoconstriction-volume analysis of the pathophysiology of hypertension and of its value as a guide to therapy.

PRA AS AN INDICATOR OF PATHOPHYSIOLOGY

The value of PRA for indicating the plasma and ECF volume characteristics of hypertensives has been examined by Schalekamp et al.[23] This report compares values for plasma and ECF volumes, for plasma aldosterone and aldosterone secretion rate in normotensive control subjects, essential hypertensives with normal PRA, and low-renin hypertensives. Despite the suppression of PRA in the last group, values for all the other functions were not significantly different from those of the normotensive or the normal-PRA hypertensive groups. The mean age of the low-renin hypertensive group was 11 years older than the other groups, and this may partly explain the hyporeninemia.

We have looked at another part of the hypothesis — whether hypervolemia in essential hypertension causes increased cardiac output and a lower vascular resistance than occurs in hypovolemic ("vasoconstricted-hyperreninemic") essential hypertension.[24, 25] We compared hemodynamic functions of two groups of essential hypertensive patients — one with hypovolemia (this is the more frequent type) and one with hypervolemia. The latter had significantly higher diastolic pressure than the former, but the same cardiac output, so that vascular resistance was higher. Thus, these studies do not support the suggestion that hyporeninemia indicates hypervolemia and high cardiac output.

PRA AS A GUIDE TO THERAPY

The proposition is that knowing PRA can indicate what treatment should specifically lower arterial pressure by interfering with the dominant pressor mechanism in any given patient. There are two questions: Is diuretic therapy more effective in patients with suppressed PRA? Is propranolol antihypertensive because it suppresses renin release, and is it the drug of choice when hyperreninemia is present?

First, in regard to *diuretic treatment*, the evidence seems mixed. Vaughan et al.[22] found that more patients with low PRA achieved substantial pressure reduction with either chlorthalidone or spironolactone than did patients with normal PRA. However, diuretic therapy was not effectively antihypertensive in every patient with suppressed PRA. Similarly, Crane, Harris, and

Johns[26] found that 77 per cent of hypertensive patients with hyporesponsive PRA responded to spironolactone therapy, compared with 38 per cent with normally responsive PRA. Adlin, Marks, and Channick[27] report similar differences in arterial pressure responses to spironolactone and hydrochlorothiazide between groups of patients with low PRA and normal PRA. Weinberger and Grim,[28] however, did not find that differences in pressure responsiveness to diuretic therapy were in any way related to "renin-profiling." In summary, one must conclude that low PRA does not predict every case of salt- and water-dependent essential hypertension.

In regard to *propranolol therapy,* Bühler et al.[21] concluded that "regardless of etiology, antihypertensive effectiveness of propranolol correlated with control renin levels and with the decrement of renin secretion." Again, there are two issues here: (1) that PRA measurement will indicate which patient should receive propranolol as specific therapy, and (2) that the antihypertensive effect of propranolol results from decreased renin release.

As far as the first issue is concerned, it seems that "hyperreninemic" hypertension is responsive to drugs (or procedures) that suppress renin, but that propranolol does not always have this effect.[29] Thus, propranolol cannot be considered an all-purpose anti-renin drug. For the second issue, it must be pointed out that many investigators have failed to find a significant relationship between the fall in arterial pressure and the decrease in PRA during propranolol therapy.[30-36] That is not surprising since propranolol is a beta-adrenergic-blocking drug and beta-adrenergic activity has functions over and above renin release.

Summary

Routine measurement of peripheral venous PRA adds information about essential hypertension because it tells something about one of the important systems that participate in arterial pressure control. However, "renin profiling" does not have the power previously ascribed to it for predicting the prognosis of treated hypertension or the responsiveness to specific antihypertensive drugs.

References

1. Brunner HR, Laragh JH, Bare L, et al: Essential hypertension: renin and aldosterone, heart attack and stroke. N Engl J Med 286:441–449, 1972.
2. Kaplan NM: The prognostic implications of plasma renin in essential hypertension. JAMA 231:167–170, 1975.
3. Doyle AE, Jerums G, Johnston CI, et al: Plasma renin levels and vascular complications in hypertension. Br Med J 2:206–207, 1973.
4. Mroczek WJ, Finnerty FA, and Catt KJ: Lack of association between plasma-renin and history of heart attack or stroke in patients with essential hypertension. Lancet 2:464–469, 1973.
5. Genest J, Boucher R, Kuchel O, et al: Renin in hypertension: how important as a risk factor? Can Med Assoc J 109:475–478, 1973.
6. Stroobandt R, Fagard R, and Amery AKPC: Are patients with essential hypertension and low renin protected against stroke and heart attack? Am Heart J 86:781–787, 1973.
7. Christlieb AR, Gleason RE, Hickler RB, et al: Renin, a risk factor for cardiovascular disease? Ann Intern Med 81:7–10, 1974.
8. Weinberger MH, Perkins BJ, and Yu P: Renin and clinical correlates in primary and secondary hypertension. In Sambhi MP (ed): Mechanisms of Hypertension. Amsterdam, Excerpta Medica, 1973, pp 332–342.

9. Gulati SC, Adlin EV, Biddle CM, et al: The occurrences of vascular complications in low renin hypertension (abstr). Ann Intern Med 78:828, 1973.
10. Laragh JH, Baer L, Brunner HR, et al: Renin, angiotensin and aldosterone system in pathogenesis and management of hypertensive vascular disease. Am J Med 52:633–652, 1972.
11. Winternitz MC, Mylon E, Waters LL, et al: Studies on the relation of the kidney to cardiovascular diseases. Yale J Biol Med 12:623–679, 1940.
12. Masson GMC, Plahl G, Corcoran AC, et al: Accelerated hypertensive vascular disease from saline and renin in nephrectomized dogs. Arch Pathol 55:85–97, 1953.
13. Masson GMC, Corcoran AC, and Page IH: Experimental production of a syndrome resembling toxemia of pregnancy. J Lab Clin Med 38:213–226, 1951.
14. Masson GMC, del Greco F, Corcoran AC, et al: Acute diffuse vascular disease elicited by renin in rats pretreated with cortisone. Arch Pathol 56:23–35, 1953.
15. Masson GMC, del Greco F, Corcoran AC, et al: Effects of renin in rats pretreated with hydrocortisone and somatotrophin. Am J Med Sci 226:296–303, 1953.
16. Masson GMC, del Greco F, Corcoran AC, et al: Pressor effects of subcutaneously injected renin in rats. Am J Physiol 180:337–340, 1955.
17. Giese J: Renin, angiotensin and hypertensive vascular damage: a review. Am J Med 55:315–332, 1973.
18. Constantinides P, and Robinson M: Ultrastructural injury of arterial endothelium. Arch Pathol 88:99–105, 1969.
19. Robertson AL, and Khairallah PA: Effects of angiotensin II and some analogues on vascular permeability in the rabbit. Circ Res 31:923–931, 1972.
20. Laragh JH: Vasoconstriction-volume analysis for understanding and treating hypertension. In Laragh JH (ed): Hypertension Manual. New York, Yorke Medical Books, 1973, pp 823–849.
21. Bühler FR, Laragh JH, Vaughan ED Jr, et al: The antihypertensive action of propranolol. In Laragh JH (ed): Hypertension Manual. New York, Yorke Medical Books, 1973, pp 873–898.
22. Vaughan ED Jr, Laragh JH, Gavras I, et al: The volume factor in low and normal renin essential hypertension. In Laragh JH (ed): Hypertension Manual. New York, Yorke Medical Books, 1973, pp 851–871.
23. Schalekamp MA, Lebel M, Beevers DG, et al: Body-fluid volume in low-renin hypertension. Lancet 2:310–311, 1974.
24. Tarazi RC: Hemodynamic role of extracellular fluid in hypertension. Circ Res 38 (Suppl II):II-73–II-83, 1976.
25. Dustan HP, Tarazi RC, and Bravo EL: Hemodynamic assessment of "volume-vasoconstriction" hypothesis in essential hypertension (abstr). Circulation 54 (Suppl II):II-97, 1976.
26. Crane MG, Harris JJ, and Johns VJ Jr: Hyporeninemic hypertension. Am J Med 52:457–466, 1972.
27. Adlin EV, Marks AD, and Channick BJ: Spironolactone and hydrochlorothiazide in essential hypertension. Arch Intern Med 130:855–858, 1972.
28. Weinberger MH, and Grim CE: Effects of spironolactone and hydrochlorothiazide on blood pressure and plasma renin activity in hypertension. In Sambhi MP (ed): Systemic Effects of Antihypertensive Agents. New York, Stratton Intercontinental Medical Book Corp, 1976, pp 481–493.
29. Robertson JIS, Bühler FR, George CF, et al: Report on Round Table on renin suppression and the hypotensive action of beta-adrenergic-blocking drugs. Clin Sci Mol Med 48:109s–115s, 1975.
30. Bravo EL, Tarazi RC, and Dustan HP: β-Adrenergic blockade in diuretic-treated patients with essential hypertension. N Engl J Med 292:66–70, 1975.
31. George CF, Lewis PJ, Steiner JA, et al: A comparison of propranolol and compound RO3-4787 in the treatment of arterial hypertension in man. Clin Sci Mol Med 48:65s–67s, 1975.
32. Geyskes GG, Boer P, Leenen FHH, et al: Effect of volume depletion and subsequent propranolol treatment on blood pressure and plasma renin activity in patients with essential and with renovascular hypertension. Clin Sci Mol Med 48:69s–71s, 1975.
33. Maggiore Q, Biagini M, Zoccali C, et al: Long-term propranolol treatment of resistant arterial hypertension in haemodialysed patients. Clin Sci Mol Med 48:73s–75s, 1975.
34. Leonetti G, Mayer G, Morganti A, et al: Blood pressure decrease and responsiveness to renin-releasing stimuli under increasing doses of propranolol in patients with essential hypertension. Clin Sci Mol Med 48:77s–79s, 1975.
35. Morgan T, Carney S, and Roberts R: Changes in plasma renin activity and blood pressure after acute and chronic administration of β-adrenergic receptor-blocking drugs. Clin Sci Mol Med 48:81s–83s, 1975.
36. Weber MA, Oates HF, and Stokes GS: Beta-adrenergic receptors and renin release: studies with beta-adrenoreceptor-blocking agents in the conscious rabbit. Clin Sci Mol Med 48:89s–91s, 1975.

Comment

Dr. Laragh presents a powerful and detailed argument supporting the thesis that he and his group have developed; namely, that hypertension is a spectrum with extreme vasoconstriction at one end and hypervolemia at the other, with varying degrees in between. Dr. Laragh proposes that renin profiling defines this state, and thus leads to more appropriate and logical management. Renin profiling refers not only to measurement of plasma renin activity, but also includes a determination of the state of salt balance as judged by a 24-hour urinary sodium assay. Thus, Laragh proposes that both renin and sodium profiling be carried out in the hypertensive patient, and not merely a determination of plasma renin activity alone.

I leave it to the reader to sort out the conflicting evidence presented by Dr. Dustan and to arrive at his/her own conclusion as to whether inappropriate renin-induced vasoconstriction results in an added adverse vasculotoxic effect in essential hypertension. If one is convinced that such is the case, determination of plasma renin activity would seem to be a reasonable routine procedure in hypertensive patients if for no other reason than that it would provide a prognostic measurement that is currently unavailable by other standard tests of patients with hypertension.

There can be little doubt that the vasoconstrictor-volume model has greatly clarified our understanding of the pathophysiology of hypertension, and it may explain some of the variability in response that is seen following treatment with particular antihypertensive agents. The question posed here, however, is whether it is necessary to characterize the renin-sodium state of the hypertensive patient in order to manage him/her appropriately. This is of considerable practical importance, since hypertension is virtually an epidemic in the United States, with recent figures suggesting that there are over 30 million patients suffering from this problem. Although renin assay and 24-hour urinary sodium determination to characterize the vasoconstriction-volume state of the hypertensive patient are relatively simple, they are not yet generally available. Thus, to suggest that they be performed routinely requires strong evidence that therapy cannot be carried out well or intelligently in their absence. The initial steps of the current stepped-care approach to the treatment of hypertension seem to me to take empirically some of this into consideration. If one starts all patients with hypertension on a diuretic agent, those who have a dominantly hypervolemic cause of their hypertensive disease should respond with a significant drop in arterial pressure. If, however, the patient fails to respond because his form of hypertension is included in the vasoconstriction end of the spectrum, with a blood volume that may even be contracted, one can then add a step-two drug, which in many centers today is propranolol. Presumably, propranolol, through its beta-adrenergic-blocking effect, would inhibit renin secretion, and arterial pressure would be lowered in patients in whom hyperreninemia is the major pathophysiologic abnormality.

Therefore, from a management standpoint, and without trying to lessen the importance of the observations made by Laragh and his associates, it seems reasonable for the general practitioner to consider the hypertensive patient a candidate for routine renin-sodium profiling whenever renovascular hypertension or adrenocortical hypertension is suspected or whenever a simple therapy trial as described above fails. Then, the physician can always take this resistant minority of patients and either empirically add other types of antihypertensive agents or, contrariwise, discontinue medication for two weeks, carry out renin-sodium profiling and/or other investigative procedures, and define better the cause of hypertension in that patient and the failure to respond to usual management. This would seem to be a practical expedient to insure that the large population of hypertensive patients is managed with antihypertensive medication and is not left untreated.

ELLIOT RAPAPORT, M.D.

Twenty-three

Should Asymptomatic Patients with Mild Hypertensive Disease Be Treated Continuously with Antihypertensive Drugs?

ASYMPTOMATIC PATIENTS WITH MILD HYPERTENSION
SHOULD BE TREATED CONTINUOUSLY
Edward D. Frohlich, M.D.

THE UNCERTAINTIES OF DRUG THERAPY IN MILD
HYPERTENSION
W. McFate Smith, M.D.

COMMENT

Asymptomatic Patients with Mild Hypertension Should Be Treated Continuously

EDWARD D. FROHLICH, M.D.

Vice President, Education and Research, Alton Ochsner
Medical Foundation; Director, Division of Hypertensive
Diseases, Ochsner Clinic, New Orleans, Louisiana

Until recent years, the efficacy of antihypertensive therapy had not been established.[1-3] Although it was easy to demonstrate benefits of treatment of patients with malignant hypertension,[4] and even of patients with moderate to severe hypertension, it was more difficult to establish benefits in patients with mild to moderate degrees of hypertensive cardiovascular disease. Even though antihypertensive drugs became available in the mid to late 1950's, years of prospective research were necessary to convince therapeutic nihilists that antihypertensive therapy significantly reduces morbidity and mortality.

The Veterans Administration Cooperative Study in Hypertension ultimately reported that antihypertensive therapy was efficacious for patients with diastolic arterial pressures ranging from 90 to over 129 mm Hg; however, the ultimate recommendations of the National High Blood Pressure Education Program were more qualified;[5] the latter study recommended antihypertensive therapy primarily for patients with persistent diastolic pressures of 105 mm Hg and greater. My own viewpoint is that, all things being equal, patients having a persistent elevation of diastolic pressure of greater than 90 mm Hg should be the beneficiaries of continuous antihypertensive therapy — whether or not they have symptoms and whether or not there is evidence of target organ involvement.

Veterans Administration Cooperative Study: Its Significance

The Veterans Administration Cooperative Study, from its very early phase to the later stages, demonstrated the efficacy of continuous antihyper-

559

Table 1.   *VA Cooperative Study[3] — Causes of Death from Complications*
of Hypertension

	NUMBER OF PATIENTS	
	Placebo Group	*Treatment Group*
Events directly related to hypertensive vascular disease		
Cerebrovascular hemorrhage	3	0
Subarachnoid hemorrhage	1	0
Dissecting aneurysm	1	0
Events associated with hypertension		
Myocardial infarction	3	2
Sudden death	8	4
Cerebrovascular thrombosis	3	1
Ruptured atherosclerotic aneurysm	0	1
Total	19	8

tensive pharmacologic therapy by demonstrating a significant reduction in morbidity and mortality, even in patients with the less severe forms of hypertensive cardiovascular disease (diastolic pressures 90 to 114 mm Hg).[3] Antihypertensive drug therapy (using the combination of a thiazide diuretic, reserpine, and hydralazine) not only significantly reduced mortality from complications of hypertension (Table 1), but also reduced morbidity from such events as congestive heart failure, hypertensive retinopathy, hypertensive encephalopathy, stroke, and aortic dissection (Table 2).[3] There were more cardiovascular and renal pathological events in the group of patients treated with placebo that did not require their removal from this double-blind study (Table 3) than in those treated with antihypertensive drugs. Furthermore, as a less solid end point, a number of patients whose

Table 2.   *VA Cooperative Study[3] — Morbid Events Requiring the Removal*
of the Patients from this Double-Blind Study

	NUMBER OF PATIENTS	
	Placebo Group	*Treatment Group*
Events directly related to hypertension	9	0
Uncontrolled congestive heart failure	5	0
Dissecting aneurysm	1	0
Subarachnoid hemorrhage	1	0
Retinal hemorrhage	1	0
Acute hypertensive encephalopathy	1	0
Treatment failures	7	1
CVA thrombosis	4	0
Progressive azotemia	1	0
Retinal hemorrhage and (?) papilledema	1	0
Retinal hemorrhage with hypertensive encephalopathy	1	0
Hypotension	0	1
Total	16	1

Table 3. *VA Cooperative Study[3] — Morbid Events Not Requiring That the Affected Patient Be Removed from the Double-Blind Study*

	NUMBER OF PATIENTS	
	Placebo Group	*Treatment Group*
Stroke (thrombosis or TIA)	8	4
Congestive heart failure	6	0
Myocardial infarction	2	5
Atrial fibrillation	2	3
Heart block	1	1
Serum creatinine (>2.0 mg per cent)	1	0
Proteinuria (persistent)	1	0
Total	21	13

arterial pressure continued to increase progressively were removed from the study lest their personal health be jeopardized by diastolic hypertension advancing to exceedingly high levels — levels at or above which the efficacy of antihypertensive therapy had been established.

Therefore, the benefit of antihypertensive therapy became well established with publication of the results of the study, and another major national program was subsequently instituted.[5] This program was designed to educate not only the professional medical community, but also the entire general population, concerning the merits of and necessity for continuous blood pressure control. This program presented facts on the following matters: the merits of determining the blood pressure of the entire population; the need for identifying all those with hypertension in the population screened; the importance of having this medical problem thoroughly evaluated once the potential patient is identified; the institution of therapy; and the importance of ongoing medical follow-up and indefinite and continuous antihypertensive therapy.

The Limitations of the VA Cooperative Study

The VA Cooperative Study, as could be expected, failed to provide all the answers to the public health problem of high blood pressure. Many who have been concerned with implementation of the findings believe that it demonstrated incontrovertibly that the higher the systolic and diastolic pressure, the worse the prognosis. Life insurance actuarial data, as well as the prospective Framingham Study, have confirmed this finding.[6, 7] However, the VA Cooperative Study did not show that reduction of arterial pressure will inevitably improve the long-term prognosis, and this must yet be shown prospectively.

Several other concepts also remain to be established. First, efficacy of therapy has not been shown in a large population of female patients. The VA Study was restricted to men, and hypertension varies in severity in men and women, depending upon age and other factors.[8] Second, the VA Cooperative Study was unable to reach any conclusions regarding hypertension (especially mild hypertension) in black patients; there were only a few blacks with mild hypertension in the study. Moreover, since hypertension in the black man seems to be more severe than in a white man of comparable age,[7] it may not be valid to advocate that only diastolic pressure in excess of 105 mm Hg should be treated in black patients. Perhaps therapy should be advocated at a lower diastolic pressure level in the black patient. Third, there were just too few subjects under 45 years of age included in the VA Study; and fourth, there were too few subjects whose pretreatment diastolic pressure was less than 105 mm Hg. This explains why the National High Blood Pressure Education task forces advocate antihypertensive therapy only for those whose diastolic pressure is higher than 105 mm Hg.[5]

From the foregoing, I believe it is legitimate to raise the following question: Is it fair that prolonged (lifelong) antihypertensive therapy should be recommended for an individual under 45 years of age if the diastolic pressure elevation is mild (i.e., between 90 and 105 mm Hg)?

The deficiencies of the VA Study underscore the need for an additional, but larger, multiclinic study involving both sexes and all races, and especially including young people and women with mild hypertension.

A final point concerning limitations of the VA Cooperative Study is that it failed to demonstrate that antihypertensive therapy is effective in preventing heart attacks. However, in fairness to the study and its experimental design, we must ask whether it is reasonable to expect that this study could have shown that. First, remember that the study also failed to demonstrate that antihypertensive therapy is *not* effective in preventing heart attacks. The average age of the men entering the study was older than 45 years, and postmortem studies in the Korean and Vietnam wars indicated that 18-year-old men had already developed atherosclerosis of the coronary arterial supply to the myocardium.[9, 10]

If the aim of the study is to confirm or deny that antihypertensive therapy prevents heart attacks, we must intelligently design a new prospective study. This study will be exceedingly hard to mount for the following reasons: First, the study will require large numbers of asymptomatic volunteer subjects (the estimated need is more than 8500 and probably more than 10,000). Second, the study will involve primarily young people, who are extremely mobile in today's American society, and this will greatly affect the ability to follow up such individuals. The study will obviously require a long follow-up period in order to demonstrate reduction in myocardial infarction rate as well as other end points related to development of atherosclerotic cardiovascular disease. Third, patient "compliance" will be difficult to achieve in the young individual who is asymptomatic and who is asked to remain on continuous drug therapy, which admittedly will be associated with certain side effects. Finally, such a prolonged study involving large numbers of patients will be extremely costly — perhaps too costly for present budgetary restrictions.

The Unresolved Questions and Personal Views

DIASTOLIC PRESSURE 90 TO 104 MM HG

Thus, although it has not been proved by prospective studies, my personal belief is that all persons whose diastolic pressure remains persistently in excess of 90 mm Hg should receive antihypertensive pharmacologic therapy. However, *if* the individual is young, *if* the individual has no evidence of target organ involvement, *if* the individual has parents whose life spans have been unrestricted, and *because* the individual is required to take drugs that have known additional (or side) effects other than the reduction of arterial pressure, we must ask whether it is reasonable to advocate prolonged therapy as a broad public health measure. To my way of thinking, it is more reasonable to permit an individual decision by the managing physician on a case-by-case basis; a public health dictum is a "horse of a different color."

MILD HYPERTENSION IN WOMEN

With respect to possible differences between the sexes in responses to antihypertensive therapy, we do not know whether treatment of hypertension, especially for diastolic pressures less than 105 mm Hg, but also those between 105 and 114 mm Hg, is as efficacious in women as it is in men. Thus, is hypertension actually of equivalent severity in men and women of the same age? Would a woman require more therapy or less therapy than a man with the same level of blood pressure? What is the impact of therapy not only on the female patient, but also on the growth and development of an unborn child? And, what about that child's later development? Are we aware of all the risks of antihypertensive therapy on a developing fetus? What do we know about effects of therapy on specific organ function of the fetus? Therefore, are these risks greater than the benefits of therapy in a mildly hypertensive woman? Information at present is obviously incomplete, and we must rely on the hope that clinical investigation will provide this necessary information in the near future.

MILD HYPERTENSION IN THE BLACK PATIENT

Do we know what recommendations should be made concerning the treatment of hypertension in the black patient? Is it fair to extrapolate information that is already known about the white patient to the black patient? If we are to assume that severity of hypertension, as well as its prevalence, is greater in the black, can we draw fundamental answers from epidemiologic experience from a different population? Perhaps treatment in the black should be initiated at a diastolic pressure of 80 or 85 mm Hg, for example, rather than at 90 or 105 mm Hg.

OTHER UNRESOLVED FACTORS

We do not know whether pharmacologic treatment of mild hypertension (for example, diastolic readings as low as 80 to 90 mm Hg or 90 to 105 mm Hg) at an earlier age will reduce the chances of later development of heart attacks. Would this form of therapeutic intervention be as good as low-sodium diet therapy at this stage? We do not know whether the benefits of therapy, already demonstrated in the VA Cooperative Study, might be offset by possible long-term adverse effects of pharmacologic therapy.

We also do not know the long-term (as long as 45 years) effects of drug therapy: What is the effect of 45 years of hypokalemia? What are the effects of 30 to 45 years of relative carbohydrate intolerance? What are the effects of long-term depletion of catecholamine stores from vital tissues (e.g., brain, nerve endings, myocardium, and so on)? What is the effect of long-term treatment by drugs that produce low-grade adrenal stimulation or inhibition, prolonged contraction of intravascular volume, or prolonged stimulation of the kidney to raise circulating plasma renin activity? In other words, are the benefits demonstrated by the VA Cooperative Study (for men with hypertension whose average age was older than 45 years and whose diastolic pressures were greater than 105 mm Hg) of sufficient magnitude to offset the risk of unwanted effects of drugs?

ALTERNATIVES TO PHARMACOLOGIC THERAPY

In 1977, a report was published by an outstanding group of physicians detailing the present state of knowledge concerning high blood pressure in the young.[11] They told us that hypertension is a far more common problem in children than had been anticipated; that pressures that are higher in childhood will also be higher in adulthood; that the blood pressure of children whose parents have high blood pressure seems to be higher than that of children whose parents have normal blood pressure; and that the most common type (if it is a type) of hypertension in childhood is essential hypertension. These findings, and previous observations on the efficacy of low-sodium diet therapy in hypertension, have prompted certain baby food companies to modify their preparations. Thus, rather than design their foods for the established tastes of mothers, they will provide foods low in sodium. Perhaps this early conditioning in infancy will modify the salt taste of the older child and adult. Perhaps this is a glimmer of light on the hypertension horizon, and these beginnings may modify population food tastes, which may in turn modify the projections for mild hypertension. Perhaps it will eventually become possible to decrease the sodium content in prepared, canned, and frozen foods for adults. Since natriuretic therapy is the generally accepted basis for continuous drug therapy in the mildly hypertensive adult patient, a novel and natural means of treatment may already be at hand.

Conclusions

The major benefit of antihypertensive therapy for severe hypertension, I am convinced, is the significant reduction of cardiovascular morbidity and mortality. I am equally convinced that the therapeutic approach advocated by the National High Blood Pressure Education Program is valid. Diastolic pressure maintained higher than 105 mm Hg must be reduced. Indeed, I personally also believe that diastolic hypertension in excess of 90 mm Hg should be treated. Our epidemiologic, insurance, prospective, and clinical investigative studies have convinced me that diastolic arterial pressure elevation higher than 90 mm Hg significantly increases the risk of cardiovascular death and morbidity, and it also compounds those identifiable risks that predispose men and women to later atherosclerotic heart disease.

However, scientifically, it remains to be demonstrated that reduction of arterial pressure of man and woman, child and adult, black and white, those under and over 45 years of age, no matter what the height of diastolic pressure in excess of 90 mm Hg, provides benefits in excess of the risk of pharmacologic therapy. This is the challenge we inherit from our previous studies. It is our responsibility to underscore these gaps in our knowledge to those agencies who are responsible for the public health and to provide the answers to these questions. Our patients and our own moral conscience demand no less.

References

1. Veterans Administration Cooperative Study Group on Antihypertensive Agents. 1962. Double-blind control study of antihypertensive agents. II. Further report on the comparative effectiveness of reserpine, reserpine and hydralazine, and three ganglion blocking agents, chlorisondamine, mecamylamine, and pentolinium tartrate. Arch Intern Med 110:222–229, 1962.
2. Veterans Administration Cooperative Study Group on Antihypertensive Agents. Effects of treatment on morbidity in hypertension. I. Results in patients with diastolic blood pressure averaging 115 through 129 mm Hg. JAMA 202:1028–1034, 1967.
3. Veterans Administration Cooperative Study Group on Antihypertensive Agents. Effects of treatment on morbidity in hypertension. II. Results in patients with diastolic blood pressures averaging 90 through 114 mm Hg. JAMA 213:1143–1152, 1970.
4. Mohler RF, and Freis ED: Five-year survival of patients with malignant hypertension treated with antihypertensive agents. Am Heart J 60:329–335, 1960.
5. National High Blood Pressure Education Program, National Heart and Lung Institute. Professional Education. Report of Task Force II to the Hypertension Information and Education Advisory Committee, September 1, 1973.
6. Kannel WB: Role of blood pressure in cardiovascular morbidity and mortality. Progr Cardiovasc Dis 17:5–24, 1974.
7. Kannel WB, McGee D, and Gordon T: A general cardiovascular profile: the Framingham study. Am J Cardiol 38:46–51, 1976.
8. Stamler J, Stamler R, Tiedlinger WF, Algera G, and Roberts RH: Community hypertension screening of 1 million Americans. Community hypertension evaluation clinic (CHEC) program, 1973–1975. JAMA 235:2299–2306, 1976.
9. Emos WF, Holmes RH, and Bryer J: Coronary disease among United States soldiers killed in action in Korea. Preliminary report. JAMA 152:1090–1093, 1953.
10. McNamara JJ, Molot MA, Stremble JF, and Cutting RT: Coronary artery disease in combat casualties in Vietnam. JAMA 216:1185–1187, 1971.
11. Report of the Task Force on Blood Pressure Control in Children. Prepared by the National Heart, Lung, and Blood Institute's Task Force on Blood Pressure Control in Children. Pediatrics 59 (Suppl):797–820, 1977.

The Uncertainties of Drug Therapy in Mild Hypertension

W. McFATE SMITH, M.D., M.P.H.

Clinical Professor of Medicine and Epidemiology,
University of California, San Francisco; Chief, Research
Branch, Division of Hospitals and Clinics, United States
Public Health Service, San Francisco, California

The controversy offered by the proposition "Asymptomatic Patients with Mild Hypertensive Disease Should Be Continuously Treated with Antihypertensive Drugs" constitutes one of modern medicine's great dilemmas. It is well established that malignant, severe, and even moderate hypertensive disease conveys mortality and major morbidity risks that are beneficially affected by drugs that lower blood pressure. In these instances, the benefits clearly outweigh the known and potential hazard, expense, and inconvenience of continuous drug therapy.

Logic suggests, indeed dictates to some, that similar benefit will accrue to patients with mild, uncomplicated, asymptomatic hypertensive disease. To date, this benefit has not been demonstrated, and given the lower level of risk to which such people are exposed, many serious therapists have been reluctant to subject them to the potential harm, inconvenience, and expense of lifelong medication.

Thus, although in one instance the hazard/benefit ratio is clearly favorable, in the other it is uncertain. The components of the hazard/benefit ratio of treating mildly elevated blood pressures should be studied critically. The potential benefit from therapy relates directly to the risk of continuing exposure to given blood pressure levels. This risk needs to be known and placed in perspective relative to more severe disease.

Risks of Mild Hypertension

Cited most often as defining the risks of mild hypertension are the actuarial studies. Here the risk for given blood pressure strata of groups of insurance applicants can be expressed as mortality ratios, survival rates, or

566

reduction of life expectancy. In this kind of analysis, since the mortality experience of a given group is attributed to their original blood pressure category, it is assumed that the mortality experience results from exposure to that blood pressure throughout their lives. However, it is reasonable to suppose that much of the adverse experience of the group resulted from those individuals whose blood pressures progressed to successively higher levels as they grew older. Since in 25 to 30 per cent of those with mildly elevated blood pressures it does show such a tendency to rise, the risk for those who remain at their original blood pressure level is overstated.[1]

In the National Pooling Project, the gradient of risk of nonfatal myocardial infarctions and all coronary deaths for men ages 40 to 49 was minor, increasing from a 10-year rate of 603 per 10,000 at diastolic pressures of < 85 mm Hg, to 707 per 10,000 for diastolic pressures of 95 to 104 mm Hg.[2] This rate is approximately 30 per cent of that for the group with pressures > 104 mm Hg.

In the Western Electric study of 1816 men followed for 17 years, whereas the total mortality rate for men with pressures of 90 to 109 mm Hg was nearly 50 per cent more than those with pressures < 90 mm Hg, in absolute terms both rates were less than one per cent per year.[3] Fifty per cent of these deaths were attributed to coronary disease. For men with higher diastolic pressures, both the relative and absolute risk rose dramatically.

Cerebrovascular complications were also of very low frequency in the studies just described, occurring rarely before the age of 60 in the Pooling Project and in only two per cent of the men in the Western Electric population over the 17 years of observation.

The experience of the control group in the 10-year Public Health Service trial[5] is also consistent with a low-risk status for those who remain in the mildly elevated blood pressure category (see Tables 2 to 4).

Thus, it appears that for mild hypertension, the target for improvement is relatively small. How much improvement can you offer an asymptomatic individual with a low-risk condition? At what hazard and cost? If one defines hypertension as that level of blood pressure above which the risk of the disease exceeds that of diagnosis and treatment, perhaps adults with diastolic blood pressures < 105 mm Hg and without other significant risk factors should not be considered "hypertensive." However, for the sake of discussion, let us accept the level of risk of mildly elevated blood pressures as something we should reverse or prevent if possible. Given this goal, it is important to bear in mind that at least half of the excess mortality associated with hypertension is due to coronary heart disease. What is the evidence of benefit?

Benefits of Treatment in Mild Hypertension

The Veterans Administration study of men with diastolic blood pressures of 90 to 114 mm Hg is most often cited as providing the data to support the logic that mild hypertensives should benefit from drug therapy, just as groups with more severe disease do. However, most interpretations of the VA study

Table 1. *Major Morbid Events*

	ACTIVE	PLACEBO
Myocardial Infarction		
Fatal	1	1
Nonfatal	6	5
Sudden Death	1	1
Stroke	0	2
	8	9

have not appreciated that there were very few mild hypertensives included. The baseline blood pressures were obtained after three days of hospitalization, so that the diastolic blood pressure range of 90 to 114 mm Hg corresponds more closely to office blood pressures of 100 to 120 mm Hg. Furthermore, over 50 per cent of the veterans had a cardiac, central nervous system, or renal abnormality at entry. One in five had either a prior myocardial infarct, stroke, or previous congestive heart failure; 21 per cent were age 60 or more. Thus, by neither blood pressure nor target organ damage criteria can they be considered "mild" hypertensives. Even so, the complication rates in the treatment and control groups were similar for the 90 to 104 mm Hg stratum. Moreover, coronary heart disease occurred equally in both groups, even when the 105 to 114 mm Hg stratum was included. The Veterans Administration investigators have themselves concluded that patients in the diastolic pressure range of 90 to 104 mm Hg derived very little benefit from therapy unless they had cardiovascular abnormalities at entry or were over 50 years of age.

The only completed controlled trial in *mild* hypertension is that conducted by the Public Health Service hospitals.[5] It began in 1966 and was concluded 10 years later after amassing nearly 2400 man-years of observation. The study population included 389 men and women with an average age of 44 years and an upper age limit of 55 years. Subjects who had discernible target organ damage or who had known or recognizable predisposition to degenerative vascular disease were excluded. Pretreatment *clinic* diastolic blood pressures were between 90 and 115 mm Hg, with over 75 per cent in the range of 90 to 104 mm Hg. The mean systolic pressure was 148 mm Hg, and the mean diastolic pressure was 99 mm Hg.

Table 2. *First Morbid Events*

	ACTIVE		PLACEBO	
	N	%	N	%
Randomized	193	100.0	196	100.0
Patients with events	59	30.6	92	46.9
Hypertensive	28	14.6	64	32.6
Atherosclerotic	31	16.1	28	14.3
BP Progression	0	0.0	12°	6.1
Patients without events or				
progression	134	69.4	97	49.5

°Includes three with concurrent events.

Table 3.   *First Morbid Event—Atherosclerotic*

	ACTIVE		PLACEBO		A/P
	N	%	N	%	
Randomized patients	193	100	196	100	
Atherosclerotic	31	16.1	27	13.8	1.17
Myocardial infarction	5	2.6	6	3.1	0.84
Death	2	1.0	1	0.5	2.00
Other CHD	23	11.9	20	10.2	1.17
Peripheral arterial insufficiency	1	0.5	0	0.0	

Lowering of blood pressure in the active-treatment group occurred promptly and was virtually complete in the first four months, with a modest further reduction over the course of follow-up. The difference in systolic pressure for the two regimens at 12 months was 18 mm Hg, and for diastolic pressure, 10 mm Hg. These group mean differences persisted or widened subsequently.

The major end points of death, stroke, and myocardial infarction were used in a sequential analysis to determine the earliest possible termination point for the study. The decisions for and against active therapy were nearly equal, with the involved end points totaling 17 (Table 1). It is apparent that the occurrence of these major morbid events was not influenced by therapy.

The *first* end point (of varying degrees of severity) manifested by each subject while on assigned medication is shown in Table 2. The rate in the group receiving active drug therapy was 30.6 per 100 (59 of 193), which was about two-thirds that of those receiving placebo, 45.9 per 100 (92 of 196). The complications are divided into those that are considered to be a consequence of the elevated blood pressure *per se* and those that are a result of the associated atherosclerotic process. All of the observed difference in incidence between the treatment and placebo groups is accounted for by reduction in "hypertensive" end points in the group receiving active hypertensive agents. Tables 3 and 4 provide a further breakdown of this classification, revealing that *those manifestations of coronary heart disease that occurred with equal frequency in the treatment groups included fatal and nonfatal myocardial infarction, angina pectoris, abnormal double Master's test, and other ECG abnormalities ascribable to coronary heart disease.* Hypervoltage and left

Table 4.   *First Morbid Event—Hypertensive*

	ACTIVE		PLACEBO		A/P
	N	%	N	%	
Randomized patients	193	100.0	196	100.0	
Hypertensive	28	14.5	63	32.1	0.45
CVA	0	0.0	2	1.0	
Hypervoltage	8	4.1	23	11.7	0.35
LVH	9	4.7	20	10.2	0.46
Cardiomegaly	11	5.7	14	7.1	0.80
Retinopathy	0	0.0	4	2.0	

ventricular hypertrophy were the most frequent end points, with the overall incidence in the active drug therapy group being less than half that of the placebo group. Congestive heart failure and renal insufficiency did not occur.

Treatment failure, defined as a progressive rise of diastolic blood pressure to levels exceeding 130 mm Hg, occurred in 12 individuals prior to the occurrence of any other morbid event. An additional 12 treatment failures occurred subsequent to earlier minor morbid events. *Treatment failures occurred only in the placebo group.*

Discussion

Caution in interpreting and applying the results of the Veterans Administration study to mild hypertension was urged by VA investigators and others soon after the initial report. Efforts were made to define the limitations of the study because of concern that unjustifiable widespread use of the antihypertensive agents would result from the justifiable acclaim that the research received. In addition to the points already reviewed here, it was emphasized that females, in whom hypertension is more common but also more benign, were excluded from the study. Even then, as well as subsequently, it was suggested that one consider withholding drugs until the average diastolic pressure *under conditions comparable to those in the Veterans Administration Study* is over 104 mm Hg.[6, 7]

It was also recommended that since the yearly mortality rate for mild hypertension over a 10-year period was approximately that of the general population and was even lower for females and young men under 25, that periodic observation alone was appropriate for such groups.[8] For middle-aged men, treatment was recommended, but a hygienic regimen was the first step in such therapy. The regimen consisted of exercise, no smoking, weight control, and a sharp reduction of dietary salt, fat, and sweets.

The Public Health Service study, although not powerful in a statistical design sense, confirms the low level of risk for mild hypertension over a 10-year period. Moreover, in subjects whose blood pressures were well controlled, no protection was demonstrated against coronary heart disease. Furthermore, not only was the total and cardiovascular mortality rate low in the control group, but morbidity (rates per year) was also of low frequency and was minor in severity. The most frequent morbid event, left ventricular hypertrophy, occurred at a rate of only 2.63 per 100 patients per year.

On the other hand, it must be noted that active drug treatment was 55 per cent effective in preventing such minor complications and completely eliminated the progressive rise of blood pressure to dangerous levels.

Conclusions

In summary, I would emphasize that the only available data *do not* support the thesis that patients with mild, uncomplicated hypertensive disease should be treated with long-term drug therapy. Under the circumstances of relatively low risk, and given the as-yet-unanswered questions about the potential long-range toxic effect of the drugs, it seems prudent to defer drug use while trying reasonable alternatives. The routine use of drugs should be reserved for moderate or severe hypertension. Certainly for the overweight individual with the salt intake of the average American diet, a hygienic program including regular exercise, weight control, reduced dietary salt, and management of other risk factors should be attempted. Implicit in such an approach is the requirement for regular follow-up to identify the earliest sign of progression of the condition.

References

1. Julius S, and Schork MA: Borderline hypertension — a critical review. J Chronic Dis 23:723–754, 1971.
2. Paul O: Risk of mild hypertension: a ten year report. Br Heart J 33 (Suppl):116–121, 1971.
3. Paul O, and Miller J: Complications of mild hypertension. Ann NY Acad Sci 304:59–63, 1978.
4. Veterans Administration Cooperative Study Group on Antihypertensive Agents: Effects of treatment on morbidity in hypertension. II. Results in patients with diastolic blood pressure averaging 90 through 114 mm Hg. JAMA 213:1143–1152, 1970.
5. Smith W: Treatment of mild hypertension. Results of a ten-year intervention trial. U.S. Public Health Service Hospitals Cooperative Study Group. Circ Res 40(Suppl I):I-98–I-105, 1977.
6. Ingelfinger FJ, Relman AS, and Finland M (eds): Controversy in Internal Medicine I. Philadelphia, WB Saunders Company, 1966.
7. Ingelfinger FJ, Ebert RV, Finland M, and Relman AS (eds): Controversies in Medicine II. Philadelphia, WB Saunders Company, 1974.
8. Proger S: Antihypertensive drugs: praise and restraint. (editorial) N Engl J Med 286:155–156, 1972.
9. Robinson SK: Identification of mild hypertension and some risk factors that influence prognosis. J Am Geriatr Soc 21(8):379–382, 1973.

Comment

This controversy highlights the paucity of data documenting the effect of antihypertensive medication in patients with mild arterial hypertension. Both Drs. Frohlich and Smith recognize that the mildly hypertensive patient is at distinctly less risk of subsequent morbid events than the patient with moderate or severe hypertension. In light of the relatively smaller risk facing the mildly hypertensive patient, it becomes reasonable to ask if we should give such asymptomatic patients long-term drugs that have side effects, some of which may be potentially serious, even if we disregard the cost factor.

Epidemiologically speaking, it may not be warranted with our present state of knowledge to undertake mass treatment of this mildly hypertensive population. However, on an individual basis, I think a strong case can be made for treatment of certain selected patients. I am particularly concerned about the young asymptomatic hypertensive. If one detects a consistently elevated diastolic blood pressure in the neighborhood of 90 to 104 mm Hg in a young patient, I would treat him/her with antihypertensive medication. The significance of this degree of elevation in a 20-year-old patient may not only portend many years of increased target organ trauma, but may also reflect a greater potential for subsequent development of more severe hypertensive disease in the future. It makes sense to me to attempt to lower this pressure into what is generally considered the normal range if this can be accomplished without overly vigorous treatment.

In contrast, a 65-year-old patient with a comparably elevated blood pressure would not normally be treated by me unless he demonstrated some target organ disease already present and attributable to this level of arterial hypertension. In any case, it is clear that more data in this whole area are necessary and desirable.

ELLIOT RAPAPORT, M.D.

573

Twenty-four

Does Measurement of Contractility Indices Aid in the Management of the Cardiac Patient?

MEASUREMENT OF CONTRACTILITY INDICES AIDS IN MANAGEMENT OF THE CARDIAC PATIENT
   Dean T. Mason, M.D., et al.

THE MEASUREMENT OF CONTRACTILITY INDICES IN THE MANAGEMENT OF CARDIAC PATIENTS: CLINICALLY USELESS
   G. E. Burch, M.D.

COMMENT

Measurement of Contractility Indices Aids in Management of the Cardiac Patient*

DEAN T. MASON, M.D.;
ANTHONY N. DEMARIA, M.D.;
WILLIAM J. BOMMER, M.D.;
JAMES A. JOYE, M.D.;
DANIEL S. BERMAN, M.D.;
GARRETT LEE, M.D.;
AND EZRA A. AMSTERDAM, M.D.

Section of Cardiovascular Medicine, Departments of
Medicine and Physiology, University of California at Davis
School of Medicine and Sacramento Medical Center, Davis
and Sacramento, California; and the Department of
Nuclear Medicine, Cedars-Sinai Medical Center, Los
Angeles, California

To clarify our interpretation of the meaning and framework of our assignment, the topic under consideration is cardiac contractility (also termed inotropic or contractile state), and our viewpoint is that accurate determination of this fundamental property of the myocardium is helpful in providing improved care of patients with heart disease. Since meaningful indices of contractility can be obtained by a variety of atraumatic modalities, as well as by cardiac catheterization, the issue is approached here from a broad base, taking into account both non-invasive and invasive techniques. The dividing line between what we judge is the antagonist's contention (i.e., that the physical examination alone is always sufficient to provide all of the information necessary about contractile state, thereby a largely subjective and qualitative estimation), and our position is that we favor the modern concept that, in addition to the useful findings provided by physical examination, the use of certain procedures developed within the past few years in appropriate patients affords needed objective and quantitative data for more precise as-

*Supported in part by Research Program Project Grant HL-14780 from the NHLBI, NIH, Bethesda, Maryland, and California Chapters of the American Heart Association.

577

sessment of contractility and cardiac function in improving patient-care decisions and management in selected situations.

Cardiac Contractility

At the onset, it is essential to define the subject under discussion, ventricular contractility. Recent findings obtained from experimental and clinical studies[1] on the control of force and velocity of ventricular contraction have clarified that the function of the intact heart is normally governed by intimate integration of four principal determinants regulating stroke volume and cardiac output: (1) preload (ventricular end-diastolic volume); (2) contractility (variable force of ventricular contraction independent of loading); (3) afterload (ventricular systolic tension during ejection); and (4) heart rate. Preload and contractility are fundamental, intrinsic mechanisms inherent in the contractile machinery of the myocardium, while afterload and heart rate are largely under extrinsic autonomic modulation. Thus, cardiac function and ventricular performance are general terms that include the combined actions of the four principal determinants (not necessarily only the contractility determinant) of cardiac output.

The disturbed mechanisms operative in all types of clinical heart disease can be evaluated and characterized by isolated or composite disorders of these four major determinants of cardiac performance.[1] The recent development of improved techniques and concepts for assessment of cardiac function by both hemodynamic methods and myocardial mechanics[2] has provided means for differential analysis of the roles of each fundamental determinant and their relationships to cardiac compensatory mechanisms governing stroke output in heart disease.

Pathophysiologic Types of Heart Disease

Clinical heart disease can be broadly classified according to three general types of cardiac functional abnormalities[1]: (1) primary contractility disturbance, as in idiopathic or ischemic myocardial disease; (2) diastolic mechanical inhibition of cardiac performance (ventricular underloading), as in restricted ventricular filling in mitral stenosis or pericardial tamponade; and (3) systolic mechanical ventricular overloading, characterized by (a) excessive pressure loading, as in aortic stenosis or essential hypertension, or (b) increased volume loading, as in mitral or aortic regurgitation.

Cardiac Compensatory Mechanisms

Congestive heart failure in systolic ventricular overloading and in primary inotropic disorders occurs when there is substantial depression of contractility.[1] Cardiac decompensation ensues when the impairment of contractile state becomes particularly severe. With systolic hemodynamic overloading or primary contractility disturbance imposed on the heart, three principal compensatory mechanisms provide a limited amount of cardiac reserve to support ventricular function for maintenance of normal resting cardiac output[1]: (1) the Frank-Starling mechanism; (2) ventricular hypertrophy; and (3) the sympathetic nervous system. However, deleterious symptoms necessarily accompany increased operation of these compensatory mechanisms, restricting the extent to which they can be employed.

An understanding of the interactions between contractile state, mechanical abnormalities, and ventricular compensatory mechanisms is essential for a rational approach to the management of congestive heart failure.[1] The abnormal mechanisms operative in each type of heart disease can be analyzed as isolated or combined disorders of the major determinants of cardiac performance. Moreover, appreciation of the determinants of cardiac function provides the physiologic basis for improved understanding of the manner in which various types of heart disease lead to disturbed pump performance and for an organized approach to therapy in the management of congestive heart failure.[3] The physiologic approach to treatment is based on therapeutic adjustment of the four major determinants of cardiac function — preload, contractility, afterload, and heart rate — to provide optimal circumstances for depressed contractile force of the failing pump to deliver normal cardiac output.

Physical Examination

Careful physical examination with cardiac history remains the fundamental basis and the best initial method for early detection of left and right heart failure. Thereby, certain physical signs themselves constitute contractility indices that relate to impaired ventricular function and operation of compensatory reserve mechanisms.[4] These physical indices of myocardial dysfunction can be obtained by analysis of the external systemic venous and arterial pulses, chest examination, cardiac auscultation, and abdominal examination.[4]

Visual inspection of the jugular veins permits a remarkably accurate estimation of central venous pressure and, in turn, right heart failure, since with elevation of right ventricular end-diastolic pressure, right atrial pressure rises. Elevated venous pressure is best observed from the right jugular veins, with the patient's head elevated so that the oscillating blood column top is easily noted. The head of the supine patient's bed is tilted upward until the jugular veins of the patient begin to empty; the pulsating meniscus represents the blood column summit. Central venous pressure (cm water) is equal to this meniscus height, measured relative to the right atrium (the zero level of the column). Column height is estimated from the superior sternal angle, since the right atrium is approximately 5 cm below the sternal angle. With the patient's head elevated 30 degrees, vertical distance from the sternal angle to the top of the blood column is normally under 3 cm. These 3 cm plus the 5 cm from the sternal angle to the right atrium equal 8 cm of blood (approximately 11 mm Hg). Central venous pressure is elevated when vertical distances from the highest point of jugular vein pulsation is more than 3 cm above the sternal angle.[4] Valuable information about cardiac function is also gained from jugular venous pulse contour analysis. The "v" wave is prominent and occurs early in tricuspid regurgitation. The "a" wave is accentuated with right ventricular hypertrophy because of the chamber's reduced compliance.

Palpable dicrotic carotid artery pulsation is often associated with left ventricular pump failure. Thus, in left ventricular failure with reduced stroke volume and diminished cardiac output, a characteristic decrease in the amplitude rate of rise of the systolic percussion wave results in increased amplitude of the subsequent dicrotic pulse, which often becomes palpable.[4] Also, in left ventricular pump failure, the ejection period of the carotid pulse may become shortened because of diminished stroke volume and elevated peripheral vascular resistance. Another useful physical index observed in the arterial pulse is pulsus alternans, alterations of strong and weak peripheral pulses occurring sequentially with each beat.[5] A sign of severe left ventricular dysfunction, pulsus alternans is the result of changes in the force of ventricular contraction caused by variations of contractility and ventricular preload, leading to the alternating magnitude and rate of rise of the carotid arterial pulse. The discrepancy between the amplitude of strong and weak beats and the duration of the phenomenon is directly related to depression of left ventricular contractility. Because of increased sympathetic activity in congestive heart failure, resting heart rate increases with excessive frequency of pulse after minimal exertion, and there is mild diastolic hypertension with narrow pulse pressure. Furthermore, the engorged pulmonary vasculature in left heart failure leads to abnormal Valsalva maneuver response.[6] Thus, the increased pulmonary reservoir maintains left ventricular filling pressure throughout the maneuver, and consequently, stroke volume ejected from the impaired left ventricle remains higher, as does systemic blood pressure. Since systemic blood pressure does not fall during the maneuver, there is neither post–Valsalva maneuver blood pressure overshoot nor reflex bradycardia. Since there is redistribution of reduced total peripheral blood flow among the body's organs in left heart failure,[2] perfusion of the cutaneous and renal circulations is diminished, which results in decreased skin temperature, heat intolerance, and often, prerenal azotemia. In addition, the distal extremities become cool, increased sweating occurs, and there may be cyanosis due to increased oxygen extraction, causing oxygen desaturation in the skin's veins.

Left ventricular failure produces a rise in left ventricular end-diastolic pressure and left atrial pressure, which is transmitted to the pulmonary capillaries via a rise in pulmonary venous pressure. When pulmonary capillary hydrostatic pressure exceeds colloid osmotic pressure, transudation of fluid into the interstitial spaces occurs, leading to increased pulmonary extravascular fluid. Interstitial edema leads to alveolar edema, with pulmonary rales detectable by chest wall auscultation. Pleural effusions are also common in chronic congestive heart failure. Hydrothorax most often occurs with right heart or biventricular failure, with increased systemic venous pressure being more important than elevated pulmonary capillary pressure in pleural effusion formation. Chronic heart failure ultimately results in progressive left ventricular hypertrophy, which can be perceived by precordial palpation. In concentric hypertrophy without dilation, left ventricular hypertrophy produces increased apical pulse amplitude in the left lateral position. In hypertrophy with reduced left ventricular compliance, palpation reveals prominent presystolic pulsation caused by left atrial contraction with diminished ventricular distensibility. In right ventricular hypertrophy, abnormal outward systolic motion occurs along the left sternal border. Left ventricular dilation is determined by precordial palpation with the apical impulse lateral to the midclavicular line. Left ventricular dilation also causes widening of the mitral valve ring and papillary muscle dysfunction, resulting in incompetence of the mitral valve leaflets, with pansystolic murmur at the cardiac apex. Similarly, right ventricular dilation can lead to tricuspid regurgitation with systolic murmur, often increasing during inspiration, at the lower left sternal border.

Impairment of ventricular contractility is usually accompanied by a low-frequency early diastolic sound (S_3), audible with the stethoscope bell placed lightly over the apex of the heart. A presystolic or fourth heart sound (S_4) during atrial contraction may also occur with ventricular dysfunction and/or decreased ventricular diastolic compliance. In sinus tachycardia, S_3 and S_4 usually merge to produce a summation gallop. Since the rate of left ventricular pressure rise is diminished during isovolumic systole with depressed contractility,[7] first-heart-sound intensity is decreased in left ventricular failure. Left ventricular ejection may also be delayed in the presence of myocardial failure, and second-heart-sound paradoxical splitting may occur.

In right heart failure, elevated right atrial pressure increases venous pressure throughout the entire systemic venous bed, thus leading to engorgement of abdominal organs, with hepatomegaly and, occasionally, splenomegaly. Severe tricuspid regurgitation may cause liver pulsation during systole. In addition, peripheral edema and ascites may occur in severe chronic right heart failure. The hepatojugular reflux maneuver may elucidate borderline right ventricular failure.

Exercise Stress Testing

Exercise stress testing provides a useful, objective, non-invasive technique by which to assess cardiac function and contractility.[2] In the absence of extra-cardiac factors limiting oxygen transport, exertional capacity is determined principally by cardiocirculatory dynamics. Therefore, measurement of exercise tolerance affords a cardiac performance index. Normally, cardiac output increases during exercise, secondary to augmentation of heart rate, myocardial contractility, and stroke volume.[2] Since the exertional cardiac output increase correlates linearly with maximal total body oxygen consumption (VO_2), the VO_2 achieved at maximal exercise is an indirect index of cardiac function.[2] Exercise stress testing may uncover abnormal cardiac function in occult heart disease, as well as quantify impaired cardiac performance in overt cardiac disorders. Dynamic treadmill or bicycle exercise is carried out, since cardiocirculatory responses with isotonic exertion are proportional to aerobic requirements. Treadmill exertion has been the predominant form of exercise stress testing performed in this country.

The most accurate method of quantifying exertional capacity is measurement of maximal total body oxygen uptake ($\dot{V}O_2$). A number of techniques can be used for collection and analysis of respired gases during exercise testing. In our laboratory, the on-line measurements of oxygen consumption and CO_2 production are performed via mass spectrometer. A popular treadmill exercise protocol for assessing maximal oxygen consumption has been developed by Bruce and associates.[8] The Bruce Test, which applies progressive increases in both treadmill speed and slope at three-minute intervals, provides a linear relationship between duration of exercise and oxygen uptake. Since close estimation of maximal total body oxygen consumption for an individual may thereby be obtained indirectly simply by determining minutes of exertion, cardiac function is evaluated in this manner. Oxygen requirements for various stages of exercise have been well established for a number of treadmill exercise protocols in addition to that developed by Bruce. We have utilized an exercise protocol known as

BRANCHING MULTISTAGE TREADMILL TEST PROTOCOL

STAGE	WALK TIME min	BRANCH I SPEED MPH	BRANCH I SPEED M/min	BRANCH I SLOPE %	BRANCH I VO₂ ml/min·Kg	BRANCH II SPEED MPH	BRANCH II SPEED M/min	BRANCH II SLOPE %	BRANCH II VO₂ ml/min·Kg	BRANCH III SPEED MPH	BRANCH III SPEED M/min	BRANCH III SLOPE %	BRANCH III VO₂ ml/min·Kg	BRANCH IV SPEED MPH	BRANCH IV SPEED M/min	BRANCH IV SLOPE %	BRANCH IV VO₂ ml/min·Kg	BRANCH V SPEED MPH	BRANCH V SPEED M/min	BRANCH V SLOPE %	BRANCH V VO₂ ml/min·Kg
1	0-2	1.97	53	0	9.5																
2	2-4	2.62	70	0	12	If below 70% MHR* at 4 minutes, follow Branch II															
3	4-6	2.62	70	3	14	3.19	85	0	14.5												
4	6-8	2.62	70	6	17	3.19	85	3.5	18	If below 70% MHR* at 8 minutes, follow Branch III											
5	8-10	2.62	70	9	20	3.19	85	6	21	3.63	97	3.5	21								
6	10-12	2.62	70	12	23	3.19	85	9	24.5	3.63	97	7	25	If below 70% MHR* at 12 minutes, follow Branch IV							
7	12-14	2.62	70	15	26	3.19	85	12	28	3.63	97	10	29	4.01	107	7.5	30				
8	14-16	2.62	70	17.5	32	3.19	85	15	32	3.63	97	13	33.5	4.01	107	12	36.5	If below 70% MHR* at 16 minutes, follow Branch V			
9	16-18	2.62	70	20	32.5	3.19	85	17.5	36.5	3.63	97	16	38.5	4.01	107	15	42.5	5.21	139	12.0	47
10	18-20	2.62	70	22	36	3.19	85	20	41	3.63	97	19	44.5	4.01	107	18	49	5.21	139	16.0	57
11	20-22					3.19	85	22	44.5	3.63	97	22	51	4.01	107	20	54	5.21	139	19.5	66.5
12	22-24													4.01	107	22	60	5.21	139	22.0	77
13	24-26																	6.20	166	22.0	85

*MHR = Maximal Heart Rate

Figure 1. Protocol for branching multistage treadmill test. As delineated, the test employs an initial two-minute period of walking, followed by successive three-minute periods of walking in which speed is constant (MPH = miles per hour; M/min = meters per minute) while treadmill's angle of elevation (slope) is gradually increased at walking stages within each branch. Work rate is progressively greater in branches I through V, resulting from moderate rise in speed of treadmill (kept constant for given branch) with gradual elevation of slope at each period of walking. If individual's heart rate is below 70 per cent of maximal predicted heart rate (70% MPH) at stage of walking indicated for given branch, protocol for next higher branch is followed. Normal values for total body oxygen consumption ($\dot{V}O_2$) are given for each stage of walking of each branch. Exercise testing of this type is not rapidly stressful and is well tolerated, allowing identification of subtle differences in physical and cardiac performance.

the Branching Multistage Treadmill Protocol.[9] The branching system utilizes increases in both treadmill speed and slope based on the individual's response to the previously applied work load (Fig. 1). Thereby, individuals who exhibit marked increases in heart rate in response to one work load are given only a small additional increment of effort, while individuals who tolerate a previously applied level of exertion without substantial change in heart rate are given a considerably greater augmentation of effort. Accordingly, by means of the branching protocol, we are able to estimate overall total body oxygen consumption within relative narrow limits. Thus, with regard to exercise protocols, we prefer the branching procedure for evaluating cardiac function ($\dot{V}O_2$), and the Bruce Test for detecting myocardial ischemia (ECG ST-segment depression). Concerning the relation of $\dot{V}O_2$ to symptomatic classification of cardiac function, maximal oxygen consumption of 14 mL O_2/kg/min or less is considered functional Class III (cardiac symptoms with ordinary activity), while maximal oxygen consumption of over 21 mL O_2/kg/min is defined as functional Class I (normal). Thus, evaluation of impairment of cardiac function by means of exercise stress testing represents an important application of this non-invasive diagnostic technique. Furthermore, assessment of exertional tolerance provides objective numerical analysis of cardiac performance initially and serially during chronic evaluation. In our hospital, graded treadmill exercise testing is a standard test performed in all patients with cardiac disease.

Systolic Time Intervals

The simultaneous recording of the electrocardiogram, phonocardiogram, and carotid arterial pulsations allows indirect determination of total electromechanical systole (Q–S_2 interval — the period from the beginning of the QRS complex to the first high-frequency vibration of the second heart sound). Included in this period are left ventricular ejection time (LVET —onset of upstroke to the incisural notch of the carotid tracing) and pre-ejection period (PEP — total electromechanical systole minus LVET) (Fig. 2).[10] Normally, the LVET is 415 ± 10 (SD) msec, and the pre-ejection period is 132 ± 12 (SD) msec. Although we have found the measurement of systolic time intervals (STI) to be less useful indices of cardiac function and contractility than the other procedures described here, the STI concept is briefly described for comprehensive understanding of techniques that may be utilized.

In patients with primary and secondary abnormalities of myocardial contractility, PEP usually lengthens, while LVET shortens, sometimes before overt congestive heart failure. Thus, the ratio of pre-ejection period to ejection time (PEP/LVET — normal 0.35 ± 0.04 [SD]) provides an index of cardiac function, permitting gross separation of patients with diminished contractility from normal patients. The PEP/LVET ratio is relatively sensitive to diminished contractile state of cardiomyopathies, systemic arterial hypertension, and chronic coronary heart disease. In valvular heart disease,

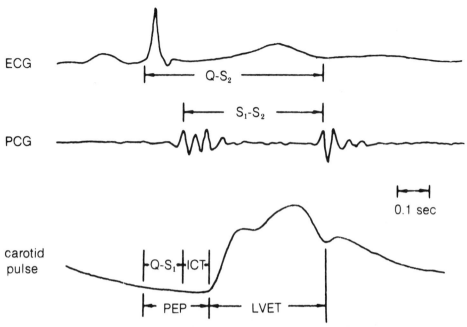

Figure 2. Systolic time intervals. Recordings of the electrocardiogram, phonocardiogram (PCG), and indirect carotid arterial pulse demonstrate the systolic time intervals (ICT = isovolumic contraction time; PEP = pre-ejection period; LVET = left ventricular ejection time).

however, the index is somewhat less accurate owing to concomitant chronic pressure and volume overload. Acute myocardial infarction usually results in normal or variable PEP, whereas LVET is abbreviated. In serial studies in individual patients, PEP is altered by acute changes of preload or afterload alone, as well as by changes in contractility. Digitalis shortens both the PEP and LVET. Leg exercise in patients with angina pectoris due to coronary disease leads to increase of LVET, which remains unchanged in normal subjects. PEP shortens with exercise in normal subjects, but remains unchanged in patients with angina pectoris. Left ventricular conduction defects produce lengthening of PEP without alterations of LVET. In these disturbances, however, determination of isovolumic contraction time as the measure of pre-ejection duration offers advantages over PEP, since the isovolumic contraction time is not influenced by variations of QRS depolarization time.

Echocardiography

The most important new examining technique in cardiovascular medicine is echocardiography. By providing acoustic images of pulsed ultrasound reflected from the interface between two structures of different densities, the echocardiogram measures dynamic movement of heart chambers and valves, gives absolute dimensions of cardiac structures, and quantifies hemodynamic and mechanical performance characteristics of the heart.[11] This technique has rapidly become an indispensable tool in non-invasive diagnostic cardiology and is employed for the study of cardiac function, identification of disease entities, and evaluation of medical treatment. Echocardiography can evaluate cardiac performance by measurement of heart chamber size; left ventricular wall thickness; derived left ventricular volumes; left ventricular wall motion; velocity of circumferential fiber shortening; and alterations of mitral valve motion, which reflect changes in left ventricular compliance. Figure 3 demonstrates the single time-motion (M-mode) sector scan of an echocardiogram taken at the level of the mid left ventricle to show the manner in which left ventricular dimensions and other variables that provide quantitative indices of cardiac function and

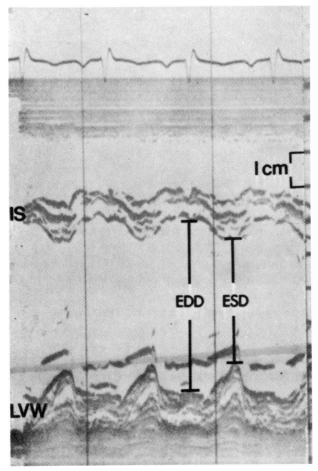

Figure 3. Normal left ventricular echogram. Left ventricular dimensions are noted on this echogram of a normal subject. Parameters of cardiac function derived from these measurements include: end-diastolic volume (EDV) = EDD³; stroke volume (SV) = EDV − ESV; mean velocity of circumferential fiber shortening (V_{CF}) = EDD − ESD/ET × EDD, where ET is ejection time. (IS = interventricular septum; EDD = end-diastolic dimension; ESD = end-systolic dimension; LVW = left ventricular posterior wall).

Echocardiographic normal values

Left ventricle, end-diastolic dimension	3.5 to 5.6 cm
Left ventricular wall thickness	0.7 to 1.1 cm
Right ventricle, end-diastolic dimension	0.7 to 2.3 cm
Left atrium dimension	1.9 to 4.0 cm
Left ventricular ejection fraction	0.66 ± 0.09 SD
Left ventricular mean velocity of circumferential fiber shortening (V_{CF})	1.26 ± 0.24 SD circ/sec

Figure 4.   Echocardiographic normal values.

contractility are obtained. Figure 4 provides normal values for certain of these important variables obtained by echocardiography.

The recent advent of two-dimensional echocardiography has enabled the evaluation of cardiac function by ultrasound with greater accuracy.[11] Accordingly, by providing an additional dimension (either superior-inferior or lateral) to the standard anteroposterior "ice-pick" view of one-dimensional echocardiography, cross-sectional echocardiography allows examination of a greater expanse of the heart. More important, by virtue of affording spatial orientation, two-dimensional echocardiography permits visualization of the heart and great vessels from new transducer positions on the thorax, thereby enabling imaging of cardiac structures heretofore impossible to image. A variety of technical approaches have been utilized in imaging the heart two-dimensionally by ultrasound. The simplest approach has been to attach a mechanical device capable of rotating the single-element ultrasound transducer rapidly through 30- to 90-degree sector arcs. When this rotating single crystal is interfaced with an electrical device capable of providing information regarding the transducer in space, a wedge-shaped, two-dimensional image is produced. A second type of approach is to arrange series of individual ultrasound transducers in linear array and to simultaneously display the echoes from each element. Finally, the more complex approach to two-dimensional cardiac imaging is the phase-array technique, by which multiple echocardiographic elements are transmitted with variable time delay, so that the ultrasound beam may be steered electronically through sector arcs of the heart (Fig. 5).[12] Each of these approaches has a unique set of advantages and limitations.

The standardly applied cross-sectional imaging devices provide sector arc images of cardiovascular structures of variable angles, ranging from 30 to 90 degrees. This fan-shaped sector arc may then be directed into the thorax from several positions. The conventional approaches to imaging the heart with two-dimensional echocardiography have included aligning the sector arc along the long axis of the left ventricle (from the aorta to the left ventricular apex) and along the short axis of the left ventricle (perpendicular to the long axis). In addition, the ability to visualize wide expanses of cardiac anatomy has enabled positioning of the ultrasound transducer at the cardiac apex, so that the fan-shaped sector arc includes all four cardiac chambers

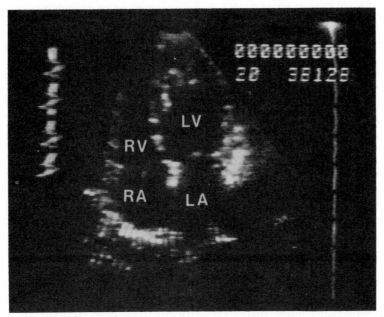

Figure 5. Hemiaxial or four-chamber view of a cross-sectional echogram in a normal patient. The ultrasound transducer has been positioned at the point of maximal apical impulse and directed superiorly, posteriorly, and medially. All four cardiac chambers, the interatrial and interventricular septa and mitral and tricuspid valves, may be simultaneously evaluated in this projection. (RA = right atrium; RV = right ventricle; LA = left atrium; LV = left ventricle).

with mitral and tricuspid valves. Such a four-chambered (hemiaxial) view is particularly helpful in imaging the entire silhouette of the left ventricle, as well as enabling the ultrasound recording of the right ventricle and right atrium (Fig. 5).[12]

The ability to image the heart with two-dimensional echocardiography has many advantages. A tomogram of the entire left ventricular silhouette may be obtained in a variety of positions, thus eliminating the potential error of recording isolated portions of the left ventricle that may not be representative of the structure and function of the whole chamber. Thereby, cross-sectional echocardiography substantially enhances the accuracy of ultrasound in the evaluation of left ventricular size, contractile pattern, function, and contractility. In our experience, various forms of segmental dyssynergy as recorded by two-dimensional echocardiography have correlated well with those observed by cineangiography or anticipated by electrocardiographic evidence of previous myocardial infarction. Furthermore, approaches are now being perfected to determine left ventricular volume from the two-dimensional echocardiogram. An important additional capability conferred by two-dimensional echocardiography has been the capacity to evaluate the structure and function of the right ventricle and right atrium.[12] Studies in our laboratory have indicated that these right-sided cardiac chambers were easily and reproducibly imaged in nearly all patients in whom the examination was attempted (Fig. 5). In addition, measurements of right ventricular and right atrial size by two-dimensional echocardiography compared favorably with those of plaster casts of these chambers obtained from necropsy specimens. Furthermore, measurements of right atrial and right ventricular size by two-dimensional echocardiography clearly distinguished patients with right ventricular volume overload from normal subjects. Accordingly, cross-sectional echocardiography has permitted evaluation of right-sided cardiac chamber dysfunction by ultrasound.

Early experience with cross-sectional echocardiography has yielded promising results concerning a new application of the technique that is of major importance in the improved evaluation of cardiac function by ultrasound. Specifically, the peripheral venous injection of almost any liquid, including the patient's own blood, is capable of producing microcavitations or microbubbles that reflect ultrasound and fill the cardiac chambers with a dense cloud of echoes.[13] These microcavitations are subsequently filtered by the pulmonary circulation and are not normally imaged in the left-sided cardiac chambers. Thereby, two-dimensional echocardiography coupled with the peripheral venous injection of a liquid material is capable of providing data regarding intracardiac flow patterns. These studies have been of marked value in the recognition of right-to-left cardiac shunts and in the detection of tricuspid regurgitation.[13] More important, however, the resultant cross-sectional echocardiograms can be subjected to analysis by analog photometry, and the appearance and decay characteristics resulting from the microcavitations representative of cardiac flow may be measured. Our early experience has indicated that such echographic dye-dilution curves are of considerable value in the non-invasive assessment of cardiac output.

Another promising new development regarding cross-sectional echocardiography relates to its valuable combination with Doppler ultrasound.[14] The Doppler shift of an ultrasound signal produced by a column of blood is related to the velocity of the blood and the angle at which the ultrasound beam strikes the column. By knowing the velocity of flow via the Doppler shift and also the cross-sectional area through which blood flow occurs, as obtained by cross-sectional echocardiography, calculation of actual blood flow through the given area of the central circulation is provided. Such techniques combining two-dimensional echocardiography and Doppler ultrasound are of considerable value in the accurate, non-invasive assessment of cardiac function and contractility indices.

Nuclear Cardiology

Non-invasive nuclear cardiology techniques have been used in three major areas in the evaluation of ventricular function: (1) determination of ejection fraction and abnormalities of regional wall motion; (2) evaluation of regional myocardial perfusion using peripheral venous injections of radioactive potassium, rubidium, or thallium (cold-spot imaging); and (3) identification of acute myocardial infarction with radiopharmaceuticals (technetium-99m pyrophosphate and related agents) that accumulate in the necrotic myocardium (hot-spot imaging). The technique of radioisotopic angiocardiography was initially developed in 1969[15] using the Anger scintillation camera. Subsequently, a non-invasive radionuclide method was described using gated cardiac blood pool imaging with the scintillation camera for estimating ejection fraction and segmental contraction. Ejection fraction can also be measured by using scintillations obtained with the camera within an area of interest encompassing the left ventricular chamber. Measurement of ejection fraction is also possible by the area-of-interest approach using a single precordial probe with a strip-chart recorder. Unlike the gated blood pool imaging methods, these latter area-counts methods fail to provide information regarding regional contraction patterns.

In our laboratories, we have developed an improved method of dual-gated blood pool imaging for measuring ejection fraction and assessing regional contraction patterns in patients (Fig. 6).[16] The validity of this imaging technique has been established by correlation with selective left ventricular cineangiography in a large group of patients (Fig. 6B), and its practicality and usefulness in directing clinical decisions have been demonstrated by our experience in several patients. With the patient in a supine position beneath the detector of a scintillation camera equipped with a high-resolution collimator and rotated 30 degrees to the right anterior oblique position, a bolus of 15 to 20 mCi of ^{99m}Tc-tagged autologous red blood cells is injected through a short plastic catheter in an antecubital vein (Fig. 6A). The scintigraphic data obtained during the initial minute after injection are collected without gating on videotape for subsequent validation of the location of the aortic and mitral annuli. After the first minute, an R-wave–triggered gating device activates the oscilloscope of the scintillation camera for a 60-msec period at end-diastole and again at end-systole (Fig. 6A). The phonocardiogram is used for the precise timing of the end-systolic gating interval,[16] which consists of the 60 msec immediately preceding the first high-frequency component of the second heart sound. End-diastole is

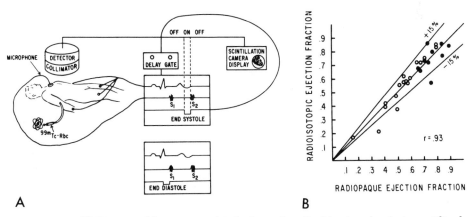

A   B

Figure 6. (A) Diagram of the scintigraphic dual-gated cardiac blood pool technique utilized. (B) Comparison of left ventricular ejection fraction measurements obtained by radioisotopic and radiopaque methods in 27 patients. Closed circles are normal contraction pattern; open circles are abnormal contraction pattern. Center line is line of identity and outlines represent 15% distribution limits.

established as the 60-msec interval immediately after the R wave and is pinpointed by setting the delay control of the gating apparatus at zero. Thus, the end-diastolic interval always occurs immediately after the QRS complex and is independent of the R-R interval. Polaroid film is used to record 500,000-count gated images of end-systole and end-diastole from 500 to 1000 cardiac cycles, requiring approximately 10 minutes per picture. After the initial end-systolic imaging, gated images can be obtained in the modified left anterior oblique position for observation of septal and posterior wall motion, or repeated right anterior oblique gated images can be obtained after the administration of sublingual nitroglycerin to assess the viability of abnormally contracting segments.[17] These procedures do not require repeated injection of the radiopharmaceutical.

The dual-gated images are interpreted by outlining the borders of the left ventricle with a paraffin pencil. In most patients, these borders, including the aortic and mitral planes, are determined by inspection of the end-systolic and end-diastolic gated images; in some patients, however, it is necessary to use the initial transit image of the left ventricle. Transparent 35-mm photographs of the outlined end-systolic and end-diastolic images and of calibration images are projected to life size, and the superimposed outlines of the left ventricle in systole and diastole are traced onto paper. From this tracing, regional contraction patterns are observed, and the end-systolic and end-diastolic volumes are determined by the area-length method. Ejection fraction is calculated by dividing stroke volume by the end-diastolic volume. Comparison of the scintigraphic method with left ventricular cineangiography in a large group of patients showed excellent correlations of ejection fraction and abnormal contraction patterns.[16] An example of the use of the dual-scintigraphic imaging technique in evaluating pump performance in a patient with pre-infarction angina before and after sublingual nitroglycerin[17] and after surgical coronary revascularization is shown in Figure 7. Gated scintigraphy documented the efficacy of surgery without the use of cardiac catheterization. With respect to abnormalities in the region of the septum, a striking example of the diagnostic capabilities of this procedure[16] is shown by the modified left anterior oblique images that were obtained in a patient with idiopathic hypertrophic subaortic stenosis (Fig. 8).

By combining a computer with a scintillation camera and gating device, it is now possible to obtain images of the cardiac blood pool during selected segments from the entire cardiac cycle. This technique is multiple-gated cardiac blood scintigraphy.[18] With the dual-gated technique[16] delineated above, scintigraphic data are obtained from only the selected end-systolic and end-diastolic portions of the cycle, and the remaining scintigraphic data are discarded. With the multiple-gated technique, in contrast, imaging is performed throughout the many different phases of the cardiac cycle.[18] The resulting information can be used to form a ventricular time-versus-activity curve (Fig. 9). Since the number of counts emitted from the blood pool radiopharmaceutical is proportional to the blood volume in a given region, the ventricular time-versus-activity curve is a relative time-versus-volume curve of the left ventricle. From this curve, ejection fraction

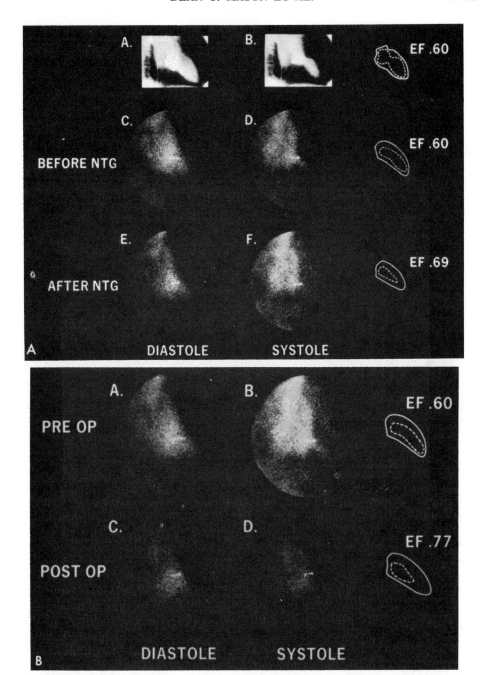

Figure 7. (Panels A and B). Scintigraphy in preinfarction angina. In Panel A, left ventricular right anterior oblique cineangiograms (top) in diastole (angiogram A) and systole (angiogram B) are compared with scintigrams in a patient with the preinfarction angina syndrome before (Panel A: images C and D; Panel B: images A and B) sublingual nitroglycerin (NTG). Illustrations on the right represent end-diastolic (solid lines) and end-systolic (broken lines) silhouettes; ejection fractions (EF) are also given. Scintigraphic images taken after nitroglycerin (Panel A: images E and F) and after successful coronary artery bypass surgery (Panel B: images C and D) reveal improvement of the hypokinetic left ventricular apex during systole, indicating ischemic involvement rather than infarction of this area.

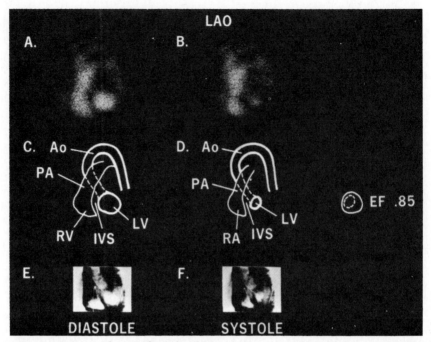

Figure 8. Scintigraphy in idiopathic hypertrophic subaortic stenosis. Biventricular left anterior oblique (LAO) cineangiograms (bottom) in a patient with idiopathic hypertrophic subaortic stenosis are here compared with scintigrams (top) at end-diastole and at end-systole: Diagrams (center) are drawn from the radionuclidic images; ejection fraction (EF) is also noted. Asymmetric thickening of the interventricular septum is clearly documented in the systolic and diastolic scintigraphic and cineangiographic pictures. (Ao = ascending aorta; PA = pulmonary artery; IVS = interventricular septum; LV = left ventricle; RA and RV = right ventricle).

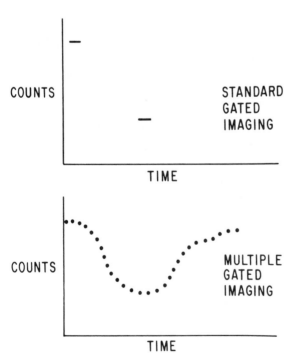

Figure 9. Comparison of multiple-gated and standard dual-gated imaging. In the dual-gated approach (top), the scintigraphic imaging data are collected only from the end-diastolic and end-systolic portions of the cardiac cycle; with multiple-gated imaging (bottom), scintigraphic data are accumulated from the entire cardiac cycle. When counts from a left ventricular region of interest are plotted against time, a time-versus-activity curve that is relative to a time-versus-volume curve of the left ventricle is formed.

can be measured by comparing the peak to the nadir, and in addition, other systolic and diastolic properties of ventricular contraction and relaxation can be observed.

With the multiple-gated scintigraphic blood pool technique, both the imaging data and electrocardiographic data (a pulse representing the R wave) are put into the dedicated minicomputer (Fig. 10A).[18] Based on the temporal relation between the scintigraphic events and the R wave, the computer places the scintigraphic data into different memory components (Fig. 10B). In our laboratory, the cardiac cycle is divided into 28 equal segments, and thereby, 28 separate images are obtained from each cardiac cycle. As in the dual-gating technique, scintigraphic data from successive beats are accumulated until the average image contains 200,000 counts in the region of the heart. Recent advances in computer programming allow

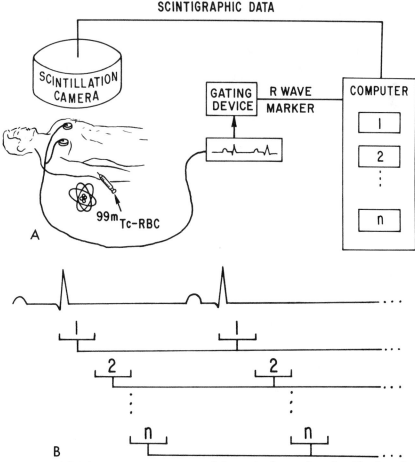

Figure 10. (A) Schematic representation of the multiple-gated cardiac blood pool scintigraphic technique. Both scintigraphic data and electrocardiographic data (an R-wave pulse) are put into the computer. (B) Diagram of the method by which the computer generates the multiple-gated images. The computer places the scintigraphic data into different memory buffers, depending on the temporal relation of these data to the R-wave marker. For each interval, scintigraphic data from successive beats are accumulated until the average image contains 200,000 counts in the region of the heart.

images for ejection fraction to be obtained from one-minute accumulation of scintigraphic data, and images for visualization of wall motion from two to three minutes of scintigraphic imaging.[18] As with the dual-gated technique, the multiple view can be obtained and the imaging procedure can be repeated after a variety of interventions, such as administration of nitroglycerin or bicycle exercise, without need for a separate injection of radiopharmaceutical. After completion of the multiple-gated scintigraphic study, the scintigraphic data are visualized on the oscilloscope of the computer by playback of the 28 different images in a movie format. This allows accurate assessment of regional wall motion. Subsequently, the computer processing of the left anterior oblique view is utilized for the semiautomatic detection of the left ventricular edge. Left ventricular ejection fraction and time-versus-activity curves are calculated from the radioactivity within the 28 computer-derived left ventricular edges. In our laboratory,[18] the technique has proved to be an accurate method for assessing regional wall motion and left ventricular ejection fraction.

The multiple-gated scintigraphic method, like the dual-gated technique,[16] is useful for the non-invasive evaluation of global and regional left ventricular function.[18] With respect to multiple-gated scintigraphy with nitroglycerin, it is possible to assess the viability of dyssynergistic segments in coronary disease with a single injection of the blood pool radiopharmaceutical in a manner similar to that utilized with contrast cineangiography. The advantage of the multiple-gated scintigraphic technique is that multiple determinations can be made, so that the peak of drug action can be observed; further scintigraphy does not cause depression of myocardial contractile state associated with contrast medium. We have determined that patients with prior infarction have no improvement in wall motion after the administration of nitroglycerin, whereas patients without prior myocardial infarction may show improvement in wall motion in akinetic segments.[18] The multiple-gated technique is also helpful in predicting the effects of coronary bypass surgery on left ventricular function. Since resolution of images is better with blood pool technetium-99m methods than with myocardial cold-spot imaging with thallium-201, the sensitivity of stress wall motion blood pool techniques appears greater than that of thallium-201 stress myocardial perfusion scintigraphy in the detection of coronary disease. Thus, gated blood pool scintigraphic evaluation of left ventricular function, both global and regional, during exercise stress and pharmacologic intervention is a valuable modality in the non-invasive assessment of chronic coronary disease and in the evaluation of cardiac function and contractility in other types of heart disease as well.

Cardiac Catheterization

The most important advance in cardiovascular medicine in the past 25 years has been the development of methods for catheterization of the human heart that can be carried out with relative ease and safety. Application of these techniques has provided an appreciation of the pathophysiologic mechanisms in heart disease and has established cardiovascular diagnosis and evaluation on a scientific basis. The ability to define precisely and to quantify even the most complex disorders has spearheaded innovative medical therapy, successful surgical treatment, and investigative interest in heart disease in general. As a result of the rapid and spectacular progress achieved in invasive techniques and procedures for the direct diagnosis of heart disease and the evaluation of cardiac function and contractility, the specialized science of cardiac catheterization is the "Supreme Court" of cardiology and the "gold standard" for verification of the accuracy and reliability of the aforementioned noninvasive methods.

It is not our intent to delineate the methods and rationale involved in the clinical assessment of heart disease and ventricular performance by cardiac catheterization. These techniques and the significance of the data obtained have been discussed in detail by us previously.[19] Suffice it to state that there are two general approaches to the evaluation of contractility and function of the heart: (1) its pump (hemodynamics) performance characteristics and (2) its muscle (mechanics) performance characteristics. In the traditional approach of pump analysis, contractile state can be estimated qualitatively by the standard hemodynamic variables of cardiac output, stroke volume, systolic ejection rate, left ventricular end-diastolic pressure, and the more complex variables of ventricular end-diastolic volume, ejection fraction, stroke work, stroke power, and ventricular mass. The accuracy of cardiac pump measurements in the evaluation of contractility is increased by determining the hemodynamic response to certain interventions such as exercise and alterations in ventricular loading. Furthermore, inotropic accuracy is improved by evaluating hemodynamic responses within the concept of the Frank-Starling principle (ventricular function curves), which relates pump performance characteristics such as cardiac output to ventricular preload (left ventricular end-diastolic pressure). Recently, it has become possible to clinically examine contractility and ventricular function by the second general approach, muscle mechanics, which describes the force, velocity, and length of the ventricular myocardium. In the quantification of contractile state, the mechanical events occurring during both the isovolumic and the ejection phases of systole have been developed along two general lines: (1) isovolumic indices utilizing dp/dt (rate of ventricular pressure rise) and (2) ejection indices employing V_{cf} (circumferential fiber shortening rate).

In the management of cardiac patients, catheterization is mandatory for the precise definition of the extent and nature of the disorder in the consideration of heart surgery. Furthermore, catheterization is often necessary for diagnosis and for evaluation of ventricular function in the proper management of the cardiac patient by medical therapy. Invasive diagnostic techniques are required for measurements of intracardiac pressures and delineation of coronary anatomy. Nevertheless, in the past decade, increasing attention has turned to the development of improved non-invasive techniques for cardiovascular evaluation. It is the value of these new non-invasive methods that we have particularly focused upon in this essay. It is clear that the recent advances in non-invasive techniques have already contributed greatly to modern cardiology, and there is considerable promise of extension of these exciting developments in the future. Some of the new non-invasive methods are able to provide more accurate information than invasive examination, such as some of the measurements obtained by echocardiography and nuclear cardiology, while other non-invasive measurements and techniques serve as valuable screening tests for the identification of patients who should undergo more precise measurement by cardiac catheterization.

ACKNOWLEDGMENTS

The authors gratefully acknowledge the technical assistance of Robert Kleckner, Alexander Neumann, Raya Drahun, and Leslie Silvernail.

References

1. Mason DT: Regulation of cardiac performance in clinical heart disease: interactions between contractile state, mechanical abnormalities and ventricular compensatory mechanisms. Am J Cardiol 32:437–448, 1973.
2. Mason DT, Spann JF Jr, Zelis R, and Amsterdam EA: Alterations of hemodynamics and myocardial mechanics in patients with congestive heart failure: pathophysiologic mechanisms and assessment of cardiac function and ventricular contractility. Progr Cardiovasc Dis 12:507–557, 1970.
3. Mason DT, Miller RR, Williams DO, DeMaria AN, Segel LD, and Amsterdam EA: Management of chronic refractory congestive heart failure. In Mason DT (ed): Congestive Heart Failure. New York, Yorke Medical Books, 1976, pp 293–312.
4. Mason DT, DeMaria AN, Amsterdam EA, Miller RR, and Berman DS: Non-invasive evaluation of ventricular function. Cardiovasc Med 1:283–301, 1976.
5. Massumi R, Zelis R, Ali N, and Mason DT: External venous and arterial pulses. In Weissler AM (ed): Noninvasive Cardiology. New York, Grune and Stratton, 1974, pp 401–442.
6. Gill JR Jr, Mason DT, and Bartter FC: Idiopathic edema resulting from occult myocardiopathy and its correction with digitalis. Am J Med 39:475–480, 1965.
7. Mason DT: Usefulness and limitations of the rate of rise of intraventricular pressure (dp/dt) in the evaluation of myocardial contractility in man. Am J Cardiol 23:516–527, 1969.
8. Bruce RA: Methods of exercise testing: step test, bicycle, treadmill, isometrics. In Amsterdam EA, Wilmore JH, and DeMaria AN (eds): Exercise in Cardiovascular Health and Disease. New York, Yorke Medical Books, 1977, pp 149–160.
9. Tonkon M, Lee G, DeMaria AN, Miller RR, and Mason DT: Effects of digitalis on the exercise electrocardiogram in normal adult subjects. Chest 72:714–718, 1977.
10. Weissler AM, Harris WS, and Shoenfeld CD: Systolic time intervals in heart failure in man. Circulation 37:149–160, 1977.
11. DeMaria AN, Neumann A, and Mason DT: Echographic evaluation of cardiac function. In Mason DT (ed): Congestive Heart Failure. New York, Yorke Medical Books, 1976, pp 191–224.
12. Bommer W, Weinnert L, Neumann A, Neef J, Mason DT, and DeMaria AN: Determination of right atrial and right ventricular size by two-dimensional echocardiography. Circulation 60:91–100, 1979.
13. Bommer W, Neumann A, Mason DT, and DeMaria AN: Application of echographic contrast studies in evaluating heart disease. In Mason DT (ed): Advances in Heart Disease, Vol. III. New York, Grune and Stratton (In press).

14. Bommer W, Neumann A, Mason DT, and DeMaria AN: Current status of pulse-Doppler ultrasound in clinical cardiology. *In* Mason DT (ed): *Advances in Heart Disease*, Vol. II. New York, Grune and Stratton, 1978.

15. Mason DT, Ashburn WL, Harbert JC, Cohen LS, and Braunwald E: Rapid sequential visualization of the heart and great vessels in man using the wide-field Anger scintillation camera: radioisotope-angiography following the injection of technetium-99m. Circulation 39:19–28, 1969.

16. Berman DS, Salel AF, DeNardo GL, Bogren HG, and Mason DT: Clinical assessment of left ventricular regional contraction patterns and ejection fraction by high-resolution gated scintigraphy. J Nucl Med 16:865–874, 1976.

17. Salel AF, Berman DS, DeNardo GL, and Mason DT: Radionuclide assessment of nitroglycerin influence on abnormal left ventricular segmental contraction in patients with coronary heart disease. Circulation 53:975–982, 1976.

18. Berman DS, Amsterdam EA, Joye JA, Glass E, Levine D, Lurie A, DeNardo GL, and Mason DT: Multiple-gated cardiac blood pool scintigraphy. Presented at the Annual Western Regional Meeting of the Society of Nuclear Medicine, Las Vegas, Nevada, October, 1977.

19. Mason DT, Miller RR, Vismara LA, Williams DO, Berman DS, Salel AF, Bogren HG, DeNardo GL, and Amsterdam EA: Clinical assessment of heart disease and ventricular performance by cardiac catheterization. *In* Mason DT (ed): *Congestive Heart Failure*. New York, Yorke Medical Books, 1976, pp 225–272.

The Measurement of Contractility Indices in the Management of Cardiac Patients: Clinically Useless*

G. E. BURCH, M.D.

Emeritus Henderson Professor, Department of Medicine,
Tulane University School of Medicine; and the Charity
Hospital of Louisiana, New Orleans, Louisiana

Any reasonable, simple, reliable, inexpensive, and innocuous procedure that can assist in establishing a diagnosis and improving management should not only be accepted in the practice of medicine, but should also be fostered and strongly recommended to the practicing physician. But when a diagnostic or therapeutic procedure does not fulfill all of the above characteristics, then the procedure must be relegated to the special centers in clinics and hospitals and to clinical research laboratories for research and management of special patients. Until a procedure is fully evaluated and accepted as beneficial to patients, the procedure should be considered experimental and, in proper accordance with this, there should be no charges rendered to the patient for its use.

Medical and cardiologic training and education should be of such nature that the performance of the heart, its maximal performance capability, and safety at maximal performance can be determined at the bedside or in the physician's private office without the use of complex laboratory procedures, even when these procedures are non-invasive. Physicians who are well trained as bedside clinicians and cardiologists can evaluate the contractibility and contractility of a patient's heart by means of simple, well-established clinical procedures, such as the history, physical examination, EKG, EPA of the chest, CBC, blood chemistries, urinalysis, and stool examination. Exami-

*Supported by the Cardiovascular Research Fund, the Rowell A. Billups Fund for Research in Heart Disease, and the Feazel Laboratory.

nation of the heart, peripheral blood vessels, and pulses and blood pressure recordings provide considerable useful information concerning cardiac contractility. These are all *necessary* procedures, in any case, for the proper study, "work-up," or evaluation of any patient, and the performance of the patient's heart can be determined with these simple procedures when they are performed carefully and knowledgeably. Therefore, the master clinician and cardiologist is forced to ask: "Why is there a need to obtain other or special laboratory measurements and subject the patient to the additional expenses when the answers are already known?" Medical care is much too expensive already. The mere fact that a laboratory or technical procedure is non-invasive is not a valid reason to use the procedure, and even to disregard the expenses to the patient. Furthermore, there is no doubt that a well-trained doctor does not need these expensive non-invasive procedures, recordings, and indices to practice excellent clinical cardiology. If some physicians have learned to practice bedside cardiology without the use of expensive non-invasive procedures, then other doctors can certainly learn to do the same. In addition, these better trained cardiologists will practice better cardiology, with less expense and stress to the patients. When obtaining the history and during the physical examination, the physician establishes the patient-doctor relationship and learns the capabilities of cardiac performance while gathering data to establish the diagnosis and to plan management.

The accuracy and reliability of the methods used to determine contractility by various recording techniques and measurements, such as ejection time, presystolic ejection time, maximal ejection rate, rate of ventricular fiber shortening, and others,[1-7] need careful and further study. Even those doctors who employ such methods in the laboratory need to determine the accuracy of measurements expressed to milliseconds. For example, Figure 1 shows a published recording of the time course of carotid artery pressure obtained by a non-invasive technique.[2] It is obvious that the onset of the pulse wave is

Figure 1. Carotid artery pulse pressure tracing (CAR) recorded simultaneously with the electrocardiogram (ECG) and phonocardiogram (PCG) and used to determine left ventricular ejection time (LVET). It is obvious that the point of onset of the carotid arterial pulse pressure is difficult to determine precisely from the curve shown. (From Meng R, Hollander C, Liebson PR, Teran JC, Barresi V, and Lurie M: The use of non-invasive methods in the evaluation of left ventricular performance in coronary artery disease. I. Relation of systolic time intervals to angiographic assessment of coronary artery disease severity. Am Heart J 90:134, 1975.)

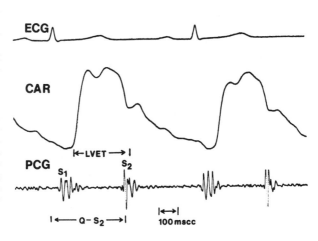

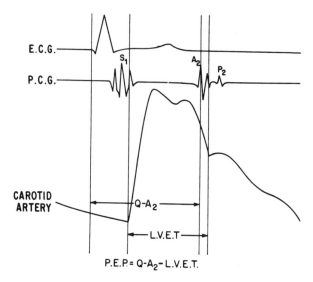

Figure 2. Diagrams of carotid artery pulse pressure curve, electrocardiogram (E.C.G.), and phonocardiogram (P.C.G.) illustrating the method used for measuring left ventricular ejection time (L.V.E.T.) and systolic time intervals. The actual recorded curves are never as sharply defined in onset as shown here. (From Crowley WF Jr, Ridgeway EC, Bough EW, Francis GS, Daniels GH, Kourides IA, Myers GS, and Maloof F: Noninvasive evaluation of cardiac function in hypothyroidism. Response to gradual thyroxine replacement. N Engl J Med 296:1, 1977.)

actually not distinctly sharp in time nor as definite as that shown in Figure 2.[3] The care and accuracy with which the measurements are made are important if the methods are to be used. It should not be assumed that the average technician is capable of obtaining and measuring recordings accurately. Surely, the pressure-volume diagrams recorded in any laboratory with the presently available methods are relatively crude, regardless of how carefully the measurements are obtained.[5, 6] Even if time courses of pressure can be recorded accurately, though this is rarely done, the time course of volume change can only be estimated roughly. The measurement of cardiac chamber volume as obtained in the laboratory is certainly unreliable and too impractical for general clinical use. The same is true for studies of the time course of intraventricular volume using x-ray techniques.[8, 9]

It is difficult to understand why so few actual recordings are published in articles based on these types of data. The authors usually present their data in table form. This type of presentation makes it impossible to judge the accuracy of the measurements or recordings reported. In some reports, only data measured from recordings are actually published. This, of course, makes it difficult for the reader to evaluate the reliability of the data. Even when original recordings are published, there is little, if any, description of the procedure or data related to the testing for accuracy or standardization of the recording methods.

The reliability of any method must be known. This is equally important for the non-invasive methods that are so strongly advocated for clinical use and that are considered so informative and superior. The measurements of the time course of the rate and magnitude of ventricular circumferential fiber shortening and systolic ejection by radionuclide angiography,[4] even with the aid of computers, are even more inaccurate. The crudeness, impracticability, and unreliability of these methods for clinical use are evident from published reports.[10] Until simple, accurate, dependable, and inexpensive recording methods become available and are proven to be superior and necessary, the physician must be trained to evaluate his patient's cardiac states at the bed-side with well-established, reliable clinical methods.

The cost to the patient for such recordings as the apexcardiogram, echo-cardiogram, treadmill exercise test, venogram, carotid arteriogram, and phon-ocardiogram is considerable — too great to be used routinely for clinical care. Furthermore, the physician often becomes so unduly involved with these recordings that he fails to give adequate attention to the patient. After all, the heart is not the entire patient. The patient tends to have several diseases and many problems that produce unhappiness, tension, and anxiety, as well as the organic diseases. Special non-invasive studies are rarely, if ever, needed in clinical cardiology, and certainly never for routine studies.

The clinical bedside study that includes a detailed history that is properly and unhurriedly obtained, a careful physical examination, CBC, urinalysis, stool examination, electrocardiogram, SMA-12, and teleoroentgenograms of the chest will suffice for almost all cardiac clinical evaluations. A master clini-cian rarely needs any other studies. It is beyond the purpose of this presenta-tion to discuss the technique for history taking or how to interpret and use the simple urinalysis, and so on. It can be stated, however, that few physicians truly understand the urine analysis or know how to use it properly to interpret the state of health of the patient and the state of health of the kidneys. In fact, I have yet to encounter a medical student or house staff physician who knows how to collect a 24-hour specimen of urine accurately. Furthermore, this procedure is usually entrusted to other people who are non-physicians and who also do not know how to collect a 24-hour specimen of urine from a patient accurately. Yet, there remains the tendency among physicians to fail to learn such simple and important aspects of clinical medicine and cardiology and, instead, to request or learn to perform the many expensive special "non-invasive" studies mentioned earlier. Until the cardiologist has learned the fundamental principles of bedside and office medicine and cardiology, such "non-invasive" and, certainly, "invasive" procedures concerned with the measurement of contractility of the heart must be ignored.

The contractility and performance of the heart as a pump can be readily determined for clinical purposes from the apex beat, heart sound, intensity of murmurs and heart sounds, the presence or absence of a protodiastolic gallop rhythm, the presence or absence of symptoms and signs of congestive heart failure, proper palpation of the peripheral arterial pulses, x-ray studies of the chest, including fluoroscopy, and electrocardiogram. Almost all of these stud-ies can be performed at the bedside. These fundamental bedside studies are excellent, simple, relatively inexpensive, and indispensable for acceptable clinical practice of cardiology.

When a diagnostic procedure is introduced into the practice of medi-cine, its usefulness should be fully established with the same criteria required for the introduction of a new drug into the practice of medicine. Until its value is properly established, the new procedure must be relegated to the laborato-ry for research or for clinical investigation. Neither the non-invasive aspect of the procedure nor the fact that patients are often impressed by gadgetry and complex apparatus can be considered justification for the use of contractility measurements when adequate and better service can be rendered to the patient with well-established clinical methods. The electrostatic machines of years ago were impressive to patients, non-invasive, and a source of income to the physician, but the medical profession, and even patients, finally forced them out of the offices of physicians.

Were contractility studies of the myocardium quantitatively reliable and sufficiently sensitive to detect myocardial disease or malfunction long before an astute clinican could detect the disturbance by simple, conventional clinical methods, then the use of methods and apparatus for measuring myocardial contractility would be justified. This is not the case, however, and certainly has not been established by any published or unpublished investigations. The existing problem in the management of cardiac patients is the inadequacy of training in bedside clinical cardiology and internal medicine. It is on this problem that the emphasis and effort in training in clinical cardiology must be focused.

References

1. McDonald IG, and Hobson ER: A comparison of the relative value of noninvasive techniques — echocardiography, systolic time intervals, and apexcardiography — in the diagnosis of primary myocardial disease. Am Heart J 88:454, 1974.
2. Meng R, Hollander C, Liebson PR, Teran JC, Barresi V, and Lurie M: The use of noninvasive methods in the evaluation of left ventricular performance in coronary artery disease. I. Relation of systolic time intervals to angiographic assessment of coronary artery disease severity. Am Heart J 90:134, 1975.
3. Crowley WF Jr, Ridgway EC, Bough EW, Francis GS, Daniels GH, Kourides IA, Myers GS, and Maloof F: Noninvasive evaluation of cardiac function in hypothyroidism: response to gradual thyroxine replacement. N Engl J Med 296:1, 1977.
4. Steele P, LeFree M, and Kirch D: Measurement of left ventricular mean circumferential fiber shortening velocity and systolic ejection rate by computerized radionuclide angiocardiography. Am J Cardiol 37:388, 1976.
5. Dodge HT, Hay RE, and Sandler H: Pressure-volume characteristics of the diastolic left ventricle of man with heart disease. Am Heart J 64:503, 1962.
6. Rackley CE, Behar VS, Whalen RE, and McIntosh HD: Biplane cineangiographic determinations of left ventricular function: pressure-volume relationships. Am Heart J 74:766, 1967.
7. Karliner JS, Gault JH, Eckberg D, Mullins CB, and Ross J Jr: Mean velocity of fiber shortening: a simplified measure of left ventricular myocardial contractility. Circulation 44:323, 1971.
8. Rackley CE, Dodge HT, Coble YD Jr, and Hay RE: A method for determining left ventricular mass in man. Circulation 29:666, 1964.
9. Sandler H, and Dodge HT: The use of single plane angiocardiograms for the calculation of left ventricular volume in man. Am Heart J 75:325, 1968.
10. Ahmad M, Dubiel JP, Logan KW, Verdon TA, and Martin RH: Limited clinical diagnostic specificity of technetium-99m stannous pyrophosphate myocardial imaging in acute myocardial infarction. Am J Cardiol 39:50, 1977.

Comment

This controversy has important ramifications for the practice of cardiology. If a variety of non-invasive and invasive tests are desirable in managing many cardiac patients, it will become standard practice for these to be obtained on most, if not all, cardiac patients. No physician can face for long the prospect of failing to order appropriate laboratory tests if it is the usual practice of his colleagues. At the same time, the indiscriminate use of various procedures that duplicate or provide information that is of dubious importance in the patient's management add unnecessarily to an already high cost of medical care.

There is little doubt in my mind that the burgeoning practice among internists toward the widespread ordering of laboratory procedures and tests has encompassed to some extent the cardiovascular field. A number of our patients have procedures ordered when the information is not necessary to the patient's management, but is obtained as further confirmation of information already provided by other modes of examination. There appears to be a desire to quantify everything, even when such information is of no real therapeutic or prognostic consequence. Furthermore, the indiscriminate use of laboratory tests tends to suppress one's thinking about the pathophysiologic mechanisms responsible for existing symptoms and signs. Overdependence of physicians on the laboratory tends to dull their clinical senses.

As in many of these controversies, I find my position to be somewhere between those taken by the authors of the articles, in this case, Dr. Burch and Dr. Mason and his colleagues. There is little doubt that M-mode echocardiography has substantially contributed to cardiovascular diagnosis and management. This non-invasive procedure provides important information in a variety of ways, and we have come to take echocardiograms on an increasing number of our cardiac patients. Similarly, nuclear cardiology is being increasingly utilized, particularly in the evaluation of patients with coronary heart disease. For example, we find ourselves frequently adding thallium perfusion studies to exercise stress testing in the evaluation of coronary heart disease.

Nevertheless, if we restrict ourselves specifically to the area of contractility indices, I tend to agree with Dr. Burch that the impreciseness of the measurements available to us greatly limits their usefulness in the ordinary management of the cardiac patient. Clearly, a patient who has signs and symptoms of congestive heart failure hardly needs the determination of a multiple-gated radionuclide ejection fraction or systolic time intervals to confirm that myocardial performance is impaired. Furthermore, the sensitivity of these tools does not justify their routine use as screening devices or means of detecting impaired cardiac contractility in an asymptomatic popula-

603

tion; nor have I found them of routine use in following the response of a patient to given interventions.

In summary, a greater restraint may be needed among some physicians relative to the use of both non-invasive and invasive procedures in attempting to judge cardiac contractility. Such tests certainly should never be substituted for careful clinical observation of the patient. Furthermore, the results of such tests, when performed, must be interpreted in light of the clinical situation.

ELLIOT RAPAPORT, M.D.

Twenty-five

Should Oral Vasodilators Be Used Routinely in the Treatment of Congestive Heart Failure?

ORAL VASODILATORS SHOULD BE USED ROUTINELY IN THE TREATMENT OF CONGESTIVE HEART FAILURE

Jay N. Cohn, M.D.

ORAL VASODILATORS SHOULD *Not* BE USED ROUTINELY IN THE TREATMENT OF CONGESTIVE HEART FAILURE

Shahbudin H. Rahimtoola, M.B., F.R.C.P.

COMMENT

Oral Vasodilators Should Be Used Routinely in the Treatment of Congestive Heart Failure

JAY N. COHN, M.D.

Professor of Medicine; Head, Cardiovascular Division,
University of Minnesota Medical School, Minneapolis,
Minnesota

Heart failure is a manifestation of impairment of cardiac performance resulting from a variety of cardiac diseases. The prognosis for long-term survival once the diagnosis of heart failure has been made is poor. In patients with structural abnormalities of the heart, cardiac symptoms may be present for years before the syndrome of heart failure develops. In primary myocardial diseases, however, heart failure may appear as the first clinical manifestation of heart disease.

Heart failure presents clinically with signs and symptoms of a low cardiac output, or an inadequate output response to exercise, and circulatory congestion. The deficiency in output, or "forward" failure, is manifested by lethargy, weakness, exertional fatigue, diaphoresis, prerenal azotemia, and even metabolic acidosis. The circulatory congestion, or "backward" failure, is characterized by dyspnea on exertion, orthopnea, paroxsymal nocturnal dyspnea, peripheral edema, ascites, and hepatic dysfunction. The goal of therapy in heart failure is to increase cardiac output, especially the output response to exertion, and simultaneously to reduce the elevated cardiac filling pressure that generates the signs and symptoms of circulatory congestion.

In physiologic terms, the goal of therapy is to shift the cardiac function curve upward and to the left, achieving a higher stroke volume with a lower ventricular filling pressure. Since the majority of diseases affecting the heart have their predominant effect on the left ventricular myocardium, it is an improvement in left ventricular function that is usually the goal of therapy. Traditional therapy for heart failure has been only partially effective. Bed rest or limited activity has been prescribed to reduce the demand for cardiac output in order to bring it more in line with a reduced output

607

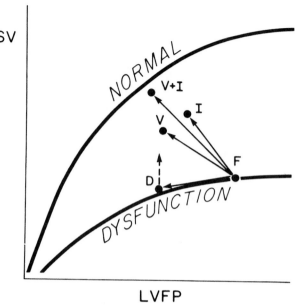

Figure 1.   Left ventricular function curve relating stroke volume to left ventricular filling pressure. Patient in heart failure may operate at point F. Diuretics (D) produce a shift to the left which may be accompanied, at least temporarily, by a fall in stroke volume. Inotropic and vasodilator agents shift the function curve upward and to the left, and the two together produce a greater increment in left ventricular performance. (Reproduced from Cohn JN, and Franciosa JA: Vasodilator therapy of cardiac failure (second of two parts). N Engl J Med 297:27–31, 1977.)

capacity of the heart. Salt restriction and diuretics have been utilized in an effort to control the circulatory congestion. Such volume depletion therapy would not, however, be expected to relieve the signs of low output, because acute reduction of cardiac filling pressure tends to move the heart's performance to the left on its function curve, resulting in a slight further reduction in stroke volume and cardiac output (Fig. 1). The long-term effects of diuretic therapy may be more beneficial, since a reduction in heart size reduces left ventricular wall tension and, thus, reduces myocardial oxygen consumption. This latter metabolic effect could improve cardiac performance if inadequate oxygen supply had been playing a role in the depressed left ventricular function. Nonetheless, the beneficial effects of diuretics on cardiac performance are mainly expressed through a reduction in filling pressure and in relief of the signs and symptoms of circulatory congestion.

The mainstay of therapy for heart failure has been digitalis, the only orally effective positive inotropic agent that has been available for clinical use. The drug usually increases the velocity of fiber shortening and shifts the cardiac function curve somewhat upward and to the left from its depressed position. However, the degree of shift is usually quite modest, and although the drug may be clinically effective in relieving some of the symptoms of heart failure, it is not usually potent enough to restore left ventricular performance to normal, except in the most mild cardiac disabilities.

What has been missing in this approach to heart failure has been an understanding of the importance of the relationship between the performance of the left ventricle and the state of the peripheral circulation. The role of the left ventricular pump is to deliver blood to the periphery for organ nutrition. The left ventricular work required to deliver this blood is primarily determined by the resistance or impedance against which the left ventricle must eject. Stroke volume ejected against a low resistance consumes considerably less energy and requires considerably less force of contraction than the same stroke volume ejected against a high resistance. Preoccupation with efforts to increase the force of contraction without consideration of the resistance residing in the peripheral circulation has deterred therapeutic advances in the management of heart failure.

Resistance in the arterial bed to left ventricular ejection is not an important determinant of cardiac output when the left ventricle is normal. The normal ventricle calls upon its reserve capacity by subtly increasing diastolic fiber length and augmenting contractile force to maintain a nearly constant stroke volume despite considerable increases in resistance. In contrast, the damaged heart loses its reserve capacity. Modest increases in resting fiber length in this situation may not appreciably augment the force of contraction, and scarred or diseased myocardium may not be capable of generating the wall tension needed to maintain a constant output in face of a heightened resistance. Consequently, cardiac output becomes inversely related to outflow resistance when the left ventricular myocardium is diseased.

Given this abnormal cardiac functional state, one might expect that outflow resistance would be endogenously adjusted to minimally necessary levels in order to preserve cardiac output in the presence of left ventricular failure. In fact, the resistance is often increased in heart failure, frequently to levels that raise the blood pressure to high-normal or hypertensive levels despite the low cardiac output. The only teleologic explanation for this apparently self-destructive peripheral vascular response is that the body has been programmed to defend against hypotension more effectively than against low cardiac output. The primitive reflexes that support blood pressure were designed to interpret a drop in cardiac output as the result of volume depletion. When the left ventricle is normal, an exaggerated rise in resistance to assure the support of blood pressure should be well tolerated. When the output falls because of heart failure, however, the reflex rise in resistance can produce a further decrement in output and a state of progressive pump failure.

In the last few years, it has become apparent that drugs that reduce left ventricular outflow resistance may be very effective in improving left ventricular performance in the failing heart. Intravenous infusion of dobutamine, a potent and quite selective inotropic drug, produces an increment in cardiac performance that is of about the same magnitude as the response to intravenous infusion of sodium nitroprusside, a potent vasodilator (Fig. 1). This response in patients with severe heart failure indicates not only that vasodilator drugs may produce a salutary effect in heart failure, but that the magnitude of the response is comparable to the magnitude of the response to the most potent inotropic agents available.

The similarity of the hemodynamic effects of vasodilator and inotropic drugs raises interesting questions about the control of cardiac output from the failing heart. When cardiac contractility is stimulated by an inotropic agent, the peripheral circulation relaxes as the cardiac output goes up, probably because of inhibition of reflex vasoconstriction resulting from the prior depression of cardiac performance. It may well be, in fact, that the increase in cardiac output is largely dependent upon this reduction in peripheral resistance. Such a thesis is supported by the similar rise in output observed when the peripheral circulation is primarily dilated with a drug that has no direct effect on the heart. Thus, the common denominator of both inotropic and vasodilator drugs is a relaxation of heightened systemic vascular resistance.

Another consideration in the comparison between inotropic and vasodilator therapy is the metabolic effects of the drugs. Myocardial oxygen consumption is primarily dependent upon wall tension, contractility, and heart rate. Inotropic drugs, by increasing contractility, tend to increase myocardial oxygen consumption, unless a concomitant reduction in rate, pressure, or chamber size counterbalances the increase. Vasodilator drugs, on the other hand, tend to reduce pressure, heart rate, and chamber size, and thus consistently reduce total myocardial oxygen consumption. The bottom line is the balance between myocardial oxygen consumption and myocardial oxygen delivery, however, and the effect of each of these groups of compounds on this balance in various clinical situations probably varies from patient to patient and is extremely difficult to measure.

The physiologic rationale for the use of vasodilator drugs in the setting of heart failure is clear. By reducing outflow resistance, a drug that dilates the arterial bed allows the damaged left ventricle to empty to a smaller end-systolic volume, resulting in a larger stroke volume and ejection fraction. Mitral regurgitation, if present, is reduced. Acute therapy with vasodilators increases cardiac output and reduces cardiac filling pressure — the therapeutic goal in the treatment of heart failure. This improved cardiac performance is accomplished with a concomitant reduction in myocardial oxygen consumption. The cost to the patient of this therapy is usually a small reduction in arterial pressure, which could in itself be harmful or beneficial, depending upon the control level of arterial pressure and the state of the coronary circulation.

The physiologic basis of vasodilator therapy is now well understood, and the salutary hemodynamic response to acute therapy with vasodilator drugs has now been well established. What has not yet been satisfactorily proved is that chronic administration of vasodilator drugs will result in a sustained improvement in left ventricular performance similar to that observed during the acute administration of nitroprusside. Furthermore, it is not known whether institution of vasodilator therapy early in the course of heart disease will prevent or forestall the development or progression of heart failure. An understanding of the answers to these unresolved questions depends upon knowledge of the natural history of heart failure as well as a thorough understanding of the unique pharmacologic effects of all vasodilator drugs that might be employed for chronic administration.

In contrast to the paucity of inotropic agents available for chronic use, a wide variety of vasodilator drugs is available, and new ones appear to be on the horizon. The efficacy of intravenous infusion of potent vasodilators, such as sodium nitroprusside and phentolamine, has been amply demonstrated in patients with heart disease related to coronary artery disease, cardiomyopathy, and valvular or structural cardiac defects. Chronic vasodilator therapy in the management of congestive heart failure is now being evaluated with trials of nitrates (isosorbide dinitrate by mouth or nitroglycerin administered in a topical ointment), hydralazine, or a combination of these agents. Other orally effective vasodilators are available and will probably also be studied for efficacy in congestive heart failure. In evaluating these different vasodilator agents, it is important to recognize that each has a rather unique spectrum of vascular effects, with varying effects on large arteries, arterioles, systemic veins, pulmonary vessels, regional vascular beds, and reflex adrenergic stimulation. Therefore, the overall hemodynamic effects of each agent tend to be different.

The only serious risk of vasodilator drugs in the management of heart failure is the fall in blood pressure that may ensue. Patients who are already hypotensive are relatively poor candidates for this therapy, although the absolute level below which a beneficial response does not occur varies from patient to patient. Another limitation is that patients with high systemic vascular resistance respond better than those with low resistance. This variation of response is hardly surprising, since the rationale of vasodilator therapy is based largely on the presence of a high systemic vascular resistance. The more intensely the systemic circulation responds to neurohumoral stimulation, the greater will be the response to the vasodilator drugs.

Thus, vasodilator drugs should have a place alongside inotropic and diuretic therapy, forming a three-pronged approach to the management of congestive heart failure (Fig. 2). But at what stage of the disease should

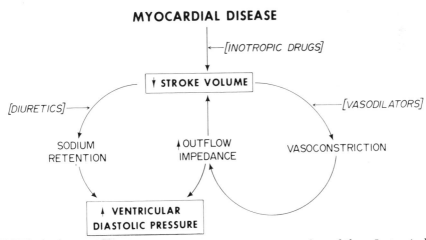

Figure 2. Sites of action of three therapeutic interventions in heart failure. Inotropic drugs support stroke volume and diuretics prevent the rise in ventricular diastolic pressure. These traditional interventions do not, however, interfere with vasoconstriction, which increases outflow resistance and leads to a reduction in stroke volume and an increase in ventricular diastolic pressure. Vasodilator drugs should be effective in dealing with this vicious cycle.

these drugs be employed? Studies to date have been confined to patients with Class III or IV (New York Heart Association) heart failure who have not responded satisfactorily to digitalis and diuretics. Because the patient is so symptomatic at this stage of the disease, it is relatively easy to assess therapeutic efficacy; but prognosis at this point is so poor that a high mortality can be expected despite treatment. It is attractive to postulate that a high outflow resistance is an important factor in the development of progressive cardiac failure. If this is the case, effective chronic vasodilator therapy introduced early in the disease could alter the natural history of heart failure. Controlled clinical trials are needed.

The safety and efficacy of chronic vasodilator therapy for heart failure have not yet been proved. Oral vasodilator drugs are available, but they may be imperfect. Large doses of nitrates are needed to produce a sustained vascular effect, but the safety and freedom from tolerance to such doses is not assured. Hydralazine appears to be very effective hemodynamically, but chronic use of this drug in patients with heart failure has not yet been thoroughly tested.

Should the physician then await the results of long-term controlled trials before utilizing this form of therapy? He must make a decision. If he agrees with the rationale behind the therapy, he may appropriately elect to add dilator drugs to the therapeutic regimen in patients with heart failure. If he is skeptical, he may elect to wait until more prospective studies are carried out. Even now, however, it seems imprudent to allow patients to slip into intractable heart failure without aggressive attempts at vasodilator therapy.

We rightfully place more stringent criteria on new therapeutic advances today than we did in the past. Rationality must be supplemented by proved efficacy in carefully designed protocols. Such restrictions have never been applied to traditional treatment, such as the use of digitalis in the treatment of heart failure. We have as yet neither the ultimate answer on efficacy nor the ultimate drug for reducing outflow resistance in congestive heart failure; but I find the physiologic rationale for vasodilator treatment so compelling that I am uncomfortable in withholding it in symptomatic patients with heart failure, except in the setting of a controlled, double-blind clinical trial designed to establish therapeutic efficacy.

Oral Vasodilators Should *Not* Be Used Routinely in the Treatment of Congestive Heart Failure

SHAHBUDIN H. RAHIMTOOLA,
M.B., F.R.C.P.

Professor of Medicine, Division of Cardiology,
Department of Medicine, University of Oregon Health
Sciences Center, Portland, Oregon

The search for new therapeutic maneuvers and their evaluation are appropriate avenues of research and investigation. However, before introducing these measures into *routine clinical use*, certain questions need to be answered. Are the new therapeutic agents (vasodilators) better than, or do they add significantly to, standard therapy (digitalis and diuretics)? There are no prospective, randomized studies that answer this question. Therefore, we have to approach the problem in a different way. We have to consider: (1) whether the standard therapy is effective, corrects a primary problem, and has stood the test of time; and (2) whether the new therapeutic agents cure the patient, correct the primary problems, are safe, have a lower complication rate, are easier to use, and have a more lasting effect. To answer these questions, it is appropriate to first review the pathophysiology of heart failure, the actions and effects of the medications that are available, and the management of the patient with heart failure.

Heart failure produces well-known symptoms and signs. These result from an abnormal elevation of systemic venous and/or pulmonary venous pressures, from an inadequate blood flow to the various tissues of the body, from excessive accumulation of sodium and water, and from changes produced in the ventricles due to dilatation and to myocardial hypertrophy and dysfunction.

613

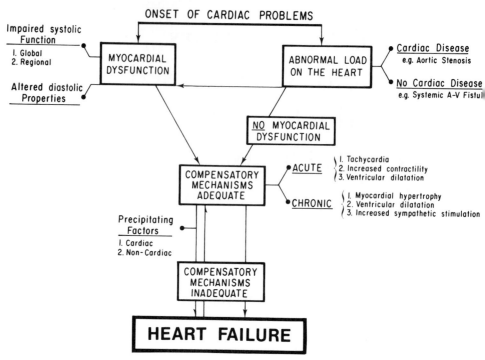

Figure 1.   Diagram of the pathophysiology of heart failure.

Pathophysiology of Heart Failure

Heart failure may result from an abnormal load on the heart, from myocardial dysfunction, or from both (Fig. 1). The abnormal load may be due to cardiac diseases, such as aortic stenosis, or to non-cardiac diseases, such as systemic arteriovenous fistulae.

MYOCARDIAL FUNCTION

The clinical syndrome of heart failure may or may not be associated with myocardial dysfunction. *Myocardial dysfunction* results from an impairment of the systolic function or from an alteration of the diastolic properties of the ventricle. Impaired systolic function may be global or regional.[1] Global myocardial dysfunction occurs with hypertensive, coronary, and valvular heart disease and with primary myocardial disease. Regional impairment of systolic function occurs classically in patients with coronary artery disease, particularly after myocardial infarction. Myocardial dysfunction due to an alteration of the diastolic properties of the left ventricle may or may not be accompanied by an impairment of systolic function (Fig. 2). Impairment of the diastolic

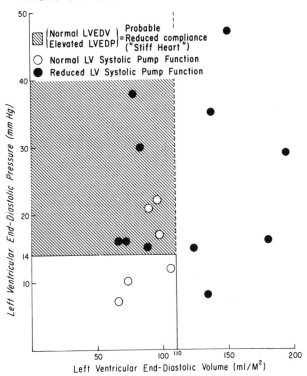

Figure 2. The relationship of left ventricular end-diastolic volume to end-diastolic pressure in patients convalescing from acute myocardial infarction (Ehsani A, et al: Arch Intern Med *135*:1539, 1975). The upper limit of normal for left ventricular end-diastolic volume is 110 cc/m² and that for left ventricular end-diastolic pressure is 14 mm Hg (two standard deviations away from the mean in "normals"). Patients with a normal end-diastolic volume and elevated end-diastolic pressure are shown in the upper left square (thatched area). Such patients probably have a reduction of left ventricular compliance and have the "stiff heart" syndrome. They may have normal left ventricular systolic pump function (open circles) or may have reduced left ventricular systolic pump function (closed circles).

properties of the heart occurs commonly after myocardial infarction, but it is also seen in diabetics and in conditions that are associated with ventricular hypertrophy. It has been called the "stiff heart" syndrome.[2]

It is interesting that the entire clinical syndrome of heart failure may occur *without myocardial dysfunction.* Some patients may have underlying heart disease, for example, mitral stenosis, acute volume overloading of the heart, such as occurs with valve regurgitation, atrial septal defects, or constrictive pericarditis. Indeed, some patients may have the clinical manifestations of heart failure, that is, edema and increased venous pressure, with or without much cardiac enlargement, and yet have no underlying heart disease. These clinical manifestations usually result from abnormal salt and water retention; from hyperkinetic circulations, such as arteriovenous fistulae; and from pressure overloading, such as with acute massive pulmonary embolism and acute, severe systemic hypertension.

COMPENSATORY MECHANISMS

When an abnormal load is placed on the heart, certain compensatory mechanisms become operational. In the *acute stage*, tachycardia, increased myocardial contractility from catecholamine stimulation, and ventricular dilatation (that is, the Frank-Starling mechanism) are available to the heart.

Although utilization of the Frank-Starling mechanism in these circumstances is extremely important and helpful, it is of limited value, because the extent to which the left ventricle can dilate acutely is restricted. It is because of the latter reason that the patient with acute severe mitral or aortic regurgitation may have a relatively normal heart size and yet be in severe pulmonary edema.

In the *chronic stage*, the heart utilizes two main compensatory mechanisms, namely, myocardial hypertrophy and ventricular dilatation. In addition, increased sympathetic stimulation may play a role. When these compensatory mechanisms prove to be inadequate, the clinical syndrome of heart failure results.

PRECIPITATING FACTORS

Certain factors that could be alleviated may contribute to the inadequacy of the compensatory mechanisms (Table 1). These factors may be *cardiac* in origin, such as arrhythmias, which may be tachyarrhythmias or bradyarrhythmias, myocardial ischemia or infarction, and an acute volume overload, such as occurs with valvular regurgitation from ruptured chordae tendineae or infective endocarditis. The precipitating factors may be *non-cardiac* in origin. These include improper use of medications, such as consumption of insufficient or excessive amounts of digitalis, diuretics, and potassium supplements; fluid overloading, particularly iatrogenic intravenous therapy; nonadherence to the dietetic recommendations; presence of associated hyperkinetic circulations, such as pregnancy, anemia, and thyrotoxicosis, which may place an undue burden on the heart; and the presence of other medical conditions, such as pulmonary embolism and respiratory infections.

EFFECTS OF HEART FAILURE

In the presence of heart failure, *cardiac output* is reduced or is inadequate for the body needs, and ventricular *filling pressure* and venous pressure are increased (Fig. 3). The reduced cardiac output affects the release

Table 1.   *Factors That Help to Precipitate Heart Failure*

CARDIAC
1. Arrhythmias
2. Myocardial ischemia or infarction
3. Others, e.g., valve regurgitation from ruptured chordae tendineae

NON-CARDIAC
1. Failure to take medications
2. Fluid overloading
3. Dietetic indiscretion, e.g., increased salt intake
4. Associated hyperkinetic circulation, e.g., pregnancy, anemia, thyrotoxicosis
5. Others, e.g., pulmonary embolism, respiratory infections

PATHOPHYSIOLOGY OF HEART FAILURE
AND EFFECTS OF VARIOUS MEDICATIONS

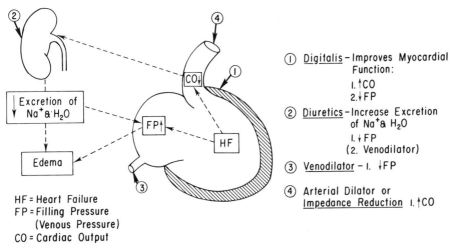

① Digitalis – Improves Myocardial
Function:
1. ↑CO
2. ↓FP

② Diuretics – Increase Excretion
of Na⁺& H₂O
I. ↓FP
(2. Venodilator)

③ Venodilator – I. ↓FP

④ Arterial Dilator or
Impedance Reduction I. ↑CO

HF = Heart Failure
FP = Filling Pressure
(Venous Pressure)
CO = Cardiac Output

Figure 3. Diagram of the results of heart failure. The effects and sites of action of the various medications are also shown.

of renal hormones and of sympathetic nervous outflow, resulting in a reduction of glomerular filtration rate and an increase of tubular reabsorption of sodium and water. The circulating blood volume is thereby increased, an attempt to correct the reduced effective arterial blood volume. However, it also increases venous pressure and contributes to edema formation.

Medications

DIGITALIS GLYCOSIDES

The first recorded use of digitalis glycosides by a physician, William Withering, was on December 8, 1775. The cardiac glycosides have four main actions: (1) electrophysiologic; (2) inotropic; (3) vascular; and (4) neural. Their *electrophysiologic effects* include a slowing of conduction through the atrioventricular node, reduction of the effective refractory period and of automaticity of the atrial muscle, and a slight reduction of the frequency of sinoatrial node impulse formation. In heart failure, the main use of their electrophysiologic effects is to control the ventricular rate in patients with atrial fibrillation, atrial flutter, and supraventricular tachycardias.

Digitalis has a positive *inotropic effect* and increases myocardial contractility of both the normal and the failing heart.[3] As a result, the force-velocity curve of the left ventricle is moved to the right, and velocity of contractile element shortening is increased. The Frank-Starling function curve is moved upward and to the left, to a new, improved ventricular function curve (Fig. 4). This is true even in patients with myocardial infarction (Fig. 5).[4, 5] Left

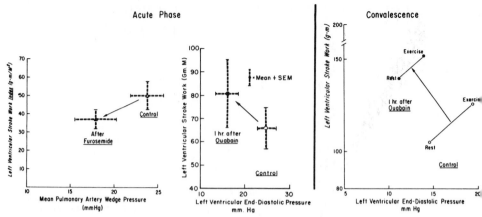

Figure 4. The effects of furosemide (left panel) and ouabain (center panel) on left ventricular (LV) function during the acute phase of myocardial infarction. Furosemide results in a fall of pulmonary artery wedge pressure and of LV stroke index (data from Kiely J, et al: Circulation 48:581, 1973). It should be remembered that in such patients mean pulmonary artery wedge pressure is frequently not the same as left ventricular end-diastolic pressure (Rahimtoola SH, et al: Circulation 46:283, 1972). After ouabain administration, the fall of LV end-diastolic pressure is accompanied by an increase of stroke work (Rahimtoola SH, et al: N Engl J Med 287:527, 1972). The right panel shows the relation of LV end-diastolic pressure to LV stroke work at rest and on exercise in the control state (open circles) and after ouabain administration (closed circles) during the convalescent phase of acute myocardial infarction (mean of four patients) (Rahimtoola SH, et al: Circulation 44:866, 1971). After ouabain, the LV function curve has moved upward and to the left. (Reproduced from Rahimtoola SH, et al: Digitalis in acute myocardial infarction. Help or hazard? Ann Intern Med 82:234, 1975. By permission.)

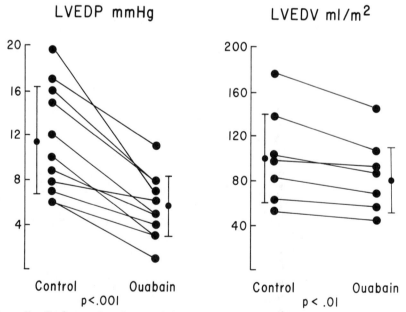

Figure 5. Ouabain reduced LV end-diastolic pressure and volume in patients with coronary artery disease even if these were normal initially. Normal LV end-diastolic pressure is ≤ 14 mm Hg and normal LV end-diastolic volume is ≤ 110 ml/m². (From DeMots H, et al: Effects of ouabain on myocardial oxygen supply and demand in patients with chronic coronary artery disease: a hemodynamic, volumetric, metabolic study in patients without heart failure. J Clin Invest 58:312, 1976. By permission.)

Myocardial Oxygen Consumption Before and ½ Hour After I.V. Ouabain (0.015 mg/kg) In Patients Not In Heart Failure

Figure 6. Ouabain results in an increase of myocardial oxygen consumption. The small increase which occurred in all patients was significant (p < 0.025). (From DeMots, H, et al: Effects of ouabain on coronary and systemic vascular resistance and myocardial oxygen consumption in patients without heart failure. Am J Cardiol 41:88, 1978. By permission.)

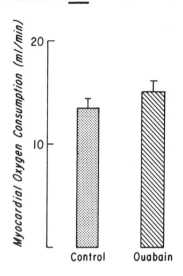

ventricular end-diastolic volume and pressure fall, and this occurs in animals[6] and in patients with normal-sized left ventricles (Fig. 6).[7] Because the output of the heart is influenced by many homeostatic mechanisms, digitalis does not increase cardiac output unless there is heart failure.

Since digitalis is a positive inotropic agent, it will increase myocardial oxygen consumption, and this has raised questions about a disproportionate increase in myocardial oxygen needs, which would be particularly detrimental to the patient with obstructive coronary artery disease and reduced coronary blood flow. However, since end-diastolic volume is also reduced, myocardial tension will be reduced, which will result in a fall in myocardial oxygen consumption unless there is a disproportionate increase in arterial pressure. The net effect of digitalis on myocardial oxygen consumption is a balance between these two opposing effects. In patients with heart failure, myocardial oxygen consumption shows no change or is reduced. Interestingly, recent data from our laboratory show that even in patients who are *not* in heart failure, the increased myocardial oxygen consumption is small, averaging 13 per cent (Fig. 7).[7, 8]

Although digitalis is not used clinically for its effects on the peripheral vessels or for its neural effects, both of these actions of the drug are important to recognize, because they may play a role in the observed effects. Digitalis acts on the *peripheral vessels* and produces both venous and arterial vasoconstriction. There are at least three mechanisms for production of arterial vasoconstriction: (1) a direct effect on the peripheral vessels;[9] (2) a neurogenically mediated effect;[10] and (3) an increased baroreceptor sensitivity. The observed effects depend on the circulatory state of the patient and on the rate of infusion of the drug. If patients are in heart failure, the vasoconstriction is

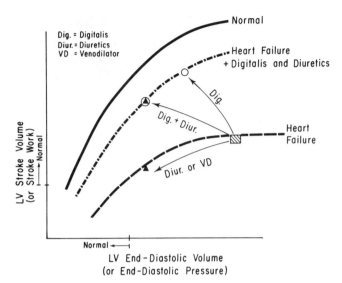

Figure 7. Diagrammatic representation of the effects of digitalis, diuretics, and venodilators on left ventricular function curve (Frank-Starling curves). Heart failure results in a severe depression of the ventricular function curve. Digitalis moves the left ventricle to an improved function curve because it is an inotropic agent. There is also a reduction in filling pressure. Diuretics, by reducing the circulating blood volume, and venodilators, by increasing the capacity of the veins, cause a reduction of end-diastolic volume and pressure. However, since these agents are not positive inotropic agents, the ventricle remains on the same function curve. A combination of digitalis and diuretics results in the ventricle operating on the same ventricular function curve as with digitalis, but at a lower filling pressure.

not seen.[9] If the patients are not in heart failure, arterial vasoconstriction occurs, but can be avoided by a slow infusion of the drug over 15 to 20 minutes.[8] Rapid injection of digitalis also produces coronary vasoconstriction, which may lead to deleterious effects in patients with coronary artery disease by producing or aggravating myocardial ischemia.[8] It is important to emphasize that these transient changes in the vascular bed and in myocardial metabolism can be practically eliminated by a slow infusion of the drug. The *neural effects* are largely vagomimetic and are responsible for the observed major electrophysiologic effects of the drug. The vagomimetic effects may, in turn, contribute to the reflex withdrawal of sympathetic tone in patients with heart failure.

In summary, the beneficial effects of digitalis in patients with heart failure result mainly from its electrophysiologic and inotropic effects. Because of its inotropic effect, cardiac output is increased and preload (end-diastolic volume and pressure) is reduced. Thus, digitalis, by acting directly on the myocardium, helps to eliminate the two main causes for the symptoms and signs of heart failure, namely, a reduced cardiac output and an increased filling pressure (Fig. 3).

DIURETICS

Diuretics increase the urinary excretion of sodium and water and, thus, lead to a reduction of circulating blood volume, venous pressure, and edema.

Intravenous furosemide is also a venodilator. Diuretics reduce ventricular preload, that is, end-diastolic volume and pressure. Since the left ventricles of many patients with heart failure are operating on the flat portion of the Frank-Starling curve, diuretics produce a small reduction or no change in cardiac output, even in patients with myocardial infarction (Fig. 5).[11] Since diuretics do not have any positive inotropic effect, the left ventricle does not move to a new function curve, and therefore, as end-diastolic volume is reduced further, diuretics will result in a fall of cardiac output. If the predominant manifestation of impaired myocardial function is an elevated filling pressure, then diuretics alone may relieve the symptoms of heart failure. However, this is rarely the case, and thus, diuretics have to be combined in most instances with a positive inotropic agent, such as digitalis. The combination of the two drugs results in a reduction of filling pressure and an increase of cardiac output, because the left ventricle has moved to a new ventricular function curve (Fig. 4).

VASODILATORS

These agents dilate the *venous* and/or the *arterial* vascular beds. Nitroglycerin appears to be a very potent venodilator and has a small effect on the arterioles, whereas phentolamine is a powerful arteriolar dilator.[12] Nitroprusside dilates the veins as well as the arterioles.[12] Venodilators produce a reduction of preload, that is, of end-diastolic volume and filling pressure (Fig. 8). Arteriolar dilators reduce left ventricular afterload and, thus, usually increase cardiac output; the reduction in filling pressure is small. Combination of the two drugs, or a drug that has both effects, reduces filling pressure and increases cardiac output. The *most dramatic effects* of arteriolar dilatation are

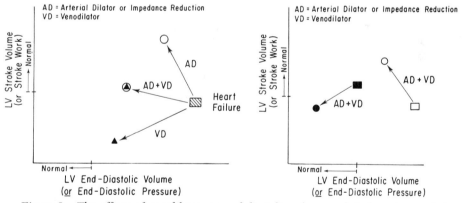

Figure 8. The effects of vasodilators on end-diastolic volume and stroke volume relationships. In the left panel are shown the effects of these drugs in heart failure. Arterial dilators usually increase cardiac output. Venodilators result in a fall of end-diastolic volume. Combination of the two drugs, or a drug with combined effects, results in a fall of filling pressure and an increase of cardiac output.

In the right panel are shown the effects of these agents with relation to the filling pressure at the initiation of therapy. In the open symbols are shown the effects of these agents when end-diastolic volume and pressure are initially increased. When filling pressure is not initially increased (closed symbols), these agents produce an undesirable effect, namely, a fall in cardiac output.

seen in patients with mitral or aortic regurgitation,[13, 14] and the most dramatic effects of venodilators are seen in patients with the "stiff heart" syndrome.

Vasodilating agents may produce an unfavorable redistribution of coronary blood flow in patients with obstructive coronary artery disease and are associated with some risk.[15] In addition, if filling pressure is not initially increased, vasodilators may have a deleterious effect (Fig. 8).

Like diuretic agents, vasodilators do not move the impaired left ventricle to a new, improved ventricular function curve. Therefore, combining an inotropic agent with a vasodilator produces more favorable effects.[16]

SUMMARY OF MEASURES THAT IMPROVE VENTRICULAR FUNCTION

The factors that determine left ventricular function are heart rate, myocardial contractility, preload, afterload, and regional wall motion. Maneuvers that alter ventricular function by changing one or more of these factors are summarized in Table 2.

Table 2. · *Measures to Improve Ventricular Function in Heart Failure*

DETERMINANT OF LEFT VENTRICULAR FUNCTION	THERAPEUTIC MANEUVER
1. Heart Rate	a. Reduce ventricular rate with digitalis, cardioversion, and antiarrhythmic agents
	b. Increase ventricular rate with pacemakers, isoproterenol
2. Myocardial Contractility	a. Increase contractility with digitalis, isoproterenol, epinephrine, norepinephrine, dopamine, dobutamine
	b. Reduce contractility with propranolol in special circumstances, such as hypertrophic cardiomyopathy with outflow obstruction and thyrotoxicosis
3. Preload	a. Reduce with digitalis, diuretics, inotropic agents, venodilators, nitroprusside, and rotating tourniquets
4. Afterload	a. Reduce with hydralazine, phentolamine, trimetaphan, and nitroprusside
5. Regional Wall Motion	Improve and protect by :
	a. Increasing arterial PO_2
	b. Decreasing MVO_2 by slowing tachycardias, reducing preload, and reducing afterload
	c. Increasing oxygen supply by correcting reduced cardiac output and hypotension
	d. Increasing coronary blood flow by coronary bypass surgery

Table 3. *Management of Heart Failure*

DIAGNOSIS
1. Of basic cardiac lesion and its severity
2. Of importance of precipitating factors

TREATMENT
1. Correct underlying cardiac lesion
2. Control precipitating factors
3. Improve myocardial function with digitalis
4. Control excess Na^+ and H_2O retention with diuretics
5. Change loading conditions of the heart: Usually, digitalis and diuretics suffice; occasionally, vasodilators are needed

PREVENTION
1. Recurrences
    Ideally, prevention of heart disease would be the most effective means of controlling heart failure

Management of the Patient with Heart Failure

Management of the patient with heart failure is a three-part process: (1) diagnosis; (2) treatment; and (3) prevention (Table 3).

DIAGNOSIS

The importance of accurately diagnosing the underlying cardiac lesions, its severity, and the precipitating factors cannot be overemphasized.

In some conditions, lack of recognition of the *underlying cardiac lesion* may preclude the use of a specific therapy that would have been beneficial to the patient. The diagnosis of congenital (Fig. 9) and valvular heart disease, especially aortic stenosis,[17] may be easily overlooked. In other situations, misdiagnosis may result in therapy that is detrimental to the patient. If digitalis is administered to a patient who has hypertrophic cardiomyopathy with outflow obstruction, his condition may deteriorate, because the outflow tract obstruction will increase. In this instance, propranolol may actually improve the patient with pulmonary edema.

It is not sufficient just to identify the pathology; the *severity* must also be estimated accurately (Fig. 10). The *precipitating factors* (Table 1) have to be identified and their importance correctly assessed (Fig. 11).

TREATMENT

As emphasized above, the underlying cardiac lesion and the factors that precipitated heart failure should be identified and treated.

Since myocardial dysfunction is usually present in heart failure, it needs to be corrected. The most practical way of doing this is with digitalis. Excessive salt and water retention is best corrected with diuretics. Combined

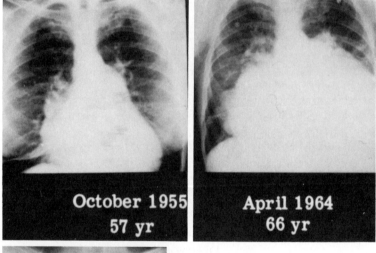

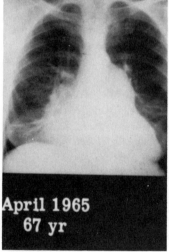

Figure 9. The chest x-ray of a woman, age 66, who was in gross congestive heart failure for many months (upper right panel). Chest x-ray 10 years prior to this when she was "asymptomatic" is shown in the upper left panel. The correct diagnosis of secundum atrial septal defect was made, and the defect was easily closed surgically; pericardial effusion was drained at surgery. This resulted in relief of the congestive heart failure state and the patient was functional Class II one year later (lower left panel). (This patient was reported previously: Rahimtoola SH, et al: Circulation 38(Suppl V): V-2, 1968.)

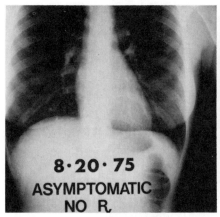

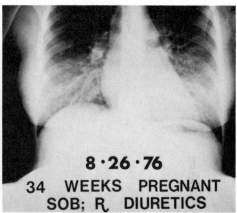

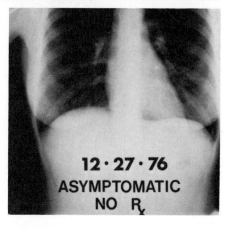

Figure 10. The chest x-rays of a patient with mitral stenosis in the third trimester of pregnancy. Because the major role of fluid overload and the minor role of mitral stenosis was correctly diagnosed, diuretics were administered and the patient returned to an asymptomatic state following delivery. (SOB = shortness of breath.)

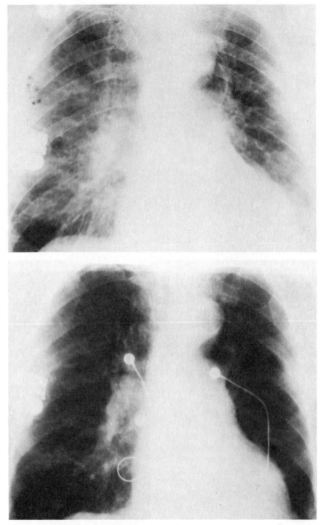

Figure 11.   A 90-year-old patient who had underlying coronary artery disease and complete atrioventricular block. Failure of the pacemaker battery pack resulted in pulmonary edema (upper panel) due to the slow heart rate of complete atrioventricular block. Replacement of the battery pack, without any other therapy, resulted in resolution of heart failure state (lower panel).

digitalis and diuretic therapy results in improvement and correction of the heart failure state in the majority of patients, even those with acute myocardial infarction (Fig. 12).

Other maneuvers that alter ventricular function can be utilized to treat heart failure (Table 2). Usually, digitalis and diuretics suffice; occasionally, oral vasodilators are needed.[18] Even in patients with systemic hypertension, usually a disease of the peripheral arterioles, the first line of therapy is usually not arteriolar dilators. Patients with systemic hypertension and severe renal vasoconstriction may have poor renal perfusion, and the heart failure state may be very difficult to control. In this instance, reduction of arteriolar tone in the kidney by arteriolar dilators may produce a dramatic effect. In

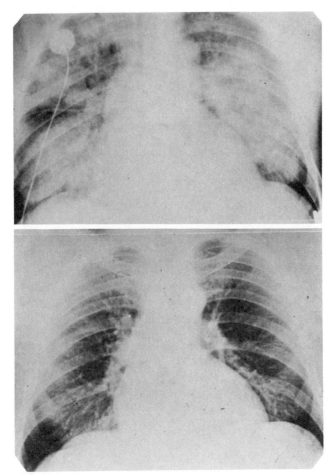

Figure 12. The upper panel shows the chest x-rays of a patient with acute myocardial infarction in severe acute pulmonary edema. Treatment with digitalis and diuretics resulted in resolution of the pulmonary edema. He was asymptomatic at time of discharge from the hospital two weeks later.

patients with acute hypertensive crisis, intravenous vasodilators may be the drugs of first choice. Patients with the "stiff heart" syndrome may need an acute sudden reduction in preload. Since the load is a temporary one, nitroglycerin may be the ideal method for reducing ventricular filling pressure, because its effects are rapid and transient (Fig. 13). Vasodilators that are correctly chosen for the desired effect may be of great value in truly resistant heart failure.

PREVENTION

It is imperative that the recurrence of heart failure be prevented. This is best accomplished by correction of the basic cardiac lesion. Unfortunately, in many patients the underlying cardiac lesions cannot be controlled, and one has to rely principally on (1) control of the precipitating factors and (2) long-

CORONARY ARTERIOGRAPHY

Right Coronary Artery   : Occluded
Left Anterior Descending : 70% stenosis
Obtuse Marginal   : 90% stenosis

Aortic Valve Area: 0.6 cm^2; 0.3 cm^2/M^2
LV End-Diastolic Volume: 66 ml/M^2
Ejection Fraction: 0.42
Mean V_{CF} : 0.92 circ/sec

LV WALL MOTION

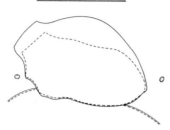

HEMODYNAMICS

Pressures (mmHg)	Rest	After LV Angio	After NTG
Brachial Artery	140/74 (100)	88/59 (75)	110/66 (86)
Left Ventricle	188/0-14	125/19-30	160/0-10
Pulmonary Artery Wedge	a=14 (7)	—	—
Pulmonary Artery	16/7 (10)	55/30 (40)	30/10 (16)
Cardiac Index (L/min/M^2)	2.0	1.6	—
Pulmonary Vascular Resistance, Units (mm Hg/L/min)	0.7	2.8	—
Heart Rate (beats/min)	84	90	96

Figure 13.   An example of a patient with probable "stiff heart" syndrome. This patient had severe calcific aortic valve stenosis and associated coronary artery disease. She had severe angina, orthopnea, and dyspnea on effort. She previously had several episodes of severe, persistent angina, and current electrocardiogram did not show evidence of myocardial infarction. However, left ventricular angiography, utilizing an external reference system (Circulation 48:1043, 1973), showed akinesis of the inferior and apical areas, suggesting that the patient had a previous myocardial infarction. At rest the left ventricular end-diastolic pressure was 14 mm Hg. After left ventricular angiography, which is known to result in an increase of circulating blood volume, the patient had a markedly abnormal response (Circulation 33:52, 1966, and 35:70, 1967). There was no increase of cardiac output. She had increases of filling pressure of the left ventricle, pulmonary artery pressure, and pulmonary vascular resistance that was persistent for a prolonged period (i.e., for over 10 to 15 minutes). At this time she became severely *symptomatic*, and administration of nitroglycerin (a venodilator) resulted in normalization of left ventricular filling pressures and improvement of left ventricular systolic pressure. She rapidly became asymptomatic. Thus, a small volume load associated with contrast angiography resulted in severe, persistent elevations of pulmonary venous pressure, probably the result of a reduced left ventricular compliance.

term therapy with digitalis and diuretics. If these do not alleviate the problem, then vasodilators may be of value.

Should Oral Vasodilators Be Used Routinely?

We can now answer the questions that were asked in the opening paragraph of this article (Table 4).

Digitalis and diuretics, standard pharmacologic therapy, are effective. The complication rates associated with their use are low and are known. They have been used in large numbers of people for long periods of time. Digitalis corrects a common primary problem in heart failure, that is, myocardial dysfunction. Digitalis is also an antiarrhythmic agent. Diuretics act on the kidney to correct the excessive Na$^+$ and water retention.

If vasodilators were to cure the patient and were not associated with severe complications, then vasodilator therapy would override the aforementioned benefits of digitalis and diuretics. However, they do not cure the patient, and their effects are short-lived. They change the loading conditions

Table 4. *Some Questions to be Considered Before Adding or Changing to Any New Therapy Intended for Routine Clinical Use*

	QUESTIONS	ANSWERS
Standard Therapy (Digitalis, Diuretics)	Is it effective ?	Yes
	Does it correct the primary problem ?	Yes
	Has it stood the test of time ?	Yes
New Therapy (Vasodilators)	Does it cure the patient ?	No
	Does it correct the primary problems ?	No
	Is it safe if used properly ?	Yes
	Does it have a lower complication rate ?	No
	Is it easier to use ?	No
	Does it have a more lasting effect ?	No

of the heart, but have no positive inotropic effect. They may increase Na^+ and water excretion, but only if they increase cardiac output. They are safe only if used properly; venodilators should not be used if filling pressures are not significantly increased, and arteriolar dilators should not be used unless cardiac output is reduced. Significant hypotension should not be allowed to occur with either form of vasodilator. Also, it should be emphasized that the effects of vasodilators have been studied in severe, but not in mild forms of heart failure. Vasodilators have no inherent antiarrhythmic properties.

The complication rate associated with chronic use of vasodilators has not been widely studied in a large number of patients who have been given these agents for a prolonged period of time. Nevertheless, complications, even with the use of appropriate doses, do occur, for example, marked unexpected hypotension with nitroglycerin and the lupus-like syndrome with hydralazine. Yet unknown complications may occur with prolonged use of the newer, or not so new, vasodilators. Vasodilators must be taken in multiple doses per day, and therefore, adherence to therapy will be more difficult. They are also expensive.

I would conclude that oral vasodilators should *not* be used routinely in the treatment of congestive heart failure. They should be reserved for the patient who does not respond to conventional therapy.

References

1. Rahimtoola SH, and Bristow JD: The problem of assessment of left ventricular performance in coronary artery disease. Chest 65:480, 1974.
2. Dodek A, Kassebaum DG, and Bristow JD: Pulmonary edema in coronary artery disease without cardiomegaly: a paradox of the stiff heart. N Engl J Med 286:1347, 1972.

3. Mason DT, and Braunwald E: Studies on digitalis. IX. Effects of ouabain on the non-failing human heart. J Clin Invest 42:1105, 1963.

4. Rahimtoola SH, Sinno MZ, Chuquimia R, Loeb HS, Rosen KM, and Gunnar RM: Effects of ouabain on impaired left ventricular function in acute myocardial infarction. N Engl J Med 287:527, 1972.

5. Rahimtoola SH, and Gunnar RM: Digitalis in acute myocardial infarction. Help or hazard? Ann Intern Med 82:234, 1975.

6. Covell JW, Braunwald E, Ross J Jr, and Sonnenblick EH: Effects of digitalis. XVI. Effects on myocardial oxygen consumption. J Clin Invest 45:1535, 1966.

7. DeMots H, Rahimtoola SH, Kremkau EL, Bennett W, and Mahler D: Effects of ouabain on myocardial oxygen supply and demand in patients with chronic coronary artery disease: a hemodynamic, volumetric, and metabolic study in patients without heart failure. J Clin Invest 58:312, 1976.

8. DeMots H, Rahimtoola SH, McAnulty JH, and Porter GA: Effects of ouabain on coronary and systemic vascular resistance and myocardial oxygen consumption in patients without heart failure. Am J Cardiol 41:88, 1978.

9. Mason DT, and Braunwald E: Studies on digitalis. X. Effects of ouabain on forearm vascular resistance and venous flow in normal subjects and in patients with heart failure. J Clin Invest 43:532, 1964.

10. Garan H, Smith TW, and Powell WJ: The central nervous system as the site of action for the coronary vasoconstrictor effects of digoxin. J Clin Invest 54:1365, 1974.

11. Kiely J, Kelly DT, Taylor DR, and Pitt B: The role of furosemide in the treatment of left ventricular dysfunction associated with acute myocardial infarction. Circulation 48:581, 1973.

12. Miller RR, Vismara LA, Williams DO, Amsterdam EA, and Mason DT: Pharmacologic mechanisms for left ventricular unloading in clinical congestive heart failure: differential effects of nitroprusside, phentolamine, and nitroglycerin on cardiac function and peripheral circulation. Circ Res 39:127, 1976.

13. Chatterjee K, Parmley WW, Swan HJC, Berman G, Forrester J, and Marcus H: Beneficial effects of vasodilator agents in severe mitral regurgitation due to dysfunction of subvalvular apparatus. Circulation 48:684, 1973.

14. Miller RR, Vismara LA, DeMaria AN, Salu AF, and Mason DT: Afterload reduction therapy with nitroprusside in severe aortic regurgitation: improved cardiac performance and reduced regurgitant volume. Am J Cardiol 38:564, 1976.

15. Gold HK, Chiariello M, Leinbach RC, Davis MA, and Maroko PR: Deleterious effects of nitroprusside on myocardial injury during acute myocardial infarction. Herz Kardiovaskulare Erkran Kungsen 1:161, 1976.

16. Miller RR, Awan NA, Joye JJ, Maxwell KS, DeMaria AN, Amsterdam EA, and Mason DT: Combined dopamine and nitroprusside therapy in congestive heart failure: greater augmentation of cardiac performance by addition of inotropic stimulation to afterload reduction. Circulation 55:881, 1977.

17. Smith N, McAnulty JH, and Rahimtoola SH: Severe aortic stenosis with impaired left ventricular function and clinical heart failure: results of valve replacement. Circulation 58:225, 1978.

18. Chatterjee K, Parmley WW, Massie B, Greenberg B, Werner J, Klausner S, and Norman A: Oral hydralazine therapy for chronic refractory heart failure. Circulation 54:879, 1976.

Comment

The introduction of oral vasodilators into the management of congestive heart failure represents a significant therapeutic advance. These agents, by altering the loading conditions of the heart both before and after contraction, can change ventricular performance acutely, in a manner that appears to benefit the patient with congestive heart failure. Arteriolar vasodilators, by decreasing the outflow resistance facing the ejecting left ventricle, produce a greater stroke output. Venodilating agents, on the other hand, reduce venous return to the heart, thus decreasing ventricular size or preload. The reduction of ventricular size also aids in reducing the wall force required to eject the ventricular output.

Pharmacologic agents that cause these beneficial pathophysiologic changes can effect acute improvement in a number of patients with severe congestive heart failure. Intractable heart failure can be reversed and diuresis produced as a result of instituting administration of these agents when other measures are no longer effective. It it nevertheless reasonable to ask whether such agents should be used routinely in the treatment of congestive heart failure. Although hemodynamic as well as clinical benefits have been shown with their acute use, data on long-term benefits are still meager. Months after institution of therapy, most of the patients I have seen seem to be doing quite well. However, as pointed out by Rahimtoola, these agents do not alter the basic pathologic state, and the long-term complications from their use are still not fully defined. Furthermore, tachyphylaxis may occur with some drugs after prolonged use, as has been noted by some with prazosin, diminishing their beneficial effects. Other agents, if used improperly, may even be harmful. For example, nitrates, which are potent venodilators, should not be given to a patient who has already had compensation restored and has a relatively low filling pressure to his left ventricle. Further diminution of this filling pressure can actually result, paradoxically, in a further diminution in cardiac output, thus harming rather than benefiting the patient.

Furthermore, since these agents do not directly affect the inotropic state of the myocardium or affect the basic underlying pathology, a serious question arises as to their value when a patient has relatively mild congestive heart failure readily controlled by the use of digitalis and diuretics.

I believe that there are sufficient data in the literature at this point to document the beneficial effects of oral vasodilators. They add another dimension to the management of congestive heart failure that has previously not been present. However, I also reserve the use of these agents for situations in which heart failure is not readily controlled by traditional means. It seems to me unnecessary, and perhaps unwise, to use agents whose long-term effects carry an unknown risk when satisfactory available agents can be used and are effective in restoring competency. On the other hand, if cardiac competency is not restored with digitalis and diuretics, oral vasodilators can be added and may be successful in restoring and maintaining cardiac competency.

ELLIOT RAPAPORT, M.D.

Twenty-six

Are His Bundle Recordings Being Overutilized in the Evaluation of Patients with Arrhythmias and Conduction Disturbances?

ARE HIS BUNDLE RECORDINGS BEING OVERUTILIZED
IN THE EVALUATION OF PATIENTS WITH ARRHYTHMIAS
AND CONDUCTION DISTURBANCES? PROTAGONISTIC VIEWPOINTS
    Alfred Pick, M.D.

HIS BUNDLE RECORDINGS ARE UNDERUTILIZED
IN THE EVALUATION OF PATIENTS WITH ARRHYTHMIAS
AND CONDUCTION DISTURBANCES
    Melvin M. Scheinman, M.D.

COMMENT

Are His Bundle Recordings Overutilized in the Evaluation of Patients with Arrhythmias and Conduction Disturbances? Protagonistic Viewpoints

ALFRED PICK, M.D.
Senior Consultant, Cardiovascular Institute; Senior
Attending Physician, Department of Medicine, Michael
Reese Hospital and Medical Center; Professor of Medicine
Emeritus, Pritzker School of Medicine, University of
Chicago, Chicago, Illinois

Having been preoccupied for many years with analysis and interpretation of complex cardiac arrhythmias in standard electrocardiograms and being asked to take a protagonistic position in the question of overutilization of His electrocardiography, I am faced with a dilemma. There can no longer be any doubt that the introduction of this technique has added new dimensions to the comprehension of electrophysiologic events in the human heart. Concepts that were derived from comparative measurements and morphologic changes in scalar electrocardiograms can now be verified by actual tracking in man of the course, direction, and sequence of depolarization of the individual cardiac chambers and the compartments of the specific cardiac conduction system.[1-3] Yet, the question can be posed in a different way. Has any of these advances fundamentally changed the ideas of genesis of cardiac arrhythmias so as to become indispensable to the practicing cardiologist for the diagnosis and differentiation of simple and com-

635

plex disorders of the cardiac rhythm encountered in routine electrocardiography and to influence a rational treatment? Or, in other words, are there justified indications to perform this invasive method to the benefit of the patient, and in which clinical settings can they safely be omitted?

There are several areas in clinical electrocardiography in which His bundle exploration may be mandatory or can be avoided by using experience and clinical judgment. A prime example is the occurrence of atrioventricular (AV) and/or intraventricular conduction disorders in the course of recent myocardial infarction, which is closely related to the decision of whether or not to apply cardiac pacing. In the case of acute anteroseptal infarction, the *development* of left bundle branch block (BBB) or anterior fascicular block in combination with right BBB can be considered to be an absolute indication for institution of at least temporary pacing, and in this case, utilizing the pacing electrode for probing the function of the atrioventricular conduction system before anchoring it within the ventricular cavity is useful and well indicated. This is not only recommended, but urgent when the partial or total left-sided intraventricular conduction defect is seen in the standard electrocardiogram to be, or to have the potential to become, associated with a first- or second-degree AV block. This frequently heralds Mobitz Type II paroxysmal or sustained complete AV block due to bilateral BBB and the danger of cardiac syncope.[4] However, the development of AV block not associated with an intraventricular conduction defect is quite a different situation. Although rare in infarction of the anterior and lateral wall, it is common in the early stages of diaphragmatic infarction, in the form of simple P-R interval prolongation and progression to second-degree Type I AV block and to complete or incomplete AV dissociation caused by simultaneous acceleration of the AV junctional escape rate, all of which are self-limited and subside spontaneously within a few days.[5] Unless the ventricular rate drops below 60 beats/min, introduction of a catheter into the ventricular cavity serves no practical purpose from the standpoint of diagnosis, prognosis, and specific management and can be, under continued monitoring of the electrocardiogram during the first week, safely omitted. Indeed, the potential risk of ventricular fibrillation by mechanical excitation of the ischemic ventricular myocardium can be avoided.

Similar considerations apply to *chronic* advanced or complete AV block. Again, rate and configuration of the ventricular complexes may *per se* be sufficient to establish the level of the conduction disturbance and the location of the spontaneous pacemaker of the ventricles. Chronic second-degree Type I block (AV nodal block) is very rare, and Type II block by itself will point to an infranodal location of the lesion. Not only in congenital but also in acquired *chronic* complete AV block, the history, especially of dizziness and syncopal attacks, will provide a better prognostic guideline and indication for permanent ventricular pacing than the precise location and magnitude of the lesion (the H-V interval).[6] When a chronic bundle branch block pattern is associated with P-R interval prolongation in the standard electrocardiogram, the response to acceleration or slowing of the atrial rate (by atropine or carotid sinus pressure), changing AV conduction to a Wenckebach periodicity, can distinguish the functional character of the

AV nodal delay from the more serious condition of Type II intrahisian AV or bilateral bundle branch block, and a diagnostic His bundle recording including atrial pacing may not add to the information obtained by the electrocardiogram.

Another more esoteric example of the redundance of His bundle recording is the case of so-called pseudo AV block of first and second degree. Recognized in clinical electrocardiograms in 1947,[7] the actual existence of this rare condition has been amply verified by electrophysiologic studies in animal experiments, at cellular levels,[8] by direct recordings from the AV conduction system in the dog,[9] and in His bundle recordings in man.[10] When *conducted* AV junctional premature beats occur simultaneously with an isolated, unexplained, sudden prolongation of the P-R interval and/or an occasional dropped ventricular complex in a standard clinical recording, the diagnosis of concealed, bidirectionally blocked, premature junctional depolarizations can be confidently made without unnecessarily submitting the patient to verification by an invasive method. However, when abrupt, unexpected changes of P-R intervals of two ranges are found without concomitant, manifest, premature AV junctional beats, dual, functionally dissociated AV nodal pathways may be present,[11, 12] and their existence should be verified by His bundle recordings, including atrial pacing.[13] Their demonstration may account for a re-entrant mechanism of undocumented paroxysms of tachycardia in the past, or predictable for the future, and indicate commencement of prophylactic antiarrhythmic therapy.

Placement of multiple exploring electrodes for simultaneous recording of action potentials of the right and left cavities of the heart[13] has proven to be invaluable in differential diagnosis of the origin and several types of mechanisms of supraventricular and idioventricular tachyarrhythmias. But has this advancement in present-day knowledge rendered criteria of routine electrocardiography entirely obsolete for the interpretation of seemingly complex disorders of cardiac rhythm? There is no question that the use of intracardiac leads is instrumental in the correction of some diagnostic errors in conventional electrocardiography. For instance, regular supraventricular escape rhythms attributed to atrial arrest may turn out in the His electrocardiogram to actually be caused by partially or completely blocked rapid atrial activity not reflected in any of the standard limb and precordial leads.[1] On the other hand, however, His electrocardiography can hardly be expected to contribute to the diagnosis of intermittent sinoatrial blocks readily recognized in the electrocardiogram. Tracing the direction of the activation front in the atria will distinguish between an atrial and AV junctional beats and rhythms, but is a His bundle recording indeed indispensable for any other purpose but to satisfy the curiosity of the clinical investigator?

With regard to supraventricular paroxysmal tachycardias, there is now a consensus established by His electrocardiography that the majority are caused by a rapid re-entry mechanism.[4] It may be limited to the AV nodal network, may or may not include the atria in the circus path or the His bundle, a total or partial AV nodal bypass, or more than a single avenue may be available for the onset of a re-entry mechanism.[14] Yet, is it necessary to verify the reciprocating character of the tachycardia in a His bundle recording when its initiation by an atrial premature beat or an interpolated ventricular premature systole, causing prolongation of the P-R interval, is recorded on the electrocardiogram? By the same token, His bundle recordings may be unnecessary with clear-cut electrocardiographic evidence of ventricular pre-excitation without, or with only rare episodes of paroxysmal tachycardia, unless a potentially life-threatening event can be anticipated on the basis of drug resistance or an anomalous shape of ventricular complexes at an extremely rapid rate — especially in combination with paroxysmal atrial fibrillation — and surgical intervention must be contemplated.[15] Similar reasoning can be applied in the still difficult differential diagnosis of other paroxysmal tachycardias with abnormal (widened) QRS complexes. Finding of a His deflection in front of the ventricular complexes at a normal H-V interval may indicate aberrant ventricular conduction of supraventricular impulses, but its foreshortening, absence, or negative value does not necessarily prove the ventricular or fascicular origin of the abnormal beats, since the position of the H deflection relative to the abnormal ventricular complexes reflects merely the difference of conduction times of the impulse toward the atria and ventricles. The persistent controversy concerning the origin and mechanism of "bidirectional" tachycardias may serve as the best example of this.[1, 17-19] However, right-sided and left-sided endocardial and epicardial exploration of the ventricular activation sequence is a *sine qua non* prerequisite for surgical attempts to abolish and/or prevent medically untreatable, life-endangering recurrence of tachycardias of ventricular origin; this is also true in the case of the ventricular pre-excitation syndrome.[15, 20]

In this short survey, some clinical situations that do not require His bundle recordings for proper treatment have been contrasted to conditions in which intracardiac exploration is mandatory but requires performance in a laboratory that is well equipped for clinical experimentation by an experienced staff of physicians and ancillary personnel. In summary, a His bundle electrocardiogram may be considered to be redundant in some disorders of impulse conduction or formation that can be readily diagnosed and prognosticated in a routine electrocardiogram, relying on a wealth of solid electrophysiologic data accumulated in the past decades by many investigators. Its role is indisputable in the solution of certain specific differential diagnostic and therapeutic problems.

References

1. Puech P, and Grolleau R (eds): *L'Activité du Faisceau de His Normale et Pathologique*. Paris, Éditions Sandoz, 1972.
2. Damato AN, Gallagher JJ, and Lau SH: Application of His bundle recordings in diagnosing conduction disorders. Progr Cardiovasc Dis 14:601, 1972.
3. Narula OS (ed): *His Bundle Electrocardiography and Clinical Electrophysiology*. Philadelphia, F. A. Davis Company, 1975.
4. Puech P: Atrioventricular block: the value of intracardiac recordings. *In* Krikler DA, and Goodwin JF (eds): *Cardiac Arrhythmias*. London, WB Saunders Company, 1975, pp 81, 116.

5. Pick A, and Langendorf R: The dual function of the A-V junction. Am Heart J 88:790, 1974.
6. Denes P, Dhingra R, Wyndham CRC, Amat-y-Leon F, Wu D, Chuquimia R, and Rosen K: Prospective observations in patients with chronic bundle branch block and marked H-V prolongation. Am J Cardiol 37:131, 1976.
7. Langendorf R, and Mehlman JS: Blocked (non-conducted) A-V nodal premature systoles imitating first and second degree A-V block. Am Heart J 34:500, 1974.
8. Moore EN, Knoeble SB, and Spear JF: Concealed conduction. Am J Cardiol 28:406, 1971.
9. Damato AN, Lau SH, and Bobb JA: Cardiac arrhythmias simulated by concealed bundle of His extrasystoles in the dog. Circ Res 28:316, 1971.
10. Rosen KM, Rahimtoola SH, and Gunnar RM: Pseudo A-V block secondary to premature nonpropagated His bundle depolarizations: documented by His bundle electrocardiography. Circulation 42:367, 1970.
11. Moe GK, Preston JB, and Burlington H: Physiologic evidence for dual A-V transmission system. Circ Res 4:357, 1956.
12. Rosen KM, Denes P, Wu D, and Dhingra RC: Electrophysiological diagnosis and manifestation of dual A-V nodal pathways. In Wellens HJJ, Janse MJ, and Lie KI (eds): The Conduction System of the Heart. Philadelphia, Lea and Febiger, 1976, p 453.
13. Curry PVL: Fundamentals of arrhythmias: Modern methods of investigation. In Puech P, and Grolleau R (eds): L'Activité du Faisceau de His Normale et Pathologique. Paris, Éditions Sandoz, 1972.
14. Kulbertus HE (ed): Re-entrant Arrhythmias: Mechanisms and Treatment. Baltimore, University Park Press, 1977, Section III, pp 117–184.
15. Gallagher JJ, Seaby WC, Anderson RW, Kasell J, Pritchett ELC, Wallace AG, and Harrison L: The surgical treatment of arrhythmias. In Kulbertus HE (ed): Re-entrant Arrhythmias: Mechanisms and Treatment. Baltimore, University Park Press, 1977, p 351.
16. Cohen HC, Gozo EG, and Pick A: Ventricular tachycardia with narrow QRS complexes (left posterior fascicular tachycardia). Circulation 45:1035, 1972.
17. Rosenbaum MB, Elizari MV, and Lazzari JO: The mechanism of bidirectional tachycardia. Am Heart J 76:4, 1969.
18. Kastor HO, and Goldreyer BN: Ventricular origin of bidirectional tachycardia. Case report of a patient nontoxic from digitalis. Circulation 48:897, 1973.
19. Cohen SI, and Youkidis P: Supraventricular origin of bidirectional tachycardia. Circulation 50:634, 1974.
20. Fontaine G, Guiradon G, Frank R, Vedel J, Grosgogeat Y, Cabrol C, and Facquet J: Stimulation studies and epicardial mapping in ventricular tachycardia: study of mechanism and selection for surgery. In Kulbertus HE (ed): Re-entrant Arrhythmias: Mechanisms and Treatment. Baltimore, University Park Press, 1977, p 334.

His Bundle Recordings Are Underutilized in the Evaluation of Patients with Arrhythmias and Conduction Disturbances*

MELVIN M. SCHEINMAN, M.D.

Professor of Medicine, Department of Medicine, University of California, San Francisco; and Chief, Electrocardiography and Clinical Cardiac Electrophysiology Section, Moffitt Hospital, San Francisco, California

The introduction by Scherlag et al.[1] of a technique for reliable recording of His bundle activity in man has greatly expanded our understanding of cardiac rhythm and conduction disturbances. Recently, we have begun to reap the clinical benefits of these studies. This article illustrates the means by which intracardiac electrophysiologic studies, including His bundle recordings, may be of important clinical value. In our view, intracardiac electrophysiologic studies are currently underutilized in most medical centers.

Clinical Application

LOCATION OF ATRIOVENTRICULAR BLOCK

The electric wave forms displayed on routine electrocardiographic recordings depend on the mass of cells undergoing depolarization, their rate of depolarization, and the lead system utilized. Consequently, in these leads, one may record atrial and ventricular depolarization and repolarization, but

*Supported in part by the National Institutes of Health, HL-20238.

640

depolarization of the common bundle and bundle branches is not recorded. However, these potentials are obtained from intracardiac electrode catheters properly positioned adjacent to these structures. This technique, therefore, enables precise location of atrioventricular (AV) conduction disturbances, which is impossible by analysis of routine electrocardiograms. The ability to locate conduction disturbances precisely is of more than just academic interest. For example, patients with infranodal block are more prone to develop Stokes-Adams attacks than are patients with a conduction block localized to the AV node. Therefore, the former are prime candidates for insertion of a permanent intracardiac pacemaker.

Mobitz I versus Mobitz II atrioventricular block

As a general rule, Mobitz I AV block indicates disease at the level of the AV node, whereas Mobitz II AV block indicates infranodal pathology. There are, however, important exceptions to this rule, as well as difficulties in distinguishing these two forms of block. Mobitz I block can occur anywhere in the cardiac conduction system, and sole reliance on surface tracings for its location may be misleading. Figure 1, for instance, shows an example of Mobitz I block occurring in the His-Purkinje system. Furthermore, other investigators have described Type II AV block in the AV node. We have observed this in patients with associated hypervagotonic states in which Type II block is characteristically associated with marked sinus slowing, as shown in Figure 2A.[2] This phenomenon could be readily reproduced by carotid massage in this patient (Fig. 2B) and was abolished by atropine.

In addition, in Type II AV block, the beat terminating the pause may often show a shorter P-R interval than subsequent conducted beats (presumably as a result of improved AV conduction following the pause). In this situation, a 3:2 Type II block would be indistinguishable from a 3:2 Type I block. El-Sherif, Scherlag, and their colleagues[3] have emphasized the difficulties in distinguishing Type I from Type II AV block in the setting of acute myocardial infarction. Classic Type II AV block patterns on routine surface recordings may, in fact, be Type I AV block in which the increment in AV conduction is in the order of only a few milliseconds, which requires rapid speed recorders to substantiate the diagnosis. They suggest that Types I and

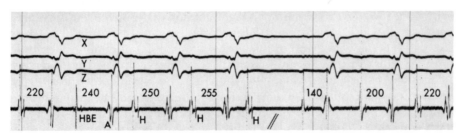

Figure 1. Simultaneous recordings of surface leads X, Y, and Z (Frank orthogonal lead system) and the His bundle electrogram (HBE). Surface leads show a right bundle branch block pattern and AV Wenckebach conduction. The Wenckebach conduction pattern is localized in the His-Purkinje system. Numerals denote progressive prolongation of infranodal conduction time.

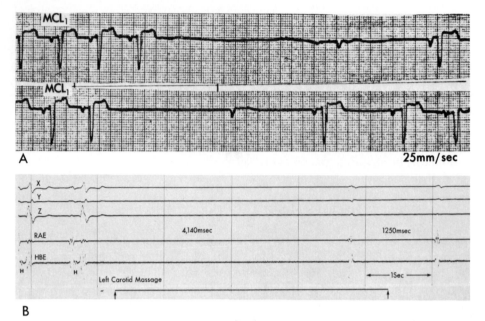

Figure 2. (A) Surface recordings (MCL₁) showing abrupt onset of sinus bradycardia and dropped P waves. The conducted beats show a fixed P-R interval. (B) Simultaneous surface X, Y, Z, and intracardiac recordings (RAE = right atrial electrogram, HBE = His bundle electrogram) during left carotid massage showing abrupt sinus bradycardia and P waves blocked in the AV node. This response was blocked by the intravenous administration of atropine.

II blocks are in reality a continuum of the same basic disorder. The implications of these findings are that His bundle recordings are an absolute requirement for precise location of the AV block.

Several additional problems are related to atypical Wenckebach cycles (maximal prolongation of AV conduction in the beat before the dropped P wave). Atypical cycles are, in fact, more common in longer Wenckebach cycles (i.e., > 4:3) and may clearly occur both at or below the AV node. Finally, analysis of surface recordings does not allow for the differentiation of Type I block from Type II block in the presence of a fixed ratio between P waves and QRS complexes (i.e., 2:1 or 3:1 block).[4]

On the other hand, it has been argued that analysis of QRS duration in addition to studying the pattern of AV conduction disturbance leads to correct location of the site of the block. Three problems are immediately evident. First, patients may have an intrahisian AV block but a normal QRS complex. Figure 3 shows an electrocardiogram of a patient with recurrent syncopal episodes and complete AV block in whom the His bundle electrocardiogram shows intrahisian block. Second, it is well recognized that asynchronous activation of the ventricles results in a bundle branch block pattern. It is conceivable that balanced disease in both right and left bundle branches may produce a perfectly normal QRS complex and first-degree AV block. Thus, the His bundle recording would be necessary for precise location of the site of the AV block. Finally, patients who have intact AV conduction but concealed

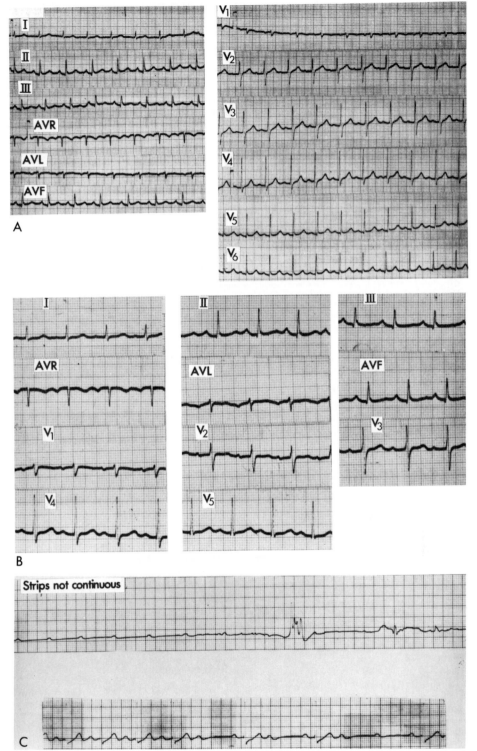

Figure 3. (A) Routine 12-lead electrocardiogram showing a normal QRS pattern and P-R interval of 0.20 second. (B) Spontaneous lengthening of the P-R interval (0.26 second) is observed. (C) The top strip shows complete AV block with ventricular asystole terminated by a blow to the chest, and the bottom strip (different lead placement) shows episodic 2:1 and 3:1 AV block.

Illustration continued on following page

643

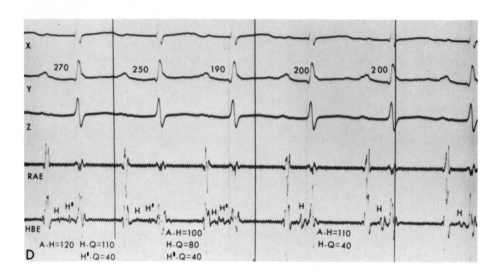

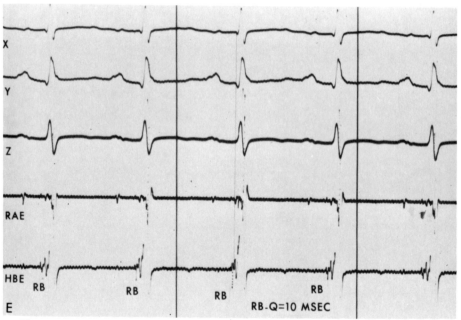

Figure 3. *Continued* (D) Simultaneous surface leads X, Y, Z, and intracardiac recordings from the right atrium (RAE) and His bundle (HBE) show marked variation in the P-R interval. The prolonged P-R interval is due to delayed conduction within the His bundle, and a split His potential (H and H′) is recorded. There is gradual fusion of these two potentials. (E) The split potentials were not His and proximal right bundle branch deflections. In this panel a discrete right bundle potential is recorded.

junctional extrasystoles may appear to have any degree of AV block. Thus, the His bundle electrocardiogram is of critical importance in establishing the proper diagnosis.

BUNDLE BRANCH BLOCK

A subset of patients with bundle branch block are at increased risk of development of high-grade AV block. High-grade AV block (and, therefore, symptoms related to this conduction disturbance) may be episodic, and normal AV conduction may be present even during prolonged electrocardiographic monitoring. In 1972, we initiated a prospective study consisting mainly of patients with transient neurologic symptoms and bundle branch block. Marked prolongation of the infranodal conduction time (H-Q interval > 70 msec) was associated with a higher incidence of progression to high-grade AV block. In addition, there was a higher incidence of sudden death in those patients with prolonged H-Q interval (> 70 msec) and New York Heart Association cardiac functional classification of III or IV.[5] Our findings suggested that insertion of a permanent intracardiac pacemaker is indicated in patients with transient neurologic symptoms and bundle branch block associated with marked prolongation of infranodal conduction time in whom no other causes for these symptoms are apparent.

Analysis of the surface electrocardiogram in the patients in our study with first-degree AV block was of limited value in predicting either the site of AV block or progression to high-grade AV block. Over 50 per cent of the patients with prolonged P-R intervals showed block at the level of the AV node. Figure 4 shows recordings from a patient with left bundle branch block and a normal P-R interval who progressed to complete AV block. Finally, there was no correlation between the type of bundle branch block pattern (i.e., unifascicular or bifascicular) and either marked prolongation of the H-Q interval or progressive AV conduction disturbances.

ARRHYTHMIA DIAGNOSIS

Proper diagnosis of a wide, complex tachycardia is perhaps one of the most difficult problems in clinical electrocardiography, because there are exceptions to all the commonly quoted rules. His bundle recording and atrial pacing are often required to make a precise diagnosis. In the absence of an accessory AV pathway, supraventricular impulses must traverse the common bundle, and hence, the QRS complex should be preceded by a His bundle deflection. Absence of a His bundle deflection, however, does not prove that the tachycardia is of ventricular origin, because this deflection may not have been recorded owing to technical difficulties. However, atrial overdrive pacing in patients with ventricular tachycardia should result in normalization (or production of a bundle branch block pattern) of the QRS complex or may yield fusion complexes, which are highly suggestive of ventricular tachycardia.

A similar and even more common problem is differentiation of aberrantly

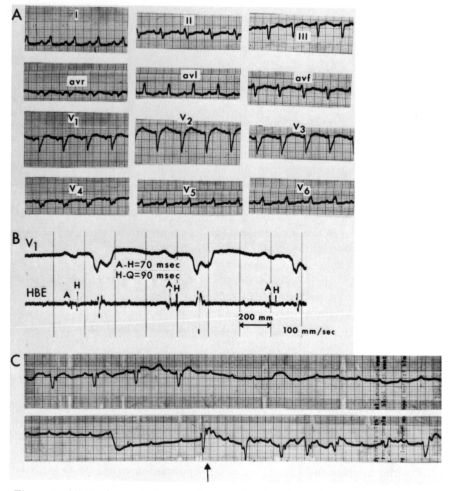

Figure 4. (A) Twelve-lead electrocardiogram showing a normal P-R interval and left bundle branch block. (B) The His bundle electrogram shows marked prolongation of infranodal conduction (H-Q = 90 msec), but the P-R interval remains normal because AV nodal conduction time (A-H) is only 70 msec. (C) Spontaneous complete AV block with ventricular asystole terminated by a junctional escape beat (arrow) was subsequently recorded.

conducted supraventricular beats from ventricular ectopy in patients with atrial fibrillation. None of the accepted rules in terms of coupling intervals, short-long cycle sequences, or QRS contour is infallible. The His bundle recordings may be of considerable value in that supraventricular beats again should be preceded by His bundle deflections. Figure 5 shows tracings from a patient with atrial fibrillation and severe congestive heart failure. The electrocardiogram while the patient was receiving digitalis showed frequent beats of both right and left bundle branch block pattern, and the patient was referred for study, as it was uncertain whether these beats were aberrantly conducted or due to digitalis-induced ventricular ectopy. His bundle recordings, however, showed that all beats were aberrantly conducted supraventricular beats, suggesting that continued use of digitalis was in order.

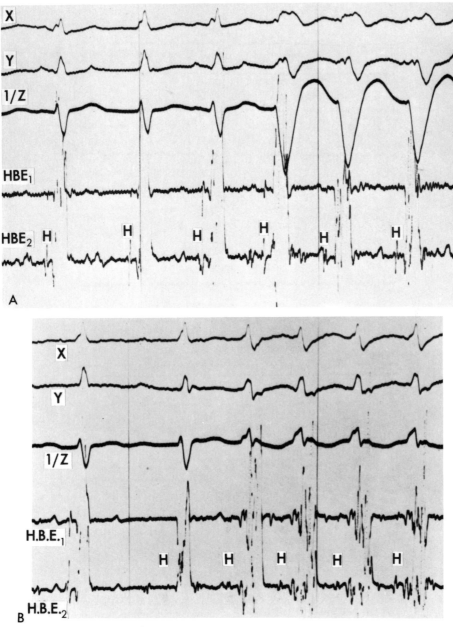

Figure 5. (A) Simultaneous recordings of surface leads X, Y, and inverse Z (1/Z) together with His bundle electrograms recorded from distal (HBE₁) and proximal (HBE₂) pairs of electrodes. The recordings show atrial fibrillation, and both normally conducted complexes (first three) and those with left bundle branch configuration (last three) are preceded by His bundle depolarization. (B) Similarly, normally conducted beats (first two) and beats with right bundle branch contour (last four) are preceded by His bundle depolarizations. Thus, beats of both right and left bundle branch contour are aberrantly conducted supraventricular complexes.

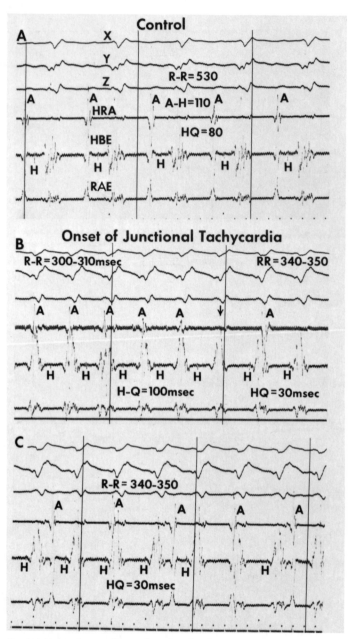

Figure 6. (A) Control recordings of surface leads X, Y, and Z together with the high right atrial (HRA) and His bundle (HBE) electrograms show a spontaneous cycle length of 530 msec and normal AV nodal conduction time (A-H = 110 msec) but prolonged infranodal conduction time (H-Q = 80 msec).

Illustration continued on opposite page

His bundle electrocardiography is of great value in the diagnosis of fascicular rhythms. Patients may present with tachycardia associated with slight prolongation of the QRS complex, and analysis of surface records might not permit differentiation between supraventricular tachycardia with minimal aberrant conduction and tachycardia originating from a fascicle of the ventricular specialized conduction system. In the latter situation, the His bundle deflection may be inscribed just before the ventricular depolarization. The abbreviated H-Q interval results from retrograde activation of the His bundle from the fascicular focus together with near-simultaneous antegrade activation of the ventricles from this same focus. Fascicular rhythms arising from the left ventricular specialized conduction system would be expected to result in a left anterior or posterior hemiblock pattern. Thus, His bundle electrocardiograms may be especially useful in diagnosing this subset of patients with ventricular tachycardia.

Figures 6A–C show the usefulness of His bundle recordings in a patient referred for evaluation of complex tachyarrhythmias. The control tracing shows a left bundle branch block pattern with prolonged infranodal conduction time. A spontaneous bout of supraventricular tachycardia was recorded that was independent of atrial depolarization (Fig. 6B). Spontaneous change to a slightly lower rate was associated with AV dissociation and marked narrowing of the H-Q interval, suggesting emergence of a lower His bundle focus (no change in surface complexes were apparent). Atrial overdrive pacing (Fig. 6D) resulted in capture with AV node Wenckebach conduction and cessation of pacing was followed by resumption of sinus rhythm. Precise location of the origin of tachycardia would have been clearly impossible by analysis of surface leads alone.

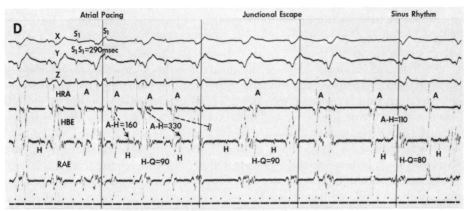

Figure 6. *Continued* (B) Spontaneous onset of tachycardia with a cycle length of 300 to 310 msec is associated with further prolongation of the H-Q interval and 1:1 ventriculoatrial conduction for the first five QRS complexes. The initial five complexes were not of atrial origin because the "antegrade" AH interval during the tachycardia should have been longer than the control A-H. In addition, atrial pacing at similar cycle lengths resulted in AV nodal Wenckebach conduction (see 6D). Furthermore, the tachycardia is clearly independent of atrial depolarization because it continues in spite of retrograde AV block (arrow).

The last two QRS complexes in B and all complexes for C (continuous recording) show emergence of a slightly slower rate with H-Q equal to 30 msec and complete AV dissociation due to the accelerated junctional rate. The last findings are interpreted as emergence of a focus lower in the His bundle (explaining the shortened H-Q interval) that discharges at a slower rate and is associated with complete retrograde block. (D) Atrial overdrive pacing (during the tachycardia) at a cycle length of 290 msec ($S_1 S_1 = 290$ msec) resulted in AV nodal Wenckebach conduction (dashed lines represent AV conduction). Termination of pacing resulted in escape of the "high" junctional focus (H-Q = 90 msec) for three beats that was followed by resumption of sinus rhythm with 1:1 AV conduction.

DIAGNOSIS AND LOCATION OF ACCESSORY PATHWAYS

Precise diagnosis and accurate location of accessory pathways assumed critical importance with the introduction of reliable surgical techniques that are effective in abolishing these pathways.[6] His bundle electrocardiograms and atrial pacing are essential for proper diagnosis. Patients with the Lown-Ganong-Levine syndrome (short P-R interval and narrow QRS complex) characteristically have a short A-H interval (< 50 msec) with less than the normally expected increase in A-H interval with atrial overdrive pacing. In contrast, patients with His-ventricular bypass tracts (Mahaim tracts) have a normal AV nodal conduction time but a short H-Q interval. With atrial pacing, the A-H interval prolongs in normal fashion, but the H-Q interval remains unchanged. On the other hand, patients with the Wolff-Parkinson-White syndrome during atrial pacing have prolongation of the A-H interval with narrowing of the H-Q interval, because the normal increment in AV nodal conduction occurs with essentially unchanged AV conduction via the bypass tract.

In addition, endocardial mapping techniques enable precise location of accessory AV pathways. This is achieved by documenting the presence of eccentric atrial activation during either ventricular pacing or supraventricular tachycardia when antegrade conduction occurs via the AV node–His axis (orthodromic conduction) and retroconduction occurs over the accessory pathway. The presence of an accessory pathway, however, does not prove its participation in the re-entrant circuit. Induction of ventricular depolarizations during orthodromic tachycardia (at a time when the His bundle is certain to be refractory), which results in foreshortening of ventriculoatrial conduction time but is associated with the same pattern of eccentric atrial activation, proves participation of an accessory pathway in the re-entrant arrhythmia.

Analyses of surface recordings alone are clearly inadequate for location of an AV accessory pathway. Classically, the Type A pattern (dominant anterior focuses in lead V_1) is thought to indicate a left-sided pathway, whereas Type B (dominant posterior forces in V_1) suggests a right-sided accessory pathway. However, investigators at Duke University have clearly shown, for example, that septal pathways may occur with either of the aforementioned surface patterns.[7] In addition, recent studies have emphasized the importance of concealed retroconduction via bypass tracts.[8] In this setting, the tachycardia proceeds antegrade through the AV node–His axis and returns to the atrium via an accessory extranodal pathway. Clearly, in this situation, the diagnosis of a bypass tract can never be made from surface electrocardiograms, because antegrade pre-excitation is never present. Finally, precise location of the pathway is further complicated by the presence of multiple accessory pathways that may confuse the interpretation of the surface leads because fusion between normal and accessory pathway(s) may be present. Figure 7 shows evidence of dual accessory AV pathways in a patient with Wolff-Parkinson-White syndrome. Quite clearly, intracardiac electrophysiologic studies are absolutely necessary for establishing proper diagnosis and locating accessory pathways.

The objective of this article is to emphasize the major clinical applications of His bundle electrocardiography. However, I would be remiss in not

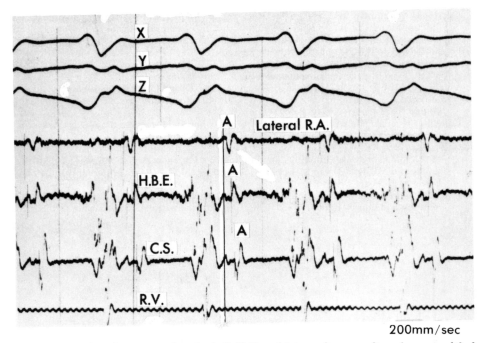

Figure 7. Simultaneous surface leads X, Y, Z, and intracardiac recordings from a modified Brockenbrough electrode catheter positioned in the lateral right atrium (RA), a septal electrogram (HBE), and a coronary sinus (CS) electrogram together with recordings from the right ventricular apex (RV) (paper speed = 200 mm/sec) show antidromic paroxysmal atrial tachycardia (antegrade conduction via the accessory pathway) with earliest atrial depolarization in the region of the lateral right atrium. During this tachycardia, one accessory pathway was used for antegrade AV conduction and a separate accessory pathway was used for ventriculoatrial conduction.

mentioning that there is currently a virtual explosion of knowledge relating to the effects of drugs on cardiac conduction and refractoriness in man. Intracardiac electrophysiologic techniques have afforded giant advances in our understanding of the mechanisms of cardiac arrhythmias and have provided deeper insights into our understanding of clinical electrocardiography. A list of the advances would include clear delineation of both AV nodal and infranodal gap phenomena, the possibility of re-entry within the His bundle, documentation of dual AV nodal conduction, and AV nodal re-entry as a cause of Wenckebach conduction in man.

In conclusion, His bundle electrocardiography plays an important role in our diagnostic armamentarium. The advances alluded to are really extensions of and a testament to the brilliant foundations constructed for us by giants of clinical electrocardiography, including my eminent protagonist.

References

1. Scherlag BJ, Lau SH, Helfant RH, Berkowitz WD, Stein E, and Damato AN: Catheter technique for recording His bundle activity in man. Circulation 39:13, 1969.

2. Massie B, Scheinman MM, Peters R, Desai J, Hirschfeld D, and O'Young J: Clinical and electrophysiologic findings in patients with paroxysmal slowing of the sinus rate and apparent Mobitz type II atrioventricular block. Circulation 58:305, 1978.
3. El-Sherif N, Scherlag BJ, and Lazzara R: Pathophysiology of second degree atrioventricular block: unified hypothesis. Am J Cardiol 35:421, 1975.
4. Zipes DP: Second-degree atrioventricular block. Circulation 60:465, 1979.
5. Scheinman MM, Peters R, Modin G, Brennan M, Meis C, and O'Young J: Prognostic value of infranodal conduction time in patients with chronic bundle branch block. Circulation 56:240, 1977.
6. Gallagher JJ, et al: The Wolff-Parkinson-White syndrome and the pre-excitation dysrhythmias: medical and surgical management. Med Clin North Am 60:101, 1976.
7. Gallagher JJ, Sealy WC, Wallace AG, and Kassell J: Correlation between catheter electrophysiologic studies and findings on mapping of ventricular excitation in the W.P.W. syndrome. *In* Wellens HJ (ed): *Conduction System of the Heart*. Philadelphia, Lea and Febiger, 1976, pp 24–48.
8. Coumel P. and Attuel P: Reciprocating tachycardia in overt and latent preexcitation: influence of functional bundle branch block on the rate of the tachycardia. Eur J Cardiol 1:423, 1973.

Comment

His bundle electrocardiography and the associated electrophysiologic studies that are performed in conjunction with it have contributed greatly to our understanding of the mechanisms and natural history of various arrhythmias and conduction disturbances. As a result, particularly in academic centers, many patients undergo His bundle catheterization with the hope that it will help in management of their particular problem.

Dr. Pick has given examples of situations in which clinical judgment, combined with classic electrocardiography and knowledge of the natural history of the process, obviates the need for performing His bundle electrocardiography. In these situations, he questions whether the His bundle study will influence clinical judgment. On the other hand, Dr. Scheinman presents examples in which electrophysiologic studies have demonstrated that the actual mechanism of a conduction disturbance or arrhythmia was different from that generally assumed on the basis of the electrocardiogram. For example, he points out that Mobitz Type I block can occur anywhere in the conduction system and, conversely, Type II Mobitz block can occur in the AV node.

I have had the pleasure of having Dr. Scheinman associated with me at San Francisco General Hospital and have admired the sophistication brought to the studies he performs and the information that he has contributed to our understanding of conduction disturbances and arrhythmias. Nevertheless, I would have to support the thesis that there is overutilization of electrophysiologic studies in clinical practice today. For example, too many asymptomatic patients have had permanent pacemakers inserted after electrophysiologic studies, based upon demonstrated electrophysiologic abnormalities, despite the fact that there is lack of proof that such management prolongs life. I question whether an elderly patient with sinus bradycardia or sinus pauses who is asymptomatic needs an electrophysiologic study. Such a patient, in my judgment, does not need a pacemaker, and therefore, why should the patient be studied for the so-called sick sinus syndrome? Even a symptomatic patient who has evidence of sick sinus syndrome electrocardiographically but is on medication known to depress sinus node function, such as propranolol, should be observed after discontinuance of the medication to see if the situation resolves before electrophysiologic study and pacemaker insertion takes place. Another example is the asymptomatic patient with bilateral bundle branch block that has not developed as part of an acute process. I believe such a patient does not need a permanent pacemaker inserted, even if a prolonged H-V interval time were demonstrated, confirming trifascicular block. Why then should the procedure be performed? Although I do not object to the performance of His bundle electrocardiography in the situation

653

of a symptomatic patient with bifascicular block in whom the symptoms are clearly documented to be syncopal episodes or frequent dizzy spells, it is clear that a permanent pacemaker is needed regardless of the His bundle findings.

In summary, His bundle electrocardiography with associated electrophysiologic studies represents a highly useful technique that often helps to clarify the mechanisms in selected cases of conduction disturbance and arrhythmias. However, it should not be a substitute for good clinical judgment based on an understanding of the natural history of the process.

ELLIOT RAPAPORT, M.D.

Twenty-seven

Is Acute Aortic Dissection a Surgical Emergency?

DISSECTING ANEURYSM OF THE AORTA
  Michael E. DeBakey, M.D.

ACUTE AORTIC DISSECTION IS *Not* A SURGICAL EMERGENCY
  Myron W. Wheat, Jr., M.D.

COMMENT

Dissecting Aneurysm of the Aorta

MICHAEL E. DEBAKEY, M.D.

President and Chancellor, Baylor College of Medicine;
Chairman, Cora and Webb Mading Department of
Surgery, Baylor College of Medicine; Director, National
Heart and Blood Vessel Research and Demonstration
Center, Baylor College of Medicine, Houston, Texas

Dissecting aneurysm of the aorta has long been recognized as a grave disease with a highly fatal course. Indeed, most studies of the natural course of the disease, including our own, have shown that more than 50 per cent of patients die within two weeks of the initial dissection and more than 75 per cent die within several months, with few surviving more than one year. Since our first successful resection of a dissecting aneurysm of the thoracic aorta in 1954, sufficient experience has accumulated to show that the highly fatal course of this disease can be favorably modified. This experience, involving about 300 cases, along with the experiences of others, has also led to the development of certain principles of treatment.

The development and introduction of highly effective antihypertensive and inotropic agents made it possible to influence the effect of pulse-wave propagation on the aortic wall and thus to influence the factors bearing on the immediate outcome in dissecting aneurysms. This is particularly true during the early treatment of the patients, that is, within the first few days after the initial episode of dissection. These drugs have made it possible to tide over many patients who might otherwise have died, allowing their condition to stabilize so that definitive surgical treatment could be accomplished under more favorable circumstances. This has led some to propose that this method of medical treatment may suffice in many patients and thus allow the dissecting aneurysm to heal itself in one way or another.

Our experience does not support this position. Indeed, our accumulated experience over a period of more than 20 years has firmly convinced us that surgical intervention should be considered the treatment of choice. Accordingly, definitive diagnosis by means of aortography should be made as expeditiously as possible and operation performed as soon as possible after adequate stabilization of the patient's condition — usually within several weeks. Surgical treatment may be necessary as an emergency, however, in patients with leaking aneurysms in whom rupture seems imminent, in those with overwhelming aortic valvular insufficiency, or in those whose

657

major branch of the aorta has been compromised. Surgical treatment is also indicated in the more chronic forms of the disease, since dissecting aneurysm is known to be progressive and may become exacerbated at any time, even after stabilization.

Our surgical experience has led us to classify dissecting aneurysms into three basic types, since the type has an important bearing on the method of surgical treatment. In Type I, the intimal tear and the dissecting process originate in the ascending aorta and extend distally for a variable distance across the aortic arch and into the descending thoracic and abdominal aorta, and sometimes into the major terminal branches. The extent of circumferential dissection varies, but it is usually incomplete. Aortic valvular insufficiency is often present.

This type of dissecting aneurysm is the most serious form of the disease, with fatal complications occurring early after onset. Indeed, many of these patients die before adequate treatment can be instituted. In our surgical experience, Type I constituted less than 15 per cent of the patients with dissecting aneurysms. It is highly important, therefore, to recognize and diagnose precisely this type of dissecting aneurysm. Medical treatment to stabilize the patient's condition should then be instituted as promptly as possible. Careful and continuous monitoring of the patient's condition should be maintained in the intensive care unit, with particular emphasis on maintaining the blood pressure as low as is consistent with adequate cerebral, cardiac, and renal function. If the patient's condition can be maintained and stabilized in this manner for 10 days to a few weeks, elective operation may then be performed. If, however, there is evidence of imminent rupture or severe aortic valvular insufficiency with progressive heart failure, emergency surgical treatment should be instituted. Surgical treatment for this type of dissecting aneurysm consists essentially in resection of the ascending aorta, with distal reapproximation of the dissected wall and replacement with a Dacron graft. If indicated, the aortic valve is replaced at the same time.

Type II dissecting aneurysm is similar to Type I in that the intimal tear and dissecting process arise in the ascending aorta, but this type differs in that the dissecting process is limited to the ascending aorta, terminating just proximal to the origin of the innominate artery. Aortic valvular insufficiency is often present in this type. In our experience, about one-fourth of the patients had Type II dissecting aneurysm, about half of whom were observed in the acute or subacute period and the other half in the more chronic stage some months, or even a few years, after onset of the disease. Aortography permits a precise diagnosis and should be done as promptly as possible. In the acute form of the disease, medical measures should be instituted in the same manner as previously described for Type I in order to stabilize the patient's condition and maintain it for about 10 days, after which surgical intervention is indicated. As in Type I, indications for emergency operation may also occur.

Surgical treatment consists essentially in resection of the ascending aorta, with a Dacron graft replacement and aortic valvular replacement, which is necessary in most patients. Aortocoronary bypass may be required in some of these patients in whom the proximal dissecting process involves the origin of the coronary arteries.

In Type III dissecting aneurysm, the intimal tear and dissecting process arise in the descending thoracic aorta, usually just distal to the origin of the left subclavian artery, and extend distally for a variable distance. In some cases, the dissecting process is limited to the descending thoracic aorta, whereas in others, it may extend below the diaphragm into the abdominal aorta. Fortunately, in most of the latter cases, the false lumen tends to be progressively smaller just above the diaphragm. In our experience, about three-fifths of the patients had Type III dissecting aneurysm; about two-thirds were observed in the acute stage of the disease and the other third in the chronic stage. Here again, precise diagnosis by aortography should be made as soon as possible, and medical treatment as previously described for Types I and II promptly instituted. After the patient's condition has been stabilized over a period of about 10 days to two weeks, surgical intervention is indicated. As in the previous types, however, emergency operation may be necessary. In our experience, about 10 per cent of patients required emergency operations, chiefly because of rupture of the aneurysm. Surgical treatment in this type consists essentially in aneurysmal resection and Dacron graft replacement. At the proximal anastomosis, the graft is attached to the normal lumen, and in those in whom the dissecting process is limited to the descending thoracic aorta, the distal anastomosis is attached to the normal aortic wall. In patients in whom the dissecting process extends below the diaphragm, the inner and outer walls of the dissection are first approximated by suture, and the anastomosis is then made to the normal lumen.

Results of treatment in our experience with this combined early medical treatment for stabilization and subsequent surgical intervention have been gratifying. In Type I, for example, the operative mortality rate was about 18 per cent, and five-year and 10-year survival rates were 50 per cent and 25 per cent, respectively. In Type II, the operative mortality rate was about 10 per cent, and five-year and 10-year survival rates were about 65 per cent and 60 per cent, respectively. In Type III, the operative mortality rate was about 12 per cent, and the five-year and 10-year survival rates were about 60 per cent and 30 per cent, respectively. In recent years, the overall operative mortality rate has been significantly reduced, and it may be expected that the late survival rates will also improve.

Acute Aortic Dissection Is *Not* a Surgical Emergency

MYRON W. WHEAT, JR., M.D.

Clinical Professor of Surgery, University of Louisville
School of Medicine, Louisville, Kentucky; Cardiovascular
Surgeon, Cardiac Surgical Associates, St. Petersburg,
Florida

Acute aortic dissection is not a surgical emergency. The designation "a surgical emergency" implies that surgery in itself is the only definitive treatment and that the sooner surgical correction is carried out, the better. Rather than a surgical emergency, acute aortic dissection is a diagnostic and therapeutic emergency.

For example, a ruptured abdominal aortic aneurysm is a true surgical emergency. In this case, unless the patient is operated on at once, with prompt proximal and distal control of bleeding and expeditious repair of the aneurysm, the mortality rate is 100 per cent. This is certainly not the case with acute dissecting aneurysm of the aorta, unless, of course, it is in the process of rupturing when seen initially; this represents only a small percentage of patients seen. Because of the potential for rapid progression of dissecting aneurysm to rupture and death, diagnosis is of paramount importance. It is equally important that the diagnosis be accurate and complete, so that the patient can be treated in the manner that will give the best opportunity for survival with the least risk in any particular circumstance.

There is one variety of acute dissecting aneurysm that is a true surgical emergency, and that is the patient with an acute Type I dissection (Fig. 1) with life-threatening aortic valve insufficiency when first seen. Although only a few such patients have been rescued, their only chance of survival is the knowledgeable cardiac surgeon who recognizes the problem and who has the courage to take the patient directly to the operating room for emergency surgical repair. Dr. Hassan Najafi[1] has reported two successful cases treated in this manner.

Short of the emergency situations of the actual rupturing aneurysm or overwhelming aortic valve insufficiency, most patients with acute dissecting aneurysms survive the initial episode, the intimal tear, and live for hours or

660

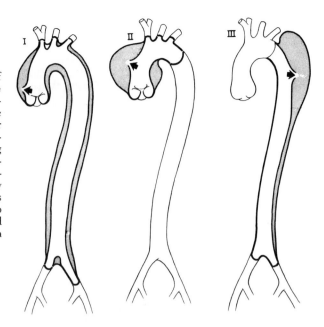

Figure 1. Classification of dissecting aneurysms of the aorta. Type I: Dissection involves ascending aorta and aortic arch and extends distally for varying distances. Type II: Dissection limited to ascending aorta. Type III: Dissection originates at or distal to left subclavian artery, extends distally for varying distances, and does not involve aorta proximal to left subclavian artery. (Modified from DeBakey ME, et al: Ann Surg *142*:586, 1955.)

days. The point is that there is time with most patients — over 90 per cent — to make a definitive diagnosis and then initiate the therapy most appropriate for that particular patient. The proper perspective for determining the treatment of a patient with an acute dissecting aneurysm of the aorta is gained from (1) knowledge of the pathogenesis of the dissecting process; (2) examination of the natural history of a series of untreated patients with acute dissecting aneurysm of the aorta; and (3) critical analysis of the treatment modalities available.

Pathogenesis of Acute Dissecting Aneurysms of the Aorta[2]

The aortas of most patients in whom a dissecting aneurysm develops show some type of medial degeneration (Fig. 2A), most commonly described as cystic medial necrosis. Atherosclerosis and syphilis are not significant factors in the etiology of acute aortic dissection. The intimal tear, which is the acute initiating factor in dissecting aneuryms of the aorta, probably is the result of a number of forces acting upon the ascending aorta and the first portion of the descending thoracic aorta.

The heart, which averages over 37 million beats per year, is suspended like the pendulum of a clock by the great vessels of the neck and moves predominantly from side to side. This motion involves primarily the ascending aorta and the first portion of the descending thoracic aorta. As a result of the continuous motion in the first portion of the aorta, the underling degeneration in the media of the aortic wall, plus the force of the blood ejected from the left ventricle, intimal tears occur most commonly in the ascending aorta in

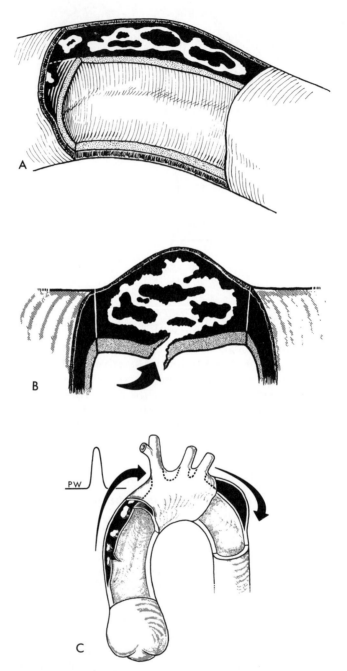

Figure 2.   Diagram of pathogenesis of dissecting aneurysms. (A) Medial degeneration in aortic wall sets the stage. (B) Combined forces acting on aortic wall produce intimal tear permitting entry of aortic bloodstream into weakened media. (C) Resulting dissecting hematoma is propagated in both directions by pulse wave produced by each myocardial contraction.

approximately two thirds of the cases. The remaining one third of the cases occur in the descending thoracic aorta, just distal to the left subclavian artery.

As the intimal tear develops (Fig. 2B), blood at systemic arterial pressure levels is immediately directed into the underlying, degenerated, medial layer, producing an acute dissecting hematoma. The dissecting hematoma, or dissecting aneurysm, is then propagated for varying distances in the wall of the aorta (Fig. 2C). The rapidity and extent of the dissection is directly related to the steepness of the pulse wave, or dp/dt max, and the extent of the medial degeneration in the aortic wall.

The forces that propagate the dissecting hematoma include blood viscosity, pressure, velocity (shearing forces), turbulence, and most important, steepness of the pulse wave, or dp/dt max. From the evidence available, the steepness of the pulse wave appears to be the most important of the forces propagating the dissecting hematoma. If this is so, the forces that cause the dissection to progress and the forces that cause the aorta to rupture must be initiated by the heart.

The major force responsible for continuation of the dissecting hematoma derives from the pulsatile nature of blood flow in large arteries. The reasoning is as follows: (1) The aorta is markedly resistant to static pressure increases. (2) Static pressure provides no pressure gradients as driving forces to induce shear stresses or other stresses on aortic tissue. (3) Experimental models, e.g., tygon-tubing aortas with rubber cement intimas, dissect only when the flow is pulsatile and not when the flow is non-pulsatile. Experiments with dog aortas confirm the relationship of pulsatile flow to dissection. (4) Protection from aortic rupture in turkeys with dissecting aneurysms can be accomplished with reserpine or with propranolol at a dosage level that does not affect the mean aortic pressure but does alter the quality of blood flow.

Another analysis of the forces that cause the progress of the dissection to continue in both a forward and retrograde direction involves continuous pressure differentials (provided by the pulsatile nature of blood flow throughout the aorta). Womersly[3] considers as a forward driving force the pressure differential along the longitudinal axis z $\frac{(dp)}{dz}$. From Figure 3A, if we assume that "z" is finite and represents the effective distance along which dissection would occur if force were applied (i.e., z equals the length of the torn intima and media), then the shape of the pressure pulse would determine the value $\Delta P = P_1 - P_2$. In Figure 3A, the pressure profile at any time is steep; and ΔP, if "z" is finite and constant, is greater than in Figure 3B, in which the shape of the pressure profile is flatter. In other words, if one could flatten the pressure curve, the driving force ΔP would be less over the effective length z. Conversely, if the pressure curve is steep (Fig. 3A), then the force driving the dissecting hematoma is increased.

From this analysis, it is apparent that if it were possible to modify the steepness of the pulse wave generated by each cardiac systole and lower the mean blood pressure, it should be possible to arrest the propagation of the dissecting hematoma. *The propagation of the dissecting hematoma* is the process that leads to death in 90 to 95 per cent of untreated patients, with

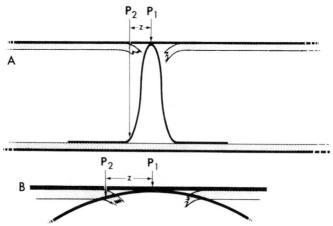

Figure 3.   Steepness of pulse wave as a factor in propagating dissecting hematoma: P_1 and P_2 represent pressures on aortic wall at these two points: z, constant and finite, equals length of torn intima and media. Driving force (ΔP) equals $P_1 - P_2$. If pressure curve is flattened as shown in B, driving force (ΔP) will be less over distance z than in A, where the pressure curve is steep.

rupture into the pericardium, producing lethal pericardial tamponade, which is most common, or rupture into the left pleural cavity, producing exsanguination. Limitation of the dissecting process should permit stabilization of the patient and provide the opportunity to make the appropriate, unhurried treatment decisions. These considerations form the basis for the application of intensive drug therapy in the management of acute dissecting aneurysms of the aorta.

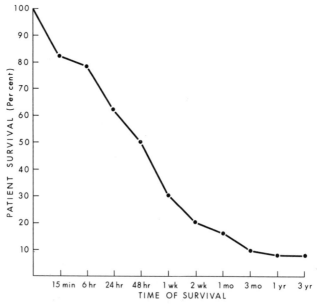

Figure 4.   Length of survival of 963 patients with acute dissecting aneurysms that were not treated.[4]

Natural History of Untreated Patients with Acute Dissecting Aneurysms of the Aorta

In 1972, Anagnostopoulos and associates[4] summarized the survival of 963 patients with acute dissecting aneurysms of the aorta who were not treated (Fig. 4). Although probably no more than five per cent die immediately at the time of the initial tear, the mortality rate may be as high as 20 per cent after six hours, 28 per cent after 24 hours, and 50 per cent within 48 hours; at the end of one week, 70 per cent of patients have died, and by three months, 90 per cent are dead. Most of the 10 per cent of patients who survive three months will survive for one to three years. The important points are: (1) Most patients with acute dissecting aneurysms of the aorta survive the initial insult and live long enough to have their dissecting process arrested or stabilized; and (2) there is time in most patients for an accurate and complete diagnosis.

Treatment Modalities

INTENSIVE DRUG THERAPY

Intensive drug therapy refers to the use of drugs or pharmacologic agents to decrease the cardiac impulse (dp/dt max) and lower the systolic blood pressure as methods of treatment of the patient with an acute dissecting aneurysm. Today, there are pharmacologic agents that can be used to dramatically lower the mean blood pressure with little effect on the heart itself. In addition, there are other agents such as propranolol, with a very marked effect on the heart by producing a negative inotropic effect with little peripheral action. By the use of these agents, singly or in combination, one can achieve the desired effects of decreasing the steepness of the pulse wave and, at the same time, dramatically lowering the static pressure of the blood, thereby significantly modifying those forces that require alteration to stabilize or arrest the progression of the dissecting hematoma. This type of approach to the treatment of the acute dissecting aneurysm has been used now for over 15 years, and the therapeutic effectiveness is well documented from a number of centers, as evidenced by the following data in Table 1.

Table 1 is a collection of the results reported from six centers since 1970. In each center, an attempt was made to use intensive drug therapy as well as surgical therapy in the treatment of acute dissecting aneurysms of the aorta. Results reported from groups using only one method or the other, or in which the treatment was incomplete or not standardized, are not included. The results show conclusively that all patients with acute dissecting aneurysms should be stabilized with intensive drug therapy, accurately diagnosed, and then treated appropriately with drugs alone or with drugs plus definitive surgery for localized, life-threatening complications of the dissecting process.

A recent report of a study, from the University of Miami,[10] in which a prospective protocol was established and adhered to, demonstrates again the

Table 1. *Summary of 240 Patients with Acute Dissecting Aneurysps Treated Medically (131) or Surgically (109)*

Author	Year Reported	ASCENDING AORTA (125 PATIENTS)				DESCENDING AORTA (115 PATIENTS)			
		Medical		*Surgical*		*Medical*		*Surgical*	
		Number	Survivors	Number	Survivors	Number	Survivors	Number	Survivors
Daily[5]	1970	9	3	14	10	5	4	7	5
Attar[6]	1971	5	0	11	5	8	4	10	4
McFarland[7]	1972	6	2	–	–	10	8	–	–
Dalen[8]	1974	9	2	22	17	6	6	8*	2
Strong[9]	1974	15	3	9	5	19	15	12	7
Bolooki[10]	1977	9	9	16	14	30	27	0	0
Total		53	19	72	51	78	64	37	18
Mortality		74%		29%		18%		52%	

*Fourteen patients were initially treated with drugs, but in eight, the progress of dissection was not controlled, which is an indication for surgical intervention. These eight patients are shown as surgically treated, since definitive surgical therapy intervened appropriately.

type of results that are possible with the appropriate application of the two treatment modalities available today. There were 25 patients with acute dissecting aneurysms of Type I. Sixteen of the 25 were stabilized, diagnosed, and operated upon promptly because of significant aortic valve insufficiency; 14 (87 per cent) survived. The remaining nine patients were treated with drugs alone; there were no in-hospital deaths, a 100 per cent survival rate, and no late deaths in a follow-up period of one to four years.

During the same period, 30 patients with Type III aneurysms were treated with intensive drug therapy; there were three in-hospital deaths — a 90 per cent survival rate. During the follow-up period, four patients required surgery, and there were no operative deaths. There were, however, three late deaths, resulting in a long-term survival rate of 80 per cent.

Based on the best available evidence, the most rational form of therapy for patients with acute dissecting aneurysms is as follows: Patients suspected of having acute dissecting aneurysms of the aorta should be admitted to an intensive care unit, where they can be monitored carefully on a minute-to-minute basis. Other cardiovascular catastrophes, such as acute myocardial infarction or cerebrovascular hemorrhage, must be ruled out by appropriate studies and consultations. It is mandatory that these patients be managed and followed on a cardiovascular surgical service. The surgeon must make the decision as to which type of therapy or combination of therapies should be used. All patients should be treated with drugs initially. However, certain patients will need to undergo surgery promptly, and the surgeon is the only one who can make the decision as to when it is appropriate to supplement drug therapy with definitive surgical intervention.

In the intensive care unit: (1) Monitor the electrocardiogram, blood pressure, and pulmonary arterial wedge pressure. Insert a Foley catheter to follow urinary output. (2) Reduce the systolic blood pressure to 100 to 120 mm Hg, if appropriate. Use sodium nitroprusside, 100 μg/ml in IV drip, during the acute phase, and continue as long as necessary. If nitroprusside is used, it is important to pretreat the patient with either intravenous propranolol or Aldomet to block the initial reflex adrenergic stimulation that produces a release of catecholamines. These catecholamines can cause an increase in the contractility of the heart, producing a steeper pulse wave secondary to the increased dp/dt max. If this pretreatment is carried out, nitroprusside is probably the agent of choice acutely. Trimethaphan, 1 to 2 mg/ml, can also be used as an IV drip without pretreatment. (3) Administer Aldomet, 250 to 500 mg IV or IM every four to six hours, with or without propranolol, 1 mg IM every four to six hours. These drugs can be used in combination, and gradually, Aldomet can be switched to an oral dosage of 250 to 500 mg every six hours in combination with propranolol, 20 mg four times daily, with good control of hypertension and cardiac impulse. (4) Guanethidine can also be used, 25 to 50 mg twice daily by mouth. Continue to monitor the electrocardiogram, blood pressure, pulses, and urinary output, and examine the stools for blood. (5) Take daily chest roentgenograms. Check for progressive mediastinal widening and pleural fluid.

Usually the blood pressure response to nitroprusside or trimethaphan is rapid and can be profound if not carefully regulated. Renal complications can be eliminated by careful monitoring of the patient. As a rule, when the blood pressure is lowered, the chest or back pain or both are dramatically relieved. Once the patient's blood pressure and pain are brought under control, indicating arrest of the progress of the dissecting hematoma, and his condition is stabilized, the diagnosis should be confirmed or ruled out by aortography. If the aortogram does not clearly delineate the site of the intimal tear or the origin of dissection, drug therapy should be continued. If the site of the intimal tear is clearly identified, the type of dissecting aneurysm found will determine the type of further treatment.

TYPES I AND II DISSECTING ANEURYSM

In this type of dissecting aneurysm, the intimal tear is in the ascending aorta or in the transverse arch with the ascending aorta involved by the dissecting hematoma. The key is involvement of the ascending aorta by the dissecting hematoma with the threat of retrograde dissection and lethal pericardial tamponade. There is good evidence from a number of centers (Table 1) that this type of aneurysm, acute as well as chronic, can be treated surgically, with a mortality rate of 10 to 30 per cent. Therefore, the patient with acute Type I or Type II aneurysm (Fig. 1) who is otherwise a good surgical risk should be taken to the operating room, and the appropriate surgery should be performed as soon as the patient's condition can be stabilized with drugs and the diagnosis has been confirmed. The improvement of surgical results in those patients with this particularly treacherous lesion is due in large part to the use of drugs to stabilize the patient's condition, arresting the progress of the dissecting hematoma, and taking the patient to surgery on a prompt, elective basis rather than as a surgical emergency.

The recent report from the University of Miami[10] emphasizes that with proper selection and careful management, only patients with Type I aneurysms who have significant aortic valve insufficiency really require surgical intervention. This type of management will not be successful, however, if applied in a nonstandardized, half-hearted manner, which is usually the case in centers reporting poor results.

TYPE III DISSECTING ANEURYSM

In this type of dissecting aneurysm, the intimal tear and dissecting hematoma are distal to the left subclavian artery. This type also includes dissections originating in the transverse arch without involvement of the ascending aorta. All patients with dissecting aneurysms originating in the descending thoracic aorta should be given drug therapy initially. If the patient's condition stabilizes, the patient is not in pain, and there is no evidence of progress of the dissection, drug therapy should be continued into the chronic long-term phase.

Surgery of the Type III aneurysm is indicated *only* when the following are present: (1) Progress of the dissecting process as shown by (a) significant increase in the size of the dissecting hematoma while the patient is receiving maximal intensive drug therapy, (b) appearance of or changing murmurs over the arterial branches of the aorta or the aortic valve area, (c) signs of compromise or occlusion of a major branch of the aorta; deepening coma; stroke; painful, cool extremity; or marked decrease in or cessation of urinary output. (2) Impending rupture of the dissecting hematoma as evidenced by (a) acute saccular aneurysm by angiocardiography, (b) significant increase in size of the aneurysm within hours, (c) blood in the pleural space or pericardium, and (d) lack of ability to control pain with intensive drug therapy. (3) Inability to bring blood pressure and pain under control within four hours with intensive drug therapy.

SUMMARY OF TREATMENT INDICATIONS FOR INTENSIVE DRUG THERAPY

1. Drug therapy is the initial treatment of choice in all acute dissecting aneurysms.
2. In Type III aneurysm, intimal tear distal to the left subclavian artery.
3. When the site of the intimal tear cannot be identified on the aortogram.
4. When the site of origin is in the transverse arch without extension of dissecting hematoma into the ascending aorta.
5. In patients who are poor surgical risks in general.
6. In stable, chronic aneurysms, with onset more than 14 days earlier.
7. In a community hospital that lacks facilities for definitive aortography and experienced cardiovascular surgical team.
8. When there is failure of opacification of the false channel.

SUMMARY OF INDICATIONS FOR DEFINITIVE SURGICAL THERAPY

1. In Types I and II aneurysms, tear in the ascending aorta or the ascending aorta is involved by the dissecting hematoma.
2. When there is aortic valve insufficiency, secondary to dissecting aneurysm.
3. When there is a localized or impending rupture.
4. When there is progress of the dissecting hematoma.
5. When there is compromise or occlusion of a major branch of the aorta.
6. In acute, saccular aneurysm.
7. If there is blood in the pleural space or pericardium or both.
8. Inability to relieve and control pain.
9. Inability to bring blood pressure and cardiac impulse under control within four hours.

A group of physicians using an approach to the treatment of acute dissecting aneurysms as outlined in this presentation should expect an overall hospital survival rate of 85 to 90 per cent. Emergency surgical intervention will be rare.

References

1. Najafi H, Dye WS, Javid H, Hunter JA, Goldin WD, and Julian OC: Acute aortic regurgitation secondary to aortic dissection. Ann Thorac Surg *14*:474, 1972.
2. Wheat MW Jr, and Palmer RF: Dissecting aneurysms of the aorta. Curr Probl Surg, July, 1971. Chicago, Year Book Medical Publishers Inc.
3. Womersly JR: Oscillatory motion of a viscous fluid in a thin-walled elastic tube. 1. The linear approximation for long waves. Philo Mag *46*:199, 1955.
4. Anagnostopoulos CE, Prabhakar MJS, and Kittle CF: Aortic dissections and dissecting aneurysms. Am J Cardiol *30*:263, 1972.
5. Daily PO, Trueblood HW, Stinson EB, Wuerflein RD, and Shumway NE: Management of acute aortic dissections. Ann Thorac Surg *10*:237, 1970.
6. Attar S, Fardin R, Ayella R, and McLaughlin JS: Medical vs. surgical treatment of acute dissecting aneurysms. Arch Surg *103*:568, 1971.
7. McFarland J, Willerson JI, Dinsmore RE, Austen WG, Buckley MJ, Sanders CA, and De Sanctis RW: The medical treatment of dissecting aortic aneurysms. N Engl J Med *286*:115, 1972.
8. Dalen JE, Alpert JS, Cohn LH, Black H, and Collins JJ: Dissection of the thoracic aorta — medical or surgical therapy? Am J Cardiol *34*:803, 1974.
9. Strong WW, Maggio RA, and Stansel HC Jr: Acute aortic dissection — twelve year medical and surgical experience. J Thorac Cardiovasc Surg *68*:815, 1974.
10. Bolooki H, Kaiser GA, and Palmer R: Current status of surgical management of acute aortic dissection: results of a prospective study of 55 patients treated during 1972–1976. *In* Bolooki H: Personal communication.

Comment

Drs. DeBakey and Wheat address an important clinical problem — the appropriate management of acute aortic dissection. Dr. DeBakey, whose pre-eminence in this field needs no elaboration, attempts to stabilize the patient initially with medical therapy but then manages all of the patients who are considered to be operable with surgery.

Dr. Wheat, who has been instrumental in demonstrating that a reduction in the force of myocardial contraction and the level of the arterial blood pressure improves the likelihood of patients with aortic dissection recovering from the initial insult, agrees that the usual so-called Type I and Type II aneurysms (tears that are initiated in and/or are limited to the ascending aorta) are best managed definitively with surgical therapy. The basic conflict appears to arise in the management of Type III dissections, i.e., those in which the intimal tear arises distal to the left subclavian artery, as well as those in patients in whom the site of the tear cannot be identified preoperatively.

There can be little doubt that the institution of combined propranolol and vasodilator therapy has materially improved the outlook of patients with acute dissections of the aorta. Many patients whose conditions in the past would have progressed to early rupture can now be stabilized by this form of management. Experience with intimal tears arising in the ascending aorta leaves little doubt that these should be managed surgically after initial stabilization. There is one exception. If a thoracic surgeon experienced in managing this problem is not immediately available, the patient should be managed medically and then transferred to an institution where a surgeon experienced in this type of problem can operate. Patients with dissections that involve the ascending aorta but in whom the actual site of intimal tear cannot be identified aortographically have a less favorable outlook. It is less preferential to manage these patients surgically; however, it probably still remains the method of choice after initial stabilization.

However, I agree with Dr. Wheat that the Type III dissection initially is best managed medically. The prognosis of patients with Type III dissections managed in this way is quite good during the first weeks and months following acute dissection. However, if the patient continues to have pain, if a spherical aneurysm appears to be developing, if the patient is becoming overly hypotensive, or if there is other evidence suggesting impending rupture, the patient should be taken to the operating room immediately.

Eventually, after many years, late deaths of medically managed Type III survivors equal the number of early surgical deaths, so that five-year survival studies comparing surgical and medical management show little difference. It would thus seem reasonable that patients with Type III dissections initially

671

be managed medically. Later, one can evaluate the desirability of attempting a definitive repair of the dissection electively in light of the patient's overall general condition and other associated problems, such as age, infirmity and other existing medical needs.

ELLIOT RAPAPORT, M.D.

Twenty-eight

Is Surgical Drainage Preferable to Needle Pericardiocentesis in Patients with Pericardial Effusion?

SURGICAL DRAINAGE IS PREFERABLE TO NEEDLE PERICARDIOCENTESIS IN PATIENTS WITH PERICARDIAL EFFUSION

    Charles E. Kossmann, M.D.

NEEDLE PERICARDIOCENTESIS IS PREFERABLE TO SURGICAL DRAINAGE IN PATIENTS WITH PERICARDIAL EFFUSION

    E. William Hancock, M.D.

COMMENT

Surgical Drainage Is Preferable to Needle Pericardiocentesis in Patients with Pericardial Effusion

CHARLES E. KOSSMANN, M.D.
Professor Emeritus of Medicine, Department of Medicine,
University of Tennessee College of Medicine, Memphis,
Tennessee

Earlier articles dealing with a method for definitive diagnosis or treatment of pericardial effusion begin with a statement of the controversial nature of the subject. One reason for controversy was stated by Kilpatrick and Chapman[1] in 1963 to the effect that "the topic in general has been plagued by astonishingly bad scholarship down through the years."

However, there are some more direct and cogent reasons. The pericardial tap is ordinarily the province of the internist or medical cardiologist, and pericardiotomy or pericardiostomy the province of the surgeon. Each sees the problem of pericardial effusion not only in terms of his own background or training but also in part, at least, in terms of the type of pericardial disease that he encounters most often. The internist or medical cardiologist sees mostly chronic serous effusions, usually as a complication of a systemic granulomatous, inflammatory, or connective tissue disease, of cardiac or renal morbidity, or of neoplasia; the surgeon, especially if on the staff of an inner-city hospital, sees mostly acute hemopericardium or pyopericardium, the result of trauma or thoracic wound infection.

The preference for pericardiocentesis over pericardiostomy with biopsy has been cyclical, depending on such variables as the completeness and frequency of reported experiences, the development of new drainage techniques both by needle[2] and by surgical exposure,[3] improvement in the clinical handling of complications of either procedure (antibiotics), new methods of management of the pericardial diseases themselves (antitubercular therapy), and the surfacing of what appear to be new disease entities of the pericardial sac (hemorrhagic effusion in patients on chronic dialysis).

675

Contributing to disagreement is the well-known but often neglected truth that experiences of one era cannot be applied to another without modification. Furthermore, the polemic nature of the subject has been determined by the absence of a long-term, controlled, prospective study by a mixed team of physicians and surgeons. The few surveys comparing the two methods are retrospective and are often dominated by the thinking of a medical or a surgical group. For all of these reasons, controversy continues.

Hazards of Pericardiocentesis

The skill of the operator in any of the procedures must be used as a factor in determining preference. As most surgical training programs are organized, it can be assumed that a partial or complete thoracotomy is, in most instances, expertly done or supervised. On the other hand, performance of a pericardiocentesis, often an emergency, may be done in the middle of the night by an operator with little experience or appreciation of the dangers of the procedure. It is surprising how few physicians know that approaching the pericardium at either sternal edge is more likely to yield right ventricular or right atrial blood than pericardial fluid unless the latter is huge in amount. Nor are many physicians familiar with the cross-sectional diagram of the heart surrounded by a large pericardial effusion published in 1926 by Conner[4] (Fig. 1), a diagram that vividly illustrates the likelihood of cardiac puncture via the parasternal route. Conner's concept of the thoracic distribution of a large pericardial effusion, though never actually proven by pericardiography or other means *in vivo*, is supported in part by cardiac ultrasonographic findings in the disease.[5] With small effusions, "fluid" is seen only posteriorly; with large effusions, it is also seen

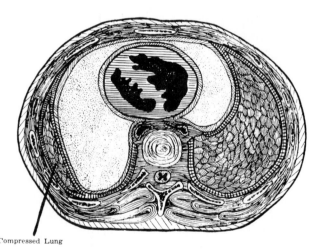

Compressed Lung

Figure 1. Transverse section of the thorax (anterior wall at top) through the cardiac ventricles illustrating L.A. Conner's concept of the locations of a large, chronic pericardial effusion (stippled area) and the compressed left lung. (From Conner LA: On diagnosis of pericardial effusion. Am Heart J *1*:421, 1926.)

anteriorly. In either instance, the width of any echo-free space is quite small, and often not large enough when converted to volumes (cube of the pericardial diameter minus the cube of the epicardial diameter) to account for the large amount of effusion seen on roentgenogram or radioisotopic scan of the intracardiac blood pool or the amount obtained by pericardio-centesis.[5]

The major concern of most cardiologists is the risk of morbidity and mortality that accompanies pericardiocentesis by any method. As with all procedures, the risk must be weighed against the urgency of the diagnostic or therapeutic objectives hoped to be achieved. Clearly, if a pulseless, clammy patient with a barely detectable blood pressure and evidence of impaired filling of the heart arrives in the emergency room with a thoracic gunshot or stab wound or anterior crushing chest trauma, pericardiocentesis for immediate relief of tamponade, and possible catheter drainage[2] to prevent recurrence, will override all other safety considerations while preparations are made to perform a thoracotomy and repair a cardiac perforation or laceration. But even under these circumstances, diagnostic skill is required, as well as speedy work-up, since the injury may not have involved the heart, but rather the pleura and lung. Pericardiocentesis may be disappointing and only add to the gravity of the situation by one of several of its complications, while pleurocentesis will yield a considerable amount of blood.

The accidents that may occur with pericardiocentesis do not seem to have been reported as frequently as they occur. This suspicion was confirmed in 1951 by Kotte and McGuire,[6] who obtained the opinions of 21 cardiologists and surgeons relative to problems experienced with pericardiocentesis. These 21 physicians had seen 18 deaths, none apparently reported, which were variously attributed to laceration of a coronary vessel, laceration of the myocardium with fatal bleeding, or ventricular fibrillation. In nonfatal cases, they also observed mild shock-like symptoms (vasovagal), ventricular tachycardia, aspiration of blood from a heart chamber, and even withdrawal of gastric juice from the stomach. Suppurative pericarditis, constrictive pericarditis, and malignancy of the pericardium appeared to increase the chances of hemorrhage when a needle was introduced into the pericardial sac.

In this survey, the physicians could not decide which needle route was the least dangerous. It appears that the xiphocostal approach of Marfan[7] is preferred over the apical or posterior routes, but minor modifications of this technique are common, especially the cephalad direction of the needle (toward the right shoulder or the left shoulder), which may account for variable adverse results with it.

A recent statement by Fowler[8] on the hazard of mortality with the procedure is that "in recent years we have observed three deaths caused by needle pericardiocentesis, despite the use of great care and supervision of the procedure by experienced personnel." Some deaths have been reported in other series, but these are usually ascribed to some factor other than the pericardial tap itself.[9, 10]

There are other hazards and shortcomings of pericardiocentesis. It has been realized for some time that tapping the pericardium for an acute inflammatory or tuberculous exudate might result in failure to acquire fluid if the gauge of the needle is not large enough for thick pus or if the fluid is eccentrically located. A tap with such exudate might theoretically contaminate adjacent structures, although reports of such a complication are difficult to find. The occurrence of arrhythmias and laceration or perforation of the myocardium and coronary vessels, particularly veins, have been discussed above. In their series of 123 patients who underwent pericardiocentesis reported by Hancock and Krikorian,[10] five developed tamponade from hemopericardium after the procedure, four of these requiring surgical relief. In at least eight others, cardiac puncture occurred without tamponade. In the report of Fredriksen and colleagues,[9] in three out of 21 pericardiocenteses, the needle entered the heart but resulted in no complications. Perforation of the stomach is an unusual complication but presumably can occur, probably more often by the subxiphoid approach than by the other routes. Pneumothorax may complicate the tap, particularly if done through the apical route. In recent years, a soft catheter left in after the pericardiocentesis has been recommended for a period of 24 to 48 hours for drainage.[2] This can result in pericardial infection, although the incidence following this particular intervention is not known. One of the greatest objections to the clinical use of pericardiocentesis is that relatively unqualified personnel often attempt it, although as noted above, even under careful and skilled supervision, accidents do occur.

Risk/Benefit of Pericardiocentesis

For purely diagnostic purposes, the removal of pericardial fluid for examination is usually disappointing, with pathognomonic findings in less than one third of the approximately 90 per cent that yield fluid at all.[10] Furthermore, a follow-up with pericardiostomy and biopsy does not seem to add a great deal.[10] There are various reports on the success of pericardiocentesis in the diagnosis of malignant involvement of the pericardium, but here the skill of another individual, the pathologist, must be evaluated. The use of continuous cardiac monitoring during pericardiocentesis and of an electrode needle for detecting an atrial or ventricular demarcation potential when the heart is touched by the needle, and the more recently suggested echocardiographic guidance of the needle,[11] have undoubtedly increased the safety of the procedure, as has the availability of continuous cardiac monitoring and defibrillatory apparatus. However, if the pericardium is thickened, as with malignancy or with nonspecific fibrous tissue as in certain stages of nonspecific or constrictive pericarditis, the needle may actually touch the pericardium and even lacerate it, causing hemorrhage without causing any displacement of the ST junction or segment[12] simply because there was only tumor tissue or fibrous tissue and no myocardium in the area that the needle lacerated.

Fear of the morbidity and mortality that pericardiocentesis can cause seems entirely justified. However, it is surprising and gratifying that more recently reported series[9, 10, 13] do not include as many cases of sudden death as might be anticipated from the report of Kotte and McGuire[6] in 1951. It may be that this represents improved overall diagnosis of effusion and its cause by non-invasive means and improved methods of handling complications of the tap, rather than any real reduction in the hazards of pericardiocentesis.

The Procedure of Choice

It has been our custom for diagnostic purposes to do an extrapleural pericardiostomy, exploring the pericardium as far as possible through a limited left thoracotomy incision[3] and taking a piece of pericardium for examination before closing the chest. In view of the frequent negative results with a simple examination of the fluid, acquisition of a piece of pericardium will often be more definitive as to whether the disease is inflammatory, granulomatous, neoplastic, or other. One benefit of the surgical approach is that it permits adequate therapeutic management of the disease with little or no increase in risk should the biopsy indicate that this is desirable. For example, if a partial thoracotomy on the left side is done through the fourth or fifth intercostal space without removal of ribs or cartilage and the biopsy on the frozen section reveals active tuberculous involvement or chronic inflammatory involvement, then the surgeon is in a position to extend the incision and increase the exposure and do a radical parietal pericardiectomy anterior to the phrenic nerves, often curing the patient of the disease process. If the patient is desperately ill, the initial part of this procedure can be done under local or intravenous anesthesia or both.

A surgical approach to the pericardium through the subxiphoid area has the disadvantage of restricting extensive exploration, if required. It limits the surgeon to taking a small piece of the pericardium and doing little else. In this regard, if malignancy of the pericardium is suspected, it can be completely absent from the anterior part of the pericardial sac but well-developed in the posterior part, since many pericardial malignancies are secondary to bronchogenic or esophageal neoplasm by direct extension to the posterior pericardium. If malignancy is suspected and the initial biopsy from the front of the pericardium is negative, a wider exploration is indicated. On the other hand, if the disease is quite definite from the clinical examination and the patient is obviously terminal, some relief may be obtained from simple pericardiocentesis with catheter drainage. A judgment on the near-terminal state of the patient with neoplastic disease is often difficult to make, and pericardiectomy may provide a surprisingly long extension of life,[13] especially if the tumor arose originally from a non-vital organ, such as the breast.

Of the drainage procedures available, the creation of a percutaneous pericardial window,[9] which was used in the past, is not recommended, because it will invariably be complicated by infection of the pericardium. On the other hand, with the ordinary thoracotomy on the left, a pleuropericardial fenestration can be created and the pericardium drained through the pleura on that side, if needed.[14] One disadvantage of this procedure is that drainage tubes must be left in the pleural cavity, the preferred route for drainage of nonspecific, inflammatory, suppurative, or tuberculous pericardial effusions. When the last is either acute or chronic, antituberculous therapy must also be instituted in the usual way over the usual period of time.

Conclusion

Pericardiocentesis is a blind and hazardous procedure that carries with it a risk of morbidity and that has a limited diagnostic yield that does not justify its use except under very special circumstances — acute tamponade or relief of chronic tamponade in patients with a terminal pericardial effusion. For the usual chronic effusion that cannot be diagnosed by noninvasive methods, a thoracotomy, either modified or complete, is the safest and most useful method. In addition to providing an adequate biopsy, it makes possible a wide exploration, if necessary, and a definitive therapy such as drainage through the pleura or pericardiectomy if the cause of the effusion on the biopsy establishes the need for either or both.

References

1. Kilpatrick, ZM, and Chapman CB: On pericardiocentesis. Am J Cardiol 16:722, 1965.
2. Schaffer AI: Pericardiocentesis with the aid of a plastic catheter and ECG monitor. Am J Cardiol 4:83, 1959.
3. Weinberg M, Fell EH, and Lynfield J: Diagnostic biopsy of the pericardium and myocardium. Arch Surg 76:825, 1958.
4. Conner LA: On the diagnosis of pericardial effusion. Am Heart J 1:421, 1926.
5. Horovitz MS, Schultz CS, Stinson, EB, Harrison DC, and Popp RL: Sensitivity and specificity of echocardiographic diagnosis of pericardial effusion. Circulation 50:239, 1974.
6. Kotte JH, and McGuire J: Pericardial paracentesis. Mod Concepts Cardiovasc Dis 20:102, 1951.
7. Marfan AB: Ponction du péricarde par l'épigastre. Ann méd chir inf 15:529, 1911.
8. Fowler NO: Pericardial disease. In Hurst JW, Logue RB, Schlant RC, Wenger NK (eds): The Heart, 3rd ed. New York, McGraw-Hill, 1974, p 1396.
9. Fredriksen RT, Cohen LS, and Mullins CB: Pericardial windows or pericardiocentesis for pericardial effusions. Am Heart J 82:158, 1971.
10. Hancock EW, and Krikorian JG: Benefits and risks of pericardiocentesis, 1970–1976. Proceedings of the Association of University Cardiologists, Phoenix, Arizona, 1977.
11. Goldberg BB, and Pollock HM: Ultrasonically guided pericardiocentesis. Am J Cardiol 31:490, 1973.
12. Sobol SM, Thomas HM Jr, and Evans RE: Myocardial laceration not demonstrated by continuous electrocardiographic monitoring occurring during pericardiocentesis. N Engl J Med 292:1222, 1975.
13. Brian S, Brufman G, Klein E, and Hochman A: The management of pericardial effusion in cancer patients. Chest 71:182, 1977.
14. Spodick DH (ed): Pericardial diseases. Cardiovasc Clin 7:1, 1976.

Needle Pericardiocentesis is Preferable to Surgical Drainage in Patients with Pericardial Effusion

E. WILLIAM HANCOCK, M.D.

Division of Cardiology, Stanford University School of
Medicine, Stanford, California

Pericardiocentesis is a widely used and accepted procedure. It is also a controversial procedure, and there is a fairly widespread resistance to its use, particularly among surgeons. Billroth[1] held that "paracentesis of the pericardium is an operation which, in my opinion, approaches very closely (what) some surgeons would term a prostitution of the surgical art and others madness."

There have been cycles of favor and disfavor for pericardiocentesis over the past century.[2] Recently, the procedure has become more popular, but this popularity is not fully reflected in current textbooks. Comprehensive descriptions of the indications, benefits, and risks of pericardiocentesis are difficult to find in the literature.

Echocardiography, generally available only since the late 1960s, greatly increased the accuracy of diagnosis of pericardial effusion, and therefore the safety of pericardiocentesis. Tuberculous and purulent bacterial pericarditis, both of which usually require surgical treatment, have become much less common. Conversely, the advent of chronic hemodialysis and aggressive radiotherapy and chemotherapy for cancer have led to a marked increase in incidence and recognition of uremic, neoplastic, and radiation-induced pericardial effusion, forms that usually do not require surgery.

681

The Uses of Pericardiocentesis

Pericardiocentesis should be used for one or more of the following purposes: (1) examination of the fluid to determine the etiology of the pericardial effusion (etiologic diagnosis); (2) physiologic measurements to determine if cardiac tamponade or another process is responsible for elevation of venous pressure or other embarrassment of cardiac function (physiologic diagnosis); (3) relief of cardiac tamponade (physiologic therapy); or (4) instillation of drugs into the pericardial space (pharmacologic therapy). Advantages and disadvantages of needle aspiration compared with surgical drainage are discussed for each of these uses and for several specific etiologic forms of pericardial disease.

ETIOLOGIC DIAGNOSIS

Examination of pericardial fluid gives specific diagnoses when specific microorganisms are identified, when cytologic study shows neoplastic cells, when the fluid is chylous, or when it is essentially whole blood. The types of pericardial disease represented by these four types of pericardial fluids are also effectively ruled out by negative examinations of the fluid, so that either a positive or negative examination is useful.

Purulent pericarditis, although relatively rare, is the most important diagnosis that is likely to be made initially and primarily from examination of pericardial fluid. This condition is often difficult to diagnose clinically and is often recognized only at postmortem examination. It often develops as a complication in severely ill patients with complex medical or surgical conditions. The index of suspicion is very important in reaching a timely diagnosis in these circumstances, and pericardiocentesis therefore has an advantage over surgery in that it is likely that a lower level of suspicion than is required for surgery would lead to the nonsurgical diagnostic procedure. Except for tuberculous pericarditis, for which a biopsy may be necessary, the diagnosis of bacterial and fungal pericarditis is made as accurately by pericardiocentesis as by surgery.

Neoplastic invasion, diagnosed by positive cytology, is the most frequent specific diagnosis to be made from examination of pericardial fluid. Occasionally, this will be a new diagnosis of neoplasm, but most often, the patient will have had a previous diagnosis of neoplastic disease, and the pericardial fluid cytology indicates whether the pericardial effusion itself is truly neoplastic. Pericardial effusions in patients with previously diagnosed neoplasms are frequently due to radiotherapy or to apparently nonspecific causes, and occasionally result from bleeding or infection secondary to bone marrow suppression. Direct neoplastic invasion is accurately reflected by the pericardial fluid cytology, with less than 10 per cent false positive or false negative results; cytology is particularly accurate in the most frequent conditions, breast and lung carcinoma, while the lymphomas and the rare pericardial mesothelioma are more likely to require biopsy. In our experience over the past six years involving 34 patients with known neoplastic disease but negative pericardial fluid cytology, in whom histologic study of the pericardium was later available, only two showed neoplastic invasion, one with Hodgkin's disease and one with mesothelioma. Thus, in the most common forms of neoplastic pericardial disease, the diagnostic accuracy of pericardiocentesis is equal to that of surgery.

Chylopericardium is readily revealed by pericardiocentesis, and surgical drainage contributes nothing more diagnostically, since the site of leakage from the thoracic duct cannot usually be identified even at thoracotomy.

Hemopericardium is usually of obvious, acute, traumatic origin, and thus is not a diagnostic problem etiologically. Occasionally, pericardiocentesis will reveal unsuspected hemopericardium. This may be from a slowly leaking aneurysm or dissection of the aorta; in such cases, full thoracotomy is promptly required, not simply a surgical drainage procedure. It may also occur as a complication of acute myocardial infarction or anticoagulant therapy, in which case any surgery should be avoided if possible. However, in contrast with hemopericardium, the finding of serosanguineous or even grossly bloody pericardial fluid is not very helpful in diagnosis, since this is not specific for tumor or tuberculosis, but also occurs in idiopathic, viral, uremic, or radiation-induced pericardial effusion. The latter forms of pericarditis give nonspecific findings both in the pericardial fluid and in biopsies of the pericardium.

For etiologic diagnosis, therefore, the advantage of pericardiocentesis over surgical drainage may be summarized as follows: (1) Nearly all the specific diagnoses that can be made from pericardial fluid or tissue can be made from examination of fluid obtained by pericardiocentesis. (2) Since surgical drainage is likely to require a higher index of diagnostic suspicion than pericardiocentesis, its routine use may lead to a damaging delay in making an important diagnosis. The simpler procedure is therefore preferable for initial use in nearly all cases.

PHYSIOLOGIC DIAGNOSIS

Elevated venous pressure and other signs of circulatory embarrassment in patients with pericardial effusion are often due to cardiac tamponade, but this should not be assumed to be the case. Such signs may also be due, entirely or in part, to visceral constrictive pericarditis, fluid overload or congestive heart failure, or superior venal caval obstruction. This type of physiologic differential diagnosis is often neglected, but it is often critically important in patients in whom drainage of pericardial effusion is under consideration.

Pericardial tamponade, due solely to fluid under pressure, is characterized by (1) equilibration of end-diastolic pressures in all of the cardiac chambers and central veins, as in any form of compressive pericardial disease (Fig. 1), and (2) elevation of intrapericardial pressure, nearly to the level of the elevated central venous pressure (Fig. 2). Successful relief of pericardial tamponade is characterized by reduction of intrapericardial pressure to normal (equivalent to intrapleural pressure), with accompanying substantial reduction of central venous pressure to normal or nearly normal levels (Fig. 2).

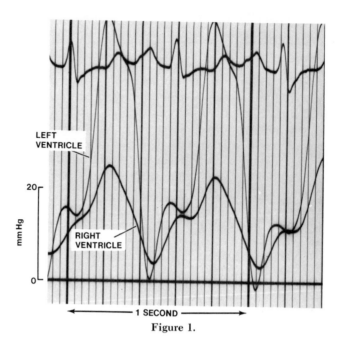

Figure 1.

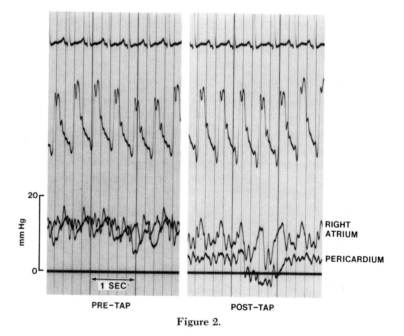

Figure 2.

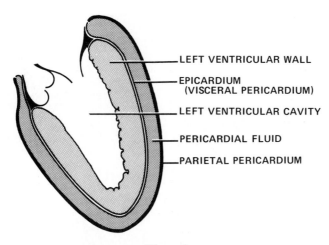

Figure 3.

It is important to recognize that the pericardium has visceral and parietal layers, just like the pleura, with the pericardial space lying between the visceral and parietal layers (Fig. 3). Constrictive pericarditis is usually thought of as the classic form in which the pericardium (parietal) is adherent, obliterating the pericardial space. It is less widely recognized that there is also an effusive-constrictive or seroconstrictive form of the disease in which there is no adherence or only partial adherence between visceral and parietal layers; pericardial effusion is present, and there is constriction of the heart by the epicardium or visceral pericardial layer. The hallmark of this condition, and the only sure method of clinical diagnosis, is the demonstration that the pericardial compressive condition remains after reduction of the intrapericardial fluid pressure to normal (Fig. 4). This condition is particularly seen in

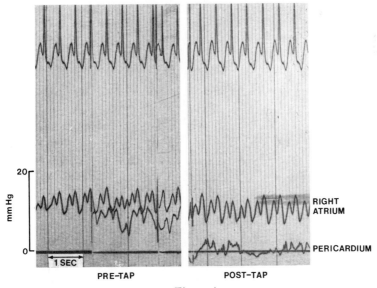

Figure 4.

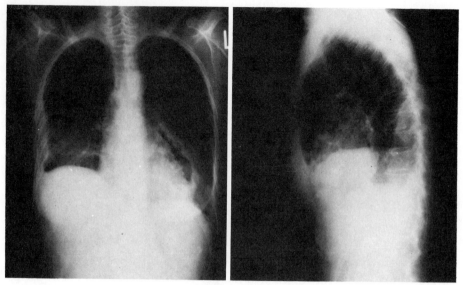

Figure 5.

idiopathic subacute pericarditis and in radiation-induced pericarditis, but it also occurs in rheumatoid, neoplastic, bacterial, and tuberculous disease. It is alleviated only by a total pericardial stripping operation, not by drainage of fluid or resection of parietal pericardium only. The pericardium is likely to be considerably thickened in these cases, sometimes with loculated effusion (Fig. 5).

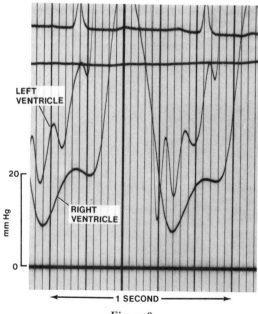

Figure 6.

Fluid overload or congestive heart failure in association with pericardial effusion is seen chiefly in uremic pericarditis, usually in patients on chronic hemodialysis. It also occurs in patients with miscellaneous forms of heart disease in whom incidental pericarditis with effusion is present. The hallmark of this condition is nonequilibration of diastolic pressures in the two sides of the heart (Fig. 6). In much of the literature on uremic pericarditis, describing many patients who have been subjected to pericardiectomy, it is likely that this physiologic differential diagnosis was not made and that in many instances true cardiac tamponade was not present or was a minor factor.

Superior venal caval obstruction in the presence of pericardial effusion occurs usually in patients with neoplastic disease and presents a difficult differential diagnosis unless right atrial pressure measurements are made. In patients with neoplastic disease, this possibility is a good reason for obtaining physiologic studies routinely when venous pressure is elevated. Drainage of a pericardial effusion in a patient whose elevated venous pressure is due to superior venal caval obstruction cannot be helpful and involves considerable risk, particularly when pericardiocentesis is attempted for a small incidental effusion or when general anesthesia is used for a surgical pericardiostomy.

RELIEF OF CARDIAC TAMPONADE

Failure to relieve cardiac tamponade by pericardiocentesis is often used as a reason for preferring surgical drainage. Certainly, there are instances when surgery is required, but not often. In our recent six-year experience, cardiac tamponade was relieved in 30 patients by single (11) or multiple (19) pericardiocenteses alone, while 14 patients required surgery. Clotted blood, organizing or highly viscid fluids, and loculated effusions cannot be aspirated adequately through a needle, but most idiopathic, uremic, and neoplastic effusions can be aspirated very efficiently.

Adequate pericardiocentesis requires a needle of at least 18 gauge, and preferably 16 gauge. The fluid must be aspirated slowly, usually over 20 to 30 minutes, for an effusion of 200 to 500 ml. Slight adjustments of needle position are often needed, and the needle may have to be reintroduced. Insertion of a plastic catheter over the needle, or over a wire guide, is useful for continued drainage and reaspiration over the next 24 to 48 hours, but the initial aspiration should be done through the needle itself, because the catheter is easily kinked and its position is difficult to adjust.

Since cardiac tamponade is a deceptive condition in which shock and death may occur seemingly unexpectedly in patients who did not appear to be in critical condition, two precautions should be emphasized. First, failure to relieve tamponade adequately by pericardiocentesis should be recognized immediately and surgical drainage resorted to promptly if a major degree of tamponade persists. Too often, the result of pericardiocentesis is assessed only subjectively by changes in symptoms or general appearance of the patient or by indirect signs, such as the degree of paradoxical pulse. The most direct and reliable assessment is the central venous pressure, preferably correlated with the intrapericardial pressure. Second, the possibility of rapid reaccumulation of fluid and recurrence of tamponade, even within hours after a successful pericardiocentesis, must also be recognized. Here again, symptoms, general appearance, and the arterial pressure are insufficient for assessment, and the central venous pressure must be monitored. If such conditions are observed, those patients needing surgical drainage can be promptly recognized, and a possible disadvantage of pericardiocentesis, namely, its role in delaying a needed surgical procedure, can be minimized.

INTRAPERICARDIAL INSTILLATION OF DRUGS

Chemotherapeutic agents for neoplasm and adrenal corticosteroids for uremic pericarditis have both been used by instillation into the pericardial space, with reportedly beneficial results. However, this type of therapy is still under investigation, and experience is limited. Pericardiocentesis, rather than surgical pericardiostomy, has usually been employed for this purpose, and it appears to be adequate.

FORMS OF PERICARDIAL DISEASE

Uremic pericarditis has become, in the era of chronic hemodialysis, one of the most frequent forms of pericardial effusion in which consideration of drainage arises. In addition to the classic uremic pericarditis, which is associated with advanced clinical uremia and is relieved by dialysis, there is a newer syndrome of pericarditis with effusion in patients who are maintained on adequate dialysis. This condition is not necessarily relieved by more intensive dialysis, and its etiology and natural history are not yet well understood. Tamponade occurs occasionally, and constriction rarely, but many patients who are suspected of having tamponade actually have fluid overload and left ventricular failure as the principal causes of circulatory embarrassment. Pericardial effusion with raised venous pressure in the patient on dialysis is the condition in which right- and left-heart catheterization combined with pericardiocentesis is most likely to be useful. Pericardiectomy has never been necessary for uremic pericarditis in our experience, and the occasional instance of cardiac tamponade has been adequately managed with pericardiocentesis alone.

Neoplastic pericardial invasion causes a form of tamponade that can usually be relieved by one or more pericardiocenteses alone. Recurrent tamponade appears to be prevented in many instances by radiotherapy, systemic chemotherapy, or by instillation of drugs into the pericardial space. Patients treated in this manner may have prolonged remissions. Avoidance of unnecessary surgery, such as pericardiostomy or pericardiectomy, is especially important in patients with neoplasm, who so often require repeated surgery and complex medical procedures during the course of their chronic illness.

Radiation pericarditis is a frequent cause of pericardial effusion in cancer patients, particularly in medical centers in which many patients with lymphoma or breast carcinoma have been treated with curative rather than palliative intent. Negative cytology in the pericardial fluid of a patient who has had 3000 to 4000 rads of radiation to the heart, particularly with no evident recurrent neoplasm elsewhere in the body, is usually sufficient to establish a presumptive diagnosis of radiation pericarditis. Tamponade in these patients can be relieved by pericardiocentesis, and if so, pericardiectomy is not indicated, despite a small risk of later constriction. Pericardial effusion accompanied by visceral constriction is particularly common in radiation disease, and the measurement of intrapericardial and central venous pressures during pericardiocentesis is especially useful in these patients. If constriction is demonstrated, a total stripping of the visceral pericardium is indicated, not a subxiphoid pericardiostomy or a partial resection of parietal pericardium only.

Purulent pericarditis usually requires surgical drainage because of the viscidity of the fluid and the tendency toward rapid development of constriction. Subxiphoid pericardiostomy is not fully adequate, however, since progression to constriction has occurred despite its use. A left thoracotomy with wide excision of parietal pericardium is the preferred surgical procedure in these cases. Pericardiocentesis is therefore preferred as the initial procedure, for acute relief of tamponade and for confirmation of the diagnosis and of the need for the more extensive surgical procedure.

Tuberculous pericarditis is very likely to require surgery because of its tendency to progress to constriction and also because the diagnosis may require biopsy of the pericardium. Thus, in patients with positive tuberculin skin tests and in circumstances otherwise suggestive of tuberculous pericarditis, a primary surgical approach to pericardial effusion should be considered. Tuberculous pericarditis has become very rare in some areas and population groups in the United States and Western Europe, but in some less developed areas of the world, it is still the most frequent cause of cardiac tamponade and constrictive pericarditis.

Traumatic hemopericardium, most often due to penetrating wounds or to complications of cardiac catheterization, also requires a different approach from most other forms of pericardial disease with effusion. Tamponade is likely to be produced by relatively small volumes of blood, often partially clotted; both of these factors make pericardiocentesis more difficult than in most other cases. Continued bleeding from a myocardial or coronary arterial laceration may require surgery in any case. Furthermore, the tamponade due to trauma is often very severe and acute, and the time occupied in preparing for and carrying out pericardiocentesis could contribute to a fatal delay of surgery. In principle, therefore, surgery is indicated in traumatic hemopericardium, but pericardiocentesis still has a place as a method of temporary relief of tamponade in some cases, and as the only procedure necessary in a few.

CONSIDERATIONS OF RISK

Since the risk of the procedure is one reason for the aversion to pericardiocentesis, it is pertinent to summarize some principles relevant to risk.

First, echocardiography should be used to confirm the presence of fluid.

The greatest risk in pericardiocentesis is when the procedure is attemped in the absence of fluid.

Second, pericardiocentesis should be performed by physicians with appropriate skill and experience, usually those with specialty training in cardiology. It should not be performed by general internists or house staff in general internal medicine unless required in a very acute emergency. Surgical pericardiostomy by an appropriately skilled surgeon may be preferable if a physician skilled in pericardiocentesis is not available.

Third, pericardiocentesis should be performed in a cardiac catheterization laboratory or similar facility in which appropriate hemodynamic instrumentation is available. This enables the effectiveness of the procedure to be documented and, particularly, permits prompt recognition and management of the complication of increased tamponade due to puncture of the heart and induced hemopericardium.

Fourth, the ECG should be monitored from the tip of the needle as a safeguard against inadvertent puncture of the heart.

If these precautions are taken, there should be no deaths attributable to pericardiocentesis, and the principal complication of cardiac puncture and hemopericardium should be reversible.

References

1. Spodick DH: Medical history of the pericardium. The hairy hearts of hoary heroes. Am J Cardiol 26:447, 1970.
2. Kilpatrick AM, and Chapman CB: On pericardiocentesis. Am J Cardiol 16:722, 1965.

Comment

The question of needle pericardiocentesis versus surgical drainage is an important and recurring problem. Both Drs. Hancock and Kossmann agree that acute tamponade with circulatory collapse should be immediately managed with needle pericardiocentesis. The critical question arises when diagnostic aspiration is desirable or only moderate hemodynamic impairment is present such that surgical intervention can be electively arranged.

I think it is clear that the risk of pericardiocentesis in terms of morbidity and mortality is significantly greater than would be anticipated from a reading of the literature. Clinical investigators and clinicians are loath to discuss, let alone report, complications resulting from their diagnostic endeavors. I suspect that most cardiologists have had experiences of serious complications, or even death, in patients in whom they have performed pericardiocentesis. Clearly, needle pericardiocentesis should not be undertaken by those inexperienced in its performance. In the hospital setting, it should generally be performed by an experienced cardiologist or by a cardiovascular surgeon, and not by the internist or medical house staff except in emergency circumstances or under the direct supervision of someone experienced in the technique.

My own reaction to the excellent arguments presented by Drs. Kossmann and Hancock is to suggest that both approaches have their places under certain circumstances. There are situations in which either the risk is sufficiently excessive or the desirability of pericardial biopsy sufficiently great to warrant surgical drainage through an extrapleural pericardiostomy using a limited left thoracotomy incision. Furthermore, in those situations in which recurrent hemopericardium may occur or in which subsequent constriction may develop, a more extensive surgical approach is desirable, namely, stripping of the pericardium rather than the creation of a simple window. It has been our experience, for example, that patients with chronic renal disease undergoing repeated hemodialysis who develop hemopericardium are prone to experience recurrent hemopericardium or eventual constrictive pericarditis. Rather than tap these patients initially, we have usually recommended surgical drainage with pericardiectomy. Our experience in this setting with window drainage has been disappointing, in that frequently these windows seal and recurrences are likely to result.

In conclusion, providing one adheres to the precautions and restraints suggested by Dr. Hancock, needle pericardiocentesis seems a reasonable approach in experienced hands when a diagnostic fluid tap is required and significant amounts of pericardial fluid are present. However, surgical drainage with associated pericardial biopsy is a useful approach that has not been carried out as often as it probably should be. Certainly, if needle pericardio-

691

centesis fails, if a serious question exists as to altered cardiothoracic anatomy, if the patient has had cardiac surgery and is likely to have adhesions, if recurrences are anticipated, if loculations are likely, or if the patient is anticoagulated or has a coagulation disorder, I would favor open biopsy and drainage.

ELLIOT RAPAPORT, M.D.

Twenty-nine

Is Palliative Surgery Preferable to Corrective Surgery in Newborns and Infants with Congenital Heart Disease and Decreased Pulmonary Blood Flow?

ON THE QUESTION OF EARLY REPAIR OF CONGENITAL
HEART DISEASE
> *Dwight C. McGoon, M.D.*

CORRECTIVE VERSUS PALLIATIVE SURGERY IN
INFANTS
> *Paul Ebert, M.D.*

COMMENT

On the Question of Early Repair of Congenital Heart Disease

DWIGHT C. McGOON, M.D.

Stuart W. Harrington Professor of Surgery, Mayo
Medical School, Rochester, Minnesota

Before beginning a specific discussion of this topic, three axiomatic principles applicable to all areas of medicine should be recalled:

First, the ultimate test of the appropriateness of any method of managing a given disease is the improvement in life expectancy and in the quality of life that it provides. This implies, therefore, the necessity of long-term follow-up, not only to establish the natural history of the condition unaltered by specific therapy, but also to provide comparisons, especially between patients managed in various specific ways. Because the whole subject of surgical treatment of the infant with CHD hardly exceeds a decade and a half, even the longest periods of follow-up are deficient in giving ultimate answers.*

Second, in comparing results of different methods of managing infants with CHD, care must be taken to determine if the comparisons are made between comparable groups. For example, instances abound in the current literature of comparisons between results of palliative operations performed some 10 or 20 years ago and results of definitive repair during the last several years. The advances in medical, surgical, and postoperative care between these two periods are disregarded.

Third, when a given method of managing a medical problem appears to have given good or highly satisfactory results thus far, considerable caution and conservatism should be exercised in replacing the "good old" method with a new and untested method of management. This is not to say that progress cannot or should not be attempted, but rather that new methods

---

*"Early" correction and "infancy" are used in this dissertation to refer to approximately the first two years of life. Specific identification will be made of subsets within this age group where indicated.

695

should be studied and tested thoroughly on a limited and local scale before well-studied and tested older methods are prematurely abandoned by the entire medical community.

Safest Age for Correction of CHD

The question is often asked, "What is the safest age for elective operations to correct CHD?" The best tests to answer such a question would be operations of great complexity and high risk, because a factor affecting mortality is more discernible in a less safe operation than in one of little risk. During the early evolution of a given operative procedure, the risk tends to be much higher than it is later. Thus, at the Mayo Clinic, we found that only partial relief of pulmonary stenosis (PS) (ratio of right ventricular to left ventricular systolic pressure of > 0.6 after repair) greatly increased the operative risk in the early experience with repair of tetralogy of Fallot as compared to our later experience when the overall risk became less.[1] Also, with reference to age as a risk factor, we found that in our earlier experience with tetralogy of Fallot, the risk of repair in infancy or early childhood was much higher than the risk of repair in children more than four years of age.[2] Furthermore, in our reports[3] on patients operated on for truncus arteriosus, the risk of repair in those less than four years of age was 2.2 times greater than that of patients between five and 12 years of age. For patients with transposition of the great arteries (TGA) with ventricular septal defect (VSD) and PS, the Rastelli operation had a mortality rate of 76 per cent in children less than four years old but of only six per cent in children five to 12 years of age. Although selection of cases may be somewhat different between these age groups, these and other experiences led to the strong impression that the most favorable age for elective cardiac operations with respect to operative risk is approximately between four and 10 or 12 years.

Categories of Patients for Choice of Management

In the practical clinical setting, there seem to be only three basic situations with respect to operative intervention for management of congenital heart disease. These are (1) operative intervention required in infancy with only direct repair available, (2) operation required in infancy with a choice between correction and early palliation with correction later, and (3) operation not required in infancy.

DIRECT SURGICAL REPAIR REQUIRED IN INFANCY

When cardiac disability due to CHD is significantly life-threatening during infancy, surgical help is required. In some cases, the only type of operative intervention available involves direct repair of the basic pathologic condition; that is, there is no applicable indirect palliative technique. Examples of this situation would be as follows: congenital aortic stenosis with cardiac failure in infancy (or any isolated valvular deformity), patent ductus arteriosus, or the rare instances when cardiac failure results from atrial septal defect in infancy, partial atrioventricular (AV) canal, or total anomalous pulmonary venous connection.

DIRECT SURGICAL REPAIR OR EARLY PALLIATION AND LATER CORRECTION REQUIRED IN INFANCY

A choice can be made between an indirect palliative approach or direct repair, the former usually involving an earlier first-stage palliation followed later by a reparative second operation. Infants exemplifying this group would be those in cardiac failure due to VSD, truncus arteriosus, or single ventricle, or those having severe cyanosis resulting from pulmonary stenosis associated with VSD (tetralogy of Fallot), with VSD and TGA, or with a single ventricle.

OPERATIVE INTERVENTION NOT REQUIRED IN INFANCY

Palliation is unnecessary in patients of this category, but rather, direct repair is elective, and a choice can be made between direct repair in infancy or at a later age. This category would include patients with any type of correctable CHD whose lives are not threatened during infancy by congestive heart failure, intense cyanosis, or pulmonary vascular obstructive disease.

Choice of Management

DIRECT REPAIR REQUIRED

Since, by definition, operative intervention in this group is indicated, and since only reparative operation is available, there is no choice in the management to be advised.

PALLIATION OR CORRECTIVE OPERATION

Currently, patients most deserving of our attention with respect to repair of CHD are those in whom operative intervention is indicated at an early age but in whom a choice must be made between a palliative and a corrective (reparative) operation. These patients have a requirement for surgical help on the basis of two separate hemodynamic presentations: (1) excessive pulmonary blood flow causing either overwork of the left ventricle and congestive heart failure or pulmonary vascular changes; and (2) decreased pulmonary blood flow with resultant intense cyanosis. It is appropriate that these categories be distinguished further as follows:

Excessive pulmonary blood flow. There are two possibilities for operative management of infants in this subgroup: either banding of the pulmonary artery or arteries (a palliative procedure) or closure of the communication between the pulmonary and systemic circulations (a reparative procedure). In keeping with the principles stated initially, the choice depends on which method will provide the greater improvement in life expectancy and the better quality of life. This decision, and others discussed herein, should be based on the *local conditions and circumstances in which the infant is being managed*, since what may be best for one group or institution may not pertain in another setting. In general, banding of the pulmonary artery (1) lacks specific guidelines as to the optimal degree of banding and is therefore an imprecise procedure; (2) results in significant operative mortality, late mortality, and increased complexity of later definitive repair; and (3) creates fibrotic changes in the pulmonary artery.

The management of specific cardiac defects requires individual discussions.

VSD. For a decade, and well before the ascendancy of profound hypothermia and circulatory arrest as a technique for operation on infants, a low operative mortality rate for correction of VSD in infancy was achieved (10 per cent from 1965 through 1969[4]), which seems clearly better than the sum of 10 to 45 per cent risk of banding and seven to 29 per cent risk of later definitive repair reported in several experiences.[5-9] It is believed that open-heart definitive repair is well tolerated in infants with VSD, because there is an immediate and notable reversal to normal of the excessive cardiac work load due to left-to-right shunting at the ventricular level. *The heart is relieved immediately*, with *ample reserve work capacity* to cope with the stress of the operative intervention itself. I have not banded a pulmonary artery in correction of VSD in the past 12 years.

Complete AV canal. If cardiac failure in infancy is primarily the result of mitral regurgitation in this condition, there is no alternative to direct repair, since banding of the pulmonary artery could not relieve mitral regurgitation or its harmful effects. If failure is primarily due to increased pulmonary blood flow, banding is a legitimate alternative, and prior to the development of techniques allowing low operative risk[10] and the successful application of these techniques even in the infant,[11] it was an attractive approach. Now, however, our practice is to perform corrective operations on all infants having intractable cardiac failure due to complete AV canal.

Single ventricle (without pulmonary stenosis). Correction of single ventricle remains in a developmental stage. Only recently are techniques being demonstrated to be apparently effective in older children, so banding remains preferable to repair in infants requiring surgical intervention for this condition.

Truncus arteriosus. Although correction of truncus arteriosus can now be accomplished at a risk of less than 10 per cent in children over four years of age, only recently has salvage of a significant percentage of infants been reported. At the Mayo Clinic, the truncus has now been repaired in 25 patients who had undergone pulmonary arterial banding in infancy.[12] Of the 17 such operations performed since the adoption of the Dacron conduit bearing a porcine valve, only one has resulted in death (six per cent). However, the initial banding of the pulmonary artery for management of truncus arteriosus is associated with a very high risk. Thus, a clear choice between early banding or early correction cannot be stated dogmatically, but it is anticipated that greater potential for improved results by the corrective approach will gradually become evident.

Decreased pulmonary blood flow. It is extremely important, in my view, that consideration of early repair in infants with this condition be sharply distinguished from such consideration in the above group with increased cardiac, and particularly systemic ventricular, work load. Indeed, in conditions characterized by decreased pulmonary blood flow, some degree of underdevelopment of the systemic ventricle is often present as a result of chronically decreased work performed by the systemic ventricle, which results from the decreased pulmonary venous return and hence decreased systemic ventricular end-diastolic volume. Complete correction in such patients does not reduce systemic ventricular work demand, but actually increases it, inherently as well as by virtue of the demands of operative stress.

Tetralogy of Fallot. For tetralogy of Fallot, in particular, uncertainty persists as to the proper choice between palliation and repair in infancy. A separate listing seems appropriate of the pros and cons of early repair as understood by the author at the time of this writing in January, 1977.

PROS

(1) The well-recognized inherent desirability of a single operation over staged procedures. Care must be taken against overemphasizing this feature, however, since it is the total days in intensive care or with intubation as well as the total risk that are the determinants of financial and emotional trauma, and not simply one versus two operations.

(2) The avoidance of risks indigenous to the child with tetralogy of Fallot, such as brain abscess or bacterial endocarditis. Our review[2] showed a 16 per cent mortality rate from diagnosis until four years of age for patients having tetralogy that was not considered sufficiently severe to require early surgical intervention.

(3) The evasion of "mutilation" of a shunt procedure. All shunts, from Blalock-Taussig or Potts through Waterston-Cooley, cause some permanent deformity, in increasing order as listed. However, the recent technique of interposing a graft of expanded Teflon between the aorta and the pulmonary artery may prove to minimize this factor.

(4) The avoidance of irreversible changes in the right ventricular myocardium that might result from a more extended period of right ventricular hypertension.

CONS

(1) The possibility of increased operative risk (as compared to the total risk of early shunt and later repair). Recent reports[13-15] of strikingly low operative risk for repair of tetralogy of Fallot in infancy obviously reduce the weight of this consideration. However, there has not been adequate time for less favorable experiences to surface, and the true risk for non-selected patients may prove to be at least 20 per cent, which is above our

personal experience of five per cent recent risk for a shunt procedure,[2] four per cent risk between shunt and four years of age,[2] and two per cent risk for complete repair after four years of age (total, 11 per cent risk).

(2) The threat of late recurrence of pulmonary stenosis after early repair. It is well known that a given stenosis may be insignificant in infancy, but *unless the stenotic segment enlarges* concomitantly with general growth, stenosis of relatively increasing severity will result. The consistent use of patch reconstruction of the right ventricular outflow tract, as practiced by Castaneda,[16] may minimize this concern, but, in any case, a follow-up of 10 or more years is required before this concern can be clarified. Indeed, since most surgeons employ outflow tract reconstruction in no more than 50 per cent of older patients, a need for consistent utilization of this step in the operation on the infant would in itself constitute a point against early correction.

(3) Less adequate intracardiac exposure in the infant than in the older child. *Relatively* larger ventriculotomies are required. Less precise repair of septal defects and increased incidence of heart block may result.

This comparison of pros and cons for early repair of tetralogy of Fallot fails to provide a clear decision. It is my judgment that correction of tetralogy in infancy has enough merit to warrant its evaluation in clinical trial, but that its use should be tested continuously in a limited experience by a few expert surgeons who are well informed in the surgical repair of tetralogy and in the demanding requirements of care of the infant after cardiac operations. It should not be advocated for general adoption until five or preferably 10 years of follow-up are available.

TGA, VSD, and PS. The profound difference in risk of the Rastelli operation in children under four years of age as compared to children over four years of age[3] leaves no question in my mind as to the preferability of an early shunt operation and later correction for this condition. Such patients are most gratifyingly palliated at low risk with a Blalock-Taussig shunt. Furthermore, such a policy minimizes the problem of an undersized conduit from the right ventricle to the pulmonary artery.

Complex defects and PS. Palliation is preferred for the infant with complex defects, such as single ventricle, double-outlet right ventricle, and corrected transposition with pulmonary stenosis, for reasons that are obvious from the preceding discussion.

Early Correction vs. Later Correction

Consideration must be given to early correction as an alternative for patients with any form of correctable CHD, even those in whom the indication for operation is not related to an urgent life-threatening condition. Two definable situations exist when such a choice is appropriate:

(1) *Conditions with poor immediate prognosis.* There are certain conditions, such as total anomalous pulmonary venous connection or severe aortic stenosis, in which the immediate prognosis is so poor that early surgical correction is required, regardless of the response to medical manage-

ment. For patients with such conditions, the risk of relapse and sudden death outweighs any advantage of prolonged delay of operation.

(2) *Severe pulmonary hypertension.* The studies of late results of repair of VSD before and after the age of two years by DuShane and Kirklin[17] clearly show a preventive effect of early correction with respect to pulmonary vascular obstructive disease. For infants with septal defects resulting in increased pulmonary blood flow and pulmonary hypertension of greater than 75 per cent of systemic pressure but not causing intractable heart failure, we perform correction electively between the ages of 18 and 24 months. An exception presently would be the child with a single ventricle, in whom successful correction at such an early age has not been demonstrated.

Comment

For the most part, this discussion had distinguished corrective operation for CHD in children before and after the age of two years. Consideration relative to "thriving" or normal development of the child has been omitted. Evidence exists that repair of CHD during childhood results in the tendency to regain losses in height and weight, and evidence is lacking that postponement of repair beyond two years of life, or even a bit longer, causes continuing physical or mental retardation. Evidence is also incomplete to assure that early correction, especially if it involves circulatory arrest, is free of permanent adverse effects, especially on the central nervous system.

Finally, with respect to the preferred type of shunt to be employed, even in infancy, my preference remains a Blalock-Taussig shunt on the side opposite the aortic arch, performed as Blalock described,[18] rather than a Potts anastomosis, which may later enlarge, or the Waterston-Cooley anastomosis, which also can become too large and can deform the right pulmonary artery. The use of grafts of expanded Teflon to establish the shunt is an attractive innovation that warrants further trial.

Summary

A trend has existed, and should continue, to apply corrective operations for congenital heart disease early in life. Consideration of the effect of this trend on life expectancy and quality of life confirms the advisability of repair during infancy for most conditions resulting in large increases in pulmonary blood flow, but leaves inconclusive the preferability of early repair of conditions accompanied by reduced pulmonary blood flow as opposed to initial palliation, when required, and later repair.

References

1. Hawe A, Rastelli GC, Ritter DG, et al: Management of the right ventricular outflow tract in severe tetralogy of Fallot. J Thorac Cardiovasc Surg 60:131, 1970.
2. Puga FJ, DuShane JW, and McGoon DC: Treatment of tetralogy of Fallot in children less than 4 years of age. J Thorac Cardiovasc Surg 64:247, 1972.
3. McGoon DC, Wallace RB, and Danielson GK: The Rastelli operation: its indications and results. J Thorac Cardiovasc Surg 65:65, 1973.
4. Ching E, DuShane JW, McGoon DC, et al: Total correction of ventricular septal defect in infancy using extracorporeal circulation: surgical considerations and results of operation. Ann Thorac Surg 12:1, 1971.
5. Bonham-Carter RE: Risks and prognosis in banding and debanding for ventricular septal defect. *In* Kidd BSL, and Keith JD (eds): *The Natural History and Progress in Treatment of Congenital Heart Defects.* Springfield, Illinois, Charles C Thomas, Publisher, 1971, pp 24–25.
6. Hallman GL, Cooley DA, and Bloodwell RC: Two-stage surgical treatment of ventricular septal defect: results of pulmonary artery banding in infants and subsequent open-heart repair. J Thorac Cardiovasc Surg 52:476, 1966.
7. Horsley BL, Zuberbuhler JR, and Bahnson HT: Factors influencing survival after banding of the pulmonary artery. Arch Surg 101:776, 1970.
8. Stark J, Tynan M, Aberdeen E, et al: Repair of intracardiac defects after previous constriction (banding) of the pulmonary artery. Surgery 67:536, 1970.
9. Hunt CE, Formanek G, Levine MA, et al: Banding of the pulmonary artery: results in 111 children. Circulation 43:395, 1971.
10. Rastelli GC, Ongley PA, Kirklin JW, et al.: Surgical repair of the complete form of persistent common atrioventricular canal. J Thorac Cardiovasc Surg 55:299, 1968.
11. McGoon DC, McMullan MH, Mair DD, et al: Correction of complete atrioventricular canal in infants. Mayo Clin Proc 48:769, 1973.
12. Parker RK, McGoon DC, Danielson GK, Wallace RB, and Mair DD: Repair of truncus arteriosus in patients with prior banding of the pulmonary artery. Surgery 78:761, 1975.
13. Barratt-Boyes BG: Primary definitive intracardiac operations in infants: tetralogy of Fallot. *In* Kirklin JW (ed): *Advances in Cardiovascular Surgery.* New York, Grune and Stratton, 1973, pp 155–169.
14. Starr A, Bonchek LI, and Sunderland CO: Total correction of tetralogy of Fallot in infancy. J Thorac Cardiovasc Surg 65:45, 1973.
15. Shirotani H, Ando F, Fukumasu H, et al: Surgical techniques in infancy: hypothermia, bypass and postoperative care. Med J Aust 2(Suppl):29, 1972.
16. Castaneda AR: Personal communication.
17. DuShane JW, and Kirklin JW: Late results of repair of ventricular septal defect in pulmonary vascular disease. *In* Kirklin JW (ed): *Advances in Cardiovascular Surgery.* New York, Grune and Stratton, 1973, pp 9–16.
18. Blalock A: The technique of creation of an artificial ductus arteriosus in the treatment of pulmonic stenosis. J Thorac Surg 16:244, 1947.

Corrective Versus Palliative Surgery in Infants

PAUL EBERT, M.D.

Professor and Chairman, Department of Surgery,
University of California Medical Center, San Francisco,
California

The question of whether to perform corrective surgery or palliative operative procedures for infants with congenital cardiac defects remains controversial. In general, the more severe the anomaly, the younger the age at which symptoms appear and thus at which the infant presents for some type of therapy. Improvements in cardiopulmonary bypass, the advent of surface hypothermia and total circulatory arrest, and more skills and expertise in postoperative management of fluids, electrolytes, and acid-base problems in small infants have made the success of total correction of congenital defects more plausible in infants. Benefits of early primary correction in terms of infant growth and psycho-social development, decreased parental anxiety, and less medical expenses are obvious. The question is whether the risk is greater at this age and whether the procedure performed can truly be considered corrective.

There are many congenital lesions, such as aortic stenosis, pulmonic stenosis, total anomalous pulmonary venous return, and cor triatriatum, for which there is no good palliative procedure available, and thus, corrective surgery must be accomplished during infancy. The operative success in these critically ill infants has increased enthusiasm to approach other specific lesions with the thought of doing corrective surgery.

Total correction versus palliation really has application for three basic lesions: ventricular septal defect, tetralogy of Fallot, and transposition of the great arteries. In these three lesions, there is an option for either palliative or corrective surgery, with both being realistic and offering immediate therapeutic benefit. In rare conditions such as truncus arteriosus, in which mortality in the first year of life is high and development of pulmonary vascular resistance great, it is obvious that the so-called corrective procedure, although possible to accomplish with a low mortality, is really only palliative, since the prosthetic conduit and heterograft valve must be changed at a later age as the child

703

grows and the size of the conduit placed in infancy becomes too small. The same argument could be made for a Fontan procedure in a child with tricuspid atresia. This "corrective" procedure is the most up-to-date method of isolating the circulation and eliminating a shunt, but if it is performed in childhood, it will undoubtably have to be altered as the child grows, owing to the limitation in size of the graft that can be placed. Similar arguments could be made for valve replacements in children with mitral insufficiency or aortic stenosis in whom total growth is as yet incomplete. The lesion may be "corrected," but subsequent operations will be required, so in many instances these would have to be considered palliative for the time.

Let us consider the three individual lesions: ventricular septal defect, tetralogy of Fallot, and transposition of the great arteries.

The question of surgical therapy for an infant with *ventricular septal defect* usually occurs when a large pulmonary flow, pulmonary pressure equal to systemic pressure, and profound heart failure are the causes of poor growth and failure to thrive. When medical management is unsuccessful, the option of either banding the pulmonary artery or closing the defect arises. Pulmonary artery banding has been successful but has many objectionable features, such as deformity of the pulmonary artery, difficulty in assessing the proper tightness of the band, right ventricular failure after banding, possible pulmonary valve incompetence, and a mortality rate associated with two procedures (banding and later correction). At the time of subsequent correction, these bands must be removed, and this increases the complexity of the subsequent total correction. If the band is left on for too long, right-to-left shunting develops, bronchial collateralization occurs, and all the undesirable effects of a right-to-left shunt are present.

Operative closure of the ventricular septal defect in infancy must be accomplished at an acceptable mortality rate, and in most situations, the mortality rate can be lower than the combined mortality rate of banding plus subsequent closure and debanding. Furthermore, a certain number of children do not survive the period between banding and corrective surgery and, thus, often are not included in series of reported cases simply because they are lost in the period between the two procedures. In infants with severe heart failure and high pulmonary flow, the ventricular septal defect is usually single, often located in the supra crista position, and thus easily accessible for operative closure through the outflow tract of the right ventricle. The actual operative approach, whether it be transventricular or transatrial, is probably of less importance than the fact that the surgeon can close this type of defect at an acceptable risk in infancy.

The majority of infants with *tetralogy of Fallot* become symptomatic at age three to six months and usually present with an acute cyanotic spell. In many instances, this represents thickening of the outflow tract of the right ventricle, with fairly good or normal pulmonary annulus and simple progression of the muscular hypertrophy. In other words, many of these infants are actually ideal candidates for total correction, since the pulmonary annulus is adequate and the majority of the obstruction is in the pulmonary outflow tract (Fig. 1). Thus, infundibular resection and closure of the ventricular septal defect without serious augmentation of the pulmonary annulus may be ac-

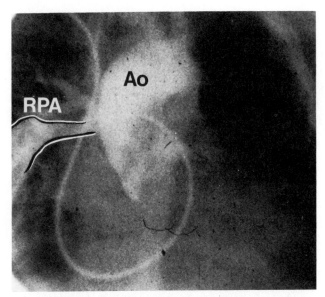

Figure 1. Aortic injection of a child having had a Waterston anastomosis performed in the first month of life. All of the flow is directed to the right pulmonary artery and none is seen going to the left pulmonary artery.

complished at this time. Once infundibular hypertrophy occurs and more right-to-left shunting is present, the aorta tends to grow, and the main pulmonary artery remains small. Thus, the same infant may be an ideal operative candidate at six months of age with an equal-sized pulmonary artery and aorta, whereas at two to three years of age, the aorta may be considerably larger than the pulmonary artery owing to the limitations of pulmonary flow.

All palliative procedures have certain complicating features. The Blalock-Taussig operation is more difficult to perform in infants, and the size of the shunt is often less than adequate. Failure of these shunts in infants less than six months of age is high, and repeated operations carry greater risks. In the very ill cyanotic infant, failure of a shunt in the immediate postoperative period may be lethal, since these infants become rapidly acidotic from hypoxia. Most ill cyanotic infants will not tolerate thoracotomy and failure of a shunt, or even an inadequate shunt, in the early postoperative period. If the size of the shunt is inadequate and flow through the shunt is low, continuing polycythemia, which is required by most cyanotic infants, further reduces flow through the shunt. The Waterston operation, although easier to perform, has the tendency to distort the pulmonary artery and increase flow to the right lung, while the left lung flow remains limited (Fig. 2). In many instances, the right pulmonary artery has become deformed or actually diseased at the site of anastomosis, and it may be smaller than the unoperated left pulmonary artery two to three years later (Fig. 3). Other shunting procedures have similar difficulties with deformity of the pulmonary artery. The descending aorta–to–left pulmonary artery shunt (Potts type) has had better bidirectional flow characteristics. This shunt, however, has more tendency to increase with time, and the likelihood of developing pulmonary vascular disease increases.

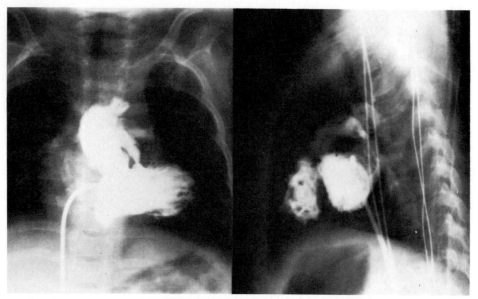

Figure 2. This is a right ventricular angiogram on a two-month-old infant with tetralogy of Fallot. There is a large ascending aorta, but a very narrow pulmonary outflow tract with valvular stenosis but a fair sized pulmonary artery. This infant has progressive cyanosis, most likely due to severe obstruction in the pulmonary outflow tract.

Obviously, elevation of pulmonary resistance is the worst complication of shunt procedures, since if it is not recognized early, definitive corrective surgery will have little chance to reverse the elevated resistance. Taking down of either the Waterston or Potts shunt can be difficult. In most instances, the right pulmonary artery in the Waterston shunt must be patched at the anastomosis site to give adequate diameter. Adhesions around the heart are present in varying degrees after an intrapericardial palliative procedure and increase the operative time for total correction.

Augmentation of the pulmonary outflow tract without closure of the ventricular septal defect makes it difficult to control the size of the pulmonary annulus and the amount of flow unless the pulmonary vessels are of diminutive size. In such instances, this form of palliation can be ideal. It is apparent that not every tetralogy of Fallot is ideal for total correction in infancy. If there is marked deformity of the pulmonary annulus and hypoplastic pulmonary arteries, then some palliative technique would seem preferable. From personal experience, opening the pulmonary annulus and enlarging the outflow tract with a small pericardial patch allows growth to the pulmonary arteries, with potential closure of the VSD in the very near future after that. The undesirable aspects of all shunts, besides the damage and deformity to the pulmonary vessels, are that these infants must remain with large right-to-left shunts and the potential complications of cerebral abscess, thrombosis, and right-to-left emboli exist. There seems little question that taking down the palliative shunt increases the complexity of the second operation.

In our own experience with 26 infants under six months of age with tetralogy of Fallot, there were two deaths, for a mortality rate of eight per

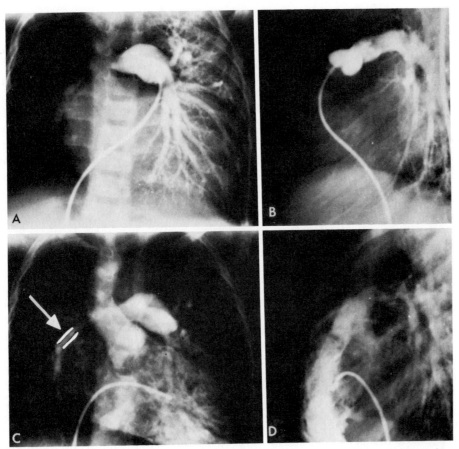

Figure 3. A sequence of angiograms on a child having a Waterston anastomosis in infancy. (A) Injection of the pulmonary artery with complete blocking of the right pulmonary artery at the right side of the anastomosis. The left pulmonary artery fills the lung without problem. (B) A lateral project of the same injection. (C) A comparative injection in the aorta and the right ventricular injection showing the unoperated main and left pulmonary artery have grown reasonably well. The right pulmonary artery distal to the Waterston shunt (arrow) is much smaller than the left, indicating some damage from the time of the initial palliative procedure. (D) The outflow tract and pulmonary annulus look to be of good size and should have been excellent for a primary operative repair.

cent. This is higher than some reported series of elective repair at an older age. These 26 infants, however, were symptomatic and would have required a palliative procedure at this same age. Thus, a combined mortality for two procedures would have to be calculated, as well as a small mortality figure that can relate to the time between the two operative procedures.

It was once thought that a palliative shunt improved the operative results at the time of total correction. The theory was that by increasing pulmonary blood flow, the lung bed was better prepared to accept the total venous return, the left ventricle was larger, and bronchial collaterals were less prominent. Although these are desirable characteristics of tetralogy of Fallot, there seems less evidence that they are necessary to achieve good operative results. The earlier total correction is easier, since extensive bronchial collaterals have not as yet developed, and thus, postoperative pulmonary complications are uncommon.

In *transposition of the great arteries*, palliative balloon septostomy has definitely increased survival. In infants that have had "unsuccessful" balloon septostomy, excluding those with ventricular septal defect and/or associated pulmonary stenosis, there is probably no acceptable palliative procedure available. The patient with straightforward transposition of the great arteries who does not improve with balloon septostomy probably has equal ventricular compliance and, thus, little likelihood of atrial shunting due to the similar filling pressures of each ventricle. In this circumstance, a Blalock-Hanlon or atrial septectomy is unlikely to improve the child, and one must be prepared to proceed with the definitive corrective procedure. With the advent of profound hypothermia and circulatory arrest, performance of an intra-atrial baffle procedure in infancy can be accomplished, and operative mortality is certainly comparable to, if not better than, elective intra-atrial baffle at a later age. The presence of pulmonary stenosis is the most unfavorable addition to the transposition complex. A direct operative approach through the pulmonary artery is usually possible in infants, unless there is atresia of the pulmonary annulus. With pulmonary atresia, a palliative procedure is usually recommended, as a conduit from the heart to the pulmonary artery will eventually be required. In most instances, the subvalvular membrane or fibromuscular rim can be excised with adequate reduction of the left ventricular pressure. In many patients with transposition of the great arteries, the pulmonary stenosis is related to marked ventricular septal hypertrophy, which blocks the exit of blood from the left ventricle. Resection of this muscle is difficult in infancy and the potential for causing left bundle branch or complete heart block exists at any age. Central shunts are difficult to perform in transposed great arteries owing to the usual direct anterior-posterior position of the aorta and pulmonary artery. Pulmonary stenosis, if severe or recurrent, may ultimately require a conduit between the heart and pulmonary artery.

Infants with pulmonary stenosis, intact ventricular septum, and atrial septal defects (ASD) without transposition have marked diminution of pulmonary blood flow. These infants often present in the first few days of life in critical condition. Direct corrective surgery is preferable, and mortality is low. Open repair of the ASD and relief of the valve stenosis can be accomplished with standard cardiopulmonary bypass.

In almost every instance, a corrective procedure offers a more definitive approach to the problem than any form of palliative surgery. The real question is whether the particular center has the skilled personnel to perform corrective surgery in infancy at a comparable mortality to children undergoing repair at one year of age or older. The majority of infants requiring surgery are under six months of age, and thus, the corrective or palliative procedure is usually accomplished within that period. If the child is over six months of age, standard techniques of cardiopulmonary bypass can most often be accomplished, and definitive surgery is more often the procedure of choice. Many can argue that surgical repair is less complete in the infant than in the older child. There is no evidence that this is true, and in most instances, there are fewer pulmonary complications from increased bronchial collateral development in cyanotic infants under six months of age than in older children who have been cyanotic for a longer period of time. Thus, the operative procedure is often technically simpler in the infant than in the older child. If comparable operative mortality figures can be attained in the specific medical center in which primary correction in infancy is performed, then there is certain to be a larger number of surviving patients, since a certain percentage of infants with congenital heart disease succumb between the time of palliative operation and subsequent total correction. With continued improvement in operative techniques, equipment, and postoperative management, it seems likely that cardiac surgery will be performed more often in infants and that the number of palliative procedures performed in children with lesions that are currently correctable is bound to decrease. If this is the case, then the benefits of the early primary correction in terms of infant growth and development and decreased parental anxiety, as well as the reduction in medical expense, are apparent.

Comment

Advances in cardiopulmonary bypass techniques have now made it feasible to attempt corrective procedures in newborns and young infants with congenital heart defects rather than waiting until two years or more have elapsed. Clearly, these skills cannot be applied in all centers, and it would be unwise to recommend definitive operative repair using cardiopulmonary bypass in lieu of traditional palliative procedures in a center that is still inexperienced in their use. As greater experience is gained with bypass techniques in the infant, an increasing tendency toward earlier definitive surgical corrections can be expected.

As stated in Dr. McGoon's excellent commentary, there is little doubt that the role of pulmonary artery banding is very limited today. Many patients who formerly would have had palliative surgery for congenital defects, resulting in increased pulmonary blood flow, should be treated with initial definitive correction at an early age.

The major area of disagreement between Dr. Ebert and Dr. McGoon concerns those patients with decreased pulmonary blood flow, particularly in tetralogy of Fallot, for whom a case can be made for an early shunt operation in cyanotic and distressed infants, with definitive repair at a later date. Dr. McGoon emphasizes the relatively low initial mortality in good centers where shunt operations are performed under these circumstances, with definitive repair postponed until patients reach an older age. On the other hand, Dr. Ebert emphasizes the success of operating on some of these infants at an early age and points out some theoretical considerations relative to the right ventricular outflow tract that suggest that earlier definitive corrective surgery may eliminate complications that can develop at a later age. It seems likely that there will be a tendency toward the use of earlier definitive correction, and Dr. McGoon agrees that more clinical trials of early definitive surgical correction of congenital heart disease in more centers over the next five to 10 years are desirable.

ELLIOT RAPAPORT, M.D.

Thirty

Should the Premature Infant with a Large Patent Ductus Arteriosus Be Managed Surgically?

THE PREMATURE INFANT WITH A LARGE PATENT
DUCTUS ARTERIOSUS SHOULD BE MANAGED
SURGICALLY

  L. Henry Edmunds, Jr., M.D.

THE PREMATURE INFANT WITH A LARGE PATENT
DUCTUS ARTERIOSUS NEED BE MANAGED
SURGICALLY ONLY OCCASIONALLY

  Abraham M. Rudolph, M.D.

COMMENT

The Premature Infant with a Large Patent Ductus Arteriosus Should Be Managed Surgically

L. HENRY EDMUNDS, JR., M.D.

William Maul Measey Professor; Chief, Cardiothoracic
Surgery, Hospital of the University of Pennsylvania,
Philadelphia, Pennsylvania

Patent ductus arteriosus (PDA) is a common lesion that develops in 10 to 20 per cent of all premature infants. The incidence is 30 to 60 per cent in those infants weighing less than 1750 grams and is also high in babies with the idiopathic respiratory distress syndrome (IRDS). Heart failure develops a few days to a few weeks after birth in 35 to 50 per cent of premature infants with PDA. In approximately 40 to 60 per cent of these infants, heart failure can be controlled by medical measures. Although the PDA eventually closes spontaneously in nearly all infants who survive, two to six per cent of all premature babies and four to 18 per cent of those weighing less than 1750 grams are candidates for therapeutic closure of the ductus arteriosus.

Premature infants with uncontrolled heart failure and minimal or no IRDS should have therapeutic closure of the PDA. Other medications are still debated. The debate centers on a possible connection between PDA and other complications of prematurity, particularly IRDS. Some clinicians recommend early therapeutic closure of the PDA in hopes of preventing or aborting IRDS and other complications of prematurity, such as necrotizing enterocolitis. Others recommend closure of the PDA only in the presence of left-to-right shunting and severe or worsening IRDS. Severe lung disease masks symptoms and signs of heart failure, and since IRDS can occur in the absence of PDA, the degree of heart failure may be difficult to assess clinically. The diagnosis of heart failure is facilitated by determining the ratio of left atrial to aortic diameters by echocardiography. At the

715

Table 1. *Premature Infants Who Had Operative Closure of the Ductus Arteriosus*

PATIENTS	IRDS	OPERATIVE RELATED DEATHS	NON-FATAL OPERATIVE COMPLICATIONS	SURVIVORS
318	243	5	5	209

present time, indications for therapeutic closure of the PDA in premature infants are clouded by the variable and unpredictable course of IRDS, by poor understanding of the relationship between PDA and other complications of prematurity, and by the tendency of the ductus to eventually close spontaneously.

Until recently, surgical ligation of the PDA was the only means to achieve therapeutic closure. The procedure is accomplished quickly and safely using a variety of light general anesthetics. Arterial and venous monitoring catheters are necessary. Either a posterolateral or anterolateral approach can be used, and the ductus can be reached transpleurally or extrapleurally. The ductus occasionally may be friable and is usually equal or larger in diameter than the aortic arch. After positive identification, the ductus is singly or doubly ligated with nonabsorbable ligatures. Operative time is usually 15 to 25 minutes. The operation is most safely carried out in the operating room as opposed to the nursery.

During the past decade, 318 premature infants, reported in 19 published articles, have had operative closure of the ductus arteriosus (Table 1). Indications for operation have varied. Birth weights ranged from 550 grams and higher, and gestational age varied between 24 and 35 weeks. The smallest survivor weighed 680 grams at birth and 700 grams at operation. Seventy-six per cent of the 318 infants had IRDS. Sixty-six per cent (209 patients) survived. Only five deaths (1.6 per cent) were related to operation or to complications of operation. One infant died of postoperative pneumothorax, another died of hemorrhage, and a third died after the left pulmonary artery was mistakenly ligated. Two infants died late from left phrenic nerve injury and chylothorax.

Atelectasis, pneumonia, pneumothorax, apneic episodes, and bradycardia were the most common postoperative complications, but they were also the most common preoperative problems. Therefore, a possible causal relationship between operation and the development of these complications cannot be determined. Pneumothorax and/or pneumomediastinum produced by high ventilatory pressures occurred most frequently when a chest tube was omitted. Only five complications among the 318 patients were clearly related to operation. One infant had temporary left vocal cord paralysis, two had hemorrhage, one developed interstitial emphysema, and another had right pleural effusion.

At the present time, two major questions regarding patent ductus arteriosus and premature infants require answers: (1) Should every PDA be therapeutically closed in premature infants in hopes of preventing or reducing some of the major complications of prematurity — IRDS, necrotizing enterocolitis and intracranial hemorrhage? If some PDAs should not be closed, then what *are* the indications for therapeutic closure of PDA in premature infants? (2) How should therapeutic closure of the PDA be accomplished — by operation or by indomethacin?

Indomethacin causes the ductus arteriosus to constrict in utero and to close in most premature human infants. A single dose (0.1 to 0.3 mg/kg) orally or rectally usually causes the ductus to close and remain closed. Repeated or higher doses are required for some infants. In some the drug is not successful. On the surface, indomethacin seems to be a miracle drug for premature infants who have PDA.

However, much more information is needed before indomethacin can be considered a safe drug for premature infants. Indomethacin is a potent, nonsteroid compound with anti-inflammatory, antipyretic, and analgesic properties. The drug inhibits prostaglandin synthesis, uncouples oxidative phosphorylation in some cells, and probably has other actions. The drug has a long half-life and is primarily excreted in the urine. Numerous toxic side effects have been reported, and indomethacin is not recommended for children under 14 years of age. Indomethacin has been associated with sudden death in five children, possibly by masking infection or activating latent infection. The drug alters polymorphonuclear cells and appears to decrease resistance to infection. Indomethacin has produced important neuropsychiatric, neurologic, visual, gastrointestinal, hematologic, and cutaneous side effects. Severe gastrointestinal bleeding, ulcer, seizures, coma, peripheral neuropathy, transverse myelitis, changes in visual acuity, and depression of bone marrow are rare but serious complications of the drug. Indomethacin is 90 per cent bound to plasma albumin and may displace albumin binding of bilirubin in neonates. In some premature infants, large doses of indomethacin (2.5 to 5 mg/kg) cause temporary oliguria, azotemia with elevation of serum creatinine, and reduction of urine sodium. In patients with liver disease and sodium retention, indomethacin depresses renal blood flow. Experience with indomethacin to date indicates that the drug has powerful actions on many different organ systems.

Indomethacin inhibits prostaglandin synthetase and presumably causes the ductus arteriosus to close by inhibiting endogenous production of prostaglandin E_1 and E_2. The prostaglandins are a family of polyenoic fatty acid compounds that are important in cell function and differentiation. Prostaglandins, found throughout the body, influence intracellular cyclic AMP by stimulating its production by adenyl cyclase. Cyclic AMP is essential for cell function, and its concentration appears to determine certain cellular activities or expressions. The prostaglandins and their precursors and intermediates form very complex and vaguely understood hormonal systems that exert powerful effects on every mammalian cell studied thus far. For instance, in cell cultures, prostaglandin E_1 induces morphologic differentiation of mouse neuroblastoma cells. Prostaglandin synthetase, which indomethacin inhibits, is responsible for the synthesis of prostaglandin precursors — the endoperoxidases from arachidonic and certain other unsaturated fatty acids. Indomethacin therefore blocks synthesis of many different normally occurring prostaglandins in addition to prostaglandin E_1 and E_2.

At the present time, not enough is known about the prostaglandins and indomethacin to risk permanent injury to the immature enzyme, cellular, and organ systems of the premature infant. Already proponents of indomethacin preclude its use in patients with hyperbilirubinemia, bleeding, thrombocytopenia, coagulation defects, or reduced renal function. Considering the ubiquity and complexity of the prostaglandins and the diverse effects of indomethacin, it is likely that this list of contraindications is incomplete. Until more is known about the use and possible long-term effects of indomethacin, surgical ligation of the PDA in premature infants is preferable. The operation is safe, as proved by the low morbidity and mortality rates. Indomethacin may eventually prove to be the "miracle drug" for closing the PDA in premature infants. Meanwhile, the surgical scar on the left chest wall seems inconsequential compared with potential drug-induced scars on the premature infant's biochemistry.

The Premature Infant with a Large Patent Ductus Arteriosus Need Be Managed Surgically Only Occasionally

ABRAHAM M. RUDOLPH, M.D.

Professor of Pediatrics, Physiology, and
Obstetrics-Gynecology and Reproductive Sciences; Neider
Professor of Pediatric Cardiology, University of California,
(San Francisco) San Francisco, California

In the normal mature infant, the ductus arteriosus usually closes by constriction within 10 to 15 hours after birth. Permanent closure is accomplished by thrombosis and fibrosis within a few days and is invariably complete by 21 days. It has been known for some time that premature infants frequently have a patent ductus arteriosus for several weeks or even months after birth. However, the high incidence of this condition in premature infants was not fully appreciated until recently. Before the introduction of continuous positive airway pressure in the management of infants with hyaline membrane disease, there was a very high early mortality of premature infants from respiratory failure, so that the presence of a patent ductus arteriosus was not recognized. With the dramatic improvement of the survival rate of premature infants in recent years, patent ductus arteriosus is a common cause of cardiorespiratory distress in the premature infant in the first few weeks after birth. The incidence of patency of the ductus arteriosus and the proportion of these infants who develop cardiopulmonary difficulties related to the ductus arteriosus vary considerably in different institutions.

Premature birth occurs in about 15 per cent of all pregnancies. At the University of California, San Francisco, we have observed an incidence of about 40 to 50 per cent of patent ductus arteriosus in infants with birth weights less than 1500 grams. In most infants with a patent ductus arteriosus,

719

there is no significant cardiorespiratory distress relating to the lesion, since the left-to-right shunt is quite small; in many, however, the ductus arteriosus causes cardiac failure or contributes to the cardiorespiratory distress associated with hyaline membrane disease and requires treatment medically. When medical measures have not been successful, surgery has been required. During the period from 1967 to 1977, 130 premature infants had surgical ligation in our hospital.

If this problem is considered on a worldwide basis, it is apparent that a significant proportion of the population would have to be subjected to surgery for ligation of the ductus arteriosus in the neonatal period. Although the surgery itself is not associated with a high risk, considerable surgical skill is required to operate on these very small infants. Also, the most serious risks are related to postoperative management of respiratory difficulties associated with the thoracotomy, particularly since many of these infants are still recovering from hyaline membrane disease. This requires great skill and advanced technology. It would be preferable, therefore, to manage premature infants with patent ductus arteriosus without resorting to surgery. Recent advances in our understanding of the physiology and pharmacologic responses of the ductus arteriosus have provided us with the means to manage the majority of premature infants with patent ductus arteriosus medically; surgery has been required in a few selected infants. It is necessary to review this information to support my contention that surgical ligation of the ductus arteriosus is indicated in premature infants only rarely.

The Ductus Arteriosus in the Fetus

During fetal life, the ductus arteriosus is widely patent, and it diverts 85 to 90 per cent of the blood ejected by the right ventricle away from the lungs to the descending aorta. It was generally believed that the ductus was held open by the pressure within the lumen and that it was passively maintained in the dilated state. Recently, several studies[1-3] have demonstrated that the ductus arteriosus is probably actively maintained in a relaxed state by the action of prostaglandins. We have demonstrated that both acetylsalicylic acid and indomethacin cause constriction of the ductus arteriosus when administered to fetal lambs in utero. These drugs inhibit synthesis of prostaglandins in body tissues and cause constriction of the ductus either by inhibiting local production of prostaglandins within the ductus arteriosus itself or by preventing its production in other tissues, thus decreasing circulating blood levels of prostaglandins. We have demonstrated that the effect is related to prostaglandin synthetase inhibition and not to a direct effect of the drugs on the ductus arteriosus, since infusion of prostaglandin E_1 overcame the constrictor effect of these drugs. The relaxant effect is produced by the E series, but not by the F series, of prostaglandins infused into the fetus. It is possible, however, that local production of thromboxanes within the wall of the ductus is responsible for the natural dilator effect during fetal life.

Postnatal Closure of the Ductus Arteriosus

The ductus arteriosus begins to constrict soon after birth and is usually functionally closed within 10 to 15 hours in the normal mature infant. Initially, the closure is produced by muscular constriction, but permanent closure occurs by thrombosis and fibrosis and is usually complete within three weeks. It has been known for some time that the ductus arteriosus is very responsive to an increase in the environmental PO_2 to which it is exposed. At the fetal arterial PO_2 of about 20 torr, the ductus is relaxed; but with an increase in PO_2 above 35 torr, it begins to constrict, and the mature ductus usually is markedly constricted at levels above 60 torr. It is not known whether the effect of oxygen is due to a direct influence on the smooth muscle or whether oxygen stimulates the release of a local vasoactive substance. Recently, it has been suggested that oxygen may alter the response of the ductus arteriosus to prostaglandins E and F. Starling and Elliott in Auckland, New Zealand, showed that isolated ductus arteriosus strips constricted with prostaglandin $F_{2-\alpha}$ in a high-oxygen environment but did not respond in low PO_2. Coceani and Olley[4] have noted that the relaxing effect of prostaglandin E on the ductus arteriosus was more prominent at a low PO_2 than at a high PO_2. From this data, an attractive theory has been proposed that when the ductus arteriosus is subject to the low PO_2 in utero, prostaglandin E produces relaxation, but prostaglandin $F_{2-\alpha}$ has no effect. After birth, with the increase in PO_2 associated with pulmonary ventilation, the relaxant effect of prostaglandins is lost, and the constrictor effect of prostaglandin $F_{2-\alpha}$ becomes dominant. However, Dr. Ronald Clyman, working in our laboratories, has not been able to confirm the observations that prostaglandin E_1 is an effective dilator only at low PO_2. Furthermore, studies in newborn infants with congenital cardiac lesions in whom arterial PO_2 is high have shown that prostaglandin E_1 is able to dilate the ductus arteriosus.

Ductus Arteriosus in Premature Infants

It is not known why there is a high incidence of persistent patency of the ductus arteriosus in premature infants. The lack of constriction is not due to inadequate smooth muscle development, since acetylcholine can produce constriction of the ductus in premature animals as well as in premature infants. Several years ago, Dr. Dorothy McMurphy, working in our laboratories, showed that isolated perfused ductus arteriosus preparations derived from fetal lambs demonstrated differences in response to increasing PO_2 in premature ductus specimens as compared with mature ductus specimens. The ductus arteriosus obtained from immature animals required a higher PO_2 to initiate constriction, and considerably higher PO_2 levels to produce significant constriction, than mature ductus. The degree of response of the ductus arteriosus to the increased PO_2 levels was directly proportional to gestational age. These findings suggested that the mechanism responsible for the persistent patency of the ductus arteriosus in premature infants was related to an immaturity of the response to increasing PO_2. Recently, however, Dr. Clyman has shown that the response of the ductus arteriosus to oxygen may be affected by light. The constrictor response of the mature ductus to oxygen is not significantly affected by exposure to light. However, the immature ductus can be constricted by oxygen in the dark, but when exposed to light, it relaxes, even in a high-oxygen environment. This information thus raises a question regarding the concept that lack of adequate constriction of the ductus arteriosus in the premature infant is related to an inadequate response to oxygen.

Clinical Features of Patent Ductus Arteriosus in Premature Infants

Associated with the fall in pulmonary vascular resistance that occurs after birth, a left-to-right shunt develops through the ductus arteriosus. This results in an increase in the volume of blood returning to the left ventricle and, thus, an increase in the output of the ventricle both to maintain an adequate systemic blood flow and to provide blood that recirculates through the lungs. Although patent ductus arteriosus in mature infants does not usually result in cardiorespiratory difficulties within the first four to eight weeks after birth, in premature infants cardiorespiratory difficulties present much earlier.

The manifestations of patent ductus arteriosus in premature infants are often different from those observed in mature babies. Frequently, an infant who has hyaline membrane disease shows temporary improvement of the respiratory distress and then has a progressive increase in systemic arterial PCO_2 and in the end-tidal pressure required to maintain effective ventilation. Often, there is no significant enlargement of the heart, but a murmur is heard at the mid to upper left sternal border. Usually, this murmur is present only during systole, but it may extend into diastole. In the presence of a large ductus arteriosus, cardiac murmurs may be absent. The roentgenologic appearance of the lungs is not helpful in determining whether there is a patent ductus arteriosus with a large left-to-right shunt, as frequently there are severe changes in the lungs associated with hyaline membrane disease. An increase in pulse volume or the development of a bounding or collapsing pulse is helpful in suggesting the presence of a patent ductus arteriosus with a large shunt and, in those infants in whom umbilical arterial pressure is being monitored, an increase in pulse pressure may suggest the development of a left-to-right shunt through the ductus arteriosus.

Recently, a close association between a patent ductus arteriosus and the development of necrotizing enterocolitis in premature infants has been described. Before gross changes occur in the bowel, with the typical radiologic appearance, suggestive signs may be evident. These include abdominal distension, delayed emptying of the stomach, and blood in the stools.

Differentiation between the respiratory distress associated with cardiac failure due to a patent ductus arteriosus and that related to hyaline membrane disease is often very difficult. The presence of a bounding pulse or wide pulse pressure and a cardiac murmur are helpful in confirming the presence of a patent ductus arteriosus but do not provide specific information regarding the magnitude of a left-to-right shunt. Echocardiography has been very useful in assessing the magnitude of a left-to-right shunt in these infants. The increase in venous return to the lungs associated with a left-to-right shunt results in an enlargement of the left atrium. By measuring the size of the left atrium and comparing it with that of the aorta by echocardiography, it is possible to evaluate the magnitude of the left-to-right shunt. Normally, the left atrial-to-aortic diameter ratio is about 0.7 to 0.8, but a large left-to-right shunt results in an increase in the ratio, and when it exceeds 1.2, the shunt is likely to be very large. It should be appreciated that a high left atrial-to-aortic diameter ratio does not specifically make the diagnosis of patent ductus arteriosus, but merely indicates the presence of a large left-to-right shunt. This could be due to a ventricular septal defect, persistent truncus arteriosus communis, or other congenital cardiac lesions that produce large shunts.

Management of Premature Infants with Patent Ductus Arteriosus

It is important to recognize that the ductus arteriosus closes spontaneously within four to eight weeks in the majority of premature infants with persistent patency. It is almost unheard of for the ductus arteriosus to remain open in these infants for more than three months. Thus, unlike in the mature infant, in whom spontaneous closure of the ductus arteriosus beyond the first week or two after birth is unusual, surgical ligation or division of the ductus arteriosus should be avoided in premature infants unless the symptoms are so severe that they cannot be managed medically. Early in the experience in managing premature infants with patent ductus arteriosus, the usual measures applied to mature infants with cardiac failure were instituted. This included administration of digoxin and diuretic agents.

Recently, it has been recognized that there are several ancillary factors that contribute to the development of symptoms in premature infants with patent ductus arteriosus. Hypoglycemia occurs commonly, particularly in infants who have cardiorespiratory distress and hypoxia. Severe hypoglycemia may interfere with myocardial performance and thus contribute to the development of cardiac failure. Similarly, hypocalcemia is a common finding in premature infants, and this, too, may contribute to a decrease in myocardial performance. Blood glucose and calcium levels should be checked repeatedly, and if they are reduced, they should be corrected promptly.

A second important factor contributing to the development of cardiac failure is excessive fluid intake. There had been a tendency in some nurseries to administer fairly large volumes of fluid in an attempt to provide adequate caloric intake and also to avoid the development of hypovolemic shock. It was not unusual for volumes of over 200 ml/kg to be administered each 24 hours. It is now recognized that fluid volumes of greater than 150 ml/kg/24 hrs should be avoided in these premature infants, as fluid overloading often contributes to the development of cardiovascular symptoms, presumably due to the development of pulmonary edema.

Another important aspect of management is to maintain the hematocrit level at about 45 per cent. There is a significant incidence of low hemoglobin and hematocrit levels in premature infants. Frequent sampling of blood for measurement of blood gases and other analyses often contributes to a reduction in hematocrit levels to 30 per cent or less. Because oxygen delivery to the tissues is dependent on the hemoglobin level as well as systemic blood flow, it is important to maintain the hematocrit at a level of about 45 per cent to aid in oxygen supply to the tissues, since systemic blood flow may be considerably reduced owing to the cardiac failure. The maintenance of hematocrit levels at about 45 per cent may have a direct effect in stimulating closure of the ductus arteriosus; it has frequently been noted that within the period of 24 to 48 hours after increasing the hematocrit level, the ductus appears to close spontaneously. Since we have adopted these measures, the incidence of severe cardiac failure in premature infants with persistent patent ductus arteriosus has been reduced considerably.

If severe cardiorespiratory distress persists, treatment with digitalis preparations and diuretic agents should be instituted. The digitalis preparation most commonly used is digoxin, but it should be administered with caution to premature infants, because there is a high incidence of toxicity associated with this drug. Our impression is that digoxin is not as effective in treating cardiac failure in premature infants as it is in mature infants. Also, there is a significant risk of toxicity, particularly the development of a prolongation of atrioventricular conduction, progressing to complete heart block. In view of the high incidence of toxicity, a lower dose of digoxin is recommended for premature infants than is usually used in mature infants. I suggest using 30 μg/kg as a digitalizing dosage to be administered in the first 24 hours in three divided doses, followed by a maintenance dosage of 10 μg/kg/24 hrs given in two equal doses. It should also be appreciated that plasma digoxin levels required to produce an increase in myocardial performance are usually higher than those required in adults. Plasma digoxin levels of 2 to 4 ng/ml, which are often associated with toxicity in adults, do not frequently result in toxicity in premature infants. Diuretic therapy is often more effective in treating the symptoms of cardiac failure in premature infants. Furosemide may be administered intramuscularly in doses of 1 mg/kg body weight, and this is usually an effective agent. In infants with repeated episodes of pulmonary edema, large doses of as much as 5 mg/kg have been used to produce a required effect. It is most important to monitor serum electrolyte levels, since premature infants are very prone to develop hypokalemia and also hyponatremia.

If the infant responds to the method of treatment outlined above, no further treatment will be required, as the ductus will close spontaneously. Previously, if there was an inadequate response to these measures, the ductus arteriosus was closed surgically, usually by ligation. Recently, there have been several reports of attempts to close the ductus by pharmacologic means in premature infants. Since prostaglandin synthesis inhibitors are capable of constricting the ductus arteriosus in fetal animals, it was thought that they may be effective in closing the ductus arteriosus in premature infants. We have used both acetylsalicylic acid and indomethacin in a series of premature infants with patent ductus arteriosus who had evidence of cardiorespiratory distress with large left-to-right shunts and inadequate response to the medical measures outlined above. These infants previously would have been subjected to surgery to close the ductus arteriosus. Acetylsalicylic acid was used in three infants. The ductus was completely constricted in one infant; in the second, there was partial constriction but marked improvement of symptoms, and surgery was not required; and in the third infant, there was no response and the ductus was ligated surgically. Indomethacin has been administered to 45 premature infants with patent ductus arteriosus. These infants also all had symptoms that had not responded to the usual medical measures. After indomethacin administration, the ductus arteriosus constricted markedly or closed completely in 33 babies; marked clinical improvement occurred in nine others, but the ductus did not close completely within 48 hours after the administration of indomethacin. However, no additional treatment was required in any of the 42 infants. In three infants, surgical ligation of the ductus was required. At the present time, indomethacin is being administered either by nasogastric tube or rectally. It is not known whether the lack of adequate response is related to lack of absorption of the drug from the gastrointestinal tract or whether it is due to ineffectiveness of the drug in closing the ductus arteriosus even with adequate plasma levels. Recently, a lyophilized preparation of indomethacin has become available, and this is being tested experimentally by intravenous administration to ensure adequate plasma levels.

Although indomethacin is apparently an extremely effective agent in inducing constriction of the ductus arteriosus in premature infants, there are several serious toxic effects that may result from the drug. A most important toxic response is the development of oliguria, or even anuria, resulting in severe nitrogen retention. The mechanism of this effect is not known; it may be due to an effect on the kidney itself or an effect on renal blood flow. It is possible that the effect may be due to stimulation of vasopressin release from the neurohypophysis. The development of a bleeding tendency is another important toxic result of indomethacin administration. We have therefore considered the presence of bleeding as a contraindication to administration of indomethacin. Since bleeding from the bowel occurs frequently in infants with necrotizing enterocolitis, and also since indomethacin may have gastrointestinal toxic effects in adults, we do not use indomethacin in infants with this complication.

The dose of indomethacin administered intragastrically or rectally that is required to close the ductus arteriosus effectively in most infants is well below that usually used in adults on an equivalent weight basis. We have used several dosage regimens, but our current approach is to administer 0.2 mg/kg in a single dose. The infant is evaluated, and if the ductus is not closed within six to eight hours or if there is not a marked reduction in left atrial-to-aortic diameter ratio, a second dose of 0.2 mg/kg is given, followed by the third dose, if necessary, after 16 hours. We do not recommend using more than three doses of 0.2 mg/kg each. Using this dosage and the precautions mentioned, we have not observed toxic effects in these infants. When effective, treatment results in a rapid reduction in left atrial-to-aortic diameter ratio and dramatic clinical improvement. In some infants, after initial closure of the ductus arteriosus, there has been clinical evidence of reopening within two to five days. In these instances, a second course of indomethacin usually has been effective in closing the ductus arteriosus. If the treatment with indomethacin is not effective, it is necessary to resort to surgical ligation of the ductus.

By using this approach to management, it has been possible to avoid surgery in the majority of premature infants with patent ductus arteriosus. Surgical ligation is required only in a few instances in which there is inadequate response to the measures outlined or in those infants in whom indomethacin therapy is considered to be contraindicated at the present time. This includes infants with bleeding tendency, necrotizing enterocolitis, markedly elevated serum bilirubin levels, or elevated serum creatinine levels. It is possible, however, that after further clinical trials have been completed, some of these contraindications may be eliminated.

Thus, although there is still an obvious need for surgical ligation of the ductus arteriosus in an occasional premature infant with persistent patency, it should be required only rarely.

References

1. Danilowicz D, Rudolph AM, and Hoffman JIE: Delayed closure of the ductus arteriosus in premature infants. Pediatrics 37:74, 1966.
2. Kitterman JA, Edmunds LH Jr, Gregory GA, Heymann MA, Tooley WH, and Rudolph AM: Patent ductus arteriosus in premature infants: incidence, relation to pulmonary disease and management. N Engl J Med 287:483, 1972.
3. Siassi B, Blanco C, Cabal LA, and Goran AG: Incidence and clinical features of patent ductus arteriosus in low birth weight infants: a prospective analysis of 150 consecutively born infants. Pediatrics 57:347, 1976.
4. Coceani F, and Olley PM: The response of the ductus arteriosus to prostaglandins. Can J Physiol Pharmacol 51:220, 1973.

Comment

The observation that indomethacin, an inhibitor of prostaglandin synthesis, constricts the ductus arteriosus in premature infants has raised the question as to whether this therapy is preferable to surgery in premature infants with a large patent ductus arteriosus. It is clear that in most premature infants, a patent ductus arteriosus eventually spontaneously closes, in contrast to the full-term infant with a persistent PDA. Thus, there would appear to be little indication for surgery as a routine simply because of the presence of a detectable patent ductus arteriosus. The controversy arises in regard to these premature infants who demonstrate distress, generally respiratory in origin, related to or contributed by a large patent ductus arteriosus. These symptoms may be directly due to heart failure or may result from pulmonary engorgement with intensification of underlying symptoms produced by a co-existing infant respiratory distress syndrome.

I am not a pediatric cardiologist and have no personal experience in managing this problem. My knowledge is limited to reports in the medical literature of use of either indomethacin or surgical ligation. However, I am unaware of any study that has demonstrated a difference in mortality from either approach. It is also clear from both Dr. Edmunds' and Dr. Rudolph's dissertations, as well as from other studies in the literature,[1] that significant toxic effects may be associated with indomethacin administration.

My own response to these discussions is to suggest that what is needed to clarify this problem is a large randomized study with concurrent controls of premature infants with symptoms related to a large patent ductus arteriosus. One such small series that has recently been reported found no difference in mortality, but did demonstrate that those infants managed surgically required fewer medications, achieved gastrointestinal function sooner, were weaned from mechanical ventilation sooner, and had a smaller hospital bill.[2] More studies of this type are clearly desirable.

In the interim, it would seem rational to manage the patient with digitalis and furosemide. If symptoms persist, a single-dose schedule with indomethacin would seem indicated if no obvious contraindication, such as a bleeding diathesis, enterocolitis, hyperbilirubinemia, or renal problems, exists. If there is not a speedy improvement or if mechanical ventilation seems necessary, surgery would appear to be desirable.

ELLIOT RAPAPORT, M.D.

References

1. Merritt TA, DiSessa TG, Feldman BH, Kirkpatrick SE, Gluck L, and Friedman WF: Closure of the patent ductus arteriosus with ligation and indomethacin: a consecutive experience. J Pediatr 93:639, 1978.
2. Cotton RB, Stahlman MT, Bender HW, Graham TP, Catterton WZ, and Kovar I: Randomized trial of early closure of symptomatic patent ductus arteriosus in small premature infants. J Pediatr 93:647, 1978.

Thirty-one

Are Tissue Valves Preferable to Mechanical Prosthetic Valves?

TISSUE VALVES ARE PREFERABLE TO MECHANICAL
PROSTHETIC VALVES
    Warren D. Hancock

CASE FOR MECHANICAL PROSTHESES FOR CARDIAC
VALVE REPLACEMENT
    Benson B. Roe, M.D.

COMMENT

Tissue Valves Are Preferable to Mechanical Prosthetic Valves

WARREN D. HANCOCK

Developer-Scientist, Hancock Laboratories, Inc., Anaheim, California

Since the introduction of the first ball-in-cage prosthesis in 1959–1960 by Harken and Starr, hundreds of thousands of lives have been prolonged by mechanical heart valve substitutes. Progressive changes and innovations have led to improved hydraulic performance, extended durability, and reduced thrombogenic potential.

Nevertheless, all mechanical valves are associated with a number of potentially serious complications: thromboembolism, thrombosis, sudden irreversible failure, hemolysis, and noise. Patients are required to maintain lifetime anticoagulation therapy, which, in itself, carries a significant morbidity and mortality. As a result of these drawbacks, surgeons and cardiologists have long been interested in the use of various types of tissue valves.

Early experience with homografts by a number of investigators demonstrated freedom from the above complications. However, availability was unreliable, and durability was uncertain and dependent on the method of preservation and the technical skill of the implanting surgeon. We were convinced that a properly preserved xenograft mounted in a stent, which would preserve the natural anatomic geometry, could be the best heart valve substitute.

In November 1969, we completed development of a method for preserving and assembling porcine aortic valves for aortic and atrioventricular valve replacement. This complex method is known as the Stabilized Glutaraldehyde Process (SGP). Initially, valves prepared by this process were mounted in rigid stents. Later, a flexible stent was introduced that minimizes stress on the valves and extends durability.

There are major differences in the clinical results with different types of mechanical valves. This is true for the various types of glutaraldehyde-preserved porcine valves as well. The tissue is simply a source of raw ma-

731

terial that can be manipulated physically and chemically so that it is transformed into a complex organic polymer with specific characteristics and a unique architecture. Unless all the physical and chemical parameters are precisely controlled, it is not possible to produce a biopolymer with optimal viscoelastic properties.

I believe tissue valves are preferable to mechanical valves on the basis of the freedom from thromboembolic complicating hemolysis and infection with their use and their hemodynamic performance and durability.

Thromboembolism

Relative freedom from thromboembolism is a critical requirement for any satisfactory heart valve substitute. Published results with mechanical prostheses show variations in thromboembolic complications from under five per cent to over 34 per cent, even when reporting data for the same type of valve. The discrepancies and variability of the data demonstrate the need for a standardized criteria of patient evaluation and data analysis.

In order to minimize variables, the experience of two major centers (Figs. 1 and 2) using similar reporting methods are presented. The actuarial curve in Figure 1 represents the comparison of thromboembolic complications of the SGP bioprosthesis and different models of the Starr-Edwards prosthesis, as evaluated by Copeland et al.[1] The follow-up information was obtained from 1128 patients who had isolated aortic valve replacements between May 1963 and April 1976. Long-term anticoagulation of patients with SGP bioprostheses was used in seven per cent of the population because of a history of previous embolism or the presence of atrial fibrillation.

Figure 2 represents an evaluation by Cohn et al.[2] of the thromboembolic complications in two groups of patients who had either an SGP bioprosthesis or the Bjork-Shiley disk valve. Long-term anticoagulation with warfarin was used in all patients receiving a Bjork-Shiley disk valve. Anticoagulants were not used in patients with the SGP bioprostheses. The results indicated that the SGP valve has a very low incidence of associated thrombotic

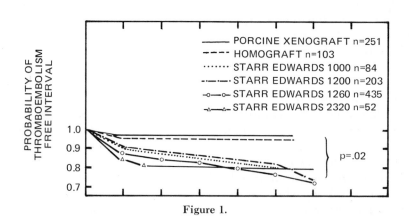

Figure 1.

RESULTS FOLLOWING AORTIC VALVE REPLACEMENT

FACTOR	HANCOCK VALVE	BJÖRK-SHILEY VALVE
Thromboemboli	1 (1.4%)	8 (11.8%)
Emboli/100 patient-years	1.0	6.1

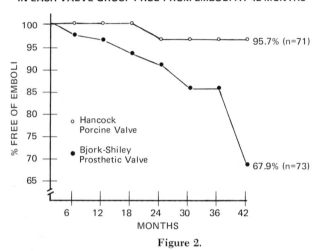

ACTUARIAL CURVES CALCULATING PERCENTAGE OF PATIENTS
IN EACH VALVE GROUP FREE FROM EMBOLI AT 42 MONTHS

Figure 2.

phenomena and does not have the disadvantage of requiring long-term anticoagulation with attendant morbidity and mortality.

Hemolysis

Chronic intravascular hemolysis is a frequent, and occasionally serious, complication of prosthetic valve replacement. Hemolysis can be severe enough to necessitate intensive iron therapy or even valve replacement. The mechanism of hemolysis is usually related to increased shear stress associated with turbulence around the prosthetic valve. Severe hemolytic anemia may develop in aortic valves with small orifices or basilar insufficiencies. Hemolysis following mitral valve replacement has been reported as high as 37.5 to 85 per cent for the Starr-Edwards 6310 and 6320 valve series, 49 per cent with the Beall prosthesis, and 15 to 35 per cent with the Bjork-Shiley prosthesis.

A hematologic study performed by Rhodes et al.[3] in 22 patients who had undergone valve replacement with an SGP bioprosthesis for periods of six to 62 months (mean 30.5 months) did not reveal hemolysis in any of the patients. Postoperative red cell indices and iron studies were normal in all

Table 1. *Preoperative and Postoperative Hematologic Parameters*

	PREOPERATIVE MEAN ± S.D.	POSTOPERATIVE MEAN ± S.D.	NORMAL VALUE
Hematocrit° [%]	39.5 ± 4.67	42.6 ± 5.76	43.5 ± 3.1
Reticulocyte index [%]	1.40 ± 1.03	1.22 ± 0.581	1.64 ± 1.08
LHD° [I.U.]	314 ± 257	204 ± 52.1	130 ± 360
Platelet blood [×10³/c.mm.]	219 ± 64	255 ± 37	248 ± 50

LDH = Lactic dehydrogenase.
°Normal values are average of male-female values.

patients (Table 1). In the same study, five patients with significantly elevated serum lactic dehydrogenase (LDH) values preoperatively returned to normal values following replacement with the SGP bioprosthesis.

Endocarditis

Infections of prosthetic heart valves are one of the most serious complications of heart surgery. Various reports show mortality rates from 50 to 100 per cent. Experience with this complication in three major centers clearly demonstrated that for prosthetic valve endocarditis, valve replacement, rather than antibiotic therapy alone, significantly reduces the mortality rate (Table 2).

Recent studies indicate that the incidence of postoperative infective endocarditis after valve replacement with an SGP bioprosthesis did not significantly differ from that reported with mechanical valves or homografts.[1, 4] However, in several instances, SGP bioprostheses survived documented bacteremia, with no signs of prosthetic dysfunction. These experiences prompted several institutions to recommend the SGP bioprosthesis as the valve of choice for patients with infective endocarditis or for patients at high risk of reinfection.

Hemodynamic Performance

The hemodynamic and clinical performance of the SGP bioprosthesis in the aortic and mitral positions indicates that it is satisfactory with regard to valvular function, effective valve area, and transvalvular gradients.

Hemodynamically, the SGP bioprosthesis compares favorably with other prosthetic devices, and in many instances is superior, particularly in patients with a small left ventricle. The mean diastolic gradient across the bioprosthesis in the mitral position of 6 mm Hg and average end-diastolic gradient of 3 mm Hg compare very favorably with gradients obtained with other mitral valve prostheses. The calculated mitral valve orifice area,

Table 2. *Outcome of Valve Replacement Versus Antibiotic Therapy Alone for Prosthetic Valve Endocarditis in Patients Surviving at Least One Week After Diagnosis**

SERIES	EARLY ONSET		LATE ONSET		TOTAL	
	Medical (death/cases)	*Valve Replacement (deaths/cases)*	*Medical (death/cases)*	*Valve Replacement (deaths/cases)*	*Medical (death/cases)*	*Valve Replacement (deaths/cases)*
Mayo Clinic	11/13	—	11/21	1/7	22/34	1/7
University of Oregon	18/21	1/1	5/16	0/5	23/37	1/6
Mass. General Hospital	7/11	2/4	4/11	1/5	11/22	3/9
TOTALS	36/45(80%)	3/5(60%)	20/48(42%)†	2/17(12%)†	56/93(60%)†	5/22(23%)†

*As compiled from three reviewed series.[1-4]
† p < 0.05

Table 3. *Prosthetic Mitral Valve Replacement: Comparison of Valve Areas and Gradients*

VALVE	CALCULATED AREA [CM²]	MEAN REST GRADIENT
Beall		7
Kay-Suzuki		5
Kay-Shiley		8.5
Bjork-Shiley		4.2
Cutter-Smeloff		6
Braunwald-Cutter	2.68	4.8
Starr-Edwards		
6000	1.9–2.9	
6120	2.39	4.6–6.0
6300	1.57	9.4
6300C	1.65–2.06	7.1–7.3
6310	2.34–2.44	4.9–6.3
Hancock	2.1	5.7
Hancock	2.15	6.5
Hancock	2.3	3.4
Hancock		2.5

averaging greater than 2.0 cm², also compares favorably with other prosthetic mitral devices (Table 3).

The hemodynamics of the aortic SGP bioprosthesis have been studied by several authors and compares well with other commonly used mechanical prostheses. The mean systolic gradients for the bioprostheses in these studies ranged from 11 to 22 mm Hg, with a peak gradient from zero to 52 mm Hg. For mechanical valves, the average gradient ranged from 14 to 19 mm Hg, with a peak gradient from zero to 55 mm Hg (Table 4).

Our experience indicates that the SGP bioprosthesis, compared with mechanical valves, is less prone to development of pannus formation, which may lead to severe narrowing of the orifice area. This may be an

Table 4. *Prosthetic Valve Gradients: Aortic Position*

VALVE	TYPE	AUTHOR	PEAK GRADIENT Range	PEAK GRADIENT Average
Starr-Edwards 2310	Ball	Winter et al.	[0–55]	16
Starr-Edwards 2310	Ball	Kloster et al.	[7–28]	15
Smeloff-Cutter	Ball	McHenry et al.	[5–27]	19
Bjork-Shiley	Disk	Bjork et al.	[9–22]	14
Bjork-Shiley	Disk	Beherndt et al.		14
Lillehei-Kaster	Disk	Mitha et al.	[4–40]	19
Hancock	Porcine	Reis et al.	[15–35]	22
Hancock	Porcine	Hannah et al.	[0–38]	16
Hancock	Porcine	Morris et al.	[17–28]	23
Hancock	Porcine	Cohn et al.	[5–32]	16
Hancock	Porcine	Blanx et al.	[3–24]	11
Hancock	Porcine	Lurie et al.	[3–52]	18.7

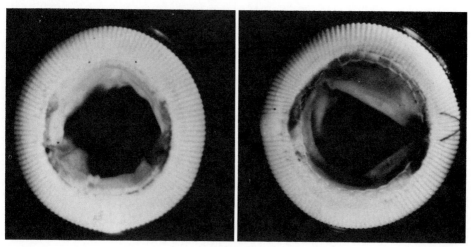

Figure 3.

important consideration, particularly for patients in whom anticoagulants are contraindicated.

Ideally, a valve substitute should not cause clinically significant gradients, even under exercise conditions. In patients with a small aortic root, this is not possible with any currently available prosthesis.

Recently, a new type of SGP aortic and pulmonary bioprosthesis with a modified orifice (MO) was introduced into clinical use. In the MO valves, the septal shelf or muscle portion of the right coronary cusp, which is relatively inflexible tissue found in porcine but not in human aortic valves, has been eliminated, allowing the cusp a complete range of motion and full orifice effect (Fig. 3). This has been achieved by excising the appropriate leaflet and replacing it with a carefully sized noncoronary leaflet from another valve. The new cusp is attached to the flexible stent in a way that ensures the structural integrity of the bioprosthesis.

Figure 4 compares the *in vitro* hydrodynamics of a size 19-mm MO bioprosthesis, a standard size 19-mm bioprosthesis and a current Bjork-Shiley model 19-mm prosthesis under physiologic flow ranges. The results showed that the MO bioprosthesis offered significant improvement.

Durability

The remaining issue is longevity. It appears the longevity of the SGP bioprosthesis is at least equal to that of the mechanical prosthesis. Follow-up periods extend beyond seven years. The five-year failure rate (cases requiring reoperation) is estimated to be about five per cent between the fifth and seventh years. This figure is based upon valves returned to the author for examination from numerous centers. The total valvular dysfunction rate appears to be approximately one in 1000 cases. Tissue dysfunction has oc-

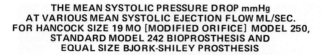

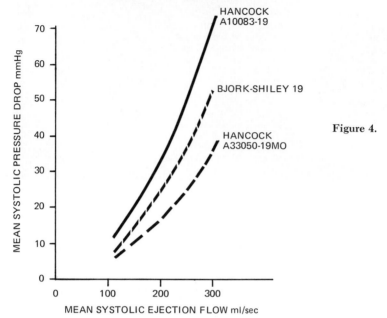

THE MEAN SYSTOLIC PRESSURE DROP mmHg
AT VARIOUS MEAN SYSTOLIC EJECTION FLOW ML/SEC.
FOR HANCOCK SIZE 19 MO [MODIFIED ORIFICE] MODEL 250,
STANDARD MODEL 242 BIOPROSTHESIS AND
EQUAL SIZE BJORK-SHILEY PROSTHESIS

HANCOCK
A10083-19

BJORK-SHILEY 19

HANCOCK
A33050-19MO

Figure 4.

MEAN SYSTOLIC PRESSURE DROP mmHg

MEAN SYSTOLIC EJECTION FLOW ml/sec

curred as little as two months and as long as 76 months after implantation. Statistically, dysfunction is not related to the duration of implantation or to location (mitral, aortic, or conduit). Documented sepsis or suspected infection, as well as metabolic disturbances, have played a role in certain cases; in others, no satisfactory explanation is available. It is important to note that the SGP bioprosthesis does not fail catastrophically. When dysfunction does occur, it almost always develops over a period of time, allowing ample opportunity for an elective replacement. This is in contrast to the mechanical prosthesis, which may fail suddenly and irreversibly.

Since it is impossible to predict accurately the expected life of any heart valve except on the actual experience in real time, this discussion has dealt with the data obtained to date. However, it is interesting to study hypothetical situations as well. This can also be highly beneficial in determining risk-to-benefit ratios and in establishing a framework from which to make intelligent decisions. Several sets of data, based upon certain hypotheses, were fed into the computer for actuarial analysis. These hypotheses were:

1. Assume a risk of death due to anticoagulant therapy or other factors of "x" rate per year.

2. Assume an expected time to replacement (reoperation) of a bioprosthesis of "x" years and a mortality at reoperation of "x" per cent.

For this computation, no other factors were considered. In other words, it would be assumed that all other factors were equal, e.g., the risk of operative mortality and non–valve-related complications. The literature indi-

CUMULATIVE INTERVAL RATES vs. YEARS AFTER OPERATION

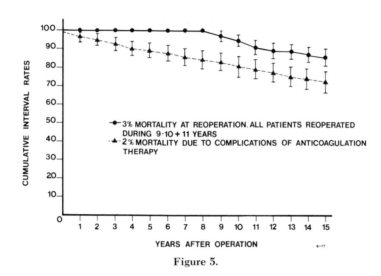

Figure 5.

cates that it would be reasonable to assume a two per cent per year mortality[1] from the complications of anticoagulation and/or catastrophic prosthetic failure. A three per cent mortality at elective reoperation for bioprosthesis replacement would be an accurate percentage for most major centers.

Under these circumstances, assuming a 10-year life for the SGP bioprosthesis, 84 per cent of the patients will be surviving for 15 years, compared with 72 per cent of the group on anticoagulation therapy (Fig. 5).

If one assumes that the deaths due to anticoagulation and associated factors are approximately equal to the risk of reoperation, the patient is at less risk with the SGP bioprosthesis, with an expected durability of five years or more. From an actuarial standpoint, if one assumes a three per cent mortality rate in the prosthetic group and an eight per cent mortality rate at reoperation with a 10-year expected life for the SGP bioprosthesis, the patient with the bioprosthesis is at less risk for the first 14 years after implantation (Fig. 5), after which the risks become approximately equal. However, the three per cent mortality rate for complications with any of the prostheses would appear to be unduly optimistic, and a 10-year life expectancy may be unduly pessimistic for the SGP bioprosthesis.

References

1. Copeland JG, Griepp RB, Stinson EB, and Shumway NE: Long-term follow-up after isolated aortic valve replacement. J Thorac Cardiovasc Surg 74:857, 1977.
2. Cohn LH, Sanders JH Jr, and Collins JJ Jr: Aortic valve replacement with the Hancock porcine xenograft. Ann Thorac Surg 22(3):221, 1976.
3. Rhodes GR, and McIntosh CL: Evaluation of hemolysis following replacement of atrioventricular valves with porcine xenograft. J Thorac Cardiovasc Surg 73(2):312, 1976.
4. Magilligan DJ, Quinn EL, and Davila JC: Bacteremia, endocarditis, and the Hancock valve. Ann Thorac Surg 24:508, 1977.

Case for Mechanical Prostheses for Cardiac Valve Replacement

BENSON B. ROE, M. D.

Professor of Surgery; Co-Chief of Cardiothoracic Surgery,
University of California, San Francisco,
San Francisco, California

Selection of the safest and most effective replacement device for diseased cardiac valves remains controversial in a highly competitive, multiple-choice marketplace 20 years since the first clinically successful valve replacements in 1960. In that interval, approximately 350,000 devices have been implanted in patients after varying degrees of testing *in vitro* and *in vivo*. A majority of these devices have been withdrawn from clinical use or continue to be employed only by their inventors. Disuse has resulted from a variety of failures, which include: (1) mechanical dysfunction from wear, breakage, or erosion;[1, 6, 7] (2) mechanical dysfunction from material distortion (liposcopic or hygroscopic swelling);[2] (3) thrombogenicity;[3] (4) tendency to disrupt from its implantation site (inadequate sewing ring); (5) spatial incompatibility (trauma or obstruction from cage);[4] (6) fragmentation of cloth covering;[5] and (7) inadequate lumen.

Accumulated clinical experience has lead to mechanical improvements and the employment of better materials. Thromboembolic complications remain unresolved, although it appears that their incidence is distinctly lower with some devices than with others, suggesting the possibility that flow patterns, surface characteristics, and methods of handling may play a significant role in the genesis of such complications.

The ideal characteristics for a prosthetic cardiac valve have so far never all been achieved. Table 1 defines the generally accepted requisites.

While currently available prostheses, both mechanical and tissue, appear to be free of toxicity and significant foreign-body reaction, their degree of durability and reliability is variable and is still largely undetermined for most models. Clark et al.[8] have reported the destructive result of high-frequency testing of various valves, and revealed that significant failure rates occur much earlier in tissue valves than in any mechanical models. Several manufacturers have been conscientious in providing information about failures, but insuffi-

740

Table 1. *Requisites of the Ideal Prosthetic Cardiac Valve*

1. *Durability*—functioning without critical wear or breakage for decades.
2. *Reliability*—functioning indefinitely without failure to open or close completely.
3. *Non-thrombogenicity*—resisting coagulation and the deposition of blood elements on its surfaces.
4. *Non-reactivity*—non-toxic and not causing foreign-body reaction.
5. *Non-carcinogenic*—containing no carcinogenic materials.
6. *Non-traumatic*—functioning without damaging blood cells or intracardiac structures.
7. *Implantation security*—providing a sewing ring or other means of attachment that will cushion the disruptive impact and will promote incorporation into the tissue.
8. *Non-obstructive*—providing an orifice that is not obstructive at normal flow rates *in vivo*.
9. *Prevention of tissue overgrowth*—providing surfaces that will resist encroachment of pseudoendothelium on the lumen.
10. *Silent*—functioning at a sound level that is not annoying or worrisome to the patient or those around him.

cient time has elapsed to assess long-term performance of the ostensible superior recent innovations. It stands to reason that the delicate cusps of "tanned" heterologous tissue will not endure forever (even the most expensive shoes will wear out), and it would be surprising if they were not subject to at least the same degenerative and calcific changes that occur in normal valves. Several case reports have revealed fibrosis and calcification of the xenograft cusps; others have shown partial disruption of the tissue from its supporting stent.[9-11] It is thus probable, if not already evident from the historic background of other tissue valves, that any virtues of the glutaraldehyde-preserved xenograft must be balanced against the risk, stress, and expense of necessary replacement after an undetermined period of perhaps 10 years. These values will weigh more heavily in one direction or the other under certain circumstances that influence the choice:

1. Age. Elderly patients who have a shorter life expectancy and less concern about future operation, who are less likely to encounter high output states that render a critical orifice obstructive, and who may be less reliable in maintaining an anticoagulant program are preferred candidates for tissue valves.

2. Occupational hazards. In cases in which exposure to frequent trauma compounds bleeding under anticoagulation, a tissue valve would be favored.

3. Cardiac arrhythmias and atherosclerotic disease. Patients who require anticoagulation to prevent thrombosis for reasons other than the prostheses would not derive the principal benefit of the tissue valve (freedom from anticoagulation) and would be better off with a mechanical device.

4. Anatomic limitations. Patients whose hearts cannot accommodate a bioprosthesis of adequate size not to be obstructive may have no alternative but to receive a mechanical model with a larger relative orifice area.

These considerations should not affect the choice of replacement device under ordinary conditions and are not germane to the controversy.

Product consistency and reliability can be provided in the manufacture of a mechanical device by the application of stringent specifications. Materials, dimensions, and tolerances are predictably identical from unit to unit. In tissue valves, on the other hand, there are a number of variables that are difficult or impossible to control. The contour and tissue strength of the valve vary among animals; and the personal judgment used in selecting those most suitable for mounting cannot be supported by valid measurements. The mounting process in the tissue valve "manufacture" must necessarily be done by hand, with techniques that require skill and precision. Although the best manufacturers are providing excellent models, it is not possible to assure product consistency from one unit to another that approaches that of a mechanical device. The extent to which these probable discrepancies may influence clinical results cannot be determined, but they must be considered as an important danger potential.

An optimal orifice is very difficult to provide. Every replacement device must include a supporting structure to contain the occluding mechanism; it must also contain either a mechanism to secure the device into the heart or an attachment to support sutures for that purpose. This structure therefore necessarily occupies some portion of the orifice area in which the device is placed. In a large orifice, this area is usually not critical, because the remaining lumen is adequate to prevent restriction of normal flows. In smaller sizes, however, the peripheral supporting structure cannot be proportionally reduced, and therefore, it occupies a progressively significant proportion of the anatomic orifice area in successively smaller sizes. Many of the early models of mechanical valves provided a relatively small and somewhat obstructive effective orifice as compared with the more recent devices such as the Bjork-Shiley tilting disc prothesis, which provides a favorable relationship between its internal diameter and its external diameter (ID–OD ratio) even down to its tiny sizes. Tissue valves mounted on cloth-covered stents, however, have proven to be significantly obstructive, with effective orifices that are notably smaller than comparably sized mechanical valves. For example, the effective orifice of a 25-mm Hancock porcine bioprosthesis is smaller than that of a 19-mm Bjork-Shiley tilting disc prosthesis. In addition to the area occupied by the stent itself, the tissue valves mounted within its orifice do not totally retract to the periphery of that lumen and present some obstruction to flow through it. Examination of the tissue valve opening in a pulse duplicator reveals the effective orifice to be triangular in shape rather than circular. In the case of mounted pig valves, the base of the septal cusp includes a block of the septal musculature that impinges on this segment of the lumen. Excessive resistance is the most serious deficiency of currently available tissue valves. Clinical reports have documented with physical findings and catheterization data that significant but inconsistent gradients exist across most tissue valves.[12-14] Calculated valve orifice areas under physiologic conditions are significantly inconsistent and unpredictable for any given valve size, substantiating the problem of reproducibility in the manufacturing process. This combination of small effective orifice and inconsistency has caused most surgeons to avoid using mounted porcine valves with external diameters less than 25 mm in adults, thereby limiting the applicability of the bioprostheses.

Thrombogenicity of the tissue cusps is predictably minimal, but the incidence of thromboembolic complication after implantation of bioprostheses is by no means zero.[15, 16] The cloth suture ring and the cloth-covered stent provide a sizable surface for potential thrombus formation unless and until they become covered with a pseudoendothelium. As a result, most surgeons keep patients anticoagulated for six to eight weeks after tissue valve implantation to reduce the thromboembolic hazard, but late embolic episodes are reported to occur at the rate of two to three per hundred patient-years.

Technical hazards and difficulties are definitely greater during the implantation process of a stented tissue valve than for most mechanical prostheses. Among these hazards are

1. The possibility of obstructing flow to one of the coronary arteries by unavoidably positioning a supportive post of an aortic replacement in front of a coronary ostium.

2. The danger of looping a suture blindly around the supporting post of a mitral replacement as the device is seated into the valva annulus. Such a suture can impair opening of the valve or even damage the cusps.

3. The time involved in washing the glutaraldehyde out of the bioprosthesis after the size is selected adds to the intracardiac operating time. This time may be critical in difficult technical situations or when multiple valve replacements are required. Since most surgeons now perform their intracardiac maneuvers under cold ischemic cardioplegia, any prolongation adds to the ischemic insult and may increase the operative risk.

4. The delicate character of the tissue cusps makes them subject to accidental damage during the implantation process compared with the almost impervious metal, pyrolite, and elastomer elements of mechanical devices.

In summary, the tissue valve's major virtue of reduced thrombogenicity and incidental benefit of noiseless operation are less important in ordinary circumstances than the proven durability and superior flow characteristics of currently available mechanical prostheses. The ease, speed, and relatively safer technical aspects of implanting a mechanical prosthesis undoubtedly contribute to somewhat better operative and long-term results.

References

1. Clark RE, et al: Quantification of wear, hemolysis, and coagulation deficits in patients with Beall mitral valves. Circulation 56(Suppl II):II-139, 1977.
2. Roberts WC, et al: Lethal ball variance in the Starr-Edwards prosthetic valve. Arch Intern Med 126:517, 1970.
3. Duvoisin GE, et al: Factors affecting thromboembolism associated with prosthetic heart valves. Circulation 35, 36(Suppl I):I-70, 1967.
4. Rahimtoola SH: The problem of valve prostheses–patient mismatch. Circulation 58:20, 1978.
5. Shah A, et al: Complications due to cloth wear in cloth-covered Starr-Edwards aortic and mitral valve prostheses and their management. Am Heart J 96:407, 1978.
6. Roe BB, et al: Occluder disruption of Wada-Cutter valve prosthesis. Ann Thorac Surg 20:256, 1975.
7. Silver MD, et al: The pathology of wear in the Beall, Model 104, heart valve prosthesis. Circulation 56:617, 1977.
8. Clark RE, et al: Durability of prosthetic heart valves. Ann Thorac Surg 26:323, 1978.
9. Fishbein MC, et al: Pathologic findings after cardiac valve replacement with glutaraldehyde fixed porcine valves. Am J Cardiol 40:331, 1977.
10. Spray TL, and Roberts WC: Structural changes in porcine xenografts used as substitute cardiac valves. Gross and histologic observations in 51 glutaraldehyde-preserved Hancock valves in 41 patients. Am J Cardiol 40:319, 1977.

11. Ashraf M, et al: Structural alterations of the porcine heterograft after various durations of implantation. Am J Cardiol 41:1185, 1978.
12. Levine FH, et al: Hemodynamic evaluation of the Hancock modified-orifice bioprosthesis in the aortic position. Circulation 59(Suppl I):I-33, 1978.
13. Lurie AJ, et al: Hemodynamic assessment of the glutaraldehyde-preserved porcine heterograft in the aortic and mitral positions. Circulation 56(Supp II):II-104, 1977.
14. Jones EL, et al: Hemodynamic and clinical evaluation of the Hancock xenograft bioprosthesis for aortic valve replacement (with emphasis on management of the small aortic root). J Thorac Cardiovasc Surg 75:300, 1978.
15. Hetzer R, et al: Thrombosis and degeneration of Hancock valves: clinical and pathological findings. Ann Thorac Surg 26:317, 1978.
16. Hetzer R, et al: Thromboembolic complications after mitral valve replacement with Hancock xenograft. J Thorac Cardiovasc Surg 75:651, 1978.

Comment

Two decades after the first successful cardiac valve replacement and after hundreds of thousands of such operations, the search for a better cardiac valve prosthesis continues. There seems little doubt that the Stabilized Glutaraldehyde Process porcine prosthesis developed by Hancock represents a significant advance. This device has gained increasing acceptance, particularly for use in the mitral area, where the ring size permits a large enough prosthesis to minimize the pressure gradient resulting from obstruction produced by the valve itself. Nevertheless, it is clear that problems still occur with the porcine xenografts. Although thromboembolic complications with the porcine valve are distinctly less common than with the usual mechanical prosthetic valve, and despite the fact that one avoids the need for anticoagulants with the porcine valve, thromboembolic complications do occur. Most of these are seen relatively early; however, we have seen a massive embolic stroke in a patient approximately four years after the implantation of a Hancock valve in the mitral position.

The Hancock valve has proved more difficult in patients who require aortic valve replacement. Frequently, the size of the outflow tract is not large enough to permit insertion of a valve of sufficient orifice area to prevent a large residual gradient. Under these circumstances, we have chosen the Bjork-Shiley valve as a highly satisfactory replacement. On the other hand, in the mitral area, we have found the Hancock valve to be the replacement device of choice. The advantage of not needing chronic anticoagulation has been particularly appealing; however, anticoagulants may still be desirable if the patient has persistent atrial fibrillation postoperatively. Although Mr. Hancock has quoted the more unfavorable literature on the thromboembolic complications of mechanical prosthetic valves today, compared with the porcine xenograft, I believe it is fair to say that the incidence of thromboembolic complications with the Hancock valve in patients who are not on anticoagulants is certainly no greater, and possibly less, than the incidence of thromboembolic complications using mechanical prosthetic valves in patients fully anticoagulated. It is also clear that unlike earlier tissue valves. the Stabilized Glutaraldehyde Process has seemingly overcome, to a very great extent, the deterioration that was seen in the early years following insertion of various tissue valves.

In summary, the introduction of the Hancock tissue valve, and more recently the Carpentier-Edwards tissue valve, represents a significant advance in the development of prosthetic valves. These valves are not yet ideal, and the search for better tissue and mechanical valves will continue. Both tissue and mechanical prosthetic valves can be placed today in either the aortic or mitral valve rings with relatively little mortality and subsequent morbidity. My own preference is to see the tissue valve placed in the mitral orifice routinely, but only in the aortic area when there is sufficient outflow tract enlargement to insure that the internal orifice area will not result in an unusual gradient across the valve.

ELLIOT RAPAPORT, M.D.

INDEX

747